This book is to be returned on or before
the last date stamped below.

ADVANCES IN NEUROLOGY

Volume 98

ADVANCES IN NEUROLOGY

Volume 98

Multiple Sclerosis and Demyelinating Diseases

Editor

Mark S. Freedman, BSc MSc, MD, CSPQ, FAAN, FRCPC

Director, Multiple Sclerosis Research Unit
University of Ottawa and the Ottawa Hospital Research Institute
The Ottawa Hospital—General Campus
Ottawa, Ontario, Canada

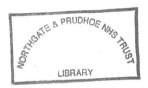
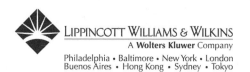
LIPPINCOTT WILLIAMS & WILKINS
A **Wolters Kluwer** Company

Philadelphia • Baltimore • New York • London
Buenos Aires • Hong Kong • Sydney • Tokyo

Acquisitions Editor: Fran DeStefano
Managing Editor: Scott Scheidt
Marketing Manager: Adam Glazer
Production Manager: Dave Murphy
Manufacturing Manager: Ben Rivera
Project Manager: Richard Hund
Design Coordinator: Teresa Mallon
Comp: SPI Publisher Services

© 2006 by Lippincott Williams & Wilkins
530 Walnut Street
Philadelphia, PA 19106
www.LWW.com

Printed in the United States

Library of Congress Cataloging-in-Publication Data

ISBN: 0781751705
ISSN: 0091-3952

Care has been taken to confirm the accuracy of the information presented and to describe generally accepted practices. However, the authors, editors, and publisher are not responsible for errors or omissions or for any consequences from application of the information in this book and make no warranty, expressed or implied, with respect to the currency, completeness, or accuracy of the contents of the publication. Application of this information in a particular situation remains the professional responsibility of the practitioner.

The authors, editor, and publisher have exerted every effort to ensure that drug selection and dosage set forth in this text are in accordance with current recommendations and practice at the time of publication. However, in view of ongoing research, changes in government regulations, and the constant flow of information relating to drug therapy and drug reactions, the reader is urged to check the package insert for each drug for any change in indications and dosage and for added warnings and precautions. This is particularly important when the recommended agent is a new or infrequently employed drug.

Some drugs and medical devices presented in this publication have Food and Drug Administration (FDA) clearance for limited use in restricted research settings. It is the responsibility of health care provides to ascertain the FDA status of each drug or device planned for use in their clinical practice.

The publishers have made every effort to trace copyright holders for borrowed material. If the have inadvertently overlooked any, they will be pleased to make the necessary arrangements at the first opportunity.

To purchase additional copies of this book, call our customer service department at (301) 223-2300 or fax orders to (301) 223-2320. Lippincott Williams & Wilkins customer service representatives are available from 8:30 am to 6:30 pm, EST, Monday through Friday, for telephone access. Visit Lippincott Williams & Wilkins on the Internet: http://www.lww.com.

10 9 8 7 6 5 4 3 2 1

Advances in Neurology Series

Dedication

This text is dedicated to the memory of Donald Winston Paty (1936-2004), devoted clinician, learned professor, and mentor to so many, whose work helped to shape the entire face of the Multiple Sclerosis network, both in Canada and worldwide.

Contents

Contributing Authors

Jack Antel, MD
Professor
Department of Neurology and Neurosurgery
McGill University
Montreal, Canada

Douglas L. Arnold, MD
Professor
Department of Neurology and Neurosurgery
McGill University
Montreal, Canada

Neurologist
Department of Neurology
Montreal Neurological Institute/Hospital
Montreal, Canada

Amit Bar-Or, MD, FRCP(C)
Assistant Professor
Director, Program in Experimental Therapeutics
Scientific Director, Clinical Research Unit
Departments of Neurology and Neurosurgery;
Microbiology and Immunology
Montreal Neurological Institute and McGill
University
Montreal, Canada

Staff Neurologist
McGill University Hospital Center
McGill University
Montreal, Canada

Gary Birnbaum, MD
Clinical Professor of Neurology
Department of Neurology
University of Minnesota
Minneapolis, Minnesota

Director
MS Treatment and Research Center
Minneapolis Clinic of Neurology
Golden Valley, Minnesota

Andrew Chojnacki, PhD
Postdoctoral Fellow
Genes and Development Research Group
Department of Cell Biology and Anatomy
University of Calgary, Faculty of Medicine
Calgary, Canda

Joy Derwenskus, DO
Deparment of Neurology
Northwestern University
Chicago, Illinois

Fellow
Department of Neurology
The Corinne Goldsmith Dickinson Center for
Multiple Sclerosis
Mount Sinai Medical Center
New York, New York

Rajas Deshpande, MD, DM
Clinical Fellow—CNS
Multiple Sclerosis (CNS) Department
London Health Sciences Center
University of Western Ontario
London, Canada

Hooman F. Farhadi, MD
Graduate Student
Department of Neurology and Neurosurgery
McGill University
Royal Victoria Hospital
Montreal, Canada

Massimo Filippi, MD
Tenure Professor
Department of Neurology
University Vita e Salute
Milan, Italy

Director
Neuroimaging Research Unit
Scientific Institute HSR
Milan, Italy

Hans-Peter Hartung, MD
Professor and Chairman
Department of Neurology
Heinrich-Heine-University Düsseldorf
Düsseldorf, Germany

Robert M. Herndon, MD
Professor
Department of Neurology
University of Mississippi Medical School
Jackson, Mississippi

Staff Physician
Department of Neurology
University Hospital
Jackson, Mississippi

Bernd C. Kieseier, MD
Assistant Professor
Department of Neurology
Heinrich-Heine-University Düsseldorf
Düsseldorf, Germany

Marcelo Kremenchutzky, MD
Assistant Professor
Clinical Neurological Sciences Department
University of Western Ontario
London, Canada

Neurologist
Multiple Sclerosis Clinic and Division of Neurology
London Health Sciences Centre—University Campus
London, Canada

David K.B. Li, MD, FRCP(C)
Professor
Department of Radiology
University of British Columbia
Vancouver, Canada

Radiologist
Department of Radiology
University of British Columbia Hospital
Vancouver, Canada

Mary Jane Li, BSc (Pharm)
Research Assistant
Department of Rediology
University of British Columbia Hospital
Vancouver, Canada

Robert P. Lisak, MD
Parker Webber Chair and Professor
Department of Neurology
Wayne State University
Detroit, Michigan

Neurologist-in-Chief
Department of Neurology
Detroit Medical Center
Detroit, Michigan

Fred D. Lublin, MD
Professor of Neurology
Department of Neurology
Mount Sinai School of Medicine
New York, New York

Attending Director
Department of Neurology
The Corinne Goldsmith Dickinson Center for
Multiple Sclerosis
Mount Sinai Medical Center
New York, New York

Claudia F. Lucchinetti, MD
Associate Professor
Department of Neurology
Mayo Clinic College of Medicine
Rochester, Minnesota

Consultant
Department of Neurology
Mayo Clinic
Rochester, Minnesota

Yazmín Morales, BA
Masters Degree Student
Clinical Research Training Program
Mayo Clinic College of Medicine
Mayo Graduate School
Rochester, Minnesota

Medical Student
Pritzker School of Medicine
University of Chicago
Chicago, Illinois

Oliver Neuhaus, MD
Resident
Department of Neurology
Heinrich Heine University
Düsseldorf, Germany

Paul O'Connor, MD, MSc, FRCP(C)
Associate Professor
Department of Medicine (Neurology)
University of Toronto
Toronto, Canada

Division Chief
Department of Neurology
St. Michael's Hospital
Toronto, Canada

Trevor Owens, PhD
Professor
Department of Neurology and Neurosurgery
McGill University
Montreal, Canada

Professor
Department of Neuroimmunology
Montreal Neurological Institute
Montreal, Canada

Joseph E. Parisi, MD
Professor of Pathology
Consultant
Department of Laboratory Medicine and Pathology,
and Neurology
Mayo Clinic
Rochester, Minnesota

Donald Paty, MD, FRCP(C)*
Division of Neurology, Department of Medicine
University of British Columbia
Vancouver, Canada

*Deceased

Alan C. Peterson, MD
Associate Professor
Departments of Human Genetics, Oncology, and
Neurology and Neurosurgery
McGill University
Montreal, Canada

Molecular Oncology Group
Royal Victoria Hospital
McGill University and Genome Quebec Innovation
Centre
Montreal, Canada

George P.A. Rice, MD
Professor
Clinical Neurological Sciences Department
University of Western Ontario
London, Canada

Multiple Sclerosis Clinic Director
Clinical Neurological Sciences—Neurology
Department
London Health Sciences Centre
London, Canada

Andrew Riddehough, BSc
Director of Operations
MS/MRI Research Group, Department of Medicine
University of British Columbia
Vancouver, Canada

Maria Assunta Rocca, MD
Research Fellow
Neuroimaging Research Unit
Scientific Institute HSR
Milan, Italy

Francesca Ruffini, PhD
Postdoctoral Fellow
Neuroscience-Neuroimmunology Unit
DIBIT-San Raffaele Hospital
Milan, Italy

A. Dessa Sadovnick, PhD
Professor
Department of Medical Genetics
University of British Columbia
Vancouver, Canada

Professor
Faculty of Medicine, Division of Neurology
Vancouver Coastal Health Authority—University of
British Columbia Hospital
Vancouver, Canada

Maria Carmela Tartaglia, MD
Resident
Department of Neurology
University of Western Ontario
London, Canada

Resident
Department of Neurology
London Health Sciences Center
London, Canada

Edward J. Thompson, DSc, MD, PhD
Professor
Department of Neuro Immunology
Institute of Neurology, Queen Square
London, England

Anthony Traboulsee, MD, FRCP(C)
Clinical Assistant Professor
Department of Medicine (Neurology)
University of British Columbia
Vancouver, Canada

Alex C. Tselis, MD, PhD
Associate Professor
Department of Neurology
Wayne State University
Detroit, Michigan

Staff Neurologist
Department of Neurology
Detroit Medical Center
Detroit, Michigan

Samuel Weiss, PhD
Professor
Department of Cell Biology and Anatomy
University of Calgary
Calgary, Canada

Dean M. Wingerchuk, MD, MSc, FRCP(C)
Associate Professor of Neurology
Department of Neurology
Mayo Clinic College of Medicine
Rochester, Minnesota

Consultant
Department of Neurology
Mayo Clinic
Scottsdale, Arizona

Jerry S. Wolinsky, MD
Bartels Family and Opal Rankin Professorships in
Neurology
Department of Neurology
The University of Texas Health Science Center at
Houston
Houston, Texas

Guojun Zhao, MD
Research Associate
Division of Neurology, Department of Medicine
University of British Columbia
Vancouver, Canada

Preface

Twenty-five years ago, Multiple Sclerosis (MS) was yet another one of those neurological enigmas—a disease of unknown cause affecting the central nervous system (CNS) of young adults, causing demyelination and axon loss. At times it resulted in severe disability, but most of the time, especially early on, "attacks" tended to resolve completely. Since there was no treatment, neurologists often just told patients recovering from their initial relapses that they had "inflammation of the nervous system" that would get better with time, and sometimes prescribed the mother of all anti-inflammatory drugs, steroids, to help speed recovery. There was hesitancy in telling patients the truth about their disease: that they might have MS, since this would just invoke fear and anxiety of the unknown.

Looking back at the veritable explosion of research into MS over the past 25 years, we have made incredible strides at defining the disease pathologically and distinguishing it from other conditions that might either mimic the clinical or paraclinical presentation of the disease. The MRI scanner has proved to be one of the single most important non-invasive advances in diagnosing the disease, with changes that could be correlated pathologically The genetics of MS has yet to be fully deciphered; however, significant leads have been generated and much has been learned from the intensive study of affected families. Natural history studies have given us the power to somewhat predict the course of illness. The ever-expanding field of immunology has revealed mechanisms of immunopathogenesis that are being proven in the field with the advent of new therapies directed at these very mechanisms. Treatments proven to alter the natural history of the disease emerged at the beginning of the last decade, creating a shift in the thinking of neurologists: you needed to tell patients they had MS so effective therapy could begin early enough to make a difference.

Yet current therapies were only modestly effective and damage to the myelin and axons continued to pile up in most patients, ultimately leading to various degrees of disability. This prompted a push to define the mechanisms of the CNS damage and to understand why innate mechanisms of repair were ineffective. Studies in these areas have revealed possible ways that we can begin to think about enhancing CNS repair or even promote regeneration.

With all of this research and development in the field of MS it is not surprising that several excellent texts are already out there. When challenged to come up with something novel for this project, I was immediately confronted with my own thought of "not another MS book that will be outdated in a year." After some serious contemplation however, I felt that a significant contribution to the field would entail a text that focused on the "hard facts," leaving behind the speculation, the "maybes" and the "could be's" for other texts and stick instead to what we truly know. The idea was to have a single "timeless" text that reviews MS and demyelinating diseases in a way that sets the scene for years to come. There will no doubt be substantial advances in the field for years to come. This new information will only complement what is found here, and will build upon the established knowledge. It is a challenge to write a chapter without speculating or putting in preliminary thoughts or ideas in the hope that these will ultimately ring true, but all too often are proven wrong some time down the road (at times even before the text reaches print). When you read an older text and see what people thought when they wrote their chapters, it's sometimes hard to imagine how they could have been so far from the truth. You then get the sense that the whole text must be outdated and therefore not of any contemporary use. I wanted this issue of "Advances" to serve as a "foundation" on which to build the true story in years to come. Therein lies the challenge: to determine what is truly fact now, supported by evidence, and what is not. What is not belongs elsewhere; the facts belong here. This was the mandate given to all of the contributors to this text; they have clearly met their obligation.

This text should prove to be a useful source to anyone involved in MS basic or clinical research or the management of MS patients. It is not comprehensive and there are areas that could have been expanded if not for limitations. All the writers of chapters are themselves renowned for their own contributions in the field of MS research and readers will appreciate the careful and accurate manner in which they've assembled their facts. Although there is still no single text written to date that encompasses everything about MS or related demyelinating diseases, this book should prove to be a solid foundation of knowledge, with information that should prove to be sound and true for years to come.

Mark S. Freedman, HBSc, MSc, MD, CSPQ, FAAN, FRCPC
Professor of Medicine (Neurology)
University of Ottawa
Ottawa, Ontario CANADA

1

The Natural History of Multiple Sclerosis

Rajas Deshpande,[1] Marcelo Kremenchutzky,[1] and George P.A. Rice[2]

[1]*Multiple Sclerosis Clinic, London Health Sciences Centre, London, Ontario, Canada;*
[2]*Clinical Neurological Sciences, London Health Sciences Centre, London, Ontario, Canada*

INTRODUCTION

Natural history studies of chronic diseases have been historically tantamount to a fundamental part of nosology, improved understanding of pathogenesis, and the practical clinical applications of predicting patients' outcomes. Needless to say, natural history data play an undeniably essential role for establishment of baselines for therapeutic adventure and development of disease-modifying therapies. Studying the patterns in the evolution, progression, and accumulation of disability in a population with multiple sclerosis (MS) helps us learn associations and behavior of the disease and to have a better understanding of the clinical course and possible outcome of a given patient. The clinical, natural history, and prognostic features of MS have been well described by several investigators, including only a few geographically defined, population-based studies extending over long periods of follow-up, discussed below under various headings. The idealized criteria for a true inception cohort laid down by Sackett et al.(1985) are being approached. Observations of this kind have also been useful in clinical trial design and interpretation(1,2).

The Multiple Sclerosis Clinic

The Multiple Sclerosis Clinic at the London Health Sciences Centre, University Campus, London, Ontario, Canada, was established in 1972 to provide long-term care for MS patients from southwestern Ontario. Although these data have limitations, the characteristics of our original clinic population have been meticulously outlined in numerous previous studies based on its patient population (3–9).

In general, primary care is delivered to patients in the immediate area and secondary care to patients in the surrounding area. Tertiary referral is provided for patients with MS from northern and southern Ontario and, to a lesser extent, for patients from adjacent regions and provinces. The subgroup from Middlesex County, which represented 90% of Middlesex County MS patients at the time of a formal prevalence study in 1988, has served as a strictly geographically based, standard population against which less strictly defined subgroups of patients can be compared (10). This subgroup has served to validate the pooling of groups for total population analysis. Yearly evaluations eliminated much of the instability that characterizes disability end-points derived from short–term periods of observation. After more than 25 years, mean follow-up there was 96.3% accuracy in the diagnosis of MS based on clinical grounds, even including cases originally designated as "possible." This entire cohort was identified before the advent of the MRI technology. Not a single case of treatable disease emerged in follow-up of those ultimately deemed not to have MS.

In the 1970s and mid-1980s, patients in the Multiple Sclerosis Clinic were seen on a yearly basis, and an effort was made to continue this for the Natural History Cohort described in detail here. Unsurprisingly, this was not possible for all patients, many of whom became severely disabled, and it was particularly difficult for those who became institutionalized. However, for this latter group, advanced disability end-points had already been reached. Information on physical status in the most severely disabled patients has often been derived from follow-up with primary care physicians, family and, as much as possible, from the patients themselves. This has included visits to patients in local nursing homes.

A change of name consequent to a change of marital status or, less often, from moving to a different country was the principal challenge. Extensive efforts, however, were made to trace patients lost to follow-up. This included repeated attempts to locate the patients, contact their family doctors, their relatives and neighbors, and local Multiple Sclerosis Society chapters, as well as the examination of telephone directories and local as well as regional hospital records. We had assistance from the Government of Ontario and its Ministry of Health, which provided access to the provincial registry of all deaths. This source identified the final outcome in the majority of patients lost to follow-up through copies of death certificates, to establish the cause of death. Necessarily, some arbitrary decisions had to be made regarding the cause of death where clinical records were suboptimal. If, however, the cause of death was listed as heart disease, cancer, or some other disorder not directly or indirectly related to or associated with MS, such patients were considered not to have died of MS irrespective of their degree of disability. Nevertheless, information on disability independent of disorders causing death was obtained and recorded.

Overall, the core of this so-called London (Ontario) Natural History Cohort is composed of some 1,000 patients and has given us over 26,000 patient-years of observation experience through three decades. Figure 1-1 summarizes schematically the most relevant characteristics of this patient group. Data from a second, similarly sized, more contemporarily seen, population-based cohort served for testing hypotheses and also for validation purposes. Most of our

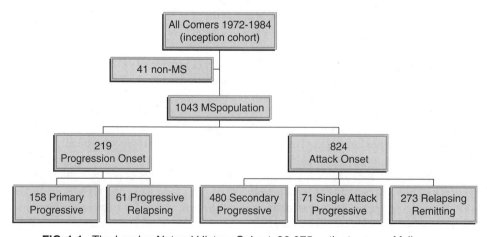

FIG. 1-1. The London Natural History Cohort: 26,075 patient-years of follow-up.

discussion in this chapter will be based on repeated critical evaluations of these observations, and further invaluable experience gathered from our additional more than 5,500 case records on file (Fig. 1-1).

Classification of Clinical Course

In the absence of specific clinical or paraclinical diagnostic markers for MS, many classifications have been proposed and followed (11), and these will be discussed elsewhere in this book. For the purpose of this discussion about the natural history of multiple sclerosis, we have chosen to follow the phenomenological classification initially suggested by McAlpine et al. (12):

- Relapsing Remitting Multiple Sclerosis (RRMS)
- Primary Progressive Multiple Sclerosis (PPMS)
- Secondary Progressive Multiple Sclerosis (SPMS)

This pragmatic classification, although somewhat arbitrary, is very useful in daily practice, while giving us the convenience of unambiguous description and rationalized interpretation of long-term clinical outcomes amongst subgroups defined by clinical features. This clinical course classification has more recently been the subject of an international survey (13) which, for the most part, served to simplify terminology. Although the recommendations made were on the basis of extensive collective experience, unanimity of opinion was not possible. We have further attempted to consolidate nomenclature and decided not to use the terms "Relapsing Progressive" and "Progressive Relapsing" as they merely represent clinical deviations of the other two (8,14,15).

Depending upon the severity, MS also has been classified as Benign (very few and far apart attacks with complete or near-complete recovery followed by clinical silence lasting years or even decades) and Malignant (acute, polysymptomatic onset with very rapid and aggressive progression to severe disability or death). The term "Active MS" has been in use to refer to ongoing disease processes seen either clinically or radiologically, while "Inactive MS" suggests silence by both criteria.

RRMS is the most common presenting form of MS, characterized by episodes of acute or subacute onset of constant neurological dysfunction (referred to as a relapse, attack, flare-up, or exacerbation), which lasts for more than 24 hours, usually resolves within weeks and remits to complete or partial recovery. Following a period of this "relapsing-remitting" course, the majority of these patients (over 80% in 25 years) will gradually but relentlessly develop attack-free worsening with progressive accumulation of disability. Accordingly, these patients, formerly in the RRMS category, evolve into and form the SPMS category.

On the other hand, PPMS subjects are characterized by a subacute or chronic onset of unremitting neurological dysfunction with gradual worsening (i.e., progression) over years, with cumulative fixed disability and hardly any reversal of acquired neurological dysfunction. Overlapping exacerbations, particularly in the late course of this type of MS, are rare but not unknown and may occur at any time, even in the early years or decades after clinical onset.

Although the above categories encompass most clinical presentations of MS, individual variations are very common. There may be attacks in PPMS, and sometimes SPMS may begin after one single attack (16). There may be relapses with very little recovery, accumulating rapid neurological disability. It is not uncommon to encounter patients who have had one or two relapses followed by a disease silence and minimal or no disability for many years.

RELAPSING REMITTING MULTIPLE SCLEROSIS

This is by far the most common initial clinical phenotype, accounting for up to about 85% of the total MS population at the onset of the disease. The mean age of symptomatic onset is 29 years, with the majority of patients in the age group between 20 and 39 years. This compares well to reports from other researchers such as the Lyon, France group where the median age of onset was 31 years (SD 10 years, range 5–67 years) (17,18).

In a study at the Mayo Clinic in Rochester, Minnesota, the median age at onset was reported to be 37.2 years (range 16.7 to 65.3) for men, 35.4 years (range 17.3 to 59.6) for women, and 36.2 years (range 16.7 to 65.3) overall (19). Approximately 10% to 15% of our patients are diagnosed before the age of 20 (mostly in their late teens, although pediatric MS is being more often recognized nowadays), whereas about 5% of patients are diagnosed above the age of 49 years.

A selective gender predilection is commonly seen in MS, as it is often reported in other autoimmune conditions. In our population the male:female ratio is 1:2 for the entire cohort and there is a much more conspicuous female preponderance amongst younger RRMS patients as compared to older, progressive MS cases (20). In a study from the Mayo Clinic, newly diagnosed MS cases over a period of 15 years (from 1985 through 2000) included 38 men and 94 women, the male:female ratio being 1:2.4. (19). Another study from Lyon, France reported a male:female ratio of 1:1.7 (17, 18).

In RRMS, the most common clinical presentation is the acute onset of sensory deficit. This may be associated with or followed by other transient neurological dysfunction. Amongst the next most common presentations, optic neuritis is remarkable. Most of the time the patient distinctly recalls the symptomatic onset, but it is not unheard of for some patients to recall this event only retrospectively after direct questioning.

The other modes of presentation in RRMS commonly include acute or subacute onset of hemi sensory deficit, acute transverse myelitis (complete or incomplete), acute ataxia, hemi paresis or a brainstem syndrome with diplopia due to internuclear ophthalmoplegia (unilateral or bilateral), vertigo, tinnitus and/or ataxia (Table 1-1).

The sharp clinician is accustomed to recognizing additional symptoms overlapping or even predating clinically evident attacks. These symptoms are often paroxysmal, and may appear in clusters. The most classic and well-recognized is an electric-shock-like or sometimes a pulling, tingling sensation running down the spine and legs on flexion of the neck (the L'hermitte symptom). Many individuals later recollect having had this symptom in the past, but neglected it at the time. The unexplained occurrence of trigeminal neuralgia (*tic doloreux*) in a young subject should also raise a suspicion of an early presentation of MS. Some patients present with frequent, transient symptoms of radicular or neuropathic pain, photopsias, painful tonic spasms, involuntary limb movements, and an MS characteristic—useless hand syndrome. Very rarely, less than 5% of patients have seizures, and still more infrequent are hemiballismus, chorea, and acute cognitive or affective syndromes.

Overwhelming fatigue, though a very common accompaniment to a presenting neurological dysfunction or a relapse, is rare as a presenting feature alone. This fatigue is usually worse in the afternoon and may be quite disabling. The transient appearance or worsening of neurodeficits (most typically visual impairment, but any functional system can be involved) on exposure to any form of heat (atmospheric, hot shower, exercise, fever, or even hot food or drinks) is known as the Uhthoff

TABLE 1-1 *Initial presentation in total clinic population*

Age at onset (yrs)	n	Percentage with initial presentation					
		Optic neuritis	Sensory	Motor (acute)	Motor (insidious)	Diplopia and/ or vertigo	Limb ataxia and/or impairment of balance
< 20	131	22.9	46.5	6.1	3.8	17.6	13.7
20–29	435	22.8	52.2	7.3	6.2	12.4	11.3
30–39	310	13.2	44.2	6.8	14.5	11.0	14.8
40–49	173	9.2	33.5	2.9	30.6	16.8	12.7
> 49	47	6.3	31.9	4.2	46.8	12.8	10.6
Total	1096	17.2	45.4	6.2	13.9	12.9	13.2

phenomenon, and is a very common accompaniment to relapses. Some or all of these symptoms mentioned above usually appear first during an attack, but may also linger on between relapses, often severe enough to dominate other symptoms.

Once the neurological dysfunction starts, it progresses briefly to its worst state (e.g., complete loss of vision in one eye or total sensory loss below a spinal level with paraplegia and loss of sphincter controls). This progression may evolve over a few days or up to a couple of weeks. After this initial stage a clinical plateau is commonplace, with stabilization of symptoms for a few weeks, usually within a month. Subsequently, recovery ensues, which can be partial or complete and commonly occurs over a few weeks. The mean duration of an attack is 42 days. Recovery is often achieved faster, better, and more completely after the first few relapses, but there are many who retain some perceivable deficit, evolving in the form of residual cumulative disability, which may be in the form of scotomas, posterior column deficits or sphincter disturbances, mild gait disturbances, or pyramidal signs.

The attack rate in the early years of MS is an important predictor of long-term outcome. In our studies, the mean annual attack rate in the first year after onset is 1.5 in the total population. However, attack rates may vary greatly in different studies, particularly when patients are specifically selected (i.e., for participation in clinical trials) or represent selected subgroups (i.e., hospitalized, etc.). Several studies serve to illustrate such variation. Goodkin et al. (21) described an average attack rate of 0.64 per year; Durelli et al. (22) described an average attack rate of 0.94 per year; Jacobs et al. (23) reported annualized attack rates of 1.20; and Johnson et al. (24) reported 2.90 attacks per year, amongst others.

Interestingly, although there may be variation when surveying untreated populations as well, figures tend to be more closely grouped. However, it is typical that after the second year there is a remarkable drop in the relapse rate. Over half a century ago, McAlpine and Compston (25) described attack rates of 1.23 in the first year and 0.42 in the second year. More recently, early studies from our London, Ontario geographically-based cohort demonstrated attack rates of 1.57 in the first year and 0.35 in the second year for the Natural History cohort (4).

The subsequent disease course is more predictable for populations than for individual patients. Relapses occur at variable frequency in various patients. The frequency of relapses varies even in a given patient at different times. However, there is a clear tendency for the frequency of relapses to be greater in the initial years, and the recovery to be more complete, too. (2,4,26,27,28).

With the passage of time, relapses tend to leave behind more neurological and functional deficits. The accumulated deficits tend to increase with each relapse, and disability accumulates. However, all progression is not secondary to relapses; there also is gradual progression independent of relapses. After this early relapsing phase, most patients enter the progressive phase of the disease. After the first decade from onset, over 50% of patients whose disease was initially relapsing-remitting enter a progressive phase of MS. Approximately a cumulative 90% develop progressive disease after 25 years of follow-up (3). It has been commented that if followed-up long enough, eventually nearly all RRMS patients will convert to the progressive form of the disease. Our personal observations have shown a mean duration of conversion from the time of the first attack to the onset of the progressive form of the disease is approximately 11 years, although it has been reported to be of up to 19 years (29,30).

After entering this phase, progression appears to be independent of, although worsened by, the accumulated neurodeficits due to relapses. Gradual, relentless worsening of predominantly the pyramidal and cerebellar systems ensues, oftentimes shadowed by sphincter and sexual dysfunction. Additionally, cortical types of deficits occasionally appear, such as various kinds of dysarthrias, memory disturbances, and frontal lobe dysfunction. Disturbances of brainstem functions, including deglutition, set in and aspiration becomes common. This phase will be discussed in more detail in the following text.

PROGRESSIVE MULTIPLE SCLEROSIS

Curiously enough, but consistently over many study-years, the progressive phase of MS has been demonstrated to have remarkable similarities in its clinical profile, independent of the clinical MS phenotype. Hence, it makes sense to discuss the natural history of the progression of MS, whether primary or secondary, under one heading, that of progressive MS. However, certain distinctions between the primary and secondary progressive MS classes, and certain facts about them, are of particular interest and are worth separate paragraphs.

Clinically, PPMS begins at a relatively later age as compared to RRMS. Its onset peaks in the late fourth decade, in contrast to early fourth decade in RRMS. The female preponderance in PPMS is not as prominent as in RRMS, with a ratio of 1.3:1. Attack-free progression appears to develop more quickly, but this may be only apparent in the early years. The progression rates are similar once progression begins (16,17).

Relapses in the preprogressive phase of SPMS do not seem to significantly impact the later speed or severity of the progressive phase. Of course, the pre-existing neurodeficits (relapse remnants) may exaggerate the disability on initial assessment. Worth noticing, though, is the fact that in individuals with one, single attack predating the progressive phase of MS, the severity of the inaugural attack may anticipate a sooner onset of attack-free progression. Involvement of more than three neurological systems due to attack is associated with earlier onset of progression (16,31).

Progressive MS presents most commonly as subtle, pyramidal-cerebellar dysfunction gradually evolving over months or years in a frank myelopathy. The diffuse involvement of these two systems, added to the transient sensory phenomena, makes it very difficult to localize the lesions. A myelopathy should raise the possibility of a diagnosis of MS even when there is no prior history of relapses. In all classes of MS, progression predominantly involves the pyramidal system, followed by the cerebellar system. This "Chronic Progressive Myelopathy" is a

characteristic presentation of most PPMS patients. Posterior columns are next in frequency of initial presentation, and cranial nerves are commonly only involved very late. In progressive MS, too, cortical and bulbar functions, and, to a greater extent, basal ganglionic functions appear preserved until very late in the disease course in most cases.

Progression does not seem to begin specifically at the sites affected by earlier relapses. The site of the original attack has been suspected of becoming a *locus minoris resistentiae* where progression begins (32). However, most researchers agree there appears to be no demonstrable relationship between the site of the initial, clinically evident expression of disease and the location of the progressive deficit. In our samples, patients with optic neuritis, brain stem, and spinal sensory MS onset are all characterized by an overwhelming predominance of distal central motor dysfunction at the outset of the progressive phase of the disease. On one hand, the distribution of sites of initial manifestations paralleled those of the general population of MS patients. On the other hand, the progressive deficit was almost exclusively localized to distal, lower-extremity, corticospinal tract fibers. (16,33).

Progression is seldom joined by overlapping relapses in its march, but when relapses occur they tend to behave like RRMS relapses, with typical temporal profiles and partial or complete recovery.

On the pyramidal-cerebellar canvas of progressive MS, sphincter and sexual dysfunction as well as posterior column sensory deficits make themselves apparent. However, the clinical picture is rarely tainted by severe visual deficits.

As disability accumulates and patients require progressively increasing support. This happens on an average about 8–12 years after the beginning of the progressive phase. At this stage, the progression seems to relatively stabilize for some time, but this appearance of stability could very well be a shortcoming of the present disability scale used (2,34). As deficits in the pyramidal and cerebellar functions are more demonstrable, once these are severely affected, it is difficult to objectively evaluate and grade progress in other neurological systems. The current disability scale largely depends on mobility to grade the disability. This is why it appears that at stages where disability is significantly affected, the patient lingers at the same score for some time in spite of progression.

The next hallmark of progression is wheelchair dependence, which usually comes after between approximately 10 and 20 years from onset of progression (2). Around this period, many medical conditions usually accompany this age group. Lack of mobility, stress of disability, and need for catheterization and resultant infections increase a patient's morbidity for life-threatening consequences.

Coexisting morbidity for strokes, cardiac, pulmonary, or renal disease may worsen the prognosis further. Falls, aspirations due to bulbar weakness, depression, memory retrieval deficits and emotional lability can be directly blamed on MS, and further complicate the scene. An Extended Disability Scale Score

(EDSS) of 10 means death due to MS, and this is usually reached after an average of 18–30 years from onset of progression (Fig. 1-2).

DISABILITY IN MULTIPLE SCLEROSIS

The Expanded Disability Scoring Scale (EDSS) has been designed to objectively evaluate MS patients (35,36). This is necessary when longitudinally evaluating patients in clinical trials for comparable outcome measures. The EDSS is based on assessment of clinical deficits in various functional systems of the central nervous system, rating them according to severity, rating the ambulation capacity and (in its absence)(the use of upper limbs, and scoring the total not by addition but by overall review of the individual system scores and deficits in ambulation and effective use of hands). The functional systems included are visual, sensory, pyramidal, cerebellar, brainstem, bowel–bladder, cerebral, and others. EDSS has 20 scoring points from 0 to 10, each point after 1 divided in two.

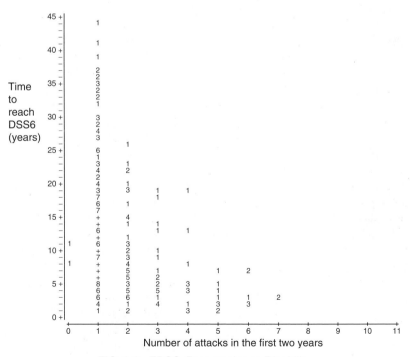

FIG. 1-2. EDSS: Progression to Disability.

The key milestones in EDSS are shown below. Please refer to the appendix at the end of the chapter for further information.

- Score 1 represents objective evidence of minimal involvement of only one functional system, with only signs and no functional disability.
- Score 3 represents moderate involvement of one functional system with or without mild involvement of others. This is associated with minimal disability.
- Score 6 means that a cane or unilateral support is required for walking. This represents ambulation disability.
- Score 8 represents wheelchair dependency, with a relatively good use of hands still maintained.
- An EDSS score of 10 represents death due to MS.

As discussed in detail later, the EDSS scale is not linear in its function. Also, with its lack of comparability of neurodeficits in various neurological systems, the scale depends heavily on ambulation as a comparable criterion. Above the score of 4, the scale mainly depends primarily on ambulation, with progression in other systems being sidelined (2). On the other hand, the scale still is the best available tool for comparable longitudinal evaluation of MS patients, as it offers hard outcome parameters eventually reached by most MS patients over the course of their disease progression.

Table 1-2 depicts results from early papers from our Natural History Cohort, where the Disability Scoring Scale (DSS) was used before its proposed extension. Anatomically similar, the DSS is comparable to EDSS with minor variations (an EDSS score of 0.5 higher than DSS has been assumed equivalent in a study) (7).

However, there is tendency to (1) progress relatively slowly from score 1 through 3, and (2) linger on for relatively longer time periods over two grades, scores 6 and 7. Obviously, these facts do not mean that the progression pace retards at these stages; they only convey a desperate need for better quantification of progression in the absence of pyramidal and cerebellar parameters. (Table 1-2).

TABLE 1-2 *Cross-section of disability at final review (2, 3)*

DSS Level	No. (%) of Patients at DSS Level[*]
1	182 (17)
2	156 (14)
3	123 (11)
4	71 (6)
5	31 (3)
6	205 (19)
7	203 (18)
8	88 (8)
9	23 (2)
10	16 (1)
Data unavailable	1
Total	1099

* These data are derived from the total population surveyed at the MS Clinic, London, Ontario.
DSS, Disability Status Scale (Kurtzke).

In RRMS, the initial deficit as already described is quite variable due to diverse neurological system involvements of different degrees. Hence, the score of 3 on the EDSS generally represents a disability level signifying moderate compromise in at least one functional system, with or without mild deficits in others. This level therefore forms a good, comparable level for natural history evaluation. The mean duration taken by the patients to reach this level is discrepant in RRMS and PPMS, quite understandably, given the late onset and probably faster early progression of PPMS (2,34,37).

The mean time for an RRMS patient to reach an EDSS score of 3 is between 6 and 8 years, while that for a PPMS patient is between 1 and 2 years. This observation may differ depending on whether the patient was observed retrospectively or prospectively (2,33,34,37).

The next level generally used for comparison is EDSS 6, and the score is reached by most RRMS patients in anywhere from 9 to 15 years, while most PPMS patients reach this score in 3 to 5 years (2) (Table 1-3, Table 1-4, Fig. 1-1).

Most RRMS patients achieve wheelchair dependency or an EDSS score of 8 in their progressive (SPMS) phase, and this varies from 18 to 30 years. PPMS patients reach this score in an average 20 years from onset of progression (2) (Fig. 1-3).

TABLE 1-3 *Time (years) from onset of multiple sclerosis to reach selected levels of disability (Median ± SE) (2, 3)*

Level of disability	Total clinic population	Seen-at-onset subgroup
DSS 3	7.69 ± 0.42	6.28 ± 0.34
DSS 6	14.97 ± 0.31	9.42 ± 0.44

Source: From Weinshenker BG, Gass B, Rice GPA, et al. The natural history of multiple sclerosis: a geographically based study. I. Clinical course and disability. *Brain* 1989;112:133-146. p 139, with permission.
DSS, Disability Status Scale (Kurtzke).

TABLE 1-4 *Median time (years) from onset of progressive multiple sclerosis to reach selected levels of disability (Median ± SE) (2, 3)*

Level of disability	Total clinic population	Middlesex county subgroup
DSS 3	1.40 ± 0.11	1.20 ± 0.33
DSS 6	4.51 ± 0.38	3.58 ± 0.52
DSS 8	24.08 ± 0.44	19.32 ± 0.46
DSS 10	-	-

Source: From Weinshenker BG, Gass B, Rice GPA, et al. The natural history of multiple sclerosis: a geographically based study. I. Clinical course and disability. *Brain* 1989;112:133-146, p 142, with permission.
DSS, Disability Status Scale (Kurtzke).

The Mayo Clinic group reported that the median time from diagnosis to EDSS scores of 3 and 6 was 17 and 24 years, respectively. Only 25% of patients with RRMS were expected to reach an EDSS score of 3 within 20 years based on Kaplan–Meier plots of time. The median time expected for SPMS patients to reach EDSS scores of 3, 6, and 8 was about 3, 10, and 38 years, respectively. The median time from diagnosis to EDSS scores of 6 and 8 for patients with PPMS was 3 and 25 years, respectively (38). In a study from Lyon, France it was reported that the median time from onset of MS to the assignment of scores of 4, 6, and 7 was 8.4 years (range 7.8–9.6 years),

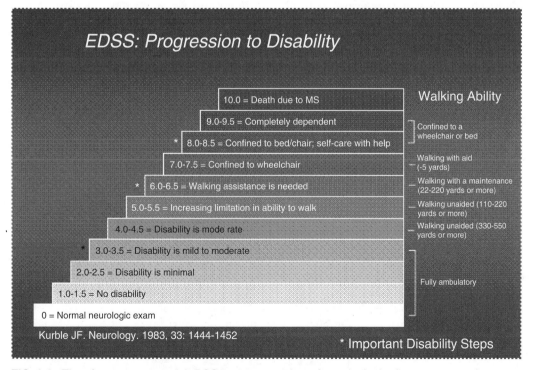

FIG. 1-3. Time from onset to reach DSS 6 versus number of attacks in the first two years after onset (+ indicates more than 10 observations at this point).

20.1 years (range 18.1–22.5 years), and 29.9 years (range 25.1–34.5 years), respectively. These observtions are analogous to the data published by our group, with minor variations. The median interval from onset of disease to reach each of these scores was significantly longer in women than in men, and in patients with a younger age of onset of MS. The interval was also longer in those with an initial RRMS course of MS, in those with complete recovery from the first relapse, and those with a longer first interattack interval. Interestingly, the median intervals to reach these target scores were significantly longer for cases with isolated optic neuritis at onset as compared to those with isolated long-track dysfunction (17).

A very useful conclusion can be drawn from these studies: Approximately 50% of patients with MS are still able to ambulate independently after 15 years of disease (2).

PREDICTORS OF PROGNOSIS, LONG-TERM OUTCOME

Given the fact that in their later course both RRMS and PPMS are progressive, and the disabilities are comparable, many predictors have been evaluated in the early course (2,4,5,31). Relapsing remitting course, early age, complete recovery from first attack, optic neuritis at onset, sensory onset, and female sex are predictors of favorable long-term outcome in MS.

The most important and reliable predictors of unfavorable, long-term outcome in MS were found, in some studies, to be: (1) attack rate in the first year of MS, and inversely, (2) shortness of first interattack interval, and (3) rate of development of early disability (EDSS 3). Late age of onset, male sex, polysymptomatic onset, incomplete recovery from first attack, and brainstem, cerebral and/or cerebellar involvement are predictive factors for an adverse outcome.

In the PPMS patients, it has been shown that an involvement of three or more neurological systems at onset, and the rapidity of early progression are adverse prognostic factors, shortening the time span to DSS 8. A shorter time of achievement of an EDSS of 3 from the onset denotes faster early accumulation of disability.

This has been associated in many studies with an earlier achievement of further milestones of disability (i.e., EDSS 6 and EDSS 8), as compared to those who had slower early accumulation of disability. A positive oligoclonal banding, though a very important aid for diagnosis, was not a significant predictor of long-term outcome.

In recent years, MRI has increasingly changed the way we evaluate MS patients, and new techniques are widening our understanding of MS in multiple dimensions. Although correlations are so far relatively poor, measures such as T2 hypointensities in gray matter, white matter atrophy, residual brain volume, spinal cord atrophy, early lesion load, and, most recently, magnetization transfer ratio analysis of normal-appearing brain tissue have all been directly associated with increased disability in MS (39). Comorbidity with other diseases definitely negatively affects long-term outcome.

MORTALITY IN MULTIPLE SCLEROSIS

Mortality in MS is not significantly different from the age-matched, general population in the early, low-disability years of MS. As the disease ages, MS-specific complications set in. The cause of death in about 50% patients with MS is due to some complication of MS, most common being pneumonia and urosepsis. In the rest of the patients, the common causes of death are the same as in general population, and include acute myocardial infarction, stroke, and malignancy. A significant minority of MS patients commit suicide, and this was found to be more common with EDSS around 5 (2).

A study of the mean time to death in MS patients revealed that the mean time to death in PPMS patients was shorter (22.3 years) as compared to non-PPMS patients. It was also stated that approximately two-thirds of patients of PPMS die due to direct complications of MS, the other one-third due to various other causes. A greater propensity of MS patients to succumb to depression, fatigue, and other medical conditions, combined with multisystem neurological deficits may be responsible for a minor shortening of total lifespan as compared to normal population, by 3 to 5 years.

There seems to be hardly any difference in the causes of mortality when RRMS (and subsequent SPMS) patients are compared with PPMS patients (Table 1-5, Table 1-6). Studies over three decades by various investigators in MS have reported the percentage of surviving patients to be between 63 and 85 at 25 years from disease onset; that percentage at 30 years was between 48 and 60.

The natural history studies, despite the limitations faced, have come a long way to contribute to our knowledge of MS. MRI studies and new immunopathogenesis study techniques have opened new avenues to better understand this disease. Intelligent and critical coupling of these two methodologies (i.e., natural history studies and newer investigations) will probably lead us to many answers about this mysterious entity called multiple sclerosis.

TABLE 1-5 *Primary causes of death for MS patients listed in 312 death certificates in the London, Ontario natural history cohort*

Cause of death	Number of deaths (n = 312)
Pneumonia	99
MS	43
Cancer	43
Heart disease	28
Septicemia	19
Respiratory failure	15
Stroke	15
Cardiac arrest	13
Suicide	6
Pulmonary embolism	4
Aspiration	3
Cachexia	3
Gastrointestinal bleeding	3
Accident	2
Dehydration	2
Respiratory arrest	2
Other* (1 case each)	12

*Other causes of death (1 case each): Acute renal failure; assisted suicide; encephalopathy; bowel infarction; cardiac arrhythmia; cardiac failure; chronic bronchitis; chronic renal failure; pyelonephritis; intestinal obstruction; head injury; pulmonary edema.

ACKNOWLEDGMENTS

For their patience and invaluable help, we would like to thank our patients and their families; the personnel at the MS Clinic at the London Health Sciences Center, London, Ontario; the MS Society of Ontario/Canada; Debra King and Linda Gibson for secretarial and manuscript assistance; Dr. Don Paty and Dr. George Ebers, along with the many others who over nearly three decades have helped with this Natural History of Multiple Sclerosis project.

TABLE 1-6 *Cause of death (underlying causes of death for some MS series in the literature) (40)*

	Number of Deaths	Mean MS-duration	MS deaths	Malignancy	Cardiovascular heart	Stroke	Suicide	Sample type
Broman 1963 (41) – Gothenburg	49	N/A	40.8%	22.4%	24.4%		6.1%	Prospective
Leibowitz 1969 (42) – Israel	73	19.8	64.4%	6.8%	20.5%	2.7%	5.4%	Population based
Malmgren 1983(43) – USA	438	22.5	53.0%	N/A				Prevalent
Phadke 1987(44) – Grampian, UK	216	24.5	61.6%	12.0%	19.0%		-	Prevalent
Hader 1988(10) – Middlesex, Ontario, Canada	45	24.7	51.1%	20.0%	11.1%	4.4%	8.8%	Population based
Citterio 1989(45) – Pavia, Italy	13	11.6	61.5%	7.6%	0	15.5%	0	Hospitalized cases
Sadovnick 1991(46) – Canada	119	19.6	47.1% [62.2%]	15.9%	10.9%	5.8%	15.1%	Two MS Clinics
Midgard 1985(47) – Norway	70	-	77.1%	15.8%	N/A			Population based
Koch-Henriksen 1998(48) – Denmark	6,068	24.5	55.4%	8.6%	17.6%		3.8%**	Population based
STAT Canada 1996(49) – Ontario, Canada	79,261	-	0.1%	27.9%	27.9%	7.6%	1.3%	General population
Natural History Cohort, London, Canada 2000	326	24.6	62.4%	12.4%	10.3%	4.5%	1.8%	population based

N/A, Not available
*, Suicides excluded from MS deaths. Altogether, they represent 6.2% of all deaths.
**, Accidents *and* suicides together.

REFERENCES

1. Cottrell DA, Kremenchutzky M, Rice GPA, et al. The natural history of multiple sclerosis: a geographically based study. V. The clinical features and natural history of primary progressive multiple sclerosis. *Brain* 1999;122: 625–639.

2. Ebers GC, Paty DW. Natural history studies and applications to clinical trials. In: Paty DW, Ebers GC, eds. *Multiple Sclerosis.* Philadelphia: F.A. Davis; 1998: 192–228.

3. Weinshenker BG, Bass B, Rice GPA, et al. The natural history of multiple sclerosis: a geographically based study. I. Clinical course and disability. *Brain* 1989;112: 133–146.

4. Weinshenker BG, Bass B, Rice GPA, et al. The natural history of multiple sclerosis: a geographically based study. II. Predictive value of the early clinical course. *Brain* 1989;112:1419–1428.

5. Weinshenker BG, Rice GPA, Noseworthy JH, et al. The natural history of multiple sclerosis: a geographically based study. III. Multivariate analysis of predictive factors and models of outcome. *Brain* 1991;114: 1045–1056.

6. Weinshenker BG, Rice GPA, Noseworthy JH, et al. The natural history of multiple sclerosis: a geographically based study. IV Applications to planning and interpretation of clinical therapeutic trials. *Brain* 1991;114: 1057–1067.

7. Cottrell DA, Kremenchutzky M, Rice GPA, et al. The natural history of multiple sclerosis: a geographically based study. VI Application to planning and interpretation of clinical therapeutic trials in primary progressive multiple sclerosis. *Brain* 1999;122:641–647.

8. Kremenchutzky M, Cottrell D, Rice GPA, et al. The natural history of multiple sclerosis: A geographically based study. VII Progressive-relapsing and relapsing-progressive multiple sclerosis: a re-evaluation. *Brain* 1999;122:1941–1949.

9. Ebers GC, Koopman WJ, Hader W, et al. The natural history of multiple sclerosis: a geographically based study. VIII. Familial multiple sclerosis. *Brain* 2000;123:641–649.

10. Hader WJ, Elliot M, Ebers GC. Epidemiology of multiple sclerosis in London and Middlesex County, Ontario, Canada. *Neurology* 1988;38:617–621.

11. Poser CM, Brinar VV. Diagnostic criteria for multiple sclerosis: an historical review. *Clin Neurol Neurosurg* 2004;106:147–158.

12. McAlpine D, Lumsden CE, Acheson ED. *Multiple Sclerosis—A Reappraisal.* Edinburgh: Livingstone; 1965.

13. Lublin FD, Reingold SC. Defining the clinical course of multiple sclerosis: results of an international survey. National Multiple Sclerosis Society (USA) Advisory Committee on Clinical Trials of New Agents in Multiple Sclerosis. *Neurology* 1996;46:907–911.

14. Andersson PB, Waubant E, Gee L, et al. Multiple sclerosis that is progressive from the time of onset: clinical characteristics and progression of disability. *Arch Neurol* 1999; Sep;56(9):1138–1142.

15. Weinshenker BG. Progressive forms of multiple sclerosis: classification streamlined or consensus overturned? *The Lancet* 15 Jan. 2000;355 (9199):162–163.

16. Kremenchutzky M, Rice GPA, Ebers GC. Secondary progressive MS following a single attack: SAP. 37th

meeting of the Canadian Congress of Neurological Sciences, Vancouver, 2002. *Can J of Neurol Sci* Vol. 29 (suppl 1); May 2002; abstract C-01:11.

17. Confavreux C, Vukusic S, Adeleine, P. Early clinical predictors and progression of irreversible disability in multiple sclerosis: an amnestic process. *Brain* 2003; 126:770–782.

18. Confavreux C, Aimard G, Devic M. Course and prognosis of multiple sclerosis assessed by the computerized data processing of 349 patients. *Brain* 1980;103: 281–300.

19. Mayr WT, Pittock SJ, McClelland RL, et al. Incidence and prevalence of multiple sclerosis in Olmsted County, Minnesota, 1985–2000. *Neurology* 2003 Nov. 25;61(10):1373–1377.

20. Runmarker B, Andersen O. Prognostic factors in a multiple sclerosis incidence cohort with twenty–five years of follow-up. *Brain* 1993;116:117–134.

21. Goodkin DE, Hertsgaard D, Rudick RA. Exacerbation rates and adherence to disease type in a prospectively followed-up population with multiple sclerosis. Implications for clinical trials. *Arch Neurol* 1989;46:1107–1112.

22. Durelli L, Bongioanni MR, Cavallo R, et al. Chronic systemic high-dose recombinant interferon alfa-2a reduces exacerbation rate, MRI signs of disease activity, and lymphocyte interferon gamma production in relapsing-remitting multiple sclerosis. *Neurology* 1994;44:406–413.

23. Jacobs LD, Cookfair DL, Rudick RA, et al. Intramuscular interferon beta-1a for disease progression in relapsing multiple sclerosis. The Multiple Sclerosis Collaborative Research Group (MSCRG). *Ann Neurol* 1996;39:285–294.

24. Johnson KP, Brooks BR, Cohen JA, et al. Copolymer 1 reduces relapse rate and improves disability in relapsing-remitting multiple sclerosis: results of a phase III multicenter, double-blind placebo-controlled trial. The Copolymer 1 Multiple Sclerosis Study Group. *Neurology* 1995;45:1268–1276.

25. McAlpine D, Compston N. Some aspects of the natural history of disseminated sclerosis: incidence, course and prognosis—factors affecting the onset and course. *QJM* 1952;21:135–167.

26. Poser CM. Exacerbations, activity and progression in multiple sclerosis. *Arch Neurol* 1980;37:471–474.

27. Poser C. The course of multiple sclerosis. *Arch Neurol* 1985;42:1035.

28. Weinshenker BG, Ebers GC. The natural history of multiple sclerosis. *Can J Neurol Sci* 1987;14:255–261.

29. Vukusic S, Confavreux C. Prognostic factors for progression of disability in the secondary progressive phase of multiple sclerosis. *J of the Neurol Sci* 2003; 206(2):135–137.

30. Minderhoud JM, Van der Hooven JH, Prange AJ. Course and prognosis of chronic progressive multiple sclerosis: results of an epidemiological study. *Acta Neurol Scand* 1988;78:10–15.

31. Poser S, Poser W, Schlaf G, et al. Prognostic indicators in multiple sclerosis. *Acta Neurol Scand* 1986;74:387–392.

32. Fog T. Topographic distribution of plaques in the spinal cord in multiple sclerosis. *Arch Neurol* 1950;63:382–414.

33. Rice GPA, Kremenchutzky M, Cottrell D, et al. Observations from the natural history cohort of London, Ontario. In: Filippi M, Comi G, eds. *Primary*

Progressive Multiple Sclerosis Series—Topics in Neuroscience. Milan: Springer-Verlag Italia; 2001: Chapter 2.

34. Paty DW, Noseworthy JH, Ebers GC. Diagnosis of multiple sclerosis. In: Paty DW, Ebers GC, eds. *Multiple Sclerosis*. Philadelphia: F.A. Davis; 1998:48–134

35. Kurtzke J. International symposium on MS—Goteberg 1972. *Ann NY Acad Sci* 1974;(suppl 58):14.

36. Kurtzke JF. On the evaluation of disability in multiple sclerosis. *Neurology* 1961;11:686–694.

37. Kurtzke JF. Clinical manifestations of multiple sclerosis. In: Vinken PJ, Bruyn GW, eds. *Handbook of Clinical Neurology*. Amsterdam: Elsevier North-Holland; 1970: 161–216.

38. Pittock SJ, Mayr WT, McClelland RL, et al. Disability profile of multiple sclerosis did not change over 10 years in a population based prevalence cohort. *Neurology* 2004;62:601–606.

39. Traboulsee A, Dehmeshki J, Peters KR, et al. Disability in multiple sclerosis is related to normal appearing brain tissue MTR histogram abnormalities. *Mult Scler* 2003;9:566–573.

40. Kremenchutzky M, Sim D, Baskerville J, et al. A study of the causes of death in multiple sclerosis patients. *Neurology* 2000;54(7) (suppl. 3A):350.

41. Broman T. Further studies concerning the natural history of multiple sclerosis. In: Pedersen E, Clausen J, Oades L, eds. *Actual problems in multiple sclerosis research*. Copenhagen: FADL's Forlag, 1963:74–76.

42. Leibowitz U, Kahana E, Alter M. Survival and death in multiple sclerosis. *Brain* 1969; 92:115–130.

43. Malmgren R, Valdiviezo N, Visscher B, et al. Underlying cause of death as recorded for multiple sclerosis patients: associated factors. *J Chron Dis* 1983;36:699–705.

44. Phadke J. Survival pattern and cause of death in patients with multiple sclerosis: results from an epidemiological survey in northeast Scotland. *J Neurol Neurosurg Psychiatry* 1987;50:523–531.

45. Citterio A, Azan G, Bergamaschi R, et al. Multiple sclerosis: disability and mortality in a cohort of clinically diagnosed patients. *Neuroepidemiology* 1989;8:249–253.

46. Sadovnick AD, Eisen K, Ebers GC, et al. Causes of death in patients attending multiple sclerosis clinics. *Neurology* 1991;41:1193–1196.

47. Midgard R, Albektsen G, Riise T, et al. Prognostic factors for survival in MS: a longitudinal, population-based study in More and Romsdal, Norway. *J Neurol Neurosurg Psychiatry* 1995;58:417–421.

48. Koch-Henriksen N, Bronnum-Hansen H, Stenager E. Underlying cause of death in Danish patients with multiple sclerosis: results from the Danish Multiple Sclerosis Registry. *J Neurol Neurosurg Psychiatry* 1998 Jul;65(1):56–59.

49. Office of the registrar, Ministry of Consumer and Commercial Relations, Ontario, Canada. Annual Report—1996.

APPENDIX I

Expanded Disability Status Scale or EDSS (Kurtzke) (29,30)
EDSS SCORE CLINICAL STATUS and DISABILITY

0 Normal neurological exam (all grade 0 in Functional Systems (FS); cerebral grade 1 acceptable.

1 No disability, minimal signs in one FS (i.e., one grade 1 excluding cerebral grade 1).

1.5 No disability, minimal signs in more than one FS (more than one grade 1 excluding cerebral grade 1).

2.0 Minimal disability in one FS (one FS grade 2, others 0 or 1).

2.5 Minimal disability in two FS (two FS grade 2, others 0 or 1).

3 Moderate disability in one FS (one FS grade 3, others 0 or 1), or mild disability in three or four FS (three or four FS grade 2, others 0 or 1).

3.5 Fully ambulatory but with moderate disability in one FS (one grade 3 and one or two FS grade 2) or two FS grade 3, others 0 or 1, or five FS grade 2, others 0 or 1.

4 Fully ambulatory without aid, self-sufficient, up and about some 12 hours per day despite relatively severe disability consisting of one FS grade 4 (others 0 or 1), or combinations of lesser grades exceeding limits of previous steps. Able to walk without aid or rest some 500 meters. (0.3 miles).

4.5 Fully ambulatory without aid, up and about much of the day, able to work a full day, may otherwise have some limitation of full activity or require minimal assistance; characterized by relatively severe disability, usually consisting of one FS grade 4 (others 0 or 1) or combinations of lesser grades exceeding limits of previous steps. Able to walk without aid or rest for some 300 meters (975 ft).

5 Ambulatory without aid or rest for about 200 meters (650 feet); disability severe enough to impair full daily activities (e.g., to work full day without special provisions). (Usual FS equivalents are one grade 5 alone, others 0 or 1; or combinations of lesser grades usually exceeding specifications for step 4.0).

5.5 Ambulatory without aid or rest for about 100 meters (325 ft); disability severe enough to impair full daily activities. (Usual FS equivalents are one grade 5 alone, others 0 or 1; or combinations of lesser grades usually exceeding specifications for step 4.0).

6 Intermittent or constant unilateral assistance (cane, crutch, brace) required to walk about 100 meters (325 ft) with or without resting. (Usual FS equivalents are combinations with more than two FS grade 3+).

6.5 Constant bilateral assistance (canes, crutches, braces) required to walk about 20 meters (65 ft). (Usual FS equivalents are combinations with more than two FS grade 3+).

7 Unable to walk beyond about 5 meters (16 ft) even with aid, essentially restricted to wheelchair; wheels self in standard wheelchair a full day and transfers alone; up and about in wheelchair some 12 hours a day. Usual FS equivalents are combinations with more than one FS grade 4+; very rarely pyramidal grade 5 alone.

7.5 Unable to take more than a few steps; restricted to wheelchair; may need aid in transfers, wheels self but cannot carry on in standard wheelchair a full day; may require motorized wheelchair; usual FS equivalents are combinations with more than one FS grade 4+.

8 Essentially restricted to bed or chair or perambulated in wheelchair; but may be out of bed much of the day; retains many self-care functions; generally has effective use of arms. Usual FS equivalents are combinations, generally grade 4+ in several systems.

8.5 Essentially restricted to bed for much of the day; has some effective use of arm(s); retains some self-care functions. Usual FS equivalents are combinations, generally grade 4+ in several systems.

9 Helpless bed patient; can communicate and eat. Usual FS equivalents are combinations, mostly grade 4.

9.5 Totally helpless bed patient; unable to communicate effectively or eat/swallow. Usual FS equivalents are combinations, almost all grade 4+.

10 Death due to MS.

2

The Genetics and Genetic Epidemiology of Multiple Sclerosis: The "Hard Facts"

A.D. Sadovnick

*Department of Medical Genetics and Faculty of Medicine, Division of Neurology,
University of British Columbia, British Columbia, Canada*

Hard facts about multiple sclerosis (MS) are difficult, if not impossible, to identify. To illustrate, concepts of pathogenesis have come, gone, and then been reintroduced, including the view that MS is an autoimmune disorder and the role of the axon in disease pathogenesis. Similarly, candidate genes and regions have been identified, replicated, and rejected on a regular basis in the MS literature.

MS is widely believed to be an autoimmune disorder (1) in which the central nervous system (CNS) myelin is attacked by the immune response, resulting in focal lesions and clinical symptomatology. The evidence for this, although circumstantially strong, remains less than definitive. This is illustrated by the presence of retinal lesions where myelin is absent and the density of lesions in the cortex, which exceed those in white matter (2). There has been recent recognition that axonal loss occurs in the acute plaque (3) and rediscovery of axonal loss in the chronic phase of the disease (4). There has been speculation that there are two phases of the disease, the first inflammatory and the second degenerative. Natural history studies have not definitively concluded whether there is (5) or is not (Kremenchutzky, Ebers, 2005, personal communication) an association between numbers of exacerbations and long-term outcome. Furthermore, those with purely progressive disease from first symptom ("primary progressive") do no better or worse than those with relapse onset when the progression phase from first symptom is compared (5). Clinical heterogeneity is obvious and recent pathologic studies indicate this may also be true, based on pathological phenotype (6). (See also Chapter 3 by Morales et al.) Given this information, it is not unexpected that the exact roles of genes and environment in the etiology, susceptibility, onset, and prognosis of MS are yet to be definitively delineated.

Debate over the roles of nature (or heredity) and nurture (or environment) in the etiology of MS began in the late 1800s when Gowers (7) stated that the familial incidence of MS was "quite exceptional," whereas Eichhorst labelled MS as an "inherited, transmissible" disease (8). Between 1921 and 1948, the medical literature reported a total of 64 sibling pairs, 13 parent–child pairs, and 15 second-and/or third-degree relative pairs concordant for MS (9). These were usually single case reports rather than large series. Although of interest, the literature on familial MS was greatly hampered by many factors, including the absence of consensus diagnostic criteria until 1965 (10), which have subsequently been updated to incorporate advances in technology and understanding about the natural history and heterogeneity of the disease (11,12).

On review, it was not unusual to find that families with more than one case of MS ("multiplex" families) actually had hereditary cerebello-pyramidal disease or hereditary spastic ataxia (13,14). One such family with 12 reportedly affected individuals (15) was later shown to have Pelizaeus–Merzbacher disease (16) rather than MS. Nevertheless, there is now strong evidence that multiplex, multigenerational MS families exist (17). It remains to be seen whether such families represent rare, autosomal dominant forms of MS, as has been found in approximately 5% of the complex disorder of Alzheimer disease (18) and had been postulated decades ago for MS (19).

Despite the problems that plagued most if not all early family studies, valiant attempts were made to explain the familial nature of MS in terms of a single-gene, "Mendelian" mode of inheritance (e.g., 9,14,19) or polygenic threshold models (e.g., 20,21). However, this research has never been conclusive, largely because family studies in MS have long been hindered by many factors, including:

1. Lack of appropriate population prevalence data
2. Absence of denominator data
3. Failure to do age-corrections
4. Publication bias toward the reporting of concordant affected relative pairs
5. Failure to recognize (or acknowledge) the skewed sex distribution
6. The extremely low penetrance necessary to account for the low frequency of familial MS

7. Absence of diagnostic criteria which included laboratory and MRI findings (e.g., 11,12)

There have been many advances in the last two decades or so which have resolved (or partially resolved) some of these problems with respect to family studies in MS. Prevalence studies have now been done in various regions of North and South America (22). While all studies are not comparable or definitive, at least there is the recognition that prevalence information is critical not only for research (e.g., baseline population risks of MS or denominators, changes in disease prevalence over time, etc.) but also for recognition of the magnitude of the MS burden to society in general and medical resources in particular. A corollary of accurately assessing prevalence is the recognition of the clinical variability of MS (23) and, hence, the need for evolving diagnostic criteria (10–12) that reflect improving technology. Similarly, recognition of the importance of age correction and skewed gender ratios is critical in determining familial risks to relatives of individuals with MS. Family studies now take into consideration factors such as the gender of individuals "affected" or "at risk," family structure, current age at present or at death and the impact thereof on "unaffected" status, diagnostic criteria, and population-specific background prevalence. Research continues and it is becoming increasingly apparent that the disease is more complex than was previously believed. Nevertheless, longitudinal, replicative, and collaborative research has finally confirmed some information that we can state, with a high degree of certainty, as "hard" facts with respect to the genetics and genetic epidemiology of MS.

GENES ARE INVOLVED IN MS SUSCEPTIBILITY

The first (and to date, only) consistent genetic association in MS has been with the HLA class I antigens A3 and B7 (24–26), later subtyped into a strong and consistent association with the HLA DR15, DQ6, and Dw2 haplotype (27–30). Nevertheless, recent work has raised questions about whether this association is in fact much more complex than originally believed (31,32).

Other than HLA, the MS literature has exploded with linkage studies, association studies, whole genome scans, SNP analyses, HapMap approaches, etc., but no definitive candidate genes or regions have been identified. An in-depth listing of the MS candidates (positive and negative) is provided by the University of California, San Francisco (32a). The failure to readily identify candidates in MS must, however, be interpreted as an indication of the complexity of the disease rather than an assumption that genes are not involved. The difficulty in identifying candidates is not unusual or specific to MS; it is also found in similar disorders such as diabetes and Alzheimer disease which, together with MS and other diseases, are now referred to as "common complex disorders."

Insight into the relative roles of genes and environment in MS has come largely from longitudinal, population-based, genetic epidemiological studies. This chapter will focus on these since, taken together, they represent "hard facts" about the relative roles of genes and environment in MS. Speculation about candidate genes and the direction for future molecular genetic research in MS is beyond the scope of this chapter. However, it must be stated that such work has to continue, although insights into future directions cannot ignore the lessons learned from the genetic epidemiology of the disease.

Familial Recurrence Risks

Using the classical genetic epidemiological approach, the first step was to determine whether relatives of MS patients had a greater risk of also developing MS compared to the background population. It was also important to adjust for the fact that the range for the MS age of onset is wide and that age must therefore be considered in the "affected" status of family members [i.e., controlling for a remaining "at risk" period if the unaffected individual is still within the usual age range for MS onset (11)]. The Canadian Network of Multiple Sclerosis Clinics (33) provided a unique opportunity to look at age-adjusted familial recurrence risks within first-degree relatives of persons with MS, compared to expectations for the general population. These risks were initially reported for the Vancouver Multiple Sclerosis Clinic (34) and longitudinal follow-up of Canadian MS patients have validated the age-correction approach used in these initial studies (35). The Canadian studies, together with those from other countries (36–38), have consistently shown that first-degree relatives of MS patients have an increased risk of developing MS (see Table 2-1).

Nature versus Nurture

The observation that a disorder occurs more often among relatives of people with MS than in the general population does not address the question about the interplay, if any, of genes and intrafamilial environment (i.e., that shared by family members such as twins, biological siblings, and non-biological siblings). Historically, especially for some psychiatric disorders, this has been addressed by looking at identical twins raised apart. However, even including the entire Canadian MS population (approximately 30,000 individuals), such twin pairs would be

TABLE 2-1 *Recurrence risks for selected relatives of persons with MS*

Relationship to person with MS	MS lifetime risk*
First-degree relative; index case only MS	3.0%
Monozygotic female co-twin	34.0%
Dizygotic co-twin	5.4%
Adopted sib	0.2%
Maternal half-sib	2.2%
Paternal half-sib	1.2%
Stepsibling	0.2%
Offspring of conjugal mating	30.5%
Offspring of consanguineous mating	9.0%
Sister of female MS patient with onset under 30 plus 1 affected parent	12.7%

*Lifetime MS risk for the general population = 0.2%.

too rare to permit any meaningful statistical analyses and conclusions. It was therefore decided to look at other special relative groups that would allow not only an estimate of the relative roles of genes and intrafamilial environment, but also replication of findings in separate samples. To this end, longitudinal, population-based studies of adoptees (39) (Figure 2-1); half-siblings (40,41) (Figure 2-2); and stepsiblings (42) (Figure 2-3); have clearly shown that it is the *biological* sharing of DNA that is responsible for the observed excess of MS among biological relatives (i.e., familial aggregation) rather than a shared family environment. This is not to say that non-genetic (environmental) factors are unimportant in susceptibility to MS or prognosis but, rather, to explain the familial aggregation of the disease (in excess over what one would expect for the general population).

In a study of 1,201 non-biological relatives of MS patients (39), only one case of MS was identified. Based on data for biological first-degree relatives, 25 cases would have been expected (34). This observed rate of 1:1,201 is what would be expected for the general population (Poisson probability = 2.5×10^{-10}).

Although the Canadian numbers are not large enough to allow an exact replication study (and as far as we are aware, no other adoption studies have been conducted on MS), ongoing ascertainment of adoptees with MS through the Canadian Collaborative Project on Genetic Susceptibility to MS (CCPGSMS) (43) has con-

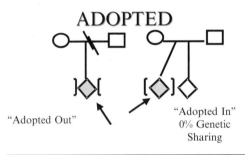

ADOPTED

"Adopted Out"

"Adopted In"
0% Genetic
Sharing

Relative		Relative	Conclude
Biological	versus	Adoptive	Genetic involvement
			Envronmental involvement

FIG. 2-1. Adoptee studies.

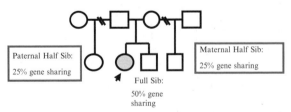

Half-Siblings and MS

Paternal Half Sib:
25% gene sharing

Maternal Half Sib:
25% gene sharing

Full Sib:
50% gene
sharing

Relative		Relative	Conclude
Half-sibling	versus	Full-sibling	Genetic involvement
Raised together	versus	Raised apart	Environment
Maternal	versus	Paternal	Maternal Effect

FIG. 2-2. Half-sibling studies.

tinued to support the findings of this adoption study. In addition, these results have been replicated through CCPGSMS studies of other specific relationships, such as half-siblings and stepsiblings.

Two half-sibling studies have been conducted as part of the CCPGSMS (40,41). Among 1,567 MS index cases, 3,436 half-siblings and 2,706 full siblings were identified. The age-adjusted, full-sibling risk was 3.11%. In contrast, the half-sibling risk in the same families was significantly lower at 1.89% (χ^2 = 7.548, df = 1, p = 0.006), but higher than expected if familial risk was simply oligogenic. Furthermore, this risk did not differ significantly regardless of whether the half-siblings were raised together (2.07%) or apart (1.97%).

Recurrence risks were examined for 687 stepsiblings of 19,746 CCPGSMS index cases, with the prior expectation that there would be no increased risk for these individuals compared to the general population, based on results of the half-sibling (40,41) and adoptee (39) data. One stepsibling with MS was identified, which was not significantly different than expected based on the general population. The stepsibling study further emphasized the importance of diagnostic criteria in family studies (42), since three additional stepsiblings were initially reported to have MS but this proved not to be the case on follow-up. (See Fig. 2-4.)

While twin studies have long been used to study the relative roles of nature and nurture, size and ascertainment constraints usually limit the results of such studies to comparison of concordance rates between monozygotic twins (who share 100% of their genetic material) and dizygotic twins (who share 50% of their genetic material) (Figure 2-4). There have been several large, population-based twin studies in MS, including those from Canada (44) and the United Kingdom (45).

In the Canadian study (44), which is the largest population-based longitudinal twin study in MS to date, bias was demonstrably minimized and an estimated 75% of all Canadian MS twin pairs were ascertained, giving a sample sufficiently large (N = 370) to permit additional, informative comparisons along with simply looking at the MZ:DZ concordance. Twinning itself was not found to affect MS prevalence and twins with MS did not differ from non-twin concordant sibling pairs for DR15 allele frequency.

Probandwise concordance rates of 25.3% (s.e. +/– 4.4) for monozygotic (MZ) twins, 5.4% (+/– 2.8) for dizygotic (DZ) twins, and 2.9% (+/– 0.6) for their non-twin siblings were found. MZ concordance was in excess of DZ concordance. The

Step-Siblings and MS

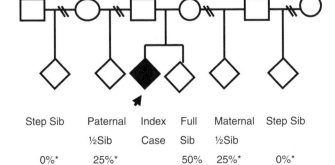

Step Sib	Paternal ½Sib	Index Case	Full Sib	Maternal ½Sib	Step Sib
0%*	25%*		50%	25%*	0%*

*% genetic sharing (identical by descent) with MS index case

FIG. 2-3. Stepsibling studies.

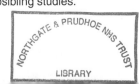

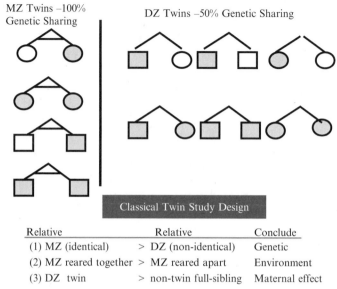

MZ Twins –100% Genetic Sharing

DZ Twins –50% Genetic Sharing

Classical Twin Study Design

Relative		Relative	Conclude
(1) MZ (identical)	>	DZ (non-identical)	Genetic
(2) MZ reared together	>	MZ reared apart	Environment
(3) DZ twin	>	non-twin full-sibling	Maternal effect

FIG. 2-4. Twin studies.

excess concordance in MZ was derived primarily from like-sexed female pairs with a probandwise concordance rate of 34 of 100 (34 +/− 5.7%) compared to 3 of 79 (3.8 +/− 2.8%) for female DZ pairs. We did not demonstrate an MZ:DZ difference in males, but the sample size was very small. Taken together, MS twin studies all clearly show that MZ concordance is consistently higher than DZ, although the MZ concordance does not approach 100%.

PARENT-OF-ORIGIN EFFECT

The preponderance of females among the general population of individuals affected with MS is well established. However, there is increasing evidence that there may be a parent-of-origin effect in MS—a maternal effect may be operative. Data for this come from the half-sibling studies (40,41) and the Canadian twin study (44).

The initial half-sibling study (40) showed a trend toward an excess of maternal half-siblings having MS compared to paternal half-siblings. However, as this was not statistically significant, it was believed to probably be an artefact. However, the second half-sibling study (41) clearly showed that MS risk for maternal half-siblings was 2.60% (37/1821), near double the

risk to paternal half-siblings of 1.26% (14/1521); $\chi^2 = 5.870$, df = 1, p = 0.015.

As part of the Canadian twin study (44), there were 238 twin index cases for whom complete family history information was available. Only full siblings raised together with the index case were included in recurrence risk calculations. The sibling recurrence risk in these families was 2.9% (s.e. = 0.6%), compared to 5.4% (+/− 2.8) for DZ twins. These data, together with the half-sibling data (and month of birth effect—*vide infra*), strongly imply a maternal effect. However, the nature of this effect (e.g., X-linkage, mitochondrial inheritance, imprinting, intrauterine exposures, maternal vitamin D levels at conception) is yet to be determined and may even be heterogeneous.

NON-GENETIC TRANSMISSION OF MS

Genetic epidemiological data, including adoptees, half-siblings, stepsiblings, and birth order studies (e.g., 39–41, 46–48) all provide evidence against the non-genetic transmission of MS in either adulthood or childhood (i.e., MS is not a transmissible disease such as AIDS). This concern is frequently raised by MS patients and their family members.

Adulthood

There does not appear to be any non-genetic sexual transmission of MS. As part of the CCPGSMS, transmission of MS among 13,128 "spouses" (the term "spouse" is being used here in a generic sense to refer to any sexual partner) of MS index cases was examined. Twenty-three couples were identified in which the spouse of an MS index case subsequently developed MS (49). This was not significantly different from expectation for the general population ($\chi^2 = 0.35$, df = 1).

Childhood

Data for half-siblings, adopted relatives and stepsiblings, taken individually and together, provide no evidence for non-genetic transmission during childhood, either through contact with an affected parent or through contact with a sibling (full, half-, step-, or adopted) who eventually developed MS (39–42).

THE NATURE OF THE ENVIRONMENTAL FACTOR(S)

Adoptee, half-sibling, and stepsibling data have clearly shown that the intrafamilial environment is not a factor in MS susceptibility (39–42). Although it is believed that the familial aggregation of MS is genetic, non-genetic (environmental) factors are still important, as illustrated by twin data in which the MZ concordance rate does not approach 100% (44,45). Taken together, the focus on the nature of the environmental factor(s) in MS is shifting away from the family and toward more population-based sources, such as climate.

A recent study of pooled data (50) from four northern MS populations found a May:November birth ratio in living incident cases from Scotland (1.89), Denmark (1.22), Sweden (1.18), and Canada (1.13), implicating a May peak and November nadir. Of interest, the birth month ratios decreased in the order of population prevalence. These data imply not only a potential parent-of-origin effect but also are consistent with previous findings of associations between higher latitudes and risk of MS; the latter findings suggest exposure to the sun may account for the geographical variation of MS (51,52). Most biologically active vitamin D is generated in the skin with exposure to ultraviolet radiation (52); an increased risk of MS related to month of birth could reflect well-documented, seasonal deficiency in maternal concentrations of vitamin D (53). It has recently been shown that vitamin D receptors are present in brain, and gestational vitamin D deficiency has striking effects on brain development in experimental animals (54).

CONCLUSION

There is still much to be learned about the roles of genes and environment in MS. However, "hard facts" to date can be summarized to include the following:

1. MS is believed to result from the interaction of genes and environment.
2. The familial aggregation of MS compared to the general population is primarily because of the sharing of genetic material.
3. The environmental component appears to be ubiquitous and acts at a population level rather than in the familial microenvironment (intrafamilial environment).
4. A number of factors may alter transmission of susceptibility, including gender and age of disease onset in family members.
5. A number of different genes will be operative—several gene regions are in play and etiologic heterogeneity cannot be ruled out. The association between MS and the MHC has long been documented but may be more complex than initially believed. Heterogeneity and complexity are to be expected.
6. MS is not a transmissible disease, either in childhood or adulthood.

Much of the information from genetic epidemiological studies is being incorporated into clinical practice with respect to genetic and reproductive counselling for MS families. This clearly shows the bridge between research and clinical practice.

ACKNOWLEDGMENTS

CCPGSMS was funded by the Multiple Sclerosis Society of Canada Research Foundation. Dr. Sadovnick is a Michael Smith Foundation Distinguished Scholar. The author thanks colleagues and collaborators for helpful discussion and collaboration. These include Professor G.C. Ebers, Dr. David Dyment, Dr. Cristen Willer, Irene Yee and members of the Canadian Collaborative Study Group including; J.J-F Oger, D.W. Paty, S.A. Hashimoto, V. Devonshire, J. Hooge, J., T. Traboulsee (Vancouver) , L. Metz (Calgary), S. Warren (Edmonton), W. Hader (Saskatoon), R.Nelson, M. Freedman (Ottawa), D. Brunet (Kingston), J. Paulseth (Hamilton), G. Rice, M. Kremenchutzky (London), P. O'Connor, T. Gray, M. Hohol (Toronto), P. Duquette, Y. Lapierre (Montreal), J.-P. Bouchard (Quebec City), T. J. Murray, V. Bhan, C. Maxner (Halifax), W. Pryse-Phillips, M. Stefanelli (St. Johns).

The author would like to thank the late Dr. Donald Winston Paty for having the foresight to enable her to integrate clinical genetics into the multidisciplinary Vancouver Multiple Sclerosis Clinic since September, 1980. At the time, this approach was very innovative, not only with respect to taking clinical genetics to a non-pediatric setting but also to even consider that genes were important in what are known as "adult onset, common complex disorders."

REFERENCES

1. Keegan BM, Noseworthy JH. Multiple sclerosis. *Ann Rev Med* 2002;53:285–302.
2. Peterson JW, Bo L, Mork S, et al. Transected neurites, apoptotic neurons, and reduced inflammation in cortical multiple sclerosis lesions. *Ann Neurol* 2001;50:389–400.
3. Ferguson B, Matyszak MK, Esiri MM, et al. Axonal damage in acute multiple sclerosis lesions. *Brain* 1997;120:393–399.
4. Trapp BD, Peterson J, Ransohof RM, et al. Axonal transection in the lesions of multiple sclerosis. *N Engl J Med* 1998;338:278–285.
5. Confavreux C, Vukusic S, Adeleine P. Early clinical predictors and progression of irreversible disability in multiple sclerosis: an amnesic process. *Brain* 2003;126:770–782.
6. Lassmann H, Bruck W, Lucchinetti C. Heterogeneity of multiple sclerosis pathogenesis: implications for diagnosis and therapy. *Trends Mol Med* 2001;7:115–121.
7. Gowers WR. *A Manual of Diseases of the Nervous System*. London: J & A Churchill; 1886.
8. Eichhorst H. Veber infantile und hereditare multiple sklerosis. *Arch Pathol Anat Physiol Klin Med* 1896;146:173–192.
9. Mackay RP. The familial occurrence of multiple sclerosis and its implications. *Research Publications, Association for Research in Nervous and Mental Diseases* 1950;28:149–177.
10. Schumacher GA, Beebe G, Kibler R, et al. Problems of experimental trials of therapy in multiple sclerosis. *Ann N Y Acad Sci* 1965;122:552–568.
11. Poser CM, Paty DW, Scheinberg L, et al. New diagnostic criteria for multiple sclerosis: guidelines for research protocols. *Ann Neurol* 1983;13:227–231.
12. McDonald WI, Compston A, Edan G, et al. Recommended diagnostic criteria for multiple sclerosis: guidelines from the International Panel on the diagnosis of multiple sclerosis. *Ann Neurol* 2001;50:121–127
13. Muller R. Genetic aspects of multiple sclerosis. *A.M.A. Archives of Neurology and Psychiatry* 1953;70:733–740.
14. Pratt R., Compston N, McAlpine D. The familial incidence of disseminated sclerosis and its significance. *Brain* 1951;74:191–232.
15. Pelizaeus F. Uber eine eigentumliche form spastischer lahmung mit cerbralerscheinungen auf hereditarer Grundlage. *Arch Psychiat Nervenkr* 1885;698–710.
16. Aicardi J. The inherited leukodystrophies: a clinical overview. *J Inherit Metab Dis* 1993;16: 733–743.
17. Dyment DA, Steckley JL, Willer CJ, et al. An extended pedigree with multiple sclerosis suggests autosomal dominant inheritance. *Brain* 2002;125:1–9.
18. Rogaeva EA, Fafel KC, Song YQ, et al. Screening for PS1 mutations in a referral-based series of AD cases. 21 novel mutations. *Neurology* 2001;57:621–625.
19. Lord D, O'Farrell AG, Staunton H, et al. The inheritance of MS susceptibility. *J Med Sci* 1990;159(suppl 8):1–20
20. MacKay RP, Myrianthopoulos NC. Multiple sclerosis in twins and their relatives: genetic analysis of family histories. *Acta Genetica* 1960;10:33–47.
21. Sadovnick AD, Spence MA, Tideman S. A goodness-of-fit test for the polygenic threshold model: application to multiple sclerosis. *Am J Med Genet* 1981;8:355–361.
22. Kurtzke JF. Multiple sclerosis in time and space—geographic clues to cause. *J Neurovirol* 2000;6 (suppl 2):S134–140.
23. Lublin FD, Reingold SC. Defining the clinical course of multiple sclerosis: results of an international survey. National Multiple Sclerosis Society (USA) Advisory Committee on Clinical Trials of New Agents in Multiple Sclerosis. *Neurology* 1996;46:907–911.
24. Naito S, Namerow N, Mickey M, et al. Multiple sclerosis: association with HL-A3. *Tissue Antigens* 1972;2:1–4.
25. Bertrams J, Kuwert E, Liedtke U. HL-A antigens and multiple sclerosis. *Tissue Antigens* 1972;2:405–408.
26. Jersild C, Svejgaard A, Fog T. HL-A antigens and multiple sclerosis. *The Lancet* 1972;2:1240–1241.
27. Hauser SL, Fleischnick E, Weiner H, et al. Extended major histocompatability complex haplotypes in patients with multiple sclerosis. *Neurology* 1989;39:275–277.
28. Cullen CG, Middletown D, Savage D, et al. HLA-DR and DQ DNA genotyping in multiple sclerosis patients in northern Ireland. *Human Immunol* 1991;30:1–6.

29. Hillert J, Olerup O. Multiple sclerosis is associated with genes within or close to the HLA-DR-DQ Subregion on a normal DR15, DQ6, Dw2 Haplotype. *Neurology* 1993;43:43–168.

30. Allen M, Sandberg-Wollheim M, Sjogren K, et al. Association of susceptibility to multiple sclerosis in Sweden with HLA class II DRB1 and DQB1 alleles. *Human Immunol* 1994;39:41–48.

31. Ligers A, Dyment A, Willer C, et al. The genetic contribution of the HLA DRB1 locus to MS susceptibility. *Am J Hum Genet*. 2001;69:900–903.

32. Dyment DA, Sadovnick AD, Willer CJ, et al. An extended genome scan in 442 Canadian multiple sclerosis affected sibships. *Human Mol Genet*. 2004, in press.

32a. University of California, San Francisco. Available at http://www.ucsf.edu/msdb/r_ms_candidate_genes.html. Accessed August 19, 2005.

33. Paty DW on behalf of the Canadian Network of Multiple Sclerosis Clinics. The Canadian experience: multiple sclerosis clinics versus traditional medical care and what made multiple sclerosis research flourish in Canada. In: *Advances in MS Research*. Fredericson S, Link H, eds. London: Martin Dunitz, 1999: 201–208.

34. Sadovnick AD, Baird PA, Ward RH. Multiple sclerosis: updated risks for relatives. *Am J Med Genet* 1988;29:533–541.

35. Ebers GC, Koopman WJ, Hader W, et al. The natural history of multiple sclerosis: a geographically based study. VIII. Familial multiple sclerosis. *Brain* 2000;123:641–649. 36. Robertson NP, Fraser M, Deans J, et al. Age-adjusted recurrence risks for relatives of patients with multiple sclerosis. *Brain* 1996;119:449–455.

37. Carton H, Vlietinck R, Debruyne J, et al. Risks of multiple sclerosis in relatives of patients in Flanders, Belgium. *J Neurol Neurosurg Psychiatry* 1997;62:329–333.

38. Montomoli C, Prokopenko I, Caria A, et al. Multiple sclerosis recurrence risk for siblings in an isolated population of Central Sardinia, Italy. *Genet Epidemiol* 2002;22:265–271.

39. Ebers GC, Sadovnick AD, Risch NJ, and the Canadian Collaborative Study Group. A genetic basis for familial aggregation in multiple sclerosis. *Nature* 1995;377:150–151.

40. Sadovnick AD, Ebers GC, Dyment D, et al. and the Canadian Collaborative Study Group. Evidence for the genetic basis of multiple sclerosis. *The Lancet* 1996: 347:1728–1730.

41. Ebers GC, Sadovnick AD, Dyment DA, et al. for the Canadian Collaborative Study Group. A parent of origin effect in multiple sclerosis: observations in half-siblings. *The Lancet* 2004;363:857–850.

42. Sadovnick D, Ebers G, Dyment DA on behalf of the Canadian Collaborative Study Group. MS in step-siblings: recurrence risk and ascertainment. (abstract) *Mult Scler* 2004;10(suppl 2):S162.

43. Sadovnick AD, Ebers GC, Risch NJ and the Canadian Collaborative Study Group. Canadian Collaborative Project on genetic susceptibility to MS, phase 2: rationale and method. *Can J Neurol Sci* 1998;25:216–221.

44. Willer CJ, Dyment DA, Sadovnick AD, et al. Twin concordance and sibling recurrence rates in multiple sclerosis. *PNAS* 2003;100:12877–12882.

45. Mumford CJ, Wood NW, Kellar-Wood H, et al. The British Isles survey of multiple sclerosis in twins. *Neurology* 1994;44:11–15.

46. Gaudet JPC, Hashimoto L, Sadovnick AD, et al. Is multiple sclerosis caused by late childhood infection: a case-control study of birth order in simplex cases of multiple sclerosis. *Acta Neurologica Scandinavica* 1995;91:19–21.

47. Gaudet JPC, Hashimoto L, Sadovnick AD, et al. A study of birth order and multiple sclerosis in multiplex families. *Neuroepidemiology* 1995;14:188–192.

48. Ahlgren C, Andersen O. No major birth order effect on the risk of multiple sclerosis. *Neuroepidemiology* 2004;23:38–41.

49. Ebers GC, Yee IML, Sadovnick AD, et al. and the Canadian Collaborative Study Group. Conjugal multiple sclerosis: population-based prevalence and recurrence risks in offspring. *Ann Neurol* 2000;48:927–931.

50. Willer CJ, Dyment DA, Sadovnick AD, et al. Timing of birth and risk of multiple sclerosis: population-based study. *BMJ* 2005;330:120-(E-pub Dec. 7, 2004).

51. Hammond SR, English DR, McLeod JG. The age-range of risk of developing multiple sclerosis: evidence from a migrant population in Australia. *Brain* 2000;123:968–974.

52. Van der Mei IA, Ponsonby AL, Dwyer T, et al. Past exposure to sun, skin phenotype, and risk of multiple sclerosis: case-control study. *BMJ* 2003;327:336.

53. Vieth R, Cole DE, Hawker GA, et al. Wintertime vitamin D insufficiency is common in young Canadian women, and their vitamin D intake does not prevent it. *Eur J Clin Nutr* 2001;55:1901–1907.

54. McGrath JJ, Feron FP, Burne TH, et al. Vitamin D3—implications for brain development. *J Steroid Biochem Mol Biol* 2004;89–90:557–660

3

The Pathology of Multiple Sclerosis: Evidence for Heterogeneity

Yazmín Morales,[1,2] Joseph E. Parisi,[3,4]
and Claudia F. Lucchinetti[4]

[1]Clinical Research Training Program (CRTP), Mayo Clinic College of Medicine,
Mayo Graduate School, Rochester, Minnesota; [2]Pritzker School of Medicine,
University of Chicago, Chicago, Illinois; [3]Department of Laboratory Medicine and
Pathology, Mayo Clinic College of Medicine, Rochester, Minnesota;
[4]Department of Neurology, Mayo Clinic College of Medicine,
Rochester, Minnesota

INTRODUCTION

Idiopathic Inflammatory Demyelinating Disorders (IIDDs)

Demyelinating disorders of the central nervous system (CNS) form a diverse group that can be divided into primary (i.e., idiopathic) and secondary types. Secondary acquired demyelinating diseases are a heterogeneous group of disorders that include viral infections, autoimmune and other inflammatory disorders, cerebral edema, ischemia, Wallerian degeneration, as well as toxic and nutritional disorders (1). The idiopathic inflammatory demyelinating diseases (IIDDs) represent a broad spectrum of disorders that vary in their clinical course, regional distribution, and pathology. This review will highlight the clinicopathologic heterogeneity within the family of IIDDs, as well as their pathogenic implications.

MULTIPLE SCLEROSIS

Heterogeneity of MS: Clinical Course and Pathology

The clinical course of multiple sclerosis (MS) is quite variable and unpredictable at onset. Natural history studies (2,3) and historical data indicate approximately 80% of MS patients present with a relapsing-remitting course of distinct relapses followed by complete, partial, or minimal recovery. The remaining 20% of patients present with primary progressive MS, characterized by the steady accumulation of irreversible neurological deficits, beginning at disease onset (2,3). Nearly 50% of all MS patients will become dependent on a walking aid and a significant percentage of these will require a wheelchair after 15 years of disease duration (2,3). While MS relapses reflect the clinical presentation of acute inflammatory focal demyelination, clinical remission early in disease is likely due to resolution of inflammation and surrounding edema, as well as remyelination. In turn, progression of neurological disabilities likely results from the accumulation of demyelinating lesions with axonal loss and gliosis (4). While MS can affect any CNS area, demyelinating lesions are most common in the periventricular white matter, cerebellum, brainstem, spinal cord, and optic nerves. These are associated with a wide spectrum of sensory, motor, and cognitive deficits (5). Permanent neurological disability in multiple sclerosis results from both incomplete recovery from relapse and disease progression (without distinct relapses).

MS Pathology: A Historical Perspective

Multiple sclerosis is a chronic neurological disease of the central nervous system (CNS) characterized by immune-mediated myelin loss with variable degrees of axonal injury. By the 19th century, the pathologic hallmarks of MS had been well-described. In particular, the gross features typical of MS, defined by sharply circumscribed gray translucent (sclerotic) plaques in CNS white matter, were characterized by Carswell (1838) (6) and Cruveiler (1841) (7). Also, the microscopic features of the MS plaque, characterized by perivascular inflammation associated with demyelination, axonal injury, and astrocytic scar formation, were first detailed by Rindficisch (1863) (8) and Charcot (1868) (9,10). By the 20th century, Kabat (1948) (11,12) had identified laboratory markers of disease, namely increases in oligoclonal immunoglobulin in the cerebrospinal

fluid (CSF) of MS patients [for reviews, refer to (13,14)]. More recently, distinct structural and immunopathological subtypes of MS were described by Lucchinetti et al. (1999–2001) (15–17). While the pathological hallmarks of MS, namely inflammation, marked myelin loss in the face of relative axonal preservation and gliosis, still define all MS lesions, there is evidence of interindividual heterogeneity (and intraindividual homogeneity) in terms of the immunological basis of demyelination, the fate of oligodendrocytes, and the extent of axonal injury and/or remyelination (see Figs. 3-1 and 3-2).

Heterogeneity of MS Histopathology

Early MS Lesions: Stages of Demyelination

Pathologically, MS is a dynamic disorder with distinct stages of demyelination. A single MS plaque may demonstrate areas at different stages of demyelination, including early and late active demyelination, as well as inactive (completely demyelinated) areas, with or without remyelination. Actively demyelinating lesions are defined by a variable inflammatory infiltrate, consisting mainly of macrophages admixed with reactive astrocytes and variable lymphocytic cuffs. The stages of demyelination can be defined using a battery of immunocytochemical stains (18), including antibodies to minor myelin proteins, namely myelin-associated glycoprotein (MAG) and myelin oligodendrocyte glycoprotein (MOG), and antibodies to major myelin proteins, namely myelin basic protein (MBP) and phospholipid protein (PLP), in addition to the standard Luxol fast blue (LFB) myelin stain. The early-active demyelinating lesion is characterized by macrophages laden with granules positive for LFB and containing both minor and major myelin proteins, and accompanied by reactive astrocytes (Fig. 3-1C). This intimate admixture of astrocytes and macrophages is a defining feature of the active lesion. Since minor myelin proteins are rapidly degraded, macrophages in the late-active lesions contain only the more slowly digested major myelin proteins (i.e., PLP and MBP). With diminishing activity, these PAS-positive, granule-laden macrophages increasingly localize to

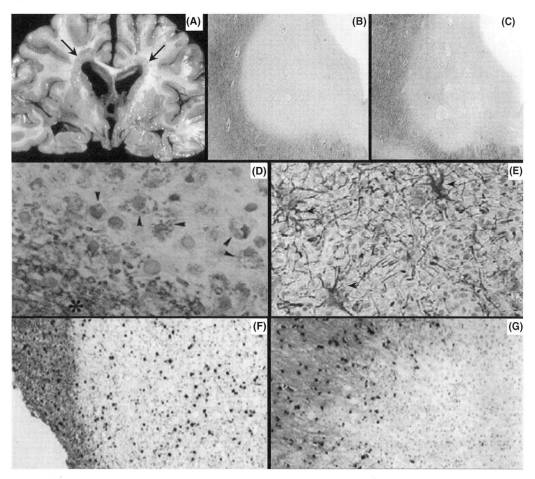

FIG. 3-1. Hallmarks of structural pathology in multiple sclerosis plaques. (**B–D, F–G** reprinted with permission from Wingerchuk DM et al. (Laboratory Investigation) 81 (3): 263–281 (2001); AOP, (doi:10.1038/labinvest.3780235); *http://www.nature.com/labinvest/* (19).)

A. Coronal macroscopic section showing brain with typical periventricular MS plaques (*arrows*). **B, C.** Photomicrographs of a chronic multiple sclerosis plaque. **B.** Well-demarcated hypocellular region of myelin loss evident in the periventricular white matter (Luxol fast blue and periodic acid-Schiff myelin stain (LFB/PAS), magnification 15×). **C.** Neurofilament (NF) staining for axons in the same lesion demonstrates a reduction in axonal density. **D.** Photomicrograph of an actively demyelinating multiple sclerosis lesion, using immunocytochemical staining of myelin oligodendrocyte glycoprotein (MOG, brown) with hematoxylin counterstaining of nuclei (blue). At the active edge of a multiple sclerosis lesion (*asterisk*), the products of myelin degradation are present in numerous macrophages (*arrowheads*) (100×). **E.** Multiple sclerosis plaque with extensive gliosis (or astrocytic scarring) consisting of a dense network of fibrillary astrocytes (*arrowheads*), stained with glial fibrillary acidic protein (GFAP). **F, G.** Photomicrographs of oligodendrocyte preservation and loss in multiple sclerosis (MS). **F.** Oligodendrocyte preservation. Many oligodendrocytes are seen adjacent to and in the center of a zone of active demyelination, stained using in *situ* hybridization for proteolipid (PLP) mRNA (black) and immunocytochemistry for PLP protein (red). **G.** Oligodendrocyte loss. In a second case, oligodendrocytes are absent from a zone of active demyelination but are preserved in the adjacent periplaque white matter.

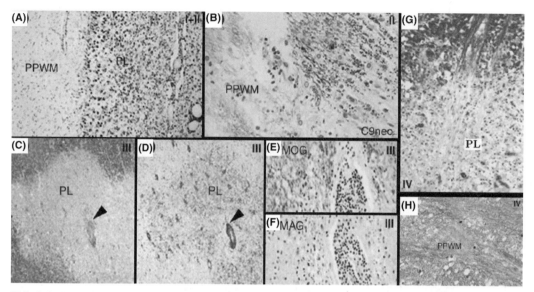

FIG. 3-2. Immunopathology patterns of early active demyelination in multiple sclerosis.
(Reprinted and altered from *Trends in Molecular Medicine*, Vol. 7(3), Lassmann H et al., Heterogeneity of multiple sclerosis pathogenesis: implications for diagnosis and therapy, pp. 115–121, (© 2001), with permission from Elsevier (20).
A. Actively demyelinating lesion following patterns I and II. The active plaque (PL) is filled with activated macrophages and microglia. There is a sharp demarcation between the actively demyelinating lesions and the periplaque white matter (PPWM), using immunochemistry staining for CD68 to identify activated macrophages/microglia (magnification 200×). **B.** Actively demyelinating plaque of pattern II that shows massive deposition of complement C9neo-antigen (brown staining) on degenerating myelin sheaths and in myelin degradation products taken up by macrophages in the zone of active demyelination (ADM). There is faint C9neo reactivity on myelin sheaths in the PPWM. Immunocytochemistry for C9neo-antigen (×500). **C:** Actively demyelinating lesion following pattern III. Myelin staining using Luxol fast blue (LFB) shows an ill-demarcated demyelinated PL. In the lesion center is an inflamed blood vessel surrounded by a small rim of preserved myelin (arrow; magnification 30×). **D.** The same lesion as shown in (**C**) stained with the leukocyte marker CD45. Myelin around the central vessel has a lower density of inflammatory cells compared to the rest of the lesion (*arrow*). In addition, this lesion has an indistinct boundary compared with the lesion in panel (**A**). Immunocytochemistry for CD45 (30×). **E.** Higher magnification of the area indicated by the arrow in panels (**C**) and (**D**) stained for myelin-oligodendrocyte glycoprotein (MOG, brown staining). There are numerous MOG-reactive fibers preserved in the lesion (300×). **F.** Higher magnification of the area indicated by the arrow in panels (**C**) and (**D**) stained for myelin associated glycoprotein (MAG). There is very little MAG immunoreactivity (300×). **G.** Actively demyelinating lesion following pattern IV. The plaque contains numerous macrophages containing myelin degradation products (stained blue with LFB) and has a sharply demarcated edge (300×). **H.** The PPWM of the lesion in (**G**). The myelin appears vacuolated and contains numerous oligodendrocytes with fragmented DNA (black nuclei) identified using an in situ tailing reaction for DNA fragmentation (400×).

perivascular areas, rather than being dispersed throughout the lesion. In the later stages of the demyelinating process, macrophages no longer contain myelin peptides or partially digested glycoproteins; thus, granules are neither LFB-nor PAS-positive. As the process continues, inflammation diminishes but glial reactivity persists. The inactive, chronic MS lesion is characterized by relative hypocellularity, containing only astrocytes and scattered perivascular chronic inflammation. [For a demyelinating stage classification scheme, refer to (18).]

Early MS: Pathology of Oligodendrocytes and Myelin

Four histopathological patterns of demyelination have been described in early active MS lesions. This classification scheme is based on several features, including (a) plaque geography, (b) extent of oligodendrocyte survival, (c) degree of remyelination, (d) evidence of complement activation, and (e) loss of myelin proteins (16). Based on a biopsy and autopsy cohort of 82 patients with early multiple sclerosis, approximately 70% of MS lesions had demyelinating patterns characterized by primary myelin destruction, designated *patterns I and II*. Both patterns I and II lesions display sharp macrophage borders at the plaque edge and the surrounding periplaque white matter (PPWM), with perivascular myelin loss and infiltration by macrophages and CD3 T-lymphocytes. Only pattern II lesions, however, exhibit immunoglobulin and complement deposition within macrophages and at sites of active myelin destruction. The remaining 30% of MS cases are characterized by primary oligodendrocyte (OLG) injury (*patterns III and IV*). Though still containing dense macrophage and T-cell infiltrates, pattern III lesions are characterized by ill-defined macrophage borders, perivascular sparing of myelin, no evidence of complement activation, a preferential loss of myelin associated glycoprotein (MAG) at the active plaque edge, and extensive OLG apoptosis with limited remyelination. Pattern IV lesions also demonstrate degeneration of oligodendrocytes in the normal-appearing periplaque white matter (PPWM), with no evidence of MAG loss or complement activation (16,19). Analysis of multiple active lesions at autopsy or of serial biopsies of the same patient revealed that the immunopathological pattern remained uniform. The presence of interindividual heterogeneity, but intraindividual homogeneity suggests the targets and immunopathogenic mechanisms leading to tissue injury in MS may be heterogeneous (16). The four immunopathological patterns of early active demyelination are summarized in Table 3-1 and Figure 3-2 (20).

In addition to the patterns of early-active demyelination, the cellular composition of tissue injury and repair evident in MS lesions is notably heterogeneous among MS patients. Various immune and toxic agents can result in injury to oligodendrocytes within MS plaques. For example, both myelin and oligodendrocytes are susceptible to damage mediated by tumor necrosis factor alpha (TNF-α) or interferon gamma (IFN-γ), reactive oxygen and nitrogen species, T-cell products (i.e., perforin or lymphotoxin) and CD8 cytotoxicity, and other inflammatory products. The wide spectrum of toxins that potentially cause injury within MS plaques also includes excitatory amino acids (i.e., glutamate), complement cascade proteins, proteolytic and lipolytic enzymes, or viral infections [for reviews, refer to (15,21)]. Dysregulation of T-lymphocyte and/or oligodendrocyte apoptosis, in particular the Fas–Fas ligand pro- and bcl2 anti-apoptosis cascades, have also been implicated in the pathogenesis of MS. These noxious stimuli may result in variable degrees of demyelination, oligodendrocyte loss, or even axonal injury in MS plaques.

Demyelinating MS lesions can be classified structurally into categories of oligodendrocyte density and degree of remyelination, as well as extent of axonal preservation, relative to the periplaque white matter. Approximately 70% of MS patients have plaques characterized by relatively preserved oligodendrocytes and extensive remyelination, referred to as *OLG category I lesions*. Preserved oligodendrocytes in these MS plaques either survived the demyelinating insult, or were recruited from OLG progenitor pools after the acute phase of demyelination (21,22). The remaining one-third of MS patients have *OLG category II lesions*, defined by reduced oligodendrocyte survival and little or no remyelination (Fig. 3-1E, F). A significant negative correlation has been shown between the density of macrophages and CD8 (cytotoxic) T-cells and the density of oligodendrocytes in MS lesions at all stages (i.e., early or late active and inactive demyelinating or remyelinating plaques). This inverse correlation may suggest

TABLE 3-1 *Summary of immunopathology patterns of early active demyelination*

EA Patterns of demyelination	Pathology	Putative mechanisms
I Macrophage Associated Demyelination	Inflammation composed of T-cells and macrophages Perivascular demyelination with radial expansion Activated macrophages and microglia associated with myelin destruction	T-cell* mediated inflammation with macrophage/microglia activation; Demyelination induced by macrophage toxins
II Antibody and Complement Associated Demyelination	Similar to pattern I lesion; Additional deposition of immuno-globulin (IgG) and activated complement at sites of active myelin destruction	T-cell* mediated inflammation with macrophage/microglia activation; Complement mediated lysis of antibody-targeted myelin
III Distal Oligodendrocyte Dystrophy	Inflammation composed of T-cells and macrophages, with perivascular sparing of myelin; Small vessel vasculitis with endothelial cell damage and microvessel thrombosis; Degeneration of distal oligodendrocyte processes (selective MAG loss), followed by oligodendrocyte apoptosis and demyelination	T-cell* mediated small vessel vasculitis with secondary ischemic damage of the white matter
IV Primary Oligodendrocyte Injury in PPWM with Secondary Macrophage Associated Demyelination	Similar to pattern I lesion; With extensive oligodendrocyte degeneration in a small rim of periplaque white matter	T-cell* mediated inflammation with macrophage/microglia activation; Demyelination induced by macrophage toxins on the background of metabolically impaired oligodendrocytes; Genetic defect of oligodendrocytes?

EA, Early Active; MAG, myelin associated glycoprotein, PPWM, periplaque white matter
*T-Cells include CD8 (cytotoxic) and CD4 (helper), both Th1 and Th2 subtypes.
[Reprinted with permission from H Lassmann et al. (2001) (20).]

that macrophages and cytotoxic T-cells play a major pathogenic role in reduced oligodendrocyte survival and remyelination (17). While OLG category I lesions are more commonly associated with patterns I or II, decreased oligodendrocyte preservation (OLG category II lesions) is typical of patterns III or IV of active demyelination (19,23). The differential preservation or loss of oligodendrocytes in acute MS lesions further supports the hypothesis of a heterogeneous pathology of demyelination and oligodendrocyte destruction or preservation within lesions (15,21).

Although the presence of remyelination in early MS lesions correlates with oligodendrocyte survival, the limited extent of remyelination in chronic MS lesions is not solely due to a lack of these cells. Chronic MS plaques with no evidence of remyelination may demonstrate variable degrees of oligodendrocyte preservation (24). While these reservoirs of "premyelinating" oligodendrocytes can potentially serve

as substrates for remyelination, these chronic lesions lack the appropriate pro-remyelinating milieu. In particular, remyelination seems to require not only the presence of healthy oligodendrocytes, but also intact interactions between axons and oligodendrocytes, growth-promoting cytokine and chemokine profiles, as well as limited fibrillary gliosis for the extension of myelin processes within the MS plaque (19,24–27).

Both the structure and immunopathology of MS lesions demonstrate high interindividual heterogeneity, but relative intraindividual homogeneity (16). Studies have shown no significant correlation between the histopathology of lesions and the clinical course and outcomes in prototypic MS. Immunopathological patterns of demyelination do not correlate with acute, relapsing-remitting, secondary progressive, primary progressive, or progressive-relapsing courses of MS. All lesions from a single individual, however, exhibit only one pattern of demyelination, similar oligodendrocyte density, and extent of remyelination, as well as comparable degrees of axonal injury (17). This suggests that fundamentally different "mechanisms and targets" of demyelination as well as tissue destruction and repair underlie distinct pathological subgroups, independent of clinical features (16,23). Finding less-invasive clinical or paraclinical surrogate markers, which accurately and reliably distinguish between pathological subtypes, can potentially guide future MS therapies targeting the distinct pathogenic processes (16,21,23,28).

Acute and Chronic MS: Remyelination

Whereas demyelination adversely affects axons, remyelination serves to restore structural and functional integrity of denuded axons. Clinically, early remyelination that precedes or prevents further axonal damage is a vital step in improving, or limiting, neurological disability in MS patients. Data on the frequency, course, or extent of remyelination in MS lesions, however, is inconclusive, whether based on pathological or radiological measures. Remyelination is in part limited by the degree of oligodendrocyte and axon preservation following the insult (21). There is marked intraindividual heterogeneity of MS lesions. not only with respect to the character of inflammatory infiltrates in the early demyelinating lesion, but also in terms of degree of oligodendrocyte survival and remyelination at all stages of demyelination (16,17). The extent of remyelination in MS lesions ranges from complete absence to partial (typically limited to the lesion edge) and, less commonly, extending throughout the whole of the previously demyelinated lesion (then designated the "shadow plaque"; see Fig. 3-3).

The ultrastructural hallmarks of remyelination include shortened internodes and decreased myelin thickness to axonal diameter ratio, relative to the surrounding normal-appearing (or periplaque) white matter (NAWM or PPWM) (21,29,30). At the light microscopic level, early remyelination is characterized by patches of thin, short, and irregularly ordered myelin sheaths, or clusters of preserved (or recruited progenitor) oligodendrocytes with short myelin processes, interspersed with the macrophage-rich infiltrate (21,31); see Fig. 3-3. The macrophages in remyelinating areas within inactive (completely) demyelinated plaques do not contain any myelin degradation products (i.e., negative for LFB, PAS, or myelin protein stains). Conversely, late remyelinating lesions are defined by little or no inflammation within areas of relatively thin, yet more densely packed and regularly organized myelin sheaths that may cover the entire length of once-denuded axons. These sharply demarcated areas of myelin pallor may also show extensive fibrillary gliosis and axonal loss, relative to the surrounding PPWM (18,21). Remyelination may be difficult to distinguish microscopically from active MS lesions with incomplete demyelination. Although both are characterized by thin, truncated, and irregularly arranged myelin sheaths, the active demyelinating lesion is characterized by T-cells and macrophages, containing granules with myelin degradation products [for a review, refer to (21)].

In addition, remyelination can be confused with secondary (Wallerian) degeneration. Although both are characterized by areas of myelin loss, Wallerian degeneration also shows a corresponding reduction in axons and lacks the T-cell infiltration evident in MS lesions [for a review, refer to (21)]. Adding to the complexity of identifying remyelinating MS lesions, active remyelination may also occur in lesions with concurrent demyelinating activity. These active demyelinating and remyelinating (ADM/RM) plaques resemble the typical remyelinating MS lesions with the addition of T-lymphocytes and macrophages containing myelin degradation products, and also display the diverse immunopathological patterns described in non-remyelinating early active demyelination lesions. Remyelination, interestingly, is more commonly associated with the early active autoimmune patterns of demyelination (patterns I and II), and less commonly in patterns III and IV, which are typically associated with significant oligodendrocyte loss. Furthermore, shadow plaques may subsequently undergo demyelination, with or without further remyelination (21,32,33).

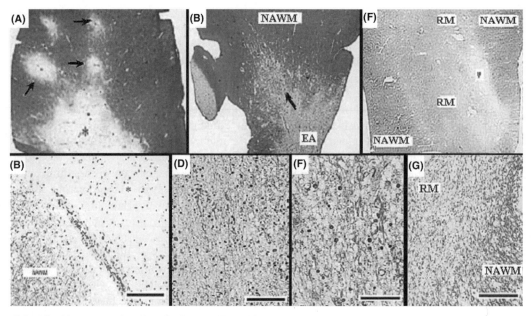

FIG. 3-3. Heterogeneity of remyelination in multiple sclerosis.
Photographs of a Luxol fast blue (LFB)-stained, paraffin-embedded brain tissue. **A.** Large demyelinated lesion (DM, *asterisk*) in the white matter and a few smaller ones (*arrows*) **B.** At higher power, the
lesion is totally demyelinated (*asterisk*) compared with the adjacent normal-appearing white matter
(NAWM) (hematoxylin-eosin (H&E); scale bar = 20 µm). **C.** Partially remyelinated lesion (*arrow*) confined to the border of an active demyelinated lesion in the white matter (*asterisk*). **D.** Photomicrograph
of the edge of the demyelinated MS lesion showing reduced LFB staining in the remyelinated (RM)
area (scale bar = 50 µm). **E.** High-power magnification shows that the axons are surrounded by thin
myelin sheaths (LFB; scale bar = 20 µm). **F.** Fully remyelinated lesion (RM), or "shadow plaque." A
sharp border is formed with the adjacent normal-appearing white matter (NAWM). Part of a ventricle
(V) is present in the lesion. **G.** The edge of the remyelinated lesion; reduced LFB staining is visible in
the RM area compared with the adjacent NAWM (scale bar = 100 µm).
[Reprinted and altered with permission from Barkhof F et al., *Arch Neurol* 2003;60(8):1073–1081, ©
2003, American Medical Association. All rights reserved (78).]

Acute and Chronic MS: Pathology of Axons

Oligodendrocytes ensheathe up to 40 adjacent
nerve axons in the CNS (5). Since myelin allows
saltatory axonal conduction to proceed,
demyelination impairs nerve conduction leading
to a wide range of neurological signs and symptoms and neurophysiological findings typical of
multiple sclerosis. Demyelinated axons propa-
gate action potentials at greatly reduced veloci-
ties, with corresponding delays in conduction of
evoked potentials (5). In addition, the hyperexcitability of demyelinated axons results in rapid
and unregulated neural firing, and may account
for the flashes of light associated with eye
movement (*phosphenes*) and electrical sensation
running down the spine or limbs associated with
neck flexion (*L'hermitte sign*) (5). Although the
frequency of firing increases, demyelinated neurons have difficulty sustaining an action potential throughout the length of the axon.
Consequently, nerves fatigue with frequent use,
leading to transient neurological deficits, often
after exercise or a hot bath (*Uhthoff phenomenon*). As a result, MS patients usually tire during
physical activity and cognitive tasks, and
recover slowly (5). Myelin sheaths also physically and electrically isolate neighboring axons.
Thus demyelination leads to *cross-talk* between
adjacent axons (*ephaptic transmission*), resulting in paroxysmal symptoms such as trigeminal

neuralgia, ataxia, dysarthria, or painful tetanic posturing of the limbs, lasting a few minutes and usually following touch or movement (5). Early clinical remission may result from reorganization at the cellular and systems level of the surviving functional pathways affected by the initial demyelination and inflammation [for a review, see (5)].

The inflammatory process of active lesions results in a toxic milieu that is further injurious to the involved tissue. Nitric oxide released by macrophages causes irreversible damage to axons and glia, in addition to promoting breakdown of the blood–brain barrier (34). Both histology and imaging show that transected axons in acute inflammatory MS plaques may undergo Wallerian degeneration during the subsequent 18 months, without extension of the lesion size or clinical deficit (5). During the acute inflammatory phase, reactive astrocytes and microglia release cytokines and growth factors that promote remyelination by surviving oligodendrocytes. Astrocytic proliferation (gliosis), however, also may in effect *shield* the chronic lesion, forming a physical barrier to further remyelination (5).

Axonal injury may be exacerbated by the loss of trophic support by myelin or glia, with resultant further axonal degeneration and accumulating clinical deficits (5). In addition to extensive oligodendrocyte loss, the extent of acute axonal injury, as defined by expression of amyloid precursor protein (APP), as well as the degree of chronic axonal loss relative to the PPWM, correlate with the degree of demyelination and character of inflammation (25,35). In particular, acute axonal injury positively correlates with the density of macrophages and CD8 cytotoxic T-lymphocytes within MS lesions, whether demyelinating, inactive, or remyelinating, but there is no correlation with expression of TNF-α or inducible nitric oxide synthase (iNOS). Acute axonal injury is most severe in secondary progressive MS compared to those with primary progressive (PPMS) or relapsing-remitting MS (RRMS) (35). The observation that acute axonal injury may occur in the absence of myelin degradation suggests that an ischemic component contributes to lesion pathogenesis (25,35).

It is thought that clinical disability occurs only after reaching a threshold of axonal loss beyond which compensatory CNS resources are exhausted (36,37). Thus, chronic progressive axonal loss may be the major cause of progressive neurological decline typical of primary progressive MS (25,35) (Fig. 3-1C). In addition to the variable patterns of demyelination and cellular composition, there is heterogeneity of MS lesions with respect to the degree of axonal damage (see Fig. 3-4).

Heterogeneity of MS Gross Pathology

Topography of MS Lesions

MS typically manifests as multifocal CNS white matter plaques of variable size and density and at different stages of demyelination. The signs and symptoms of MS reflect the multifocal localization, severity of inflammation, and extent of demyelination. Magnetic resonance imaging (MRI) studies show MS lesions almost always involve the cerebrum, with or without corresponding clinical signs and symptoms. Though

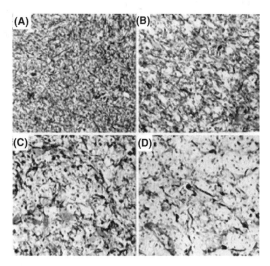

FIG. 3-4. Axonal pathology in multiple sclerosis. **A.** Normal axonal density within the normal-appearing white matter of an MS patient. **B–D.** Heterogeneity in degree of axonal loss in MS lesions ranging from minor **(B)**, moderate **(C)** and massive **(D)**. Sections are stained with Bielschowsky's silver impregnation stain.

randomly dispersed throughout the CNS white matter, MS plaques are frequently found in the periventricular white matter, especially the angles of the lateral ventricles and the floor of the fourth ventricle, as well as the deep white matter tracts (Fig. 3-1A). The anterior visual system, brain stem, and cerebellum are common sites of MS lesions. Corresponding findings include impaired coordinated movement of the eyes, limbs, as well as bulbar and axial muscles. Involvement of the spinal cord, another frequent site of MS plaques, leads to motor, sensory, and autonomic dysfunction (5).

Normal-Appearing White Matter

In addition to focal demyelinated lesions in MS, there is significant evidence of disseminated global abnormalities in normal-appearing white matter (NAWM), based on neuroimaging and pathological studies. Magnetic resonance spectroscopy (MRS) studies of the NAWM of primary progressive MS reveals reduced *N*-acetylaspartate (NAA), a marker of neurodegeneration, as well as elevated creatine, which usually serves as an internal control, with reduced NAA or choline to creatine ratios (38–40). These magnetic transfer ratios, which serve as markers of myelin integrity, also are reduced in the NAWM of progressive versus relapsing MS (41–45). Brain atrophy also increases with duration of disease, in part due to accumulating lesion load and Wallerian degeneration (44). Pathologically, the NAWM in MS is characterized by patchy mild inflammation, consisting mainly of CD8 (cytotoxic) T-cells, gliosis, microglial activation, axonal injury, and neurodegeneration (41,43). However, the degree to which the pathology of the NAWM evident in chronic MS results in active demyelination, rather than an innate white matter abnormality in MS patients, is inconclusive.

Cortical and Deep Gray Matter Pathology in MS

Since myelinated axons are present in gray matter, inflammatory demyelinating lesions also can be found in the cortical and subcortical gray mat-

ter (46,47). One hundred and ten specimens from 50 patients with 112 cortical MS lesions were histopathologically characterized and compared to white matter plaques (48). Although many cerebral cortical lesions are extensions of juxtacortical white matter plaques (i.e., *type I lesions*, 34%), some intracortical lesions have a perivenular distribution that is independent (and anatomically separate from) white matter plaques (i.e., *type II*, 16%). The majority of intracortical lesions, however, consist of a band-like demyelination within layers 3 or 4 of the cortex, extending from the pial surface and encompassing entire or even multiple gyri (i.e., *type III*, 50%). Individual MS brains often had all three types of cortical lesions (48). Furthermore, compared to white matter lesions, cortical plaques are relatively hypocellular, with 6 and 13 times fewer CD68 microglia/macrophages and CD3 T-lymphocytes, respectively (48). Similar to white matter plaques, the extent of axonal injury in cortical lesions varies greatly. There is evidence of increased neurodegeneration (e.g., neuronal apoptosis) within cortical lesions (48). Compared to most white matter lesions, cortical plaques, on average, have relatively less tissue injury, with evidence of increased neuron, axon, and oligodendrocyte preservation (48). Thus, since cortical pathology may not be readily identified on MRI and/or autopsy inspection, cortical MS lesions are more common than previously thought (48,49).

SPECTRUM OF IDIOPATHIC INFLAMMATORY DEMYELINATING DISORDERS

MS is only one member of a heterogeneous family of idiopathic inflammatory demyelinating diseases (IIDDs). The IIDDs consist of a wide spectrum of disorders, which include tumefactive MS, fulminant variants of MS (such as the Marburg variant of acute MS and Balò concentric sclerosis) and acute disseminated encephalomyelitis (ADEM). While the monosymptomatic IIDDs include transverse myelitis or isolated optic neuritis or brainstem demyelination, the recurrent disorders with a restricted topographical distribution include Devic neuromyelitis optica (NMO) and relapsing myelitis. The literature on the classification of these syndromes is often confusing. Some studies emphasize specific clinical or pathologic features to distinguish between these syndromes. However, there are examples of transitional cases that defy a specific terminology (refer to Tables 3-2 and 3-3, and Fig. 3-5).

Tumefactive Multiple Sclerosis

Occasionally, prototypic MS presents as a localized mass that clinically and radiologically is indistinguishable from a tumor (50); refer to Fig. 3-5A. Unifocal or multifocal enhancing lesions are seen on MRI and are associated with increased intracranial pressure and cerebral edema. Clinically, headache, altered mental status and cognition, aphasia, seizures, and localized signs and symptoms result. Consequently, tumefactive MS lesions are frequently biopsied. Pathologically, the hypercellular actively demyelinating MS lesion may be confused with CNS tumors. (The dense mononuclear cell infiltrates may suggest CNS lymphoma.) Creutzfeldt-Peters cells (astrocytes with fragmented nuclear inclusions) resemble mitoses and may be mistaken for atypical glial cells (Fig. 3-5A). However, unlike CNS tumors, MS lesions are characterized by numerous, granule-laden macrophages intimately admixed with reactive astrocytes. Tumefactive MS is more commonly associated with a juxtacortical enhancing open-ring at the periphery of the plaque, open to the cortex and extending into the subcortical white matter (51,52). Distinguishing tumefactive MS from CNS neoplasm is vital, since radiation and other antineoplastic therapies are exceedingly detrimental, especially in the demyelinated brain (53).

Marburg Variant of Multiple Sclerosis (Marburg MS)

First described in 1906 by Otto Marburg (54–56), Marburg MS is characterized as a truly fulminant subtype of acute MS, associated with rapid progression and death within a year from presentation. In contrast to prototypic MS, the Marburg variant is typically monophasic and almost always rapidly progressive and fatal. Relative to prototypic MS and ADEM, lesions in Marburg MS are more destructive, defined by massive macrophage infiltration, severe acute axonal injury, and extensive necrosis. Topographically, Marburg MS consists of multifocal (disseminated) lesions that may subsequently fuse to form large white matter plaques or diffuse demyelination, both in the central and peripheral nervous system. To date, there are no CSF or other laboratory measures, or clinical and radiological findings, that accurately and reliably distinguish the Marburg variant of MS from acute disseminated encephalomyelitis (ADEM), especially in protracted cases (refer to Tables 3-2 and 3-3; also Fig. 3-5B).

Balò Concentric Sclerosis (Balò)

First described by J.M. Balò in 1928, Balò concentric sclerosis (BCS) is defined by alternating bands of preserved myelin and demyelination with a characteristic concentric pattern, evident on pathological specimens and on T2 weighted MRI (57–59). The pathogenesis of the concentric pattern of demyelination is unclear. A study of 12 autopsies with BCS demonstrated that macrophages and microglia within the active demyelinating concentric bands expressed higher levels of inducible nitric oxide synthase (iNOS). In addition, oligodendrocytes, as well as some macrophages and astrocytes at the edge of the active regions and in the outermost band of preserved myelin, also had increased expression of hypoxia-inducible factor 1α (HIF-1α) and heat shock protein 70 (hsp70). The presence of these *hypoxic preconditioning* proteins suggests hypoxia may play an important role in mediating tissue injury and contributing to the concentricity typical of BCS. Due to neuroprotective effects of HIF-1α and hsp70, the rim of periplaque tissue expressing these proteins may be resistant to further hypoxia-like injury in an expanding lesion and, therefore, remains as a rim of preserved myelinated tissue (Fig. 3-5C).

BCS is more commonly reported in Asia, in particular the Philippines and China, and usually presents between 20 to 50 years of age.

TABLE 3-2 Spectrum of IIDD: comparison of clinical features

Clinical Characteristics	Prototypic MS (a)	Acute MS Variants				
		Marburg's (b)	Balò's (c)	ADEM (d)	Devic's NMO (e)	Tumefactive MS (f)
Age at Onset	30 (15–40) years	20–50 years	20–50 years	Mainly childhood, but 10% > 16 years	40 (5–65 years)	30 (15–40) years
Demographics	Most common in northern Europe	Limited data	Common in Asia: China and Philippines	Limited data	Common in Asia and Africa	Same as prototypic MS
Gender (F:M) Clinical Course	2:1 / 80% RR +/– SP 20% PP	Limited data / Monophasic, +/– rapidly progressive	Limited data / Acute onset, monophasic, +/– rapidly progressive	Equal / Acute onset, monophasic; 70% with prior viral/bacterial infection, or vaccination	7:1 (relapsing form) / Acute onset; 20% monophasic, 80% relapsing	1:1 / May remain isolated single event or develop RRMS
Short-Term and Long-Term Prognosis	Highly variable 20% benign MS 50% progressive disability by 10 and walking aid by 15 years after onset; 4-fold mortality rate with progressive MS; average life-expectancy overall	Fulminant meningism, altered consciousness, +/–seizures and increased intracranial pressure; often fatal in = 1 year	Fulminant; meningism, altered consciousness, +/–seizures and increased intracranial pressure; often fatal in = 1 year	Moderate to severe meningism, fever, altered consciousness, and headache; 70% with prodrome and immune trigger. Most with complete resolution; < 50% with residual deficits; 10–20% with no change	Typically severe: ↓↓ visual acuity, uni/bilateral blindness, hemi/paraplegia, death (respiratory compromise). Variable, but usually poor: > 50% blind/gait aid after 5 years; < 80% 5 yr survival	Highly variable
Biomarker(?) CSF Pleocytosis	None / Usually ≤ 50 cells/mm2	None / Same as prototypic MS	None / Same as prototypic MS	None / Raised in 30–80%; (> 50 cells/mm2)	NMO IgG / Usually 50–100 cells/mm2	None / Same as prototypic MS
Protein Level	Normal in 75%, rarely > 1 g/L			Raised in 30–60%	Frequently raised up to 1.5 g/L	
Intrathecal Ig with OCBs	Raised in ≥ 60% 80% OCB+			Raised in 5–60%	< 35% OCB+	

MS, multiple sclerosis; ADEM, acute disseminated encephalomyelitis; MRI, magnetic resonance imaging; Ig, Immunoglobulin; OCB, oligoclonal band

Sources: a Weinshenker (1995) (2), Lucchinetti et al. (2001, 2003) (15,23); b Genain et al. (1999) (76), Storch et al. (1998) (74); c Karaarslan et al. (2001) (58), Galluci et al. (2001) (57), Stadelmann et al. (submitted) (77); d Wingerchuk (2003) (63); e deSeze et al. (2002) (71), Fardet et al. (2003) (70), Lucchinetti et al. (2002) (72), Wingerchuk et al. (1999) (73); f Kepes (1993) (50), Masdeu et al. (1996, 2000) (51,52).

TABLE 3-3 Spectrum of IIDD: comparison of pathological and radiological features

Characteristic Pathology	Acute MS Variants					
	Prototypic MS (a)	Marburg's (b)	Balo's (c)	ADEM (d)	Devic's NMO (e)	Tumefactive MS (f)
Refer to:	Figure 3-5E	Figure 3-5B	Figure 3-5C	Figure 3-5D	Figure 3-5E	Figure 3-5A
Inflammation	Many macrophage/microglia; T-cells (perivenular and parenchymal); +/– complement and Ig deposition—i.e., in early active demyelinating pattern II (*Table 1*)	Same as prototypic MS, plus notable neutrophils; may find activated complement and Ig deposition (pattern II)	Same as prototypic MS, except concentric rings of on-off inflammation; MAG loss (pattern III)	Limited to perivenular mononuclear cells, +/– microglia at lesion edge	Many perivascular macrophage/microglia, B cells, eosinophils; ring and rosette pattern of complement and Ig deposition	Same as prototypic MS; confused with gliomas due to Creutzfeld-Peters astrocytes, but distinguished by macrophage infiltrate and border
Topography	Mainly WM, but also cortex and DGM; common at angles of lateral and floor of 4th ventricle	Mainly cerebral white matter tracts; +/– encompassing entire cerebral hemispheres	Mainly cerebral white matter tracts; +/– encompassing entire cerebral hemispheres	Disseminated or multifocal perivenular lesions; ≥ 90% in cerebral subcortical WM (periventricular in 30–60%); ≥ 90% DGM; ≥ 65% Spinal cord	Both WM and GM; optic nerves and/or spinal cord	Juxtacortical +/– extending into cortex
MRI Findings	Usually small, uni- or multifocal circumscribed (+/– enhancing) lesions	Severe edema and necrosis; +/– encompassing entire cerebral hemispheres, with mass effect	Severe edema and necrosis; +/– encompassing entire cerebral hemispheres, +/– mass effect	Minimal enhancement; perivenular or diffuse edema +/– multifocal lesions; no necrosis or atrophy	Edema, necrosis and cavitation; spinal cord lesions frequently extend > 3 vertebrae; Bilateral optic neuritis is common	Tumor-like, enhancing open-ring, protrudes into subcortical WM and opens to cortex, mass effect/edema

MS, multiple sclerosis; ADEM, acute disseminated encephalomyelitis; MRI, magnetic resonance imaging; Ig, Immunoglobulin; WM, white matter; DGM, deep gray matter

Sources: **a** Weinshenker (1995) (2), Lucchinetti et al. (2001, 2003) (15,23); **b** Genain et al. (1999) (76), Storch et al. (1998) (74); **c** Karaarslan et al. (2001) (58), Galluci et al. (2001) (57), Stadelmann et al. (submitted) (77); **d** Wingerchuk (2003) (63); **e** deSeze et al. (2002) (71), Fardet et al. (2003) (70), Lucchinetti et al. (2002) (72), Wingerchuk et al. (1999) (73); **f** Kepes (1993) (50), Masdeu et al. (1996, 2000) (51,52).

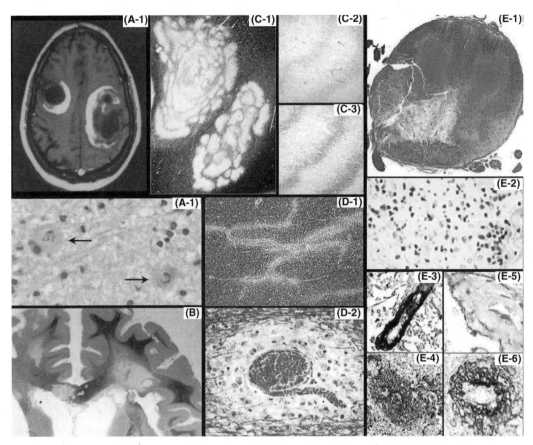

FIG. 3-5. Spectrum of idiopathic inflammatory demyelinating diseases (IIDDs): Comparison of gross and microscopic pathology. **A.** Tumefactive MS. **(A-1)** Open-ring enhancement of demyelinating lesion circumscribed to the subcortical white matter medially, lateral cleft corresponding to cortex, and mimicking tumor on gadolinium-enhanced, T1-weighted magnetic resonance imaging (MRI); **(A-2)** Creutzfeldt-Peters cells—astrocytes with nuclear inclusions (*arrows*)—in an early active demyelinating lesion; often confused with glial neoplasms. **B.** Marburg's Variant of MS. Coronal macroscopic section of with large confluent lesions with extensive demyelination, which may result in mass effect and herniation; Luxol fast blue and PAS (LFB-PAS). **C.** Balò's concentric sclerosis (BCS). Unique pathology consisting of alternating rims of myelinated and demyelinated tissue as seen in stained macroscopic **(C-1)** and microscopic **(C-2)** using LFB-PAS myelin stains (100×); similar pattern evident with axonal density **(C-3)**; neurofilament stain(NF), 100×. **D.** Acute disseminated encephalomyelitis (ADEM): Characteristic perivenular inflammation (**D-1:** Mallor myelin stain, ×200) and demyelination. (D-2: LFB, ×40ø) with surrounding normal-appearing white matter (NAWM). **E.** Devic's neuromyelitis optica (NMO). **(E-1)** Spinal cord cross-section demonstrating extensive demyelination involving both the grey and white matter (LFB-PAS, 10×). **(E-2)** Inflammatory infiltrate in NMO consists of numerous perivascular eosinophils and granulocytes, also throughout the lesion; haematoxylin–eosin (H&E) stain, 600×). Intact perivascular and parenchymal eosinophils are present within the lesion. **(E-3 through E-6)** Evidence for humoral immunity in NMO. Actively demyelinating NMO lesions show massive deposition of complement C9neo-antigen (brown) in a rim pattern on the outer surface of thickened blood vessels, as well as in a rosette perivascular pattern. **(E-3)** There is pronounced perivascular immunoglobulin (human Ig) reactivity. **(E-4)** Immunocytochemistry for IgM demonstrates a rosette perivascular staining pattern. Staining for complement activation with C9neo-antigen (red) demonstrates this rim **(E-5)** and rosette **(E-6)** pattern of staining (400×).

[**D-1** and **D-2** reprinted and altered with permission from Prineas JW et al. (2002) (79); **E** reprinted and altered from Lucchinetti CF et al., A role for humoral mechanisms in the pathogenesis of Devic's neuromyelitis optica. *Brain* 2002,125(7):1450–1461, by permission of Oxford University Press.]

Clinically, it is indistinguishable from fulminant variants of MS, which are characterized by an acute monophasic progressive course often fatal within weeks to months from onset (59–61). Typical neurological deficits include headache, altered mental status and cognition, aphasia, seizures, and increased intracranial pressure. However, these cerebral symptoms are common to most fulminant idiopathic inflammatory demyelinating diseases. Pathologically, the early active concentric lesions in BCS are characterized by primary oligodendrocyte apoptosis and selective MAG loss, as seen in pattern III cases of prototypic MS (described previously). Although clinically similar to the Marburg variant, Balò can be considered a fulminant subtype of MS, predominantly distinguished on pathologic and/or radiologic features (refer to Tables 3-2 and 3-3; also Fig. 3-5C).

Acute Disseminated Encephalomyelitis (ADEM)

The distinction between fulminant variants of multiple sclerosis (MS) and acute disseminated encephalomyelitis (ADEM) can often only be established by observing the subsequent natural history, or by pathological confirmation. (See Tables 3-2 and 3-3; also Fig. 3-5D). Unlike prototypic MS and its variants, ADEM typically is a monophasic process, affecting both male and female patients equally, and is associated with a more favorable long-term prognosis. As in MS, ADEM can cause a wide spectrum of focal and multifocal neurological disability depending on severity and location of demyelinating lesions and associated edema. Yet, unlike prototypic MS, ADEM is frequently associated with signs of acute meningoencephalopathy, including meningism, depressed level of consciousness, focal or generalized seizures, and even psychosis. However, these symptoms may also be associated with the more fulminant variants of MS, such as Marburg's and Balò's [for reviews, see (62,63)].

Acute disseminated encephalomyelitis is characterized by focal or multifocal (disseminated) inflammation of the CNS, usually one to six weeks after an immunological trigger. Clinically,

there is rapid onset of symptoms, reaching climax of disability within days. The acute phase is preceded by a prodromal phase usually consisting of fever, malaise, and myalgia, though less commonly in adults with ADEM. In particular, about 70% of patients report a preceding viral or bacterial infection or recent history of vaccination. Some of the viral infections associated with (postinfectious) ADEM include measles, mumps, rubella, varicella-zoster, Epstein Barr virus, cytomegalovirus, herpes simplex virus, Hepatitis A, and coxsackie virus. Infrequently, ADEM can also be triggered by bacterial infections, namely *mycoplasma pneumoniae*, and rarely *Borrelia burgdorferi*, *Leptospira*, and Group A (beta-hemolytic) *Streptococci*. Similarly, some vaccinations have been associated with (postvaccinial) ADEM, mainly rabies, but also pertussis, diphtheria, measles, mumps, rubella, and influenza [for review, see (62,63)].

Pathologically, ADEM shows perivenular inflammation and limited demyelination with relative sparing of axons. In particular, the perivascular Virchow–Robin spaces show extensive mononuclear cell (and often neutrophil) infiltration associated with a diffuse, often symmetric, demyelination (Fig. 3-5D). Unlike prototypic MS, the perivenular lesions in ADEM typically show similar stages of demyelination at a given time. While usually affecting the white matter in the cerebrum, cerebellum, and brain stem, ADEM may also involve the deep gray matter. In contrast to the marked gliosis characteristic of most other idiopathic inflammatory demyelinating diseases, reactive astrocytes are rare in ADEM lesions. Similarly, though extensive axonal loss may be evident in prototypic and variants of MS as well as Devic neuromyelitis optica (Devic NMO), axons are relatively preserved despite the extensive perivenular demyelination in ADEM. Finally, unlike many of the IIDDs, namely Marburg and Devic NMO, ADEM has a favorable prognosis, with most patients experiencing complete clinical remission and resolution of lesions, while 10% to 20% retain some degree of neurological disability [for reviews, see (62–66)].

No radiological finding or biological marker can consistently or definitively distinguish between ADEM and the wide spectrum of idiopathic inflammatory demyelinating diseases. Though a diagnosis is typically not feasible upon presentation, ADEM, with its monophasic course, is effectively ruled out upon a second (distant) demyelinating event. Compared to prototypic MS, ADEM is more commonly associated with a viral prodrome, encephalopathy, multifocal and deep gray matter lesions (i.e., thalami), and no oligoclonal bands but greater lymphocytic pleocytosis in the CSF [for reviews, see (62–66)]. However, despite these distinctions, a definitive diagnosis of ADEM may not be possible until months or years after the initial demyelinating event. Although cases of relapsing ADEM have been reported (67–69), these series are not based on reliable pathological confirmation of ADEM [for review, refer to (63)]. The limited extent of perivenular demyelination is the pathological hallmark of ADEM, which distinguishes it from the confluent lesions typical of MS. However, some patients have lesions with histologic features of both ADEM and MS. The presence of these transitional forms suggests a spectrum of inflammatory demyelinating diseases, which may share a common pathogenetic relationship.

Devic Neuromyelitis Optica

Devic neuromyelitis optica (Devic NMO) is an acute neurological disease characterized by necrotizing immune-mediated demyelination of the optic nerves (optic neuritis) and spinal cord (transverse myelitis), either simultaneously or days to weeks apart (57,70–73). First described in 1894, Devic NMO is more common among young adults in Asian and African populations, effecting men and women in equal frequency and ranging from 5 to 65 years at onset (57). Patients with Devic NMO (unlike those with MS) overall have a poor prognosis, often leading to unilateral or bilateral blindness, hemi- to paraplegia and/or death, mainly due to respiratory compromise caused by spinal cord lesions across multiple thoracic vertebrae. Furthermore, historical observations suggest that two-thirds of patients will relapse within one year, and most (if not all) relapse within three years of the first

attack. In contrast to prototypic MS, there is a highly variable but usually minimal and transient response to immunotherapy (73).

De Seze et al. (2002) (71) and Fardet et al. (2003) (70) characterized Devic NMO in terms of clinical, laboratory, MRI and outcome profiles and modified the diagnostic criteria proposed by Wingerchuk et al. (1999) (73). The clinical diagnosis of Devic NMO requires all absolute criteria and one major or two minor supportive criteria. The absolute criteria include optic neuritis and/or acute myelitis (occurring independently or in combination), as well as no evidence of clinical disease outside the optic nerve or spinal cord (in contrast to multiple sclerosis). The major supportive criteria include negative brain MRI at onset, spinal cord MRI with signal abnormality extending over three or more vertebral segments, and CSF pleocytosis (> 50 WBC/mm^3 or > 5 neutrophils/mm^3). Whereas the minor supportive criteria include bilateral optic neuritis, severe optic neuritis with fixed decreased visual acuity ($< 20/200$) in at least one eye, and severe, fixed, attack-related weakness in one or more limbs. These clinical criteria initially aided in differentiating between patients with Devic NMO and those with prototypic MS presenting with optic neuritis, acute myelitis, or both.

The histopathological characteristics of NMO have been described relative to prototypic MS and other acute CNS disorders (72) [refer to Table 3-3 and Fig. 3-5E]. In particular, NMO resembles an aggressive humoral EAE (anti-MOG) autoimmune rat model of MS (74) and is characterized by severe myelin and axonal destruction of both white and gray matter. Devic NMO is clinically and pathologically distinct from MS (see Tables 3-2 and 3-3 for comparison with MS). Nine autopsy specimens from patients with NMO were histopathologically characterized and compared to 73 patients with MS (72). Acute NMO lesions consisted of a prominent macrophage and microglial infiltration with necrosis of optic nerve and spinal cord white and gray matter. In addition, there was extensive perivascular inflammation, consisting of macrophages, microglia, B-cells, eosinophils, granulocytes, and prominent complement and antibody deposition. Furthermore, the deposition of complement and antibody formed perivascular ring and rosette patterns (Fig. 3-5E). While acute MS lesions also show prominent macrophage and/or microglial infiltrate, the inflammation is usually localized to the white matter, rarely consists of eosinophils and granulocytes, and infrequently results in the severe necrosis evident in NMO lesions. Furthermore, although pattern II MS lesions demonstrate complement activation and Ig deposition at sites of active myelin destruction, it is in a distribution distinct from the prominent perivascular complement activation seen in NMO lesions. Chronic NMO lesions typically result in severe scarring, cavitation, and atrophy.

The perivascular patterns of inflammation in acute NMO lesions suggest a humorally mediated autoimmune disorder possibly targeting the perivascular region and resulting in specific damage to the optic nerves and/or spinal cord. These central nervous system regions may be preferentially targeted due to increased permeability of the blood–brain barrier (BBB) to circulating pathogenic autoantibodies relative to other CNS regions. This is further supported by the recent discovery of an "NMO IgG" serological autoantibody biomarker that stains CNS vessels as well as pial and subpial regions (75). The identity of the antigen is still unknown. However, a validated NMO-IgG assay has been described, which is both specific (91% or 100%) and sensitive (73% or 58%) for Devic NMO in North America or optical–spinal MS in Japan, respectively. The NMO-IgG marker is a useful marker to help accurately diagnose, prognosticate, and treat patients with NMO. Furthermore, it will be a useful assay that more reliably differentiates NMO from MS, especially in those patients presenting with lesions limited to the optic nerves and/or the spinal cord (75).

SUMMARY

Heterogeneity of Idiopathic Inflammatory Demyelinating Disorders (IIDDs)

The idiopathic inflammatory demyelinating diseases (IIDDs) consist of a broad spectrum of disorders that vary in their clinical course, regional distribution, and pathology. Though pathology of these demyelinating disorders demonstrates extensive interindividual heterogeneity, there is notable homogeneity within individual patients. The relation between the diverse underlying pathology of IIDDs and the various clinical, paraclinical, and radiological findings is unclear. Finding less-invasive clinical or paraclinical surrogate markers, which accurately and reliably predict the underlying distinct pathologies within the family of IIDDs, can potentially guide future therapies that better target specific pathogenic mechanisms (16,21,23,28).

ACKNOWLEDGMENTS

Yazmin Morales acknowledges the Clinical Research Training Program (CRTP) and the Initiative for Minority Student Development (IMSD) Program at the Mayo Clinic, Rochester, MN, and the financial support from the NIGMS (NIH grant R25 GM55252). Dr. Claudia Lucchinetti acknowledges the financial support of the U.S. National Multiple Sclerosis Society (US NMSS grant RG3185-A-2).

REFERENCES

1. Agius LM. Towards a pathogenetic definition of multiple sclerosis in terms of integrative transformation of generic pathologic processes. *Med Hypotheses* 2003;61(2):177–181.
2. Weinshenker BG. The natural history of multiple sclerosis. *Neurol Clin* 1995;13(1):119–146.
3. Weinshenker BG, Bass B, Rice GP, et al. The natural history of multiple sclerosis: a geographically based study. I. Clinical course and disability. *Brain* 1989;112:133–146.
4. Prineas JW. The neuropathology of multiple sclerosis. In: BG Vinken P, Klawans H, eds. *Handbook of Clinical Neurology*. New York: Elsevier Science Publishers, 1985:213–257.
5. Compston A, Coles A. Multiple sclerosis. *The Lancet* 2002;359(9313):1221–1231.
6. Carswell R. *Pathological anatomy: illustrations on elementary forms of disease*. London: Logman, 1838.
7. Cruveilier J. *Anatomie pathologique du corps humain; ou description, avec figures lithographiées et coloriées, des diverses alterations morbides dont le corps humain est susceptible*. Vol. II. Paris: Baillière, 1829–1842.
8. Rindficisch E. Histologisches detail zu der grauen degeneration von gehirn und ruckenmark. *Arch Pathol Anat Physiol* 1863;26:474–483.

9. Charcot JM. Histologie de la sclerose en plaques. *Gaz Hop civils et militaires* 1868;140,141,143:554–555, 557–558,566.

10. Charcot JM. *Lecons sur les maladies du systeme nerveux faites a la salpetriere*. Paris: Cert et fils, 1880.

11. Kabat EA, Freedman DA, Murray JP, et al. A study of the crystalline albumin, gamma globulin and the total protein in the cerebrospinal fluid of one hundred cases of multiple sclerosis and other diseases. *Am J Med Sci* 1950;219:5564.

12. Kabat EA, Glusman M, Knaub V. Quantitative estimation of the albumin and gamma globulin in normal and pathologic cerebrospinal fluid by immunochemical methods. *Am J Med Sci* 1948;4:653–662.

13. Lassmann H. The pathology of multiple sclerosis and its evolution. *Philos Trans R Soc Lond B Biol Sci* 1999;354(1390):1635–1640.

14. Hafler DA. Multiple sclerosis. *J Clin Invest* 2004; 113(6):788–794.

15. Lucchinetti CF, Brück W, Noseworthy J. Multiple sclerosis: recent developments in neuropathology, pathogenesis, magnetic resonance imaging studies and treatment. *Curr Opin Neurol* 2001;14:259–269.

16. Lucchinetti CF, Brück W, Parisi J, et al. Heterogeneity of multiple sclerosis lesions: implications for the pathogenesis of demyelination. *Ann Neurol* 2001;47: 707–717.

17. Lucchinetti CF, Brück W, Parisi J, et al. A quantitative analysis of oligodendrocytes in multiple sclerosis lesions: A study of 113 cases. *Brain* 1999;122(12): 2279–2295.

18. Bruck W, Porada P, Poser S, et al. Monocyte/ macrophage differentiation in early multiple sclerosis lesions. *Ann Neurol* 1995;38(5):788–796.

19. Wingerchuk DM, Lucchinetti CF, Noseworthy JH. Multiple sclerosis: current pathophysiological concepts. *Laboratory Investigation* 2001;81(3):263–281.

20. Lassmann H, Bruck W, Lucchinetti C. Heterogeneity of multiple sclerosis pathogenesis: implications for diagnosis and therapy. *Trends in Molecular Medicine* 2001;7(3):115–121.

21. Bruck W, Kuhlmann T, Stadelmann C. Remyelination in multiple sclerosis. *J Neurol Sci*. 2003;206(2):181–185.

22. Buntinx M, Stinissen P, Steels P, et al. Immune-mediated oligodendrocyte injury in multiple sclerosis: molecular mechanisms and therapeutic interventions. *Crit Rev Immunol*. 2002;22(5–6):391–424.

23. Lucchinetti CF, Brück W, Lassmann H. Pathology and pathogenesis of multiple sclerosis. In: N.J. McDonald WI, ed. *Blue Books of Practical Neurology: Multiple Sclerosis*. 2nd ed. New York: Elsevier Science, 2003.

24. Chang A, Tourtellotte WW, Rudick R, et al. Premyelinating oligodendrocytes in chronic lesions of multiple sclerosis. *NEJM N Engl J Med* 2002;346(3): 165–173.

25. Bitsch A, Schuchardt J, Bunkowski S, et al. Acute axonal injury in multiple sclerosis: correlation with demyelination and inflammation. *Brain* 2000;123(6): 1174–1183.

26. Martin R. Immunology of multiple sclerosis, In: N.J. McDonald WI, ed. *Blue Books of Practical Neurology: Multiple Sclerosis*. 2nd ed. New York: Elsevier Science, 2003.

27. Martino G, Adorini L, Rieckmann P, et al. Inflammation in multiple sclerosis: the good, the bad, and the complex. *Lancet Neurology* 2002;1(8):499–509.

28. Bruck W, Neubert K, Berger T, et al. Clinical, radiological, immunological and pathological findings in inflammatory CNS demyelination—possible markers for an antibody-mediated process. *Mult Scler* 2001;7(3): 173–177.

29. Raine CS, Wu E. Multiple sclerosis: remyelination in acute lesions. *J Neuropathol Exp Neurol* 1993;52(3): 199–204.

30. Perier O, Gregoire A. Electron microscopic features of multiple sclerosis lesions. *Brain* 1965;88(5):937–952.

31. Mews I, Bergmann M, Bunkowski S, et al. Oligodendrocyte and axon pathology in clinically silent multiple sclerosis lesions. *Mult Scler* 1998;4(2): 55–62.

32. Prineas JW, Barnard RO, Kwon EE, Sharer LR, Cho ES. Multiple sclerosis: remyelination of nascent lesions. *Ann Neurol* 1993;33(2):137–151.

33. Prineas JW, Barnard RO, Revesz T, et al. Multiple sclerosis: pathology of recurrent lesions. *Brain* 1993;116(Pt 3):681–693.

34. Smith KJ, Lassmann H. The role of nitric oxide in multiple sclerosis. *Lancet Neurology* 2002;1(4):232–241.

35. Kuhlmann T, Lingfeld G, Bitsch A, et al. Acute axonal damage in multiple sclerosis is most extensive in early disease stages and decreases over time. *Brain* 2002;125(10):2202–2212.

36. Bjartmar C, Wujek JR, Trapp BD. Axonal loss in the pathology of MS: consequences for understanding the progressive phase of the disease. *J Neurol Sci* 2003;206(2):165–171.

37. Bjartmar C, Trapp BD. Axonal and neuronal degeneration in multiple sclerosis: mechanisms and functional consequences. *Curr Opin Neurol* 2001;14(3):271–278.

38. Suhy J, Rooney WD, Goodkin DE, et al. 1H MRSI comparison of white matter and lesions in primary progressive and relapsing-remitting MS. *Mult Scler* 2000;6(3):148–155.

39. Leary SM, Davie CA, Parker GJ, et al. 1H magnetic resonance spectroscopy of normal appearing white matter in primary progressive multiple sclerosis. *J Neurol* 1999;246(11):1023–1026.

40. Davie CA, Barker GJ, Thompson AJ, et al. 1H magnetic resonance spectroscopy of chronic cerebral white matter lesions and normal appearing white matter in multiple sclerosis. *J Neurol Neurosurg Psychiatry* 1997;63(6): 736–742.

41. Evangelou N, Esiri MM, Smith S, et al. Quantitative pathological evidence for axonal loss in normal appearing white matter in multiple sclerosis. *Ann Neurol* 2000;47(3):391–395.

42. Dehmeshki J, Silver NC, Leary SM, et al. Magnetisation transfer ratio histogram analysis of primary progressive and other multiple sclerosis subgroups. *Journal of the Neurological Sciences* 2001;185(1):11–17.

43. Kornek B, Storch MK, Weissert R, et al. Multiple sclerosis and chronic autoimmune encephalomyelitis : a comparative quantitative study of axonal injury in active, inactive, and remyelinated lesions. *Am J Pathol* 2000;157(1):267–276.

44. Pelletier J, Suchet L, Witjas T, et al. A longitudinal study of callosal atrophy and interhemispheric dysfunction in relapsing-remitting multiple sclerosis. *Arch Neurol* 2001;58(1):105–111.

45. Tortorella C, Viti B, Bozzali M, et al. A magnetization transfer histogram study of normal-appearing brain tissue in MS. *Neurology* 2000;54(1):186–193.

46. Lumsden C. The neuropathology of multiple sclerosis, In: B.G. Vinken P, ed. *Handbook of Clinical Neurology*. New York: Elsevier, 1970:217–309.

47. Cifelli A, Arridge M, Jezzard P, et al. Thalamic neurodegeneration in multiple sclerosis. *Ann Neurol* 2002;52(5):650–653.

48. Peterson JW, Bo L, Mork S, et al. Transected neurites, apoptotic neurons, and reduced inflammation in cortical multiple sclerosis lesions. *Ann Neurol* 2001;50(3):389–400.

49. Kidd D, Barkhof F, McConnell R, et al. Cortical lesions in multiple sclerosis. *Brain* 1999;122(1):17–26.

50. Kepes JJ. Large focal tumor-like demyelinating lesions of the brain: intermediate entity between multiple sclerosis and acute disseminated encephalomyelitis? A study of 31 patients. *Ann Neurol* 1993;33(1):18–27.

51. Masdeu JC, Moreira J, Trasi S, et al. The open ring. A new imaging sign in demyelinating disease. *J Neuroimaging* 1996;6(2):104–107.

52. Masdeu JC, Quinto C, Olivera C, et al. Open-ring imaging sign: highly specific for atypical brain demyelination. *Neurology* 2000;54(7):1427–1433.

53. Murphy CB, Hashimoto SA, Graeb D, et al. Clinical exacerbation of multiple sclerosis following radiotherapy. *Arch Neurol* 2003;60(2):273–275.

54. Marburg O. New studies in multiple sclerosis, II, Parencephalomyelitis periaxialis scleroticans (acute multiple sclerosis) in various infectious diseases. New York: *J Mount Sinai Hosp* 1942;9:640.

55. Marburg O. Zur Sklerosefrage. *Mitt Ges Inn Med Wien* 1912;11(202).

56. Marburg O. Multiple sklerose. In: Lewandowsky M, ed. *Handbuch der Neurologie*. Vol. 2/1. Berlin: Springer, 1911:911.

57. Gallucci M, Caulo M, Cerone G, et al. Acquired inflammatory white matter disease. *Childs Nerv Syst* 2001;17(4–5):202–210.

58. Karaarslan E, Altintas A, Senol U, et al. Balo's concentric sclerosis: clinical and radiologic features of five cases. *AJNR Am J Neuroradiol* 2001;22(7):1362–1367.

59. Marburg O. Die sogenannte "akute multiple sklerose" *J Psychiatric Neurology* 1906;40(1):211–312.

60. Courville C. Concentric sclerosis, In: B. PVaG, ed. *Handbook of Clnical Neurology*. Amsterdam: Elsevier, 1970;437–451.

61. Kuroiwa Y. Clinical and epidemiological aspects of multiple sclerosis in Japan. *Japanese J Med* 1982;21(2):135–140.

62. Murthy JM. Acute disseminated encephalomyelitis. *Neurology India* 2002;50(3):238–243.

63. Wingerchuk DM. Postinfectious encephalomyelitis. *Curr Neurol Neurosci Rep* 2003;3(3):256–264.

64. Hynson JL, Kornberg AJ, Coleman LT, et al. Clinical and neuroradiologic features of acute disseminated encephalomyelitis in children. *Neurology* 2001;56(10):1308–1312.

65. Dale RC. Acute disseminated encephalomyelitis. *Semin Pediatric Infectious Disease* 2003;14(2):90–95.

66. Dale RC, de Sousa C, Chong WK, et al. Acute disseminated encephalomyelitis, multiphasic disseminated encephalomyelitis and multiple sclerosis in children. *Brain* 2000;123(12):2407–2422.

67. Durston JH, Milnes JN. Relapsing encephalomyelitis. *Brain* 1970;93(4):715–730.

68. Cohen O, Steiner-Birmanns B, Biran I, et al. Recurrence of acute disseminated encephalomyelitis at the previously affected brain site. *Arch Neurol* 2001;58(5):797–801.

69. Miller HG, Evans MJ. Prognosis in acute disseminated encephalomyelitis; with a note on neuromyelitis optica. *Q J Med* 1953;22(87):347–379.

70. Fardet L, Genereau T, Mikaeloff Y, et al. Devic's neuromyelitis optica: study of nine cases. *Acta Neurol Scand* 2003;108(3):193–200.

71. de Seze J, Stojkovic T, Ferriby D, et al. Devic's neuromyelitis optica: clinical, laboratory, MRI and outcome profile. *J Neurol Sci* 2002;197(1–2):57–61.

72. Lucchinetti CF, Mandler RN, McGavern D, et al. A role for humoral mechanisms in the pathogenesis of Devic's neuromyelitis optica. *Brain* 2002;125(7):1450–1461.

73. Wingerchuk DM, Hogancamp WF, O'Brien PC, et al. The clinical course of neuromyelitis optica (Devic's syndrome). *Neurology* 1999;53(5):1107-.

74. Storch MK, Piddlesden S, Haltia M, et al. Multiple sclerosis: in situ evidence for antibody- and complement-mediated demyelination. *Ann Neurol* 1998;43(4): 465–471.

75. Lennon VA, Wingerchuk DM, Kryzer TJ, et al. A serum antibody marker of neuromyelitis optica. *The Lancet* 2004;364(9451):2106–2112.

76. Genain CP, Cannella B, Hauser SL, et al. Identification of autoantibodies associated with myelin damage in multiple sclerosis. *Nature Medicine* 1999;5(2):170–175.

77. Stadelmann C, Ludwin SK, Tabira T, et al. Hypoxic preconditioning explains concentric lesions in Balo's type of multiple sclerosis. *Brain* 2004; 128(5): 979–987.

78. Barkhof F, Bruck W, De Groot CJA, et al. Remyelinated lesions in multiple sclerosis: magnetic resonance image appearance. *Arch Neurol* 2003;60(8):1073–1081.

79. Prineas JW, McDonald WI, Franklin JM. Demyelinating diseases. In: L.P. Graham DI, ed. *Greenfield's Neuropathology*. 7th ed. Vol. 2. New York: Arnold, 2002: 471–550.

4

Immunobiology of Oligodendrocytes in Multiple Sclerosis

Francesca Ruffini,[1] Andrew Chojnacki,[2] Samuel Weiss,[3] and Jack P. Antel[4]

[1]Neuroscience-Neuroimmunology Unit, DIBIT-San Raffaele Hospital, Milan, Italy; [2]Genes and Development Research Group, Department of Cell Biology and Anatomy, University of Calgary, Faculty of Medicine, Calgary, Alberta, Canada; [3]Department of Cell Biology and Anatomy, University of Calgary, Calgary, Alberta, Canada; [4]Department of Neurology and Neurosurgery, McGill University, Montreal, Quebec, Canada

The clinical and pathologic features of multiple sclerosis (MS) began to be described in the mid-1800s and by the 1870s had been synthesized into a recognizable entity by Charcot and colleagues [reviewed in (1)]. Charcot emphasized the loss of the myelin sheath with relative, but not absolute, preservation of axons. He referred to the observation by Reinfleisch in 1863 of inflammation around a vessel in the center of MS plaques; this can be viewed as the beginning of the continuing debate of the relative contributions of immune-mediated versus "neurodegenerative" processes as a basis for the disease pathology. More recent analysis of the status of myelin and their cells of origin the oligodendrocytes (OLGs) raise a number of new issues regarding the status of these cells throughout the evolution of the MS disease process, including at times of initial exacerbation or subsequent relapse, recovery from relapses, and secondary progression with acquisition of fixed neurologic deficits. Injury and repair processes may be ongoing at the same time.

BASIS OF INJURY OF OLGS/MYELIN IN ACUTE LESIONS (EXCERBATIONS/RELAPSES)

Consensus regarding the status of OLGs in the earliest phases of MS lesion development has not yet been achieved, due in part to the lack of indications to surgically sample developing lesions. The usual pathologic definitions of early, active lesions have been based on extent of inflammation and active myelin breakdown. Luchinetti et al. have shown case-case heterogeneity with regard to whether the OLGs are relatively preserved or lost in such early lesions (2). The former would suggest a primary insult of the myelin membrane; the latter may implicate a primary insult of the cell body (oligodendrogliopathy). The latter is supported by observations of cases with relatively selective loss of MAG, a molecule expressed at the adaxonal region and consistent with a dying back phenomenon (3). Some of these cases feature OLGs undergoing programmed cell death (apoptosis). Most of these pathologic features are observed in specific models of experimental autoimmune encephalomyelitis (EAE), the most frequently studied animal disorder of immune-mediated CNS demyelinating disease (4). Barnett and Prineas have now described lesions in very acute cases of MS in which OLG apoptosis preceded development of an inflammatory response; such changes are unlike any observed in any current immune-mediated animal model of MS (5). Demyelination and inflammation occurred subsequent to the initial cell death, suggesting an as yet unidentified primary derangement within the OLGs themselves.

Potential mechanisms of immune-mediated OLG/myelin injury in MS—evidence that myelin-directed immune responses could initiate an inflammatory-demyelinating syndrome of the CNS—were first observed following introduction of the Pasteur rabies vaccine, a preparation that contained CNS tissue [reviewed in (6)]. This human disease complication led to development of the animal model EAE. Adoptive transfer studies in EAE have established the capacity of myelin-specific CD4 T cells to migrate and persist in the CNS. T-cells reactive with nonmyelin antigens (e.g., ove-albumin) can access the CNS but do not persist. Thus, myelin antigen presentation within the CNS is an essential event. One speculates as to the source of myelin antigens that the very first autoreactive cells would encounter when entering a presumed normal CNS. There does appear to be a

physiologic rate of turnover of the myelin membrane, although the OLGs themselves are long-lived. These auto-reactive T-cells initiate an inflammatory cascade that includes constituents of both the adaptive and innate (macrophages and microglia) immune systems [reviewed in (7)]. We will consider the contribution of these different constituents and their products to the overall tissue injury that involves OGCs/myelin and neurons/axons. We postulate that the selective OLG/myelin injury in the early MS lesion could reflect the properties of either the immune effectors or the target cells (OLGs).

Effector-Determined Selectivity

The immune system can be considered in terms of adaptive and innate constituents. The T-cells and B-cells of the adaptive immune system have receptors with a high degree of diversity, consequent to the process of rearrangement of the genes that contribute to their structure. This diversity allows for recognition of a vast array of target-specific determinants.

The role of CD4 αβ T-cells, particularly those with a Th1 phenotype, in the EAE model underlies the attempts to demonstrate whether such T-cells are direct mediators of OLG/myelin injury. Myelin-reactive CD4 αβ T-cell lines are shown to possess cytotoxic potential in in vitro assays (8,9). In the context of specific myelin/OGC-directed injury, this would require expression of MHC class II molecules on the OLGs. To date, most studies indicate a lack of such expression. In vitro studies indicate that human OLGs are not susceptible to MHC class II restricted lysis by myelin-reactive CD4 αβ T-cells, although these cells can mediate nonrestricted lysis if they up-regulate the NK-cell-associated surface antigen CD56 (8,9). Such up-regulation is generated in vitro by exposing T-cell lines to cytokines (e.g., IL-2) expected to be present in an inflammatory milieu. CD56-directed antibodies, however, do not completely eliminate this cytotoxicity implicating other ligands as being involved in the requisite adhesion process. An increased array of such molecules, previously associated with cellular interactions within the immune system or within the CNS, is shown to be expressed by cells of both systems, making them candidate molecules for promoting immune-neural interactions or actually mediating injury (10). Such molecules include ICAM/LFA-1, netrins, and semaphorins. Immune-derived semaphorins (CD100) are shown in vitro to mediate collapse of processes and apoptosis of OLGs (11). These observations support the concept that the myelin specificity of αβ T-cells would determine their specific persistence in the CNS but that their injury contribution could reflect non antigen and MHC restricted effector mechanisms.

CD8 αβ T-cells are the classic cytotoxic cell population. These cells are prominent in the parenchyma in both MS and EAE lesions (12). The observed restricted heterogeneity of the T-cell receptor repertoire of these cells has implicated them as being antigen-restricted, although the identity(ies) of such antigen(s) remains to be established (12). OLGs derived from the adult human CNS express MHC class I molecules that can be recognized by CD8 αβ T-cells. Our studies using CD8 αβ T-cells reactive to a specific peptide sequence of myelin basic protein (MBP) indicated that such cells can induce MHC class 1-restricted cytotoxicity of OGCs (13). CD8 αβ T-cells are also shown to physically attach to and resect axons, which under conditions of impaired nerve conduction do express MHC class I molecules (14). To be shown is whether axonal resection is MHC class I-restricted or whether such restrictions are bypassed as discussed above for CD4 αβ T-cells. Giuliani et al. showed that CD8 αβ T-cells and CD4 αβ T-cells when polyclonally activated (anti-CD3 antibody) in short-term (3 day) cultures, mediate neuronal but not OLG cytotoxicity (15).

Antibody-Mediated Immune Responses

For B-cells, the Ig molecule itself serves as the antigen receptor. Myelin- and OGCs-directed antibodies have been detected in serum and cerebrospinal fluid (CSF) of MS patients (16,17). The determinants recognized can be protein, carbohydrates, or lipids. Confirmation is pending regarding whether such antibodies predict the subsequent development of recurrent disease in patients who present with clinically isolated syndromes compatible with CNS inflammatory disease (18). Anti-MOG and anti-MBP antibodies have also been detected within active MS lesion

sites (19). Sera derived from a proportion of MS patients are now shown to bind to cell lines with OLG or neuronal properties (20). However, in vitro studies of primary human OGCs have not yet shown that serum or CSF from MS patients can selectively bind to or induce injury of these cells, even in presence of complement.

The potential interaction of antibody with cells of the innate immune system, present in the inflammatory environment of MS lesions, provides a means whereby nonspecific effector responses could be directed to a specific target [reviewed in (7)]. Members of the innate immune system include γδ T-cells, NK cells, and microglia/macrophages. These cells can all effect tissue injury by release of an array of mediators (discussed below) but, due to their limited receptor heterogeneity, would not be expected to recognize targets with the specificity of the adaptive immune system constituents. Recruitment of these nonspecific effectors to a specific target could, however, result from antibody binding to the specific target via the variable regions of the Ig molecule and to the Fc receptors that are expressed on the nonspecific effectors via the Fc portion of the molecule. This process is referred to as antibody-dependent cell cytotoxicity (ADCC).

Target-Determined Selectivity

Relatively selective target injury, as observed in MS, mediated by "nonspecific" effector cells and soluble molecules could reflect differential susceptibility of individual cell types to such mediators. In the case of receptor-dependent mediated injury, such susceptibility could reflect either differential expression of the required receptors on the target cell surface or differences in the intracellular signaling cascades induced by engagement of the receptors.

Tumor Necrosis Family Receptor (TNF-R) Superfamily

The potential contribution to OGC/myelin injury by ligands signaling through receptors belonging to the TNF-R superfamily provides a prototype of target-determined selectivity of injury related to differential receptor expression or signaling. These molecules have all been detected in the inflammatory environment of MS and/or EAE lesions (21–23).

TNF/TNF-R

TNF itself has long been implicated as mediating OLG injury in vitro and in vivo in transgenic animal models in which TNF is overexpressed at high levels within the CNS [reviewed in (24)]. A review of the in vitro studies indicates that significant cell death of mature bovine and human OGCs requires prolonged exposure (days) to relatively high concentrations of TNF (25,26). Animal models in which TNF or one or more of its receptors are totally ablated by gene deletion approaches indicate that TNF can also have a protective role and even promote remyelination [reviewed in (24)]. TNF induces rapid activation of a number of intracellular signaling pathways, raising the issue as to whether the net functional effect represents the balance of injury and protective signaling pathways. Injury-associated signaling pathways include the caspase cascade and the JNK pathway. The NFκB pathway is the suggested protective pathway (26).

Fas Ligand/Fas

Human OGCs in vitro, especially when exposed to IFNγ, and in situ in active MS lesions, express Fas (27). Fas-expressing OGCs in vitro undergo caspase-dependent cell death within 4 to 6 hours following exposure to Fas ligand or activating anti-Fas antibody. In our experience, fetal human neurons do not express comparable levels of Fas (as did the OLGs) and are not as susceptible to Fas-mediated injury (28,29). Giuliani et al. did find that the cytotoxicity of such of neurons mediated by polyclonally activated T-cells, as previously mentioned, was at least partially inhibited by anti-Fas antibody (15). Fetal human CNS-derived astrocytes express fas even under basal culture conditions but are still resistant to fas-signaled injury. Our studies suggest that such resistance reflects the presence of intracellular molecules (e.g., FLIP) that inhibit the caspase cascade from completing the death program (29).

TRAIL/DR4/5

Addition of tumor necrosis factor-related apoptosis-inducing ligand (TRAIL) to hippocampal slice cultures induces apoptotic death of neural cells in situ but the injury in this model does not appear to be cell-type-specific (30). The soluble products of Th1 (but not Th2) T-cell lines, as well as IFNγ, up-regulate expression of TRAIL receptors on human OLGs (31). The cells, however, remain resistant to TRAIL-mediated injury unless protein synthesis is inhibited (32). Such injury can be prevented by use of an array of caspase inhibitors (33). Our model, in which p53 overexpression in human OLGs results in these cells becoming susceptible to TRAIL-mediated apoptosis, is described in a later section (33).

Pro-Nerve Growth Factor (NGF)/P75

Although NGF is usually considered as mediating a trophic effect, NGF was initially reported to induce cell death in rodent OLGs in vitro, although we could not confirm this using the adult human OLGs (34,35). The injury effect was attributed to the nature of the NGF receptors expressed by the OLGs, namely, the low-affinity p75 NGF receptor and not the high-affinity trkA receptor. More recent studies indicate that such p75-mediated signaling can be attributed to pro-NGF (36).

Cell-Mediated Constituents of the Innate Immune System

Although γδ T-cells and NK cells are highly cytotoxic to human OGCs, and to multiple other cell types in vitro, resistant cell types are recognized [reviewed in (7)]. Members of the heat shock protein family remain candidates as the recognition molecules for γδ T-cells; one such member, αβ crystallin is considered a putative autoantigen in MS (37). Selectivity for NK cell-mediated injury could also be conferred by the array of activating and inhibitory receptors expressed by individual neural cells. Previously discussed was the capacity of αβ T-cells to acquire NK cell type properties. Microglia/macrophages are implicated as sources of an array of potential effector molecules, including proteases and nitric oxide/peroxynitrite glutamate (see below), to which different neural cell populations may be relatively more susceptible or resistant.

Excitotoxic Injury

The excitatory neurotransmitter glutamate is implicated as contributing to the tissue injury of MS. Glutamate is elevated in the cerebrospinal fluid of MS patients (38,39). MS lesions feature high levels of glutaminase in microglia and macrophages and decreased expression of glutamine synthetase and glutamate dehydrogenase, the enzymes that break down glutamate, in OLGs (40). In EAE, blocking of AMPA/kainate receptors with specific antagonists ameliorates disease outcome and promotes OLG survival (41,42). Rodent OLGs are shown to express ionotropic receptors of the AMPA and kainate subclass and are vulnerable to injury mediated by their overactivation (42–49).We have found, however, that human adult OLGs in vitro and in situ, unlike either their rodent counterparts or neurons, express only low levels of ionotropic glutamate receptors and are resistant to excitotoxicity mediated by high and sustained doses of AMPA or kainate (50).

Myelin Repair and Recovery in MS (Recovery from Relapse)

Histologic- and MR-based studies establish that a limited extent of remyelination can occur in MS. Remyelination is most apparent in the active MS lesion, indicating that demyelination and remyelination are occurring concurrently in the same lesions. Potential sources of remyelination are the previously myelinating OLGs or progenitor cells that would be recruited to the lesions. Many acutely demyelinated MS lesions contain preserved or even increased numbers of mature, presumably previously myelinating OLGs. In a variety of toxin- or virus-induced experimental animal models of demyelination, complete remyelination is a characteristic feature. Such remyelination is ascribed to recruitment of progenitor cells that differentiate into myelinating OLGs rather than to new myelin production by previously myelinating, mature OLGs (51–57). As summarized in Table 4-1 and discussed below, a number of variables can contribute to the contrasting extent of remyelination observed between the human disease MS and its animal models.

There are many potential sources of progenitor cells that could be used in the remyelination of MS lesions. Potential sources include embryonic stem cells (ESC), bone marrow-derived stem cells, neural stem cells (NSCs), and OLG progenitor cells (Table 4-2).

Embryonic stem cells have the intrinsic capacity to generate any of the cell types from the ectodermal, mesodermal, and endodermal germ layers, as well as primordial germ cells. Under the appropriate growth conditions, ESC can give rise to primitive NSCs that can generate NSCs similar to those isolated directly from the CNS (58), in that they are self-renewing and can generate neurons, astrocytes, and oligodendrocytes. The generation and differentiation of OLGs from ESC appears to follow the same developmental pattern seen in vivo (59). Thus, it may be possible to derive OLGs from recently generated human ESC (60,61). Immunosuppressive drugs would be required for allogenically derived OLGs, but this concern may be circumvented by the isolation of ESC derived from a blastocyst created by the nuclear transfer of a patient's genetic material to an enucleated oocyte (62). This approach assumes no intrinsic defect in the patient's progenitor cell population. As promising as ESC may be for the generation of OLGs, current ethical concerns question their availability and practical usefulness.

TABLE 4-1 *Determinants of progenitor cell-mediated remyelination in MS*

- Adequate numbers of pluripotential or myelin lineage committed progenitor cells
- Retained intrinsic survival and differentiation capacity of cells
- Receipt of requisite survival and differentiation factors—trophic factors, hormones
- Balance of environmental molecules that promote or inhibit migration of progenitor cells
- Balance of "positive" and inhibitory signaling pathways that regulate myelination
- Integrity of axons
- Impact of disease injury mediators

TABLE 4-2   *Oligodendrocyte progenitor cells lineage and their presence in MS lesions*

A. Progenitor cell development

Pluripotential Stem Cells	Neural Restricted Stem Cells (Neuron/Glia)	Gliai restricted Progenitors	Myelin Progenitors
	A2B5		
Nestin		NG2	
	PSN CAM		

B. Oligodendrocyte (OGC) progenitor lineage

		MOG/MBP/MAG	
	O4		
PDGF Ra		GalC	
A2B5			PLP
	NG2	(DM20)	(Full Length)

C. OGCs progenitor survival and differentiation factors

FGF-2   PDGF   NT-3   T3   SHh   IGF   GGF   CNTF

D. Progenitor cells in MS lesions

Wolswijk ('89) Chronic lesions	**04+/GalC-/NG2-**, non proliferating
Scolding ('89) Acute/chronic lesions	**PDGF Ra+**, clusters in acute lesion, no increase vs NAWM
Chang ('00) Active/chronic lesions	**NG2+PDGF Ra+**, decrease vs NAWM
Dawson ('00) Chronic lesions	**NG2+**, more immature appearance than NAWM
Maeda ('01) Active lesions	**PDGF Ra+**, proliferating and increased vs chronic and NAWM
Chang ('02) Chronic lesions	**PLP+**, premyelinating OLGs

Bone marrow-derived stem cells have also been demonstrated to be a source of neural cells (63,64), in addition to muscle (65) and liver cells (66–68), but whether or not this reflects their intrinsic potential or spontaneous cell fusion is undetermined (69–73). Nevertheless, the small contribution of bone marrow-derived cells to neural tissues (< 2%) questions whether this avenue for generating myelinating cells would prove fruitful.

NSCs have the capacity to generate OLGs, in addition to neurons and astrocytes, and have been found in the rodent embryonic and adult forebrain (74–76) as well as in human embryonic (77–80) and adult forebrains (81–84). Mouse embryonic NSCs generate OLG progenitors when passaged into platelet-derived growth factor (PDGF; Chojnacki and Weiss unpublished), an OLG progenitor mitogen (85–87). Whereas rodent NSCs continue to generate

OLGs after repeated passages (74,76,88), human NSCs, and particularly embryonic compared to adult NSCs, appear limited in their capacity to generate OLGs (78,81). This difference may not be intrinsic to human NSCs but, rather, may be the result of different environmental requirements for the generation of OLGs. The progeny of murine NSCs readily differentiate into OLGs on a poly-ornithine substrate (76), whereas a laminin substrate was found to be essential for the generation of OLGs from adult human NSCs (84). Nevertheless, only a small proportion of the cells generated by the expansion of human NSCs differentiate into OLGs (77,78,81,89), with the remainder either remaining undifferentiated or differentiating into neurons and astrocytes. Currently, there is debate as to whether or not OLG progenitors actually generate astrocytes in vivo (as they do in vitro) and there are even proposals that OLGs and neurons are generated by a common progenitor (90–92). This dispute stems mainly from the observations that the generation of neurons and OLGs, but not astrocytes, is disrupted in loss-of-function mutations of the basic helix-loop-helix transcription factors *Olig1/2* (93,94).

Properties of Rodent OLG Progenitors

On the basis of PDGFRα expression, the first OLG progenitors appear at E12.5 in the ventral spinal cord (95,96) and in the mantle of the medial ganglionic eminence of the forebrain (97–99), also known as the anterior entopeduncular area (AEP). Examination of the appearance of OLG progenitor antigens (96,100), and cell labeling experiments (101) indicate that OLG progenitors migrate dorsally to populate the entire spinal cord. Through the use of homotopic quail-chick chimeras, OLG progenitors have also been shown to migrate extensively from the ventrally located AEP to populate the entire forebrain (102). Netrins can direct the migration of spinal OLG progenitors away from the ventral ventricular zone (103), and the chemokine CXCL1 (GROα) (104) mediates the end of their migration. The extraordinary motility of OLG progenitors has also been demonstrated for optic nerve OLG progenitors, in vivo and in vitro (105,106). Netrins

are also chemorepulsive for O-2A progenitors (107). Therefore, the cues involved in guiding the migration of OLG progenitors may be conserved along the rostral/caudal extent of the CNS.

The ventral origin of OLGs suggests that local factors control their specification. In Danforth's short-tail, heterozygous mice, where both notochord and floorplate are missing in the caudal spinal cord, OLGs fail to appear (108). However, OLG production can be rescued by culturing spinal cord explants from these animals in the presence of Sonic hedgehog (SHH). These findings led to the later discoveries that inhibition of SHH prevents OLG progenitor specification in the chick (109). Induction of OLG cell fate is regulated by the SHH-regulated gene *Olig2*; given that no OLGs are produced in the spinal cord when *Olig2* function is ablated (93,94). In the forebrain, overexpression of SHH or its downstream target, *Olig1*, can induce ectopic OLG production (110), and *Olig2* is also the primary mediator of SHH signaling in the specification of OLG progenitors, given the loss of forebrain OLGs in *Olig2* null mice (94). In addition, *neuregulin-1* appears to be necessary in the generation of OLGs, as no OLGs are produced in explants of *neuregulin-1* null mice spinal cords (111). Notch signaling also appears to be required for the specification of OLGs (112).

Once specified, PDGF-A is pivotal in expanding the population of OLG progenitors. Findings that PDGF-AA stimulated the proliferation of O-2A progenitors in vitro (87,113) suggested its involvement in regulating their expansion in vivo. Subsequently, it was found that OLG progenitors express PDGFRα in vivo (96), and that mice null for PDGF-A were severely hypomyelinated (85); confirming a critical role for PDGF-A in their expansion. The proliferation of OLG progenitors can also be enhanced in vitro by fibroblast growth factor-2 (FGF-2) (114,115). Signaling by FGF-2, in combination with PDGF, inhibits the differentiation of O-2A progenitors in vitro, which normally lose responsiveness to PDGF-AA after several rounds of cell division and differentiate (114). Similarly to FGF-2, neurotrophin-3 (NT-3) also promotes the expansion and inhibits the differentiation of O-2A progenitors in combination with PDGF (116). Thus, the expansion of OLG progenitors appears to be regulated by multiple factors.

Expansion of the OLG progenitor population does not necessarily lead to an increase in myelinating cells. Early reports suggested that PDGF is a survival factor for OLG progenitors, but not for more mature OLGs (117), and this was confirmed in transgenic mice where the neuron-specific enolase promoter drove the expression of PDGF-A (118). In these animals, the OLG progenitor population was expanded but these cells died at an early stage of differentiation, leaving a normal complement of mature OLGs in the adult (118). Thus, although the expansion and survival of OLG progenitors can be induced by PDGF-AA, continued survival and differentiation is required to increase the total myelinating population. Ciliary neurotrophic factor (CNTF) (119), NT-3, insulin, insulin-like growth factors (IGFs)-1 and -2 (120), and FGF-2 (117) promote the survival of mature OLGs, and survival is further enhanced when cultures are treated with NT-3, CNTF, and insulin/ IGF-1/2 in combination (120). It is noteworthy that transgenic mice that continuously express IGF-1 under the metallothionein-I promoter fully recover from cuprizone-mediated demyelination of the corpus callosum after 5 weeks (121). This effect was attributed to negligible levels of apoptosis, in contrast to wild-type mice, which suffered from near complete demyelination after 5 weeks. Also, both CNTF and the leukemia inhibitory factor receptor signaling (required also for CNTF signaling) have been demonstrated to limit demyelination in EAE by promoting the survival of OLGs (122,123).

The differentiation of OLG progenitors can be monitored by the sequential appearance and disappearance of distinct antigens and is correlated with distinct cell morphologies (124,125). OLG progenitors initially have a bipolar morphology and express A2B5, PDGFRα and NG2 (96,126,127). Differentiation proceeds with the initiation of O4 expression and a change from bipolar to a multipolar, branched cell morphology (128). Next, the expression of A2B5, PDGFRα, and NG2 are reduced, which is associated with the appearance of myelin sheaths extending from

OLG processes. Myelinating OLGs lose NG2 and O4 expression and begin to sequentially express galactocerebroside GalC, CNPase followed by MAG , PLP, and MBP (129–132).

Several factors have been implicated in regulating OLG differentiation. BMPs can promote differentiation of bipotent astrocyte/OLG progenitors of the cortex into astrocytes at the expense of OLGs (133). Myelination is accelerated in hyperthyroid animals and delayed in hypothyroid animals (134–137), and in vitro, triiodothyronine (T3) promotes the differentiation of OLGs from O-2A progenitors (138). CNTF has been shown to promote the survival and differentiation of OLG progenitors (139–141). Neuregulin/glial growth factor prevents early OLG progenitors from differentiating and has been demonstrated to dedifferentiate mature OLGs (142). However, their differentiation into GalC-immunoreactive OLGs is prevented in mice null for *ErbB2*, a receptor for the neuregulins (143). This suggests that signaling mediated by *ErB2* is required for OLG differentiation, whereas another neuregulin receptor may mediate the effects of glial growth factor in preventing OLG differentiation. Thus, OLG differentiation is regulated by multiple signaling pathways.

Axons also have a marked influence on myelination. Recently, nerve growth factor has been found to inhibit the myelination of dorsal root ganglion neurons by OLGs, while having the opposite effect on Schwann cell myelination (144). Interestingly, nerve growth factor appears to modify axonal signals that control myelination, rather than directly affecting OLGs or Schwann cells. Neuregulin type III, released by axons, regulates Schwann cell myelin sheath thickness (145), but whether neuregulin has the same effect on OLGs is not known. Cell contact-mediated signaling initiated by axons and through the *Notch* receptor also regulates the differentiation of OLGs. OLGs and their O-2A progenitors express *Notch1* while retinal ganglion cell axons express *Jagged1* (146), a ligand for *Notch1*. *Jagged1* expression decreases with myelination, suggesting that activation of *Notch* signaling by *Jagged1* negatively regulates the onset of myelination. Wang and colleagues (146) also found that activation of *Notch* signaling with a soluble form of *Delta1* ligand or by coculturing O-2A progenitors on *Jagged1*-expressing cells inhibited the differentiation of oligodendrocytes. Also, Kondo and Raff (147) demonstrated that overexpression of *Hes5*, a downstream mediator of *Notch* signaling, inhibited O-2A differentiation induced by mitogen withdrawal or treatment with T3. In predominantly nonmyelinating areas of MS plaques, hypertrophic astrocytes express *Jagged1* near cells with an immature OLG morphology, which express *Hes5* and *Notch* (148). In contrast, remyelinating areas lack *Jagged1* expression, which supports the contention that *Notch* signaling, initiated by Jagged1, inhibits OLG differentiation in vivo. On the other hand, *Notch* signaling initiated by the novel *Notch* ligand, F3/contactin, expressed on axons, can also promote the differentiation of OLGs (149). Therefore, axons, through both cell-contact-dependent and independent mechanisms, tightly regulate the timing and quality of myelination.

Properties of Human OLG Progenitors

OLG progenitors isolated from the fetal CNS have been found to express A2B5, O4, PDGFRα, NG2, OLIG1, and DLX-2 in vitro (150–153). However, A2B5 is also expressed by neurons and astrocytes (153), and NG2 is expressed by microglia (154). Even PDGFRα has been co-localized with neuronal antigens (89). Thus, no human OLG progenitor-specific antigen has been described. Despite the lack of specific human fetal OLG progenitor antigens, isolation of fetal OLG progenitors by magnetic sorting for A2B5, followed by negative selection against PSA-NCAM+ neurons using fluorescence-activated sorting (FACS), has led to the efficient isolation of fetal OLG progenitors (155). However, the paucity of antigens that specifically label OLG progenitors makes it difficult to be certain of the ontogeny and potential of OLG progenitors in vivo.

Little is known about the factors that drive the expansion, differentiation, and survival of human fetal OLG progenitors. The proliferation of OLG progenitors from fetal human spinal cord is promoted by PDGF, NT-3, and glial growth factor 2 (150). Studies of human fetal NSCs suggest that

T3 and PDGF can also promote the appearance of O4+ preOLGs and increase the branched morphology of the OLGs (89). The maturation of OLG progenitors to CNPase+ OLGs is promoted by IGF-1 (150), in contrast to its survival effects on OLGs in rodents (120). In agreement with Roy et al., we find that fetal A2B5 cells differentiate more robustly in the presence of PDGF and NT3. More work is needed to confirm and expand what is known about the factors that promote OLG progenitor expansion, differentiation, and survival.

Regarding OLG precursors in the adult human CNS, Nishiyama et al. identified a relative abundance of NG2-expresing cells in the normal adult CNS (156). OLG progenitors can also be isolated from the human adult forebrain. Armstrong and colleagues isolated O4+, A2B5-pre-OLGs from the white matter of adult partial temporal lobe resections, but rat astrocyte-conditioned medium, PDGF, IGF-1, and FGF-2 could not induce their proliferation (157). Similar to the effects of IGF-1 on fetal OLGs, IGF-1 induced the differentiation of preOLGs to GalC-expressing OLGs. Proliferating O-2A progenitor-like cells can also be isolated from the white matter of adult humans. These progenitors express A2B5, but not O4, GalC, or GFAP, and can differentiate into A2B5+ astrocytes or A2B5+, GalC+ OLGs. Again, neither PDGF, FGF-2, IGF-1, NGF, nor NT-3 induced proliferation (158). However, astrocyte monolayers could induce 25% of the A2B5 population to proliferate.

Further evidence that A2B5+ cells in adult human white matter are OLG progenitors comes from observations that white matter cells transfected with plasmids that induce green fluorescent protein expression under the human early promoter for the OLG protein cCNPase label A2B5+ cells (159). When isolated to near purity, these cells were found to be mitotically active and differentiated largely into OLGs, with a minority differentiating into astrocytes and neurons. Whether or not the proliferation of these OLG progenitors is due to the PDGF, FGF-2, and NT-3 in the medium was not tested. As with rodent OLGs, CNTF may also be a survival factor for human OLGs, considering that a null mutation allele of the CNTF gene is associated with early-onset MS (160).

The potential use of fetal and adult human OLG progenitors in remyelination has been tested in transplant paradigms. Fetal and adult human OLG progenitors have been xenografted intracallosally into "shiverer" mice, which fail to develop MBP or compact myelin (155). Both fetal and adult OLG progenitors were able to efficiently remyelinate the forebrains of shiverer mice. Transplantation also revealed differences in the properties of fetal and adult progenitors. Whereas fetal cells were highly migratory, their maturation into myelinating OLGs was slow, and they generated astrocytes as readily as OLG. In comparison, adult-derived progenitors were less migratory, matured more quickly and in higher proportions, and did not generate astrocytes. Furthermore, progenitors from adult OGC myelinated more axons per cell than did fetal-derived progenitors. Neither fetal nor adult progenitors generated neurons, in contrast with the in vitro results mentioned above. The ability of adult human OLG progenitors to remyelinate the lysolecithin-demyelinated rat brain has also been examined (161). Interestingly, the progenitors failed to migrate when injected into normal brains, and even within demyelinated brains they avoided areas of normal myelin. Astrocytes (but not neurons) were also derived from adult human OLG progenitors in this model. This suggests that astrocytic differentiation of adult human OLG progenitors is dependent on environmental cues present in the lysolecithin model of demyelination and not the shiverer mouse model.

Our analysis of A2B5+ cells isolated from the adult CNS by magnetic bead-based immunosorting (155, 161) and maintained in relatively basal medium (DMEM-F12 supplemented with N1 (Sigma) plus FGF and T3) (see next section) indicates that a relatively greater proportion of A2B5+ cells isolated from the adult CNS are committed to the OLG lineage compared to A2B5+ cells isolated from the fetal CNS (10). The adult CNS-derived A2B5 cells have lower rates of survival and cell cycling. These observations suggest that while putative progenitor cells exist in the adult CNS, concern remains regard-ing their intrinsic potential to carry out robust remyelination.

As summarized in Table 4-2D, cells expressing specific surface markers of immature OLG (O4, NG2, PLP, PDGFα-R) or morphologic features characteristic of myelin progenitor cells are described in MS lesions. Phenotypic profiles of such cells include O4+ GalC-NG2-(162), PDGF-Rα+ GalC− (163,164), PDGF-Rα+, NG2+ (165), and PLP+ preOLGs (166). Current consensus would suggest that although such cells are present in the regions of MS lesions, their numbers are not significantly increased or decreased in these regions (Table 4-2), nor are they either actively proliferating or, conversely, undergoing apoptosis. As mentioned, a number of pathologic descriptions of MS lesions describe increased number of OLG at the lesion margins. In late, chronic MS lesions where remyelination is less widespread than in early lesions, the number of progenitors as well as the number of mature OLGs is decreased compared to the early, active lesions (167).

The extent of remyelination achieved in MS via progenitor cells is likely to reflect additional environmental factors related to guiding or inhibiting access of progenitor cells to the demyelinated region [(10) and Table 4-1]. Potential sources of molecules supporting or inhibiting progenitor migration in MS would include intact myelin or debris, inflammatory cells, and the acute or chronic glial scar. With further regard to inflammatory mediators, Aarum et al. reported that migration and differentiation of neural progenitor cells can be directed by soluble factors released by microglia (168). Neural progenitor cells express receptors that permit response to chemoattractant molecules produced by inflammatory cells or by activated glial cells. The chemokine receptor CXCR2 controls positioning of OGC progenitors in developing spinal cord by arresting their migration (169). In adult CNS, netrin-1 is a component of myelinating OGCs and is found in periaxonal myelin, the interface between the axolemma and the inner face of the myelin sheath. Netrin-1 can also be detected in the adult spleen, although the precise cellular elements expressing this molecule are not yet defined (10).

Even if potential remyelinating cells reach the lesion site, successful remyelination will be dependent on the presence and molecular integrity of the axons. In the CNS as well as the PNS, remyelinated nerve sheaths are thinner and shorter than the original sheaths, suggesting that some developmental factors regulating myelin thickness during development are absent or non-functional during remyelination in adults (170). One notes that OLG progenitors and mature human OLGs in vitro are able to survive, differentiate, and extend processes expressing all the myelin proteins, even in absence of neurons.

The above discussion has focused on the role of progenitor cells as mediators of remyelination. The extensive rodent-based studies suggest that any contribution of previously myelinating OLG seems relatively unimportant. One notes, however, differences in biologic properties of mature human and rodent OLG. OLG isolated from the adult human CNS are post-mitotic cells that, under relatively basal culture conditions (unlike their rodent counterparts), will survive indefinitely and extend extensive processes. The isolation procedure in which the cells are separated from any axonal process and their process are lost or retracted could itself be considered as a model of demyelination, and thus the process outgrowth as "remyelination." One further considers that focal demyelination could reflect loss of only one of up to 50 axonal segments that are myelinated by a single OLG. If the cell maintains some of its myelin segments, the question raised is why the cell does not reextend a process to replace the individual segment(s) that has (have) been lost. Of interest, studies of MBP expression in mouse toxin models indicate that remyelination involves activation of a different set of myelin gene promoters versus initially myelinating cells (171).

OLG/MYELIN AND AXON LOSS IN PROGRESSIVE MS

In the more advanced disease stages the extent of myelin and OLGs loss is more apparent, raising the issue of whether this reflects continued injury of these cells. This later disease stage also features continued axonal loss, raising the issue of how OLG/myelin and axonal loss impact on one another.

Mature OLG Injury

Although this presentation has focused on the initial injury to OLG/myelin in MS being immune-mediated, speculation exists as to whether initial events may relate to other types of insults, including infections, trauma, and ischemia. Both immune and nonimmune-mediated insults to the OLGs could induce a series of sublethal injury responses in OGCs that would result in their becoming susceptible to subsequent immune-mediated injury. A variety of types of insults can up-regulate expression of the transcription factor, p53. We have found that low levels of p53 overexpression, insufficient to result in cell death, results in up-regulation of fas and TRAIL receptors, making the OLGs susceptible to injury mediated by the ligands for these receptors (33). Amongst neural cells, OLGs seem especially likely to up-regulate expression of inducible stress proteins (inducible HSP) in response to sublethal injury (172). We refer to such a sequence of events as a two-hit hypothesis, as similarly proposed by McNamara and colleagues who implicated sequential glutamate- and complement-mediated injury in contributing to neuronal injury in epilepsy models (173).

Progenitor Cell Injury

The observations that progenitor cell numbers may be decreased rather than increased in acute/active MS lesions and that OLG numbers and the extent of remyelination are decreased in chronic MS lesions, raises the issue of whether the progenitor cells are themselves subject to injury as part of the MS disease. The most direct negative effect of the inflammatory response on progenitor cell-dependent remyelination would be the occurrence of immune-mediated injury to the progenitor cells. Imitola et al. have shown that that the pluripotential neural progenitor cells found in the subventricular regions can be induced by inflammatory mediators to express CD86 (a classic immune co-stimulatory molecule), and that such expression makes these cells vulnerable to T-cell-mediated injury (174). Some reports indicate that MS sera or CSF contains antibodies that react with cell lines used as models of OLG progenitors or that react with a specific OLG progenitor-associated molecule (AN2), now recognized to be the equivalent to NG2 (172). Rosenbluth et al. showed that implanting a hybridoma secreting IgM antibodies that recognize the sulfatide O4 expressed by OLG lineage progenitor cells produced focal demyelination and that remyelination occurred only when the hybridoma degenerated (175). Giraudon et al. recently showed that activated T-cells induced apoptotic death of multipotential neural progenitor cells and immature OLG (11). This injury could be inhibited with antibodies directed against sCD100/semaphorin 4D released by activated T-cells and reproduced with rsCD100. This semaphorin was shown to collapse OLG process extension and to trigger apoptosis, most likely through receptors of the plexin family. Current data further suggest that only immature (and not mature) OLGs express receptors for glutamate, a mediator implicated in causing tissue injury in EAE and MS (176,177). Microglia/macrophages that dominate the late active lesion of MS would be a potential source of glutamate. Immune constituents could also have positive effects on progenitor cell-mediated remyelination. Germ line anti-IgM antibodies can bind OLG progenitors and promote remyelination (178,179).

Axon Degeneration Secondary to Demyelination

Axonal degeneration is recognized to occur in a number of genetic dysmyelinating mutant models, implicating OLGs/myelin as providing a source of trophic support for axons. Focal demyelination of axons, as occurs in MS, has been shown to result in expression of voltage-gated sodium channels along the entire course of the demyelinated segment rather than being confined to the nodes of Ranvier. Craner et al. demonstrated diffuse distribution of Na(v)1.2 and Na(v)1.6 channels along extensive regions of demyelinated axons within acute MS plaques.

Na(v)1.6, which is known to produce a persistent sodium current, and the Na(+)/Ca(2+) exchanger, which can be driven by persistent sodium current to import damaging levels of calcium into axons, were co-localized with beta-amyloid progenitor protein, a marker of axonal injury, in such acute MS lesions (180). Their conclusion was that the coexpression of Na(v)1.6 and Na(+)/Ca(2+) exchanger is associated with axonal degeneration in MS.

An ongoing challenge is to translate the emerging insights regarding the biologic processes underlying myelin/OLG injury and repair into therapies that will impact on the neurologic deficits associated with MS. Currently, approved MS therapies are all aimed at modulating systemic immune activity or the access of immune mediators to the CNS. The therapeutic potential of agents that can access the CNS and that would either directly protect OLGs/myelin from the injury processes described in this review or prevent the consequences of demyelination on axonal survival and function remains to be tested. A number of therapeutic approaches aimed at promoting remyelination are already being explored in experimental models. These include enhancing the extent of remyelination mediated by endogenous progenitor cells and supplying (via systemic administration or intrathecal transplants) exogenous sources of cells capable of myelination. The apparent presence of myelin progenitor cells in the adult human CNS, as well as the persistence of previously myelinating OLGs in at least some MS cases early in the disease process, hold out hope that therapies aimed at enhancing endogenous myelin repair will be applicable to adult human disease. Myelin repair via exogenous cell sources will need to overcome barriers of how to administer such cells so that they reach multifocal sites of injury. The above therapeutic strategies can be complemented by those aimed at promoting neuron/axon survival and function. As has been the case with immune-directed therapies, implementation of neuroprotection and repair therapies in MS will be dependent on development of clinical and imaging-based methods to evaluate the effectiveness of such therapies.

REFERENCES

1. Antel J, Arnold D. 2004. Multiple Sclerosis. In: *Neuroglia*, 2nd edition. Antel J, Arnold D, eds. Oxford and New York: Oxford University Press, 2005:489–500.
2. Lucchinetti C, Bruck W, Parisi J, et al. Heterogeneity of multiple sclerosis lesions: implications for the pathogenesis of demyelination. *Ann Neurol* 2000;47: 707–717.
3. Rodriguez M, Scheithauer BW, Forbes G, et al. Oligodendrocyte injury is an early event in lesions of multiple sclerosis. *Mayo Clin Proc* 1993;68:627–636.
4. Owens T, Wekerle H, Antel J. Genetic models for CNS inflammation. *Nat Med* 2001;7:161–166.
5. Barnett MH, Prineas JW. Relapsing and remitting multiple sclerosis: pathology of the newly forming lesion. *Ann Neurol* 2004;55:458–468.
6. Waksman, B. Historical Perspective and Overview. In: *Clinical Neuroimmunology*. Antel J, Birnbaum G, Hartung H-P, eds. Oxford: Blackwell Science, Inc., 1998:391–404.
7. Pouly S, Antel JP. Multiple sclerosis and central nervous system demyelination. *J Autoimmun* 1999;13:297–306.
8. Vergelli M, Hemmer B, Muraro PA, et al. Human autoreactive CD4+ T-cell clones use perforin- or fas/fas ligand-mediated pathways for target-cell lysis. *J Immunol* 1997;158:2756–2761.
9. Antel JP, McCrea E, Ladiwala U, et al. Non-MHC-restricted cell-mediated lysis of human oligodendrocytes in vitro: relation with CD56 expression. *J Immunol* 1998;160:1606–1611.
10. Ruffini F, Kennedy TE, Antel JP. Inflammation and remyelination in the central nervous system: a tale of two systems. *Am J Pathol* 2004;164:1519–1522.
11. Giraudon P, Vincent P, Vuaillat C, et al. Semaphorin CD100 from activated T lymphocytes induces process extension collapse in oligodendrocytes and death of immature neural cells. *J Immunol* 2004;172: 1246–1255.
12. Babbe H, Roers A, Waisman A, et al. Clonal expansions of CD8(+) T-cells dominate the T-cell infiltrate in active multiple sclerosis lesions as shown by micromanipulation and single cell polymerase chain reaction. *J Exp Med* 2000;192:393–404.
13. Jurewicz A, Biddison WE, Antel JP. MHC class I-restricted lysis of human oligodendrocytes by myelin basic protein peptide-specific CD8 T lymphocytes. *J Immunol* 1998;160:3056–3059.
14. Neumann H, Cavalie A, Jenne DE, et al. Induction of MHC class I genes in neurons. *Science* 1995;269: 549–552.
15. Giuliani F, Goodyer CG, Antel JP, et al. Vulnerability of human neurons to T-cell-mediated cytotoxicity. *J Immunol* 2003;171:368–379.
16. Egg R, Reindl M, Deisenhammer F, et al. Anti-MOG and anti-MBP antibody subclasses in multiple sclerosis. *Mult Scler* 2001;7:285–289.
17. O'Connor KC, Chitnis T, Griffin DE, et al. Myelin basic protein-reactive autoantibodies in the serum and cerebrospinal fluid of multiple sclerosis patients are characterized by low-affinity interactions. *J Neuroimmunol* 2003;136:140–148.
18. Berger T, Rubner P, Schautzer F, et al. Antimyelin antibodies as a predictor of clinically definite multiple sclerosis after a first demyelinating event. *N Engl J Med* 2003;349:139–145.
19. Genain CP, Cannella B, Hauser SL, et al. Identification of autoantibodies associated with myelin damage in multiple sclerosis. *Nat Med* 1999;5: 170–175.
20. Lily O, Palace J, Vincent A. Serum autoantibodies to cell surface determinants in multiple sclerosis: a flow cytometric study. *Brain* 2004;127:269–279.
21. Raine CS, Bonetti B, Cannella B. Multiple sclerosis: expression of molecules of the tumor necrosis factor ligand and receptor families in relationship to the demyelinated plaque. *Rev Neurol (Paris)* 1998;154:577–585.
22. Dorr J, Bechmann I, Waiczies S, et al. Lack of tumor necrosis factor-related apoptosis-inducing ligand but presence of its receptors in the human brain. *J Neurosci* 2002;22:RC209.
23. Dowling P, Shang G, Raval S, et al. Involvement of the CD95 (APO-1/Fas) receptor/ligand system in multiple sclerosis brain. *J Exp Med* 1996;184:1513–1518.
24. Finsen B, Antel J, Owens T. TNFalpha: kill or cure for demyelinating disease? *Mol Psychiatry* 2002;7: 820–821.
25. Jurewicz A, Matysiak M, Tybor K, et al. TNF-induced death of adult human oligodendrocytes is mediated by c-jun NH2-terminal kinase-3. *Brain* 2003;126: 1358–1370.
26. D'Souza S, Alinauskas K, McCrea E, et al. Differential susceptibility of human CNS-derived cell populations to TNF-dependent and independent immune-mediated injury. *J Neurosci* 1995;15:7293–7300.
27. Pouly S, Becher B, Blain M, et al. Interferon-gamma modulates human oligodendrocyte susceptibility to Fas-mediated apoptosis. *J Neuropathol Exp Neurol* 2000;59:280–286.
28. Becher B, D'Souza SD, Troutt AB, et al. Fas expression on human fetal astrocytes without susceptibility to fas-mediated cytotoxicity. *Neuroscience* 1998;84:627–634.
29. Wosik K, Becher B, Ezman A, et al.. Caspase 8 expression and signaling in Fas injury-resistant human fetal astrocytes. *Glia* 2001;33:217–224.
30. Nitsch R, Pohl EE, Smorodchenko A, et al. Direct impact of T-cells on neurons revealed by two-photon microscopy in living brain tissue. *J Neurosci* 2004;24: 2458–2464.
31. Wosik K, Seguin R, Pouly S, et al. Interferon β (IFNβ) modulates death receptor DR4 and DR5 expression on oligodendrocytes and their ligand TRAIL on T-cells. *Neurology* 2001;56(8)A381:4–24.
32. Matysiak M, Jurewicz A, Jaskolski D, et al. TRAIL induces death of human oligodendrocytes isolated from adult brain. *Brain* 2002;125:2469–2480.
33. Wosik K, Antel J, Kuhlmann T, et al. Oligodendrocyte injury in multiple sclerosis: a role for p53. *J Neurochem* 2003;85:635–644.
34. Casaccia-Bonnefil P, Carter BD, Dobrowsky RT, et al. Death of oligodendrocytes mediated by the interaction of nerve growth factor with its receptor p75. *Nature* 1996;383:716–719.
35. Ladiwala U, Lachance C, Simoneau SJ, et al. p75 neurotrophin receptor expression on adult human oligodendrocytes: signaling without cell death in response to NGF. *J Neurosci* 1998;18:1297–1304.
36. Beattie MS, Harrington AW, Lee R, et al. ProNGF induces p75-mediated death of oligodendrocytes following spinal cord injury. *Neuron* 2002;36:375–386.
37. Bajramovic JJ, Plomp AC, Goes A, et al. Presentation of alpha B-crystallin to T-cells in active multiple sclerosis

lesions: an early event following inflammatory demyelination. *J Immunol* 2000;164:4359–4366.

38. Stover J F, Pleines UE, Morganti-Kossmann MC, et al. Neurotransmitters in cerebrospinal fluid reflect pathological activity. *Eur J Clin Invest* 1997;27:1038–1043.

39. Stover JF, Lowitzsch K, Kempski OS. Cerebrospinal fluid hypoxanthine, xanthine and uric acid levels may reflect glutamate-mediated excitotoxicity in different neurological diseases. *Neurosci Lett* 1997;238:25–28.

40. Werner P, Pitt D, Raine CS. Multiple sclerosis: altered glutamate homeostasis in lesions correlates with oligodendrocyte and axonal damage. *Ann Neurol* 2001;50: 169–180.

41. Pitt D, Werner P, Raine CS. Glutamate excitotoxicity in a model of multiple sclerosis. *Nat Med* 2000;6:67–70.

42. Smith T, Groom A, Zhu B, et al. Autoimmune encephalomyelitis ameliorated by AMPA antagonists. *Nat Med* 2000;6:62–66.

43. Yoshioka A, Bacskai B, Pleasure D. Pathophysiology of oligodendroglial excitotoxicity. *J Neurosci Res* 1996;46:427–437.

44. Matute C, Sanchez-Gomez MV, Martinez-Millan L, et al. Glutamate receptor-mediated toxicity in optic nerve oligodendrocytes. *Proc Natl Acad Sci USA* 1997;94:8830–8835.

45. Matute C. Characteristics of acute and chronic kainate excitotoxic damage to the optic nerve. *Proc Natl Acad Sci USA* 1998;95:10229–10234.

46. McDonald JW, Althomsons SP, Hyrc KL, et al. Oligodendrocytes from forebrain are highly vulnerable to AMPA/kainate receptor-mediated excitotoxicity. *Nat Med* 1998;4:291–297.

47. Sanchez-Gomez MV, Matute C. AMPA and kainate receptors each mediate excitotoxicity in oligodendroglial cultures. *Neurobiol Dis* 1999;6:475–485.

48. Kavanaugh B, Beesley J, Itoh T, et al. Neurotrophin-3 (NT-3) diminishes susceptibility of the oligodendroglial lineage to AMPA glutamate receptor-mediated excitotoxicity. *J Neurosci Res* 2000;60:725–732.

49. Alberdi E, Sanchez-Gomez MV, Marino A, et al. Ca(2+) influx through AMPA or kainate receptors alone is sufficient to initiate excitotoxicity in cultured oligodendrocytes. *Neurobiol Dis* 2002;9:234–243.

50. Wosik K, Ruffini F, Almazan G, et al. Resistance of human adult oligodendrocytes to AMPA/kainate receptor mediated glutamate injury. *Brain*. 2004; in press.

51. Rodriguez M, Pierce ML, Thiemann RL. Immunoglobulins stimulate central-nervous-system remyelination–electron-microscopic and morphometric analysis of proliferating cells. *Laboratory Investigation* 1991;64:358–370.

52. Carroll WM, Jennings AR. Early recruitment of oligodendrocyte precursors in CNS demyelination. *Brain* 1994;117:563–578.

53. Gensert JM, Goldman JE. Endogenous progenitors remyelinate demyelinated axons in the adult CNS. *Neuron* 1997;19:197–203.

54. Franklin RJM, Gilson JM, Blakemore WF. Local recruitment of remyelinating cells in the repair of demyelination in the central nervous system. *J Neurosci Res* 1997;50:337–344.

55. Keirstead HS, Levine JM, Blakemore WF. Response of the oligodendrocyte progenitor cell population (defined by NG2 labelling) to demyelination of the adult spinal cord. *Glia* 1998;22:161–170.

56. Redwine JM, Armstrong RC. In vivo proliferation of oligodendrocyte progenitors expressing PDGF alpha R during early remyelination. *J Neurobio* 1998;37:413–428.

57. Di Bello IC, Dawson MRL, Levine JM, et al. Generation of oligodendroglial progenitors in acute inflammatory demyelinating lesions of the rat brain stem is associated with demyelination rather than inflammation. *J Neurocytol* 1999;28: 365–381.

58. Tropepe V, Hitoshi S, Sirard C, et al. Direct neural fate specification from embryonic stem cells: a primitive mammalian neural stem cell stage acquired through a default mechanism. *Neuron* 2001;30:65–78.

59. Billon N, Jolicoeur C, Ying QL, et al. Normal timing of oligodendrocyte development from genetically engineered, lineage-selectable mouse ES cells. *J Cell Sci* 2002;115:3657–3665.

60. Thomson JA, Itskovitz-Eldor J, Shapiro SS, et al. Embryonic stem cell lines derived from human blastocysts. *Science* 1998;282:1145–1147.

61. Shamblott MJ, Axelman J, Wang S, et al. Derivation of pluripotent stem cells from cultured human primordial germ cells. *Proc Natl Acad Sci USA* 1998;95: 13726–13731.

62. Wilmut I, Schnieke AE, McWhir J, et al. Viable offspring derived from fetal and adult mammalian cells. *Nature* 1997;385:810–813.

63. Mezey E, Chandross KJ, Harta G, et al. Turning blood into brain: cells bearing neuronal antigens generated in vivo from bone marrow. *Science* 2000;290: 1779–1782.

64. Brazelton TR, Rossi FM, Keshet GI, et al. From marrow to brain: expression of neuronal phenotypes in adult mice. *Science* 2000;290:1775–1779.

65. Ferrari G, Cusella-De Angelis G, Coletta M, et al. Muscle regeneration by bone marrow-derived myogenic progenitors. *Science* 1998;279:1528–1530.

66. Petersen BE, Bowen WC, Patrene KD, et al. Bone marrow as a potential source of hepatic oval cells. *Science* 1999;284:1168–1170.

67. Theise ND, Nimmakayalu M, Gardner R, et al. Liver from bone marrow in humans. *Hepatology* 2000;32: 11–16.

68. Lagasse E, Connors H, Al-Dhalimy M, et al. Purified hematopoietic stem cells can differentiate into hepatocytes in vivo. *Nat Med* 2000;6:1229–1234.

69. Terada N, Hamazaki T, Oka M, et al. Bone marrow cells adopt the phenotype of other cells by spontaneous cell fusion. *Nature* 2002;416:542–545.

70. Spees JL, Olson SD, Ylostalo J, et al. Differentiation, cell fusion, and nuclear fusion during ex vivo repair of epithelium by human adult stem cells from bone marrow stroma. *Proc Natl Acad Sci USA* 2003;100: 2397–2402.

71. Vassilopoulos G, Wang PR, Russell DW. Transplanted bone marrow regenerates liver by cell fusion. *Nature* 2003;422:901–904.

72. Jang YY, Collector MI, Baylin SB, et al. Hematopoietic stem cells convert into liver cells within days without fusion. *Nat Cell Biol* 2004;6:532–539.

73. Harris RG, Herzog EL, Bruscia EM, et al. Lack of a fusion requirement for development of bone marrow-derived epithelia. *Science* 2004;305:90–93.

74. Palmer TD, Takahashi J, Gage FH. The adult rat hippocampus contains primordial neural stem cells. *Mol Cell Neurosci* 1997;8:389–404.

75. Reynolds BA, Weiss S. Generation of neurons and astrocytes from isolated cells of the adult mammalian central nervous system *Science* 1992;255: 1707–1710.

76. Reynolds BA,. Weiss S. Clonal and population analyses demonstrate that an EGF-responsive mammalian embryonic CNS precursor is a stem cell. *Dev Biol* 1996;175:1–13.

77. Carpenter MK, Cui X, Hu ZY, et al. In vitro expansion of a multipotent population of human neural progenitor cells. *Exp Neurol* 1999;158:265–278.

78. Svendsen CN, ter Borg MG, Armstrong RJ, et al. A new method for the rapid and long term growth of human neural precursor cells. *J Neurosci Methods* 1998; 85(2):141–152.

79. Flax JD, Aurora S, Yang C, et al. Engraftable human neural stem cells respond to developmental cues, replace neurons, and express foreign genes. *Nat Biotechnol* 1998;16:1033–1039.

80. Vescovi AL, Parati EA, Gritti A, et al. Isolation and cloning of multipotential stem cells from the embryonic human CNS and establishment of transplantable human neural stem cell lines by epigenetic stimulation. *Exp Neurol* 1999;156:71–83.

81. Palmer TD, Schwartz PH, Taupin P, et al. Cell culture. Progenitor cells from human brain after death. *Nature* 2001;411:42–43.

82. Kirschenbaum B, Nedergaard M, Preuss A, et al. In vitro neuronal production and differentiation by precursor cells derived from the adult human forebrain. *Cereb Cortex* 1994;4:576–589.

83. Johansson CB, Svensson M, Wallstedt L, et al. Neural stem cells in the adult human brain. *Exp Cell Res* 1999;253:733–736.

84. Arsenijevic Y, Villemure, JG, Brunet JF, et al. Isolation of multipotent neural precursors residing in the cortex of the adult human brain. *Exp Neurol* 2001;170:48–62.

85. Fruttiger M, Karlsson L, Hall AC, et al. Defective oligodendrocyte development and severe hypomyelination in PDGF-A knockout mice. *Development* 1999;126: 457–467.

86. Richardson WD, Pringle N, Mosley MJ, et al. A role for platelet-derived growth factor in normal gliogenesis in the central nervous system. *Cell* 1988;53:309–319.

87. Pringle N, Collarini EJ, Mosley MJ, et al. PDGF A chain homodimers drive proliferation of bipotential (O-2A) glial progenitor cells in the developing rat optic nerve. *Embo J* 1989;8:1049–1056.

88. Weiss S, Dunne C, Hewson J, et al. Multipotent CNS stem cells are present in the adult mammalian spinal cord and ventricular neuroaxis. *J Neurosci* 1996;16: 7599–7609.

89. Murray K, Dubois-Dalcq M. Emergence of oligodendrocytes from human neural spheres. *J Neurosci Res* 1997;50:146–156.

90. Liu Y, Rao M. Oligodendrocytes, GRPs and MNOPs. *Trends Neurosci* 2003;26:410–412.

91. Noble M, Proschel C, Mayer-Proschel M. Getting a GR(i)P on oligodendrocyte development. *Dev Biol* 2004;265:33–52.

92. Rowitch DH. Glial specification in the vertebrate neural tube. *Nat Rev Neurosci* 2004;5:409–419.

93. Zhou Q. Anderson DJ. The bHLH transcription factors OLIG2 and OLIG1 couple neuronal and glial subtype specification. *Cell* 2002;109:61–73.

94. Lu QR, Sun T, Zhu Z, et al. Common developmental requirement for Olig function indicates a motor neuron/oligodendrocyte connection. *Cell* 2002;109:75–86.

95. Lu QR, Yuk D, Alberta JA, et al. Sonic hedgehog–regulated oligodendrocyte lineage genes encoding bHLH proteins in the mammalian central nervous system. *Neuron* 2000;25:317–329.

96. Pringle NP, Richardson WD. A singularity of PDGF alpha-receptor expression in the dorsoventral axis of the neural tube may define the origin of the oligodendrocyte lineage. *Development* 1993;117:525–533.

97. Puelles L, Kuwana E, Puelles E, et al. Pallial and subpallial derivatives in the embryonic chick and mouse telencephalon, traced by the expression of the genes Dlx-2, Emx-1, Nkx-2.1, Pax-6, and Tbr-1. *J Comp Neurol* 2000;424:409–438.

98. Nery S, Wichterle H, Fishell G. Sonic hedgehog contributes to oligodendrocyte specification in the mammalian forebrain. *Development* 2001;128:527–540.

99. Tekki-Kessaris N, Woodruff R, Hall AC, et al.. Hedgehog-dependent oligodendrocyte lineage specification in the telencephalon. *Development* 2001;128: 2545–2554.

100. Ono K, Bansal R, Payne J, et al. Early development and dispersal of oligodendrocyte precursors in the embryonic chick spinal cord. *Development* 1995;121:1743–1754.

101. Warf BC, Fok-Seang J, Miller RH. Evidence for the ventral origin of oligodendrocyte precursors in the rat spinal cord. *J Neurosci* 1991;11:2477–2488.

102. Olivier C, Cobos I, Perez Villegas EM, et al. Monofocal origin of telencephalic oligodendrocytes in the anterior entopeduncular area of the chick embryo. *Development* 2001;128:1757–1769.

103. Tsai HH, Tessier-Lavigne M, Miller RH. Netrin 1 mediates spinal cord oligodendrocyte precursor dispersal. *Development* 2003;130:2095–2105.

104. Tsai HH, Frost E, To V, et al. The chemokine receptor CXCR2 controls positioning of oligodendrocyte precursors in developing spinal cord by arresting their migration. *Cell* 2002;110:373–383.

105. Small RK, Riddle P, Noble M. Evidence for migration of oligodendrocyte-type-2 astrocyte progenitor cells into the developing rat optic nerve. *Nature* 1987;328: 155–1557.

106. Ono K, Yasui Y, Rutishauser U, et al. Focal ventricular origin and migration of oligodendrocyte precursors into the chick optic nerve. *Neuron* 1997; 19:283–292.

107. Sugimoto Y, Taniguchi M, Yagi T, et al. Guidance of glial precursor cell migration by secreted cues in the developing optic nerve. *Development* 2001;128: 3321–3330.

108. Pringle NP, Yu WP, Guthrie S, et al. Determination of neuroepithelial cell fate: induction of the oligodendrocyte lineage by ventral midline cells and sonic hedgehog. *Dev Biol* 1996;177:30–42.

109. Orentas DM, Hayes JE, Dyer KL, et al. Sonic hedgehog signaling is required during the appearance of spinal cord oligodendrocyte precursors. *Development* 1999;126:2419–2429.

110. Alberta JA, Park SK, Mora SK, et al. Sonic hedgehog is required during an early phase of oligodendrocyte development in mammalian brain. *Mol Cell Neurosci* 2001;18:434–441.

111. Vartanian T, Fischbach G, Miller R. Failure of spinal cord oligodendrocyte development in mice lacking neuregulin. *Proc Natl Acad Sci USA* 1999;96: 731–735.

112. Park HC, Appel B. Delta-Notch signaling regulates oligodendrocyte specification. *Development* 2003; 130:3747–3755.

113. Raff MC, Lillien LE, Richardson WD, et al. Platelet-derived growth factor from astrocytes drives the clock that times oligodendrocyte development in culture. *Nature* 1988;333:562–565.

114. Bogler O, Wren D, Barnett SC, et al. Cooperation between two growth factors promotes extended self-renewal and inhibits differentiation of oligodendro-cyte-type-2 astrocyte (O-2A) progenitor cells. *Proc Natl Acad Sci USA* 1990;87:6368–6372.

115. McKinnon RD, Matsui T, Dubois-Dalcq M, et al. FGF modulates the PDGF-driven pathway of oligodendro-cyte development. *Neuron* 1990;5:603–614.

116. Barres BA, Raff MC, Gaese F, et al. A crucial role for neurotrophin-3 in oligodendrocyte development. *Nature* 1994;367:371–375.

117. Barres BA, Hart IK, Coles HS, et al. Cell death and control of cell survival in the oligodendrocyte lineage. *Cell* 1992;70:31–46.

118. Calver AR, Hall AC, Yu WP, et al. Oligodendrocyte population dynamics and the role of PDGF in vivo. *Neuron* 1998;20:869–882.

119. Louis JC, Magal E, Takayama S, et al. CNTF protec-tion of oligodendrocytes against natural and tumor necrosis factor-induced death. *Science* 1993;259: 689–692.

120. Barres BA, Schmid R, Sendtner M, et al. Multiple extra-cellular signals are required for long-term oligodendro-cyte survival. *Development* 1993;118: 283–295.

121. Mason JL, Ye P, Suzuki K, et al. Insulin-like growth factor-1 inhibits mature oligodendrocyte apoptosis during primary demyelination. *J Neurosci* 2000;20: 5703–5708.

122. Linker RA, Maurer M, Gaupp S, et al. CNTF is a major protective factor in demyelinating CNS disease: a neurotrophic cytokine as modulator in neuroinflam-mation. *Nat Med* 2002;8:620–624.

123. Butzkueven HJ, Zhang G, Soilu-Hanninen M, et al. LIF receptor signaling limits immune-mediated demyelination by enhancing oligodendrocyte survival. *Nat Med* 2002;8:613–619.

124. Zhang SC. Defining glial cells during CNS develop-ment. *Nat Rev Neurosci* 2001;2:840–843.

125. Miller RH, Hayes JE, Dyer KL, et al. Mechanisms of oligodendrocyte commitment in the vertebrate CNS. *Int J Dev Neurosci* 1999;17:753–763.

126. Nishiyama A, Lin XH, Giese N, et al. Co-localization of NG2 proteoglycan and PDGF alpha-receptor on O2A progenitor cells in the developing rat brain. *J Neurosci Res* 1996;43:299–314.

127. Abney ER, Williams BP, Raff MC. Tracing the devel-opment of oligodendrocytes from precursor cells using monoclonal antibodies, fluorescence-activated cell sorting, and cell culture. *Dev Biol* 1983;100:166–171.

128. Sommer I, Schachner M. Monoclonal antibodies (O1 to O4) to oligodendrocyte cell surfaces: an immunocy-tological study in the central nervous system. *Dev Biol* 1981;83:311–327.

129. Sommer I, Schachner M. Cell that are O4 antigen-pos-itive and O1 antigen-negative differentiate into O1

130. Campagnoni AT. Molecular biology of myelin pro-teins from the central nervous system. *J Neurochem* 1988;51:1–14.

131. Lemke G. Unwrapping the genes of myelin. *Neuron* 1988;1:535–43.

132. Zurbriggen A, Vandevelde M, Steck A, et al. Myelin-associated glycoprotein is produced before myelin basic protein in cultured oligodendrocytes. *J Neuroimmunol* 1984;6:41–49.

133. Mabie PC, Mehler MF, Marmur R, et al. Bone mor-phogenetic proteins induce astroglial differentiation of oligodendroglial-astroglial progenitor cells. *J Neurosci* 1997;17:4112–4120.

134. Marta CB, Adamo AM, Soto EF, et al. Sustained neonatal hyperthyroidism in the rat affects myelination in the central nervous system. *J Neurosci Res* 1998;53:251–259.

135. Rodriguez-Pena A, Ibarrola N, Iniguez MA, et al. Neonatal hypothyroidism affects the timely expression of myelin-associated glycoprotein in the rat brain. *J Clin Invest* 1993;91:812–818.

136. Dussault JH, Ruel J. Thyroid hormones and brain development. *Annu Rev Physiol* 1987;49:321–334.

137. Walters SN,. Morell P. Effects of altered thyroid states on myelinogenesis. *J Neurochem* 1981;36:1792–1801.

138. Barres BA, Lazar MA, Raff MC. A novel role for thy-roid hormone, glucocorticoids and retinoic acid in tim-ing oligodendrocyte development. *Development* 1994;120:1097–1108.

139. Mayer M, Bhakoo K, Noble M. Ciliary neurotrophic factor and leukemia inhibitory factor promote the gen-eration, maturation and survival of oligodendrocytes in vitro. *Development* 1994;120:143–153.

140. Barres BA, Burne JF, Holtmann B, et al. Ciliary neu-rotrophic factor enhances the rate of oligodendrocyte generation. *Mol Cell Neurosci* 1996;8:146–156.

141. Stankoff B, Aigrot MS, Noel F, et al. Ciliary neu-rotrophic factor (CNTF) enhances myelin formation: a novel role for CNTF and CNTF-related molecules. *J Neurosci* 2002;22:9221–9227.

142. Canoll PD, Musacchio JM, Hardy R, et al. GGF/neureg-ulin is a neuronal signal that promotes the proliferation and survival and inhibits the differentiation of oligoden-drocyte progenitors. *Neuron* 1996;17:229–243.

143. Park SK, Miller R, Krane I, et al. The erbB2 gene is required for the development of terminally differenti-ated spinal cord oligodendrocytes. *J Cell Biol* 2001;154:1245–1258.

144. Chan JR, Watkins TA, Cosgaya JM, et al. NGF controls axonal receptivity to myelination by Schwann cells or oligodendrocytes. *Neuron* 2004;43:183–191.

145. Michailov GV, Sereda MW, Brinkmann BG, et al. Axonal neuregulin-1 regulates myelin sheath thick-ness. *Science* 2004;304:700–703.

146. Wang S, Sdrulla AD, diSibio G, et al. Notch receptor activation inhibits oligodendrocyte differentiation. *Neuron* 1998;21:63–75.

147. Kondo T, Raff M. Basic helix-loop-helix proteins and the timing of oligodendrocyte differentiation. *Development* 2000;127:2989–2998.

148. John GR, Shankar SL, Shafit-Zagardo B, et al. Multiple sclerosis: re-expression of a developmental

pathway that restricts oligodendrocyte maturation. *Nat Med.* 2002;8:1115–1121.

149. Hu QD, Ang BT, Karsak M, et al. F3/contactin acts as a functional ligand for Notch during oligodendrocyte maturation. *Cell* 2003;115:163–175.

150. Wilson HC, Onischke C, Raine CS. Human oligodendrocyte precursor cells in vitro: phenotypic analysis and differential response to growth factors. *Glia* 2003;44:153–165.

151. Rivkin MJ, Flax J, Mozell R, et al. Oligodendroglial development in human fetal cerebrum. *Ann Neurol* 1995;38:92–101.

152. Zhang SC, Ge B, Duncan ID. Tracing human oligodendroglial development in vitro. *J Neurosci Res* 2000;59:421–429.

153. Satoh J, Kim SU. Ganglioside markers GD3, GD2, and A2B5 in fetal human neurons and glial cells in culture. *Dev Neurosci* 1995;17:137–148.

154. Pouly S, Becher B, Blain M, et al. Expression of a homologue of rat NG2 on human microglia. *Glia* 1999;27:259–268.

155. Windrem MS, Nunes MC, Rashbaum WK, et al. Fetal and adult human oligodendrocyte progenitor cell isolates myelinate the congenitally dysmyelinated brain. *Nat Med* 2004;10:93–97.

156. Nishiyama A, Chang A, Trapp BD. NG2+ glial cells: a novel glial cell population in the adult brain. *J Neuropathol Exp Neurol* 1999;58:1113–1124.

157. Armstrong RC, Dorn HH, Kufta CV, et al. Pre-oligodendrocytes from adult human CNS. *J Neurosci* 1992;12:1538–1547.

158. Scolding NJ, Rayner PJ, Sussman J, et al. A proliferative adult human oligodendrocyte progenitor. *Neuroreport* 1995;6:441–445.

159. Roy NS, Wang S, Harrison-Restelli C, et al. Identification, isolation, and promoter-defined separation of mitotic oligodendrocyte progenitor cells from the adult human subcortical white matter. *J Neurosci* 1999;19:9986–9995.

160. Giess R, Maurer M, Linker R, et al. Association of a null mutation in the CNTF gene with early onset of multiple sclerosis. *Arch Neurol* 2002;59:407–409.

161. Windrem MS, Roy NS, Wang J, et al. Progenitor cells derived from the adult human subcortical white matter disperse and differentiate as oligodendrocytes within demyelinated lesions of the rat brain. *J Neurosci Res* 2002;69:966–975.

162. Wolswijk G. Oligodendrocyte precursor cells in chronic multiple sclerosis lesions. *Mult Scler* 1997;3:168–169.

163. Scolding N, Franklin R, Stevens S, et al. Oligodendrocyte progenitors are present in the normal adult human CNS and in the lesions of multiple sclerosis. *Brain* 1998;121(Pt 12):2221–2228.

164. Maeda Y, Solanky M, Menonna J, et al. Platelet-derived growth factor-alpha receptor-positive oligodendroglia are frequent in multiple sclerosis lesions. *Ann Neurol* 2001;49:776–785.

165. Chang A, Nishiyama A, Peterson J, et al. NG2-positive oligodendrocyte progenitor cells in adult human brain and multiple sclerosis lesions. *J Neurosci* 2000;20:6404–6412.

166. Chang A, Tourtellotte WW, Rudick R, et al. Premyelinating oligodendrocytes in chronic lesions of multiple sclerosis. *N Engl J Med* 2002;346:165–173.

167. Prineas JW, Kwon EE, Cho ES, et al. Immunopathology of secondary-progressive multiple sclerosis. *Ann Neurol* 2001;50:646–657.

168. Aarum J, Sandberg K, Haeberlein SL, et al. Migration and differentiation of neural precursor cells can be directed by microglia. *Proc Natl Acad Sci USA* 2003;100:15983–15988.

169. Filipovic R, Jakovcevski I, Zecevic N. GRO-alpha and CXCR2 in the human fetal brain and multiple sclerosis lesions. *Dev Neurosci* 2003;25:279–290.

170. French-Constant C, Colognato H, Franklin RJ. Neuroscience. The mysteries of myelin unwrapped. *Science* 2004;304:688–689.

171. Farhadi HF, Lepage P, Forghani R, et al. A combinatorial network of evolutionarily conserved myelin basic protein regulatory sequences confers distinct glial-specific phenotypes. *J Neurosci* 2003;23:10214–10223.

172. D'Souza SD, Bonetti B, Balasingam V, et al. Multiple sclerosis: Fas signaling in oligodendrocyte cell death. *J Exp Med* 1996;184:2361–2370.

173. Xiong ZQ, McNamara JO. Fleeting activation of ionotropic glutamate receptors sensitizes cortical neurons to complement attack. *Neuron* 2002;36:363–374.

174. Imitola J, Comabella M, Chandraker AK, et al. Neural stem/progenitor cells express costimulatory molecules that are differentially regulated by inflammatory and apoptotic stimuli. *Am J Pathol* 2004;164:1615–1625.

175. Rosenbluth J, Schiff R, Liang WL, et al. Antibody-mediated CNS demyelination II. Focal spinal cord lesions induced by implantation of an IgM antisulfatide-secreting hybridoma. *J Neurocytol* 2003;32: 265–276.

176. Rosenberg PA, Dai W, Gan XD, et al. Mature myelin basic protein-expressing oligodendrocytes are insensitive to kainate toxicity. *J Neurosci Res* 2003;71: 237–245.

177. Back SA, Han BH, Luo NL, et al. Selective vulnerability of late oligodendrocyte progenitors to hypoxia-ischemia. *J Neurosci* 2002;22:455–463.

178. Warrington AE, Bieber AJ, Van K, et al. Neuron-binding human monoclonal antibodies support central nervous system neurite extension. *J Neuropathol Exp Neurol* 2004;63:461–473.

179. Ciric B, Howe CL, Paz SM, et al. Human monoclonal IgM antibody promotes CNS myelin repair independent of Fc function. *Brain Pathol* 2003;13:608–616.

180. Craner MJ, Newcombe J, Black JA, et al. Molecular changes in neurons in multiple sclerosis: altered axonal expression of Nav1.2 and Nav1.6 sodium channels and Na+/Ca2+ exchanger. *Proc Natl Acad Sci USA* 2004;101:8168–8173.

5

The Myelin Basic Protein Gene: A Prototype for Combinatorial Mammalian Transcriptional Regulation

Hooman F. Farhadi[1] and Alan C. Peterson[2]

[1]*Department of Neurology and Neurosurgery, McGill University, Montreal, Quebec, Canada;*
[2]*Departments of Human Genetics/Oncology/Neurology and Neurosurgery, McGill University, Molecular Oncology Group—Royal Victoria Hospital, McGill University and Genome Quebec Innovation Centre, Montreal, Quebec, Canada*

In this chapter, we review recent investigations that expose the strategies adopted by evolution to control the complex gene expression programs realized by the "myelin gene family." We focus on the mechanism controlling transcriptional regulation of one family member, the myelin basic protein (MBP) gene. Regulatory activity at the MBP locus arises from widely dispersed enhancer modules consisting of short, noncoding sequences that are highly conserved throughout mammals and in most nonmammalian vertebrates. Each confers a discrete regulatory subprogram to the overall MBP expression phenotype. Expression in oligodendrocytes is conferred through multiple proximal modules and independently through the proximal promoter, while Schwann cells rely upon a far-upstream module. Beyond their well-characterized, autonomous functions, such modules also engage in combinatorial relationships to refine both cell-type specificity and quantitative expression phenotypes. Of relevance to myelin cell biology, this combinatorial organization underlies an unsuspected maturation program in which the transcription factor repertoire regulating MBP expression evolves with age. Thus, the combination and/or relative activity of transcription factors engaged during primary myelin elaboration is not present in mature myelin-maintaining oligodendrocytes or, most remarkably, in remyelinating oligodendrocytes in mature animals. Should this circumstance also exist in humans, fundamental characteristics of the cells targeted in adult MS lesions, as well as those attempting myelin repair, are specific to the mature nervous system.

INTERDEPENDENCE OF AXONS AND THEIR MYELINATING GLIA

Myelin formation represents a relatively recent evolutionary adaptation of vertebrates. The electrical insulation afforded by compacted myelin membranes in the central and peripheral nervous systems allows for rapid and energy efficient conduction over long distances while respecting necessary size constraints. Within fast-conducting, myelinated fibers, the morphological and functional phenotypes of axons and their supporting glia develop and are maintained through continuous bidirectional signaling.

Significant differences exist in the way that myelinating glia interact with axons in the central and peripheral nervous systems. Whereas a single oligodendrocyte may myelinate scores of different axons, a myelinating Schwann cell associates with a single axon. The correlation between the caliber of the innervating axon and myelination is much tighter in the peripheral nervous system (PNS) than in the central nervous system (CNS) (3,76). When Schwann cells are isolated from the innervating axon, either through denervation in vivo or isolation in culture, they revert to a nonmyelinating phenotype and down-regulate the genes for the major myelin-associated proteins to low basal levels (55,56,93). Isolated oligodendrocytes, on the other hand, continue to extend their processes and induce and maintain ~30% of the normal level of expression of myelin genes (1,10,115).

Despite these differences, myelin formation and maintenance is the final step in the maturation of both oligodendrocytes and Schwann cells, and involves a complex and tightly regulated process that is supported by an intimate axon–glial physical interrelationship. The synthesis and assembly of myelin-specific components in all terminally differentiating glial cells must be precisely orchestrated to give rise to myelin. On the one hand, myelination leads to local changes in the cytoarchitecture and functional properties of the axon, including the phosphorylation status of the axonal cytoskeleton and the rate of slow anterograde axonal transport (2,11,23,52). Also, the clustering of sodium and potassium channels at the node and the juxtaparanode, respectively, is dependent on oligodendrocytes (8,49,81) and Schwann cells (5,48).

Conversely, axons also appear to control multiple features of their myelin sheaths (64,71). Part of the control that axons exert over glial cells appears to be mediated through the coordinated regulation of genes encoding myelin-specific proteins. Early in vitro experiments showed that, in addition to neurons being mitogenic for oligodendrocytes and Schwann cells (27,110), isolation of glial cells from axons results in a down-regulation of myelin-specific genes with only partial restoration of expression in co-cultures (22,59). In vivo differentiation of oligodendrocytes in the optic nerve is closely related to axonal integrity (50,62,95). Furthermore, modulation of myelin protein gene expression by axons is also observed under various experimental conditions, such as following nerve transection (55,62,85).

It seems likely that both soluble and cell-mediated signals from adjacent axons are integrated into the developmental profile of oligodendrocyte precursors, resulting in cell differentiation, up-regulation of myelin gene expression, and formation of mature myelin. For instance, oligodendrocyte maturation and survival is influenced by neuregulins expressed on axons (30,97). Neuregulin exposure induces morphological changes in cultured oligodendrocytes (17) In the absence of the neuregulin receptor ErbB2, while many oligodendrocyte precursors develop, few of these cells mature; those that do mature fail to interact with axons and do not produce myelin (51,73). In the PNS, axonally derived neuregulin promotes differentiation along a glial path (12,84) and has recently been shown to function as a key regulator of myelin sheath thickness in vivo (64). Moreover, nerve growth factor (NGF) has recently been shown to mediate potent, but inverse, effects on myelination by Schwann cells and oligodendrocytes, likely through changes in the axonal signals that control myelination (19).

Other candidates for axonally derived soluble factors include fibroblast growth factors (80), thyroid hormone (9), and adenosine (90). In particular, adenosine released in an activity-dependent manner by dorsal root ganglia axons promotes differentiation of oligodendrocyte precursors into MBP-expressing cells containing multiple processes and forming compact myelin sheaths. Myelination also appears to be regulated by electrical activity alone (24,89). Treatment of CNS explant cultures with tetrodotoxin results in significantly fewer myelin internodes transiently, while treatment with scorpion toxin (a selective sodium channel activator) results in a significant increase. Finally, axonal cell surface molecules such as L1, MAG, NCAM, and N-cadherin may also regulate formation of the myelin sheath (61).

POTENTIAL MBP TRANSCRIPTIONAL REGULATORS

Glial cells and their progenitors have historically been characterized primarily by their morphologies and expression of a small number of lineage and myelin markers. However, exciting insight into the regulatory machinery and the signalling pathways that control their major expression features is rapidly emerging (101). Despite the fact that only few such factors are well-characterized, they are providing progressively greater insight into the requirements for lineage specification, progression, and terminal differentiation (4,91). Notably, as the number of factors implicated in myelin cell biology grows, insights into unanticipated spatial and temporal oligodendrocyte heterogeneity have emerged; where both the Nkx6 transcription factor and the Sonic hedgehog signalling system were thought to be essential for the origin of the oligodendrocyte lineage, recent investigations demonstrate that oligodendrocytes appearing later in the dorsal spinal cord share no such requirements (15,97).

MYELIN PROTEIN GENE PROMOTER ANALYSIS

A comprehensive catalogue of the transcription factors controlling oligodendrocyte gene expression in all developmental states would certainly provide a foundation upon which novel therapeutic interventions could be developed. While many difficulties are yet to be addressed before we achieve such understanding, genome-wide strategies capable of evaluating the transcription factor repertoire are currently under development and in limited application. Importantly, transcriptional regulation in complex organisms is not a simple matter of turning a gene on at the right time in the right cell type. Rather, the basic mechanism emerging involves scores of factor–DNA element interactions that may be engaged to effect positive, negative, or neutral consequences on gene output. Furthermore, not all relevant interactions are likely to occur in the cells positively regulating the locus; active silencing in inappropriate cell types or at specific stages of lineage progression also may be required. Thus, to complement the insights expected from genome-wide molecular and computational approaches, it is essential that multiple model loci are sufficiently well-characterized to expose the actual structure and function relationships within their *cis*-linked regulatory sequences. It is our goal to introduce a myelin gene into this model locus category.

The promoters of myelin protein genes have been analyzed using in vitro preparations, and several regulatory sequences that identify transcription factors regulating myelin formation have emerged (14,20,45,66,68,69,74,87,102, 103). However, since no in vitro model fully recapitulates the myelinating glial phenotype and, given the apparent importance of bidirectional signalling with intact axons, reliable dissection of control mechanisms with in vitro techniques has proved difficult.

Ideally, direct insight into the complex in vivo axon–glia relationships should be achievable through mouse transgenic technology. Following this strategy, several laboratories have investigated the regulatory capacity of sequences flanking representative myelin protein gene members. Transgenic mice have been derived bearing reporter constructs regulated by various lengths of 5′ flanking sequence from the *proteolipid protein*, MBP, *protein zero*, *peripheral myelin protein 22*, and *2′, 3′ cyclic-nucleotide 3′-phosphodiesterase* genes. Targeting to oligodendrocytes and/or Schwann cells has been demonstrated with varying efficiency (34,40,41, 60,63,105,112).

Unfortunately, until recently, reliable and efficient identification of *cis*-regulatory sequences using classic transgenic methodologies has been limited. Variability in transcriptional efficiency attributable to unpredictable transgene copy numbers, and local chromatin effects at the site of integration, combined to confound the interpretation of regulatory phenotypes and have precluded fine structure analysis. To resolve these

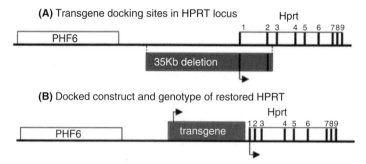

FIG. 5-1. Diagram depicting deletion in the HPRT locus where constructs are docked and the genotype of the transgene locus following homologous recombination of the construct bearing targeting vector. Hypoxanthine-aminopterin-thymidine (HAT) selection following transfection with appropriate targeting vectors allows survival only of clones in which homologous recombination has simultaneously restored deleted HPRT expression and inserted a single copy of the experimental construct, at a known site and orientation 5′ of the HPRT locus (13). *PHF6* indicates the next 5′ locus.

issues and to locate and characterize the elements regulating in vivo transcription of the MBP locus, we employed a recently described controlled transgenesis strategy wherein constructs insert in single copy at the hypoxanthine-guanine phosphoribosyltransferase (HPRT) locus. Controlling transgene genotype in this manner allows for high-resolution, interconstruct, qualitative and quantitative comparisons (13,21,98) (Fig 5-1).

Several features of MBP and its regulatory phenotype make it an ideal candidate gene for elucidating mechanisms underlying axon-glia interactions. As a major component of the major dense line, MBP plays an essential and rate-limiting role in CNS myelin formation (53,79). Also, it is a well-characterized experimental autoantigen with potential roles at multiple levels in immune-mediated mechanisms of myelin destruction (58). It is present in both CNS and PNS myelin, where it accounts for 5% to 15% and 30% to 40% of myelin protein content, respectively (42,43,65). MBP appears to be differentially regulated throughout oligodendrocyte lineage progression, achieving highest expression levels in terminally differentiated myelinating cells with modestly reduced levels maintained throughout maturity into senescence. Expression also appears to be tightly regulated under numerous experimental conditions

involving demyelination and remyelination (55,111). Both oligodendrocytes and Schwann cells regulate the appearance of MBP primarily at the transcriptional level (106), with such expression coordinated in time and place with other myelin-related genes in both cell types in response to axonal cues (37,70). Finally, MBP is a potential susceptibility gene for MS in the context of a small, Finnish population (77), raising the intriguing possibility that dysregulated MBP expression may be a component in MS onset.

Investigations using classic transgenic preparations have shown that the proximal MBP promoter targets developmentally appropriate temporal expression to oligodendrocytes but not Schwann cells (34,39,40), while 5′ flanking sequences extending to approximately −6 kb or −9 kb yield more robust expression (29,35). Additionally, the 9-kb sequence also targets expression to developing, mature, and remyelinating Schwann cells.

COMBINATORIAL CONTROL OF TRANSCRIPTION

Transcriptional regulation in multicellular organisms is complex and, for each locus, occurs through the coordinated action of multiple transcription factors acting on large numbers of regulatory elements. A common theme of such regulatory mechanisms is a combinatorial organization (44,113). A combinatorial strategy allows the organism to dynamically control gene expression in response to a variety of environmental or developmental signals through different combinations of a limited number of transcriptional regulators.

The *cis*-regulatory system of the developmentally regulated *endo16* gene of the sea urchin has been investigated to perhaps greater depth than any other locus, and thus serves as a useful model (113,114). Its major regulatory sequence is contained within approximately 2,300 bp and consists of several clusters of target sites that operate as separable, modular, regulatory units that execute distinct qualitative or quantitative functions. Through a detailed spatiotemporal analysis of endoderm reporter expression in numerous lines bearing different permutations of normal or mutated enhancer elements, Davidson and colleagues successfully developed a quantitative computational model that appropriately reflects the integrated output of defined regulatory sequences. Of significance, most *endo16* elements confer only small quantitative effects that, in aggregate, determine the integrated expression programming.

Although the analysis of *endo16* greatly enhanced our ability to contemplate the fine structure of the regulatory networks functioning in vertebrate and mammalian systems, elucidating the transcriptional regulatory network in such higher-order organisms represents a much more daunting task; each experimental approach, either computational or functional, provides only partial answers (31,32,104). Currently, a synthesis of multiple approaches is being employed that includes genomic sequence annotation, cross-species sequence comparisons, functional analysis of reporter constructs, and abstract model-building.

Patterns of gene regulation and the corresponding regulatory controls are often conserved across species, and cross-species sequence comparison has emerged as a means to reveal functionally relevant regulatory sequences. Relying on the principle that selective pressure over functional regulatory sequences causes them to evolve more slowly than surrounding unselected sequences, these so-called phylogenetic footprints are expected to confer various regulatory functions (18,83). In this regard, the mouse genome has received considerable attention, given that its genomic sequences are now easily accessible and that there is a wealth of similarity to many human-relevant biological and disease processes (including myelination and inherited and acquired myelin diseases). Using recently developed computational methods and evolving genomic databases from an increasing number of species, interspecies sequence comparisons are being performed in an efficient and comprehensive manner (26,36,86,99,100,107). Although the general usefulness of human–mouse sequence comparisons as a systematic guide to functionally relevant regulatory sequences remains untested, evolutionarily conserved sequences (in the range of hundreds of base pairs) are associated with many loci and, to date, many such conserved, noncoding sequences have been assigned regulatory functions (29,38,57,72,75,94).

EVIDENCE FOR COMBINATORIAL CONTROL OF MBP TRANSCRIPTION

The MBP transcriptional unit maps to chromosome 18 in both mouse and human, where it is distributed over a length of approximately 32 kb and 45 kb, respectively. Interestingly, it is contained within a much larger transcriptional unit (spanning 105 kb in mouse and 179 kb in human) that includes the gene *Golli* (gene expressed in the oligodendrocyte lineage). The first three MBP exons and the proximal MBP promoter contribute to translated *Golli* exons (16,78). While noncoding domains have an average level of human–mouse conservation approximating 30% to 40%, with an upper limit near 80% (46), the MBP genomic domain fortuitously appears to have undergone evolutionary change at a comparatively greater tempo, revealing an overall level of conservation at the lower end of this scale. Given this circumstance, functional domains should be clearly recognized as conserved sequence blocks lying amongst highly substituted, nonfunctional adjacent sequences. Therefore, in our initial attempts to highlight MBP regulatory sequences through phylogenetic footprints, we used thresholds of identity of 75% over a prespecified minimum length (100 bp) to define sequence conservation. We scanned 25 kb of human and 12 kb of mouse 5′ flanking orthologous sequences and identified four islands of marked sequence conservation (termed modules 1 to 4). All modules were ligated into reporter genes that were introduced, in single-copy, 5′ of the HPRT locus and investigated for *cis*-regulatory activity in subsequent lines of transgenic mice (29) (Fig. 5-1).

A diverse range of in vivo expression phenotypes, including different cell specificities, developmental programming, and expression levels was observed (Figs. 5-2 and 5-3). From these observations, it became evident that the MBP regulatory mechanism controls transcription through a combination of seemingly autonomous modular contributions that are overlaid with functions derived from integrated arrangements (Fig 5-4).

Amongst the multiple subprograms that were discerned, perhaps the most striking is the requirement of module 3 for high-level expression in mature mice. This observation requires that the MBP relevant transcription factor repertoire of mature oligodendrocytes differs from that of the less-mature oligodendrocytes in preweaning mice, either as a response to an intrinsic developmental program or as a change secondary to extrinsic differences in the environment provided in the juvenile versus the mature brain. In

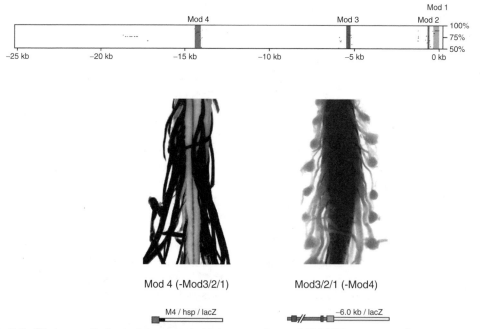

Mod 4 (-Mod3/2/1)   Mod3/2/1 (-Mod4)

FIG. 5-2. Phylogenetic footprints revealed by comparison of 5′ MBP sequence from mouse and human. The human sequence is displayed on the x axis while the percent identity, measured in a 100-bp window, is indicated on the y axis. In the proximal promoter sequence, extensive and high levels of conservation are encountered that, in this analysis, define two separable modules. More upstream is module 3 and farther upstream yet is module 4. Whole mount histochemical preparations displayed below show that module 4 containing constructs express in Schwann cells, and not oligodendrocytes, while constructs bearing the more 3′ modules are expressed in oligodendrocytes only. In both constructs, *LacZ* is the reporter gene. In the Mod3/2/1 construct, MBP 5′ flanking sequence was ligated directly to *LacZ* while in the module 4 construct, a minimal 300-bp heat shock protein promoter was introduced between module 4 and the *LacZ* reporter.

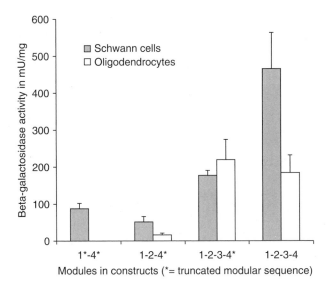

FIG. 5-3. Sciatic nerve and cervical spinal cord samples were obtained from transgenic mice containing constructs bearing different combinations of MBP regulatory modules. Samples were recovered at postnatal day 18 when myelin elaboration, MBP, and construct expression are at, or near, maximal levels. As constructs were docked in an X chromosome site, for one potentially active construct copy to be available in all cells, analyzed mice were either transgene-bearing males or homozygous females. Mice analyzed in this study were derived from intercrosses between C57Bl/6, 129PAS, and 129OLA inbred strains and, therefore, had variable genetic backgrounds. Truncated modules are indicated by ˙. Bars represent means and error bars SD.

either case, this observation defines a novel level of temporal oligodendrocyte heterogeneity.

To explore the potential origin of such age-associated heterogeneity, we investigated the regulatory phenotype of oligodendrocytes remyelinating in the mature nervous system. Transgene expression was evaluated in mice bearing constructs containing only modules 1 and 2 (29). In response to intrathecal injection of saporin conjugated to the beta subunit of cholera toxin, oligodendrocytes mount a significant remyelination response (47) but, surprisingly, we obtained no evidence indicative of transgene expression in newly myelinating oligodendro-

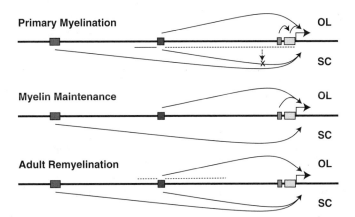

FIG. 5-4. The 5′ flanking region of the mouse MBP locus along with its four regions of high interspecies conservation (colored rectangles) are shown. The positive relationships defined so far that can drive expression in developing, mature, and remyelinating cells are represented as solid arrows. Those above the flanking sequence positively regulate expression in oligodendrocytes, while solid arrows below positively regulate expression in Schwann cells. Dotted lines represent the general location of various negative regulatory activities. (From Farhadi HF, Lepage P, Forghani R, et al. A combinatorial network of evolutionarily conserved myelin basic protein regulatory sequences confers distinct glial-specific phenotypes. *J Neurosci* 2003;23(32):10214-10223, with permission.)

cytes bearing these constructs devoid of module 3. In contrast, observations from randomly targeted MBP-LacZ transgenic lines regulated by 5′ flanking sequences containing module 3, reveal that adult, newly myelinating oligodendrocytes do express their transgene reporter coincident with new myelin deposition (33).

From these observations, it is apparent that at least part of the regulatory mechanism used to control MBP transcription during primary development is not in service during myelin repair in the mature CNS. In the context of MS lesions, while some controversy exists regarding the density of the progenitor population in regions of demyelination (54,109,116), it is nevertheless clear that such cells possess atypical myelination capabilities. In this regard, oligodendrocyte precursors have clearly been identified lying directly within chronic plaques of MS patients (108). Why these cells do not aggressively repair the demyelinated lesions, and why those oligodendrocytes that eventually do enter an active myelination program slowly elaborate only thin myelin, remain largely unanswered questions. The differences observed in the MBP transcriptional mechanism operating in primary development and in oligodendrocytes remyelinating in the mature brain may contribute to the protracted and incomplete process of remyelination often observed in the diseased or injured adult CNS.

To identify the regulatory sequences and factors that confer the module 3 expression phenotype, and in an effort to characterize the regulatory cascade functioning during adult myelin maintenance and regeneration, an intense analysis of module 3 elements and their relationship to expression in mature and remyelinating oligodendrocytes is currently underway (28). In the initial round of investigations, we focused on Nkx6.2/Gtx, an oligodendrocyte-specific homeodomain protein known to avidly bind TAAT-containing consensus sites (6,7) and that is coordinately expressed with several myelin-specific mRNAs in multiple cell states (88). While a module 3 construct bearing mutations in two of three Nkx6.2/Gtx consensus sites retains continuous oligodendrocyte targeting activity, quantitative analysis revealed a significant decrease in transcriptional efficiency

(29). Thus, this transcription factor (or related homeodomain proteins) appears to function within a complex framework finely modifying module 3 output.

Taken together, observations summarized in this chapter demonstrate that different combinations of regulatory sequences control MBP expression during development, myelin maintenance, and remyelination. Though the picture is far from complete and notable exceptions are emerging, vast numbers of positive cis-regulatory elements account for the major spatiotemporal features of MBP expression. The specific temporal, spatial, and quantitative output from the MBP gene is determined by the particular combination of evolutionarily conserved cis-regulatory binding sites that are engaging transcription factors. To arrive at a more complete picture of this complex cis-regulatory circuitry, the fine structure of individual enhancers as well as more in-depth analysis of modular interactions and negative regulatory activities will be required. Fortunately, the HPRT-based, controlled strategy of transgenesis is sufficiently robust to reveal the role played by individual elements and, consequently, is ideally suited to support such investigations (25). Additionally, initial in vitro experiments, including transfection analysis, DNase I footprinting, and electrophoretic mobility shift assays, are underway by our group and others (92) using the conserved MBP modular sequences.

CONCLUSION

Although nothing of therapeutic relevance for patients with MS has emerged so far from past and current investments in basic gene regulation mechanisms, this endeavor appears poised to yield insights with practical consequences. The convergence of recent discoveries in genome organization, along with the unexpected developments of strategies to modulate gene output (82) suggest that opportunities to control the stability and/or responsiveness of myelin-forming cells, in clinically meaningful ways, is within reach. Beyond this emerging potential, greater understanding of the mechanisms regulating gene expression is, of itself, offering a disease-relevant window into the myelination program in effect at different stages of oligodendrocyte maturation. By achieving insight into the molecular mechanisms regulating myelin formation and repair, we anticipate that novel opportunities to stabilize myelin in the diseased CNS and to promote repair following demyelinating episodes will become evident.

ACKNOWLEDGMENTS

The investigations discussed in this chapter were supported by the Canadian Multiple Sclerosis Society and Foundation, the Canadian Institutes for Health Research (CIHR), and Genome Canada/Genome Quebec. Hooman F. Farhadi was supported through a CIHR Doctoral Fellowship. We thank our many laboratory colleagues who made the investigations described in this chapter possible. In particular, we thank Dr Eric Denarier, Dr. Hana Friedman, and Dr. Melissa Beaudouin for help with figures and helpful comments on the manuscript.

REFERENCES

1. Abney ER, Bartlett PP, Raff MC. Astrocytes, ependymal cells, and oligodendrocytes develop on schedule in dissociated cell cultures of embryonic rat brain. *Dev Biol* 1981;83(2):301–310.
2. Aguayo AJ, Bray GM, Perkins SC. Axon-Schwann cell relationships in neuropathies of mutant mice. *Ann N Y Acad Sci* 1979;317:512–531.
3. Aguayo AJ, Kasarjian J, Skamene E, et al. Myelination of mouse axons by Schwann cells transplanted from normal and abnormal human nerves. *Nature* 1977;268(5622):753–755.
4. Arnett HA, Fancy SP, Alberta JA, et al. bHLH transcription factor Olig1 is required to repair demyelinated lesions in the CNS. *Science* 2004;306(5704): 2111–2115.
5. Arroyo EJ, Xu YT, Zhou L, et al. Myelinating Schwann cells determine the internodal localization of Kv1.1, Kv1.2, Kvbeta2, and Caspr. *J Neurocytol* 1999;28 (4-5):333–347.
6. Awatramani R, Beesley J, Yang H, et al. Gtx, an oligodendrocyte-specific homeodomain protein, has repressor activity. *J Neurosci Res* 2000;61(4):376–387.
7. Awatramani R, Scherer S, Grinspan J, et al. Evidence that the homeodomain protein Gtx is involved in the regulation of oligodendrocyte myelination. *J Neurosci* 1997;17(17):6657–6668.
8. Baba H, Akita H, Ishibashi T, et al.Completion of myelin compaction, but not the attachment of oligodendroglial processes triggers K(+) channel clustering. *J Neurosci Res* 1999;58(6):752–764.
9. Barres BA, Lazar MA, Raff MC, et al. A novel role for thyroid hormone, glucocorticoids and retinoic acid in timing oligodendrocyte development. *Development* 1994;120(5):1097–1108.
10. Bradel EJ, Prince FP. Cultured neonatal rat oligodendrocytes elaborate myelin membrane in the absence of neurons. *J Neurosci Res* 1983;9(4):381–392.
11. Brady ST, Witt AS, Kirkpatrick LL, et al. Formation of compact myelin is required for maturation of the axonal cytoskeleton. *J Neurosci.* 1999;19(17):7278–7288.
12. Britsch S, Li L, Kirchhoff S, et al. The ErbB2 and ErbB3 receptors and their ligand, neuregulin-1, are essential for development of the sympathetic nervous system. *Genes Dev* 1998;12(12):1825–1836.
13. Bronson SK, Plaehn EG, Kluckman KD, et al. Single-copy transgenic mice with chosen-site integration. *Proc Natl Acad Sci U S A* 1996;93(17):9067–9072.
14. Brown AM., Lemke G. Multiple regulatory elements control transcription of the peripheral myelin protein zero gene. *J Biol Chem* 1997;272(46):28939–28947.
15. Cai J, Qi Y, Hu X, et al. Generation of oligodendrocyte precursor cells from mouse dorsal spinal cord independent of Nkx6 regulation and Shh signaling. *Neuron* 2005;45(1):41–53.
16. Campagnoni AT, Pribyl TM, Campagnoni CW, et al. Structure and developmental regulation of Golli-mbp, a 105-kilobase gene that encompasses the myelin basic protein gene and is expressed in cells in the oligodendrocyte lineage in the brain. *J Biol Chem* 1993;268(7):4930–4938.
17. Canoll PD, Kraemer R, Teng KK, et al. GGF/neuregulin induces a phenotypic reversion of oligodendrocytes. *Mol Cell Neurosci* 1999;13(2):79–94.
18. Cawley S, Bekiranov S, Ng HH, et al. Unbiased mapping of transcription factor binding sites along human chromosomes 21 and 22 points to widespread regulation of noncoding RNAs. *Cell* 2004;116(4):499–509.
19. Chan JR, Watkins TA, Cosgaya JM, et al. NGF controls axonal receptivity to myelination by Schwann cells or oligodendrocytes. *Neuron* 2004;43(2):183–191.
20. Clark RE, Jr., Miskimins WK, Miskimins R. Cyclic AMP inducibility of the myelin basic protein gene promoter requires the NF1 site. *Int J Dev Neurosci* 2002;20(2):103–111.
21. Cvetkovic B, Yang B, Williamson RA, et al. Appropriate tissue- and cell-specific expression of a single copy human angiotensinogen transgene specifically targeted upstream of the HPRT locus by homologous recombination. *J Biol Chem* 2000;275(2): 1073–1078.
22. David S, Miller RH, Patel R, et al. Effects of neonatal transection on glial cell development in the rat optic nerve: evidence that the oligodendrocyte-type 2 astrocyte cell lineage depends on axons for its survival. *J Neurocytol* 1984;13(6):961–74.
23. de Waegh SM, Lee VM, Brady ST. Local modulation of neurofilament phosphorylation, axonal caliber, and slow axonal transport by myelinating Schwann cells. *Cell* 1992;68(3):451–463.
24. Demerens C, Stankoff B., Logak M., et al. Induction of myelination in the central nervous system by electrical activity. *Proc Natl Acad Sci U S A* 1996;93(18): 9887–9892.
25. Denarier E, Forghani R, Farhadi HF, et al. Functional organization of a Schwann cell enhancer, Submitted to *J Neurosci.*

26. Dermitzakis ET, Reymond A, Lyle R, et al. Numerous potentially functional but non-genic conserved sequences on human chromosome 21. *Nature* 2002;420(6915):578–582.

27. DeVries GH, Salzer JL, Bunge RP. Axolemma-enriched fractions isolated from PNS and CNS are mitogenic for cultured Schwann cells. *Brain Res* 1982;255(2): 295–299.

28. Dionne N, Denarier E, Dib S, et al. Functional dissection of evolutionarily conserved enhancers of the myelin basic protein gene, Cold Spring Harb Meeting, March 17–20, 2005.

29. Farhadi HF, Lepage P, Forghani R, et al. A Combinatorial Network of Evolutionarily Conserved Myelin Basic Protein Regulatory Sequences Confers Distinct Glial-Specific Phenotypes. *J Neurosci* 2003;23(32):10214–10223.

30. Fernandez PA, Tang DG, Cheng L, et al. Evidence that axon-derived neuregulin promotes oligodendrocyte survival in the developing rat optic nerve. *Neuron* 2000;28(1):81–90.

31. Fickett JW, Hatzigeorgiou AG. Eukaryotic promoter recognition. *Genome Res* 1997;7(9):861–878.

32. Fickett JW, Wasserman WW. Discovery and modeling of transcriptional regulatory regions. *Curr Opin Biotechnol* 2000;11(1):19–24.

33. Finsen B, Peterson AC. Remyelination is not a simple recapitulation of primary myelination. *Soc Neurosci Abstr* 2001;31:104–113.

34. Foran DR, Peterson AC. Myelin acquisition in the central nervous system of the mouse revealed by an MBP-Lac Z transgene. *J Neurosci* 1992;12(12):4890–4897.

35. Forghani R, Garofalo L, Foran DR, et al. A distal upstream enhancer from the myelin basic protein gene regulates expression in myelin-forming schwann cells. *J Neurosci* 2001; 21(11):3780–3787.

36. Frazer KA, Elnitski L, Church DM, et al. Cross-species sequence comparisons: a review of methods and available resources. *Genome Res* 2003; 13(1):1–12.

37. Gordon MN, Kumar S, Espinosa de los Monteros, A, et al. Developmental regulation of myelin-associated genes in the normal and the myelin deficient mutant rat. *Adv Exp Med Biol* 1990;265:11–22.

38. Gottgens B, Barton LM, Gilbert JG, et al. Analysis of vertebrate SCL loci identifies conserved enhancers. *Nat Biotechnol* 2000;18(2):181–186.

39. Goujet-Zalc C, Babinet C, Monge M, et al. The proximal region of the MBP gene promoter is sufficient to induce oligodendroglial-specific expression in transgenic mice. *Eur J Neurosci* 1993;5(6):624–632.

40. Gow A, Friedrich VL, Jr., Lazzarini RA. Myelin basic protein gene contains separate enhancers for oligodendrocyte and Schwann cell expression, *J Cell Biol* 1992; 119(3):605–616.

41. Gravel M, Di Polo A, Valera PB, et al. Four-kilobase sequence of the mouse CNP gene directs spatial and temporal expression of lacZ in transgenic mice. *J Neurosci Res* 1998;53(4):393–404.

42. Greenfield S, Brostoff S, Eylar EH, et al. Protein composition of myelin of the peripheral nervous system. *J Neurochem* 1973;20(4):1207–1216.

43. Hahn AF, Whitaker JN, Kachar B, et al. P2, P1, and P0 myelin protein expression in developing rat sixth nerve: a quantitative immunocytochemical study. *J Comp Neurol* 1987;260(4):501–512.

44. Halfon MS, Carmena A, Gisselbrecht S, et al. Ras pathway specificity is determined by the integration of multiple signal-activated and tissue-restricted transcription factors. *Cell* 2000;103(1):63–74.

45. He X, Gerrero R, Simmons DM, et al. Tst-1, a member of the POU domain gene family, binds the promoter of the gene encoding the cell surface adhesion molecule P0. *Mol Cell Biol* 1991;11(3):1739–1744.

46. JareborgN, BirneyE, Durbin R. Comparative analysis of noncoding regions of 77 orthologous mouse and human gene pairs. *Genome Res* 1999;9(9):815–824.

47. Jasmin L, Janni G, Moallem TM, et al. Schwann cells are removed from the spinal cord after effecting recovery from paraplegia. *J Neurosci* 2000; 20(24): 9215–9223.

48. Joe EH, Angelides K. Clustering of voltage-dependent sodium channels on axons depends on Schwann cell contact. *Nature* 1992;356(6367):333–335.

49. Kaplan MR, Meyer-Franke A, Lambert S, et al. Induction of sodium channel clustering by oligodendrocytes. *Nature* 1997;386(6626):724–728.

50. Kidd GJ, Hauer PE, Trapp BD. Axons modulate myelin protein messenger RNA levels during central nervous system myelination in vivo. *J Neurosci Res* 1990;26(4):409–418.

51. Kim JY, Sun Q, Oglesbee M, Yoon SO. The role of ErbB2 signaling in the onset of terminal differentiation of oligodendrocytes in vivo. *J Neurosci* 2003;23(13): 5561–5571.

52. Kirkpatrick LL, Witt AS, PayneHR, et al. Changes in microtubule stability and density in myelin-deficient shiverer mouse CNS axons. *J Neurosci* 2001;21(7): 2288–2297.

53. Kirschner DA, Ganser AL. Compact myelin exists in the absence of basic protein in the shiverer mutant mouse. *Nature* 1980;283(5743):207–210.

54. Lassmann H, Bruck W, Lucchinetti C, et al. Remyelination in multiple sclerosis. *Mult Scler* 1997;3(2):133–136.

55. LeBlanc AC, Poduslo JF. Axonal modulation of myelin gene expression in the peripheral nerve. *J Neurosci Res* 1990;26(3):317–326.

56. Lemke G, Chao M. Axons regulate Schwann cell expression of the major myelin and NGF receptor genes, *Development* 1988;102(3):499–504.

57. Loots GG, Locksley RM, Blankespoor CM, et al. Identification of a coordinate regulator of interleukins 4, 13, and 5 by cross-species sequence comparisons. *Science* 2000;288(5463):136–140.

58. Lutton JD, Winston R, Rodman TC. Multiple sclerosis: etiological mechanisms and future directions. *Exp Biol Med (Maywood)* 2004;229(1):12–20.

59. Macklin WB, Weill CL, Deininger PL. Expression of myelin proteolipid and basic protein mRNAs in cultured cells. *J Neurosci Res* 1986;16(1):203–217.

60. Maier M, Berger P, Nave KA, et al. Identification of the regulatory region of the peripheral myelin protein 22 (PMP22) gene that directs temporal and spatial expression in development and regeneration of peripheral nerves. *Mol Cell Neurosci* 2002;20(1):93–109.

61. Martini R. Expression and functional roles of neural cell surface molecules and extracellular matrix components during development and regeneration of peripheral nerves, *J Neurocytol* 1994;23(1):1–28.

62. McPhilemy K, Mitchell LS, Griffiths IR, et al. Effect of optic nerve transection upon myelin protein gene expression by oligodendrocytes: evidence for axonal influences on gene expression, *J Neurocytol* 1990; 19(4):494–503.

63. Messing A, Behringer RR, Hammang JP, et al. P0 promoter directs expression of reporter and toxin genes to Schwann cells of transgenic mice, *Neuron* 1992; 8(3):507–520.

64. Michailov GV, Sereda MW, Brinkmann BG, et al. Axonal neuregulin-1 regulates myelin sheath thickness. *Science* 2004;304(5671):700–703.

65. Milek DJ, Sarvas HO, Greenfield S, et al. An immunological characterization of the basic proteins of rodent sciatic nerve myelin. *Brain Res* 208(2):387–396.

66. Miskimins R, Srinivasan R, Marin-Husstege M, et al. p27(Kip1) enhances myelin basic protein gene promoter activity. *J Neurosci Res* 2002;67(1):100–105.

67. Monuki ES, Kuhn R, Lemke G. Repression of the myelin P0 gene by the POU transcription factor SCIP. *Mech Dev* 1993;42(1-2):15–32.

68. Monuki ES, Kuhn R, Weinmaster G, et al. Expression and activity of the POU transcription factor SCIP. *Science* 1990;249(4974):1300-1303.

69. Monuki ES, Weinmaster G, Kuhn R, et al. SCIP: a glial POU domain gene regulated by cyclic AMP. *Neuron* 1989;3(6):783–793.

70. Notterpek L, Snipes GJ, Shooter EM. Temporal expression pattern of peripheral myelin protein 22 during in vivo and in vitro myelination. *Glia* 1999;25(4): 358–369.

71. Notterpek LM, Rome LH. Functional evidence for the role of axolemma in CNS myelination. *Neuron* 1994;13(2):473–485.

72. Oeltjen JC, Malley TM, Muzny DM, et al. 1997, Large-scale comparative sequence analysis of the human and murine Bruton's tyrosine kinase loci reveals conserved regulatory domains. *Genome Res* 1997;7(4):315–329.

73. Park SK, Miller R, Krane I, et al. The erbB2 gene is required for the development of terminally differentiated spinal cord oligodendrocytes. *J Cell Biol* 2001;154(6):1245–1258.

74. Peirano RI, Wegner M. The glial transcription factor Sox10 binds to DNA both as monomer and dimer with different functional consequences. *Nucleic Acids Res* 2000;28(16):3047–3055.

75. Pennacchio LA, Olivier M, Hubacek JA, et al. An apolipoprotein influencing triglycerides in humans and mice revealed by comparative sequencing. *Science* 2001;294(5540):169–173.

76. Peters A, Josephson K, Vincent SL. Effects of aging on the neuroglial cells and pericytes within area 17 of the rhesus monkey cerebral cortex. *Anat Rec* 1991; 229(3):384–398.

77. Pihlaja H, Rantamaki T, Wikstrom J, et al. Linkage disequilibrium between the MBP tetranucleotide repeat and multiple sclerosis is restricted to a geographically defined subpopulation in Finland. *Genes Immun* 2003;4(2):138–146.

78. Pribyl TM, Campagnoni CW, Kampf K, et al. The human myelin basic protein gene is included within a 179-kilobase transcription unit: expression in the immune and central nervous systems. *Proc Natl Acad Sci U S A* 1993;90(22):10695–10699.

79. Privat A, Jacque C, Bourre JM, et al. Absence of the major dense line in myelin of the mutant mouse "shiverer." *Neurosci Lett* 1979;12(1):107–112.

80. Qian X, Davis AA, Goderie SK, et al. FGF2 concentration regulates the generation of neurons and glia from multipotent cortical stem cells. *Neuron* 1997;18(1): 81–93.

81. Rasband MN, Peles E, Trimmer JS, et al. Dependence of nodal sodium channel clustering on paranodal axoglial contact in the developing CNS. *J Neurosci* 1999; 19(17):7516–7528.

82. Rao M, Sockanathan S. Molecular mechanisms of RNAi: implications for development and disease. *Birth Defects Res C Embryo Today* 2005;75(1): 28–42.

83. Saluja SK, Kohane I. Localization and characterization of mouse-human alignments within the human genome. Does evolutionary conservation suggest functional importance? *AMIA Annu Symp Proc* 2003;994.

84. Sandrock AW, Jr, Dryer SE, Rosen KM, et al. Maintenance of acetylcholine receptor number by neuregulins at the neuromuscular junction in vivo. *Science* 1997;276(5312):599–603.

85. Scherer SS, Vogelbacker HH, Kamholz J. Axons modulate the expression of proteolipid protein in the CNS. *J Neurosci Res* 1992;32(2):138–148.

86. Schwartz S, Zhang Z, Frazer KA, et al. PipMaker–a web server for aligning two genomic DNA sequences. *Genome Res* 2000;10(4):577–586.

87. Shy ME, Shi Y, Wrabetz L, et al. Axon-Schwann cell interactions regulate the expression of c-jun in Schwann cells. *J Neurosci Res* 1996;43(5):511–525.

88. Sim FJ, Hinks GL, Franklin RJ. The re-expression of the homeodomain transcription factor Gtx during remyelination of experimentally induced demyelinating lesions in young and old rat brain. *Neuroscience* 2000;100(1):131–139.

89. Stevens B, Fields RD. Response of Schwann cells to action potentials in development. *Science* 2000; 287(5461):2267–2271.

90. Stevens B, Porta S, Haak LL, et al. Adenosine: a neuron-glial transmitter promoting myelination in the CNS in response to action potentials. *Neuron* 2002;36(5): 855–868.

91. Stolt CC, Rehberg S, Ader M, et al. Terminal differentiation of myelin-forming oligodendrocytes depends on the transcription factor Sox10. *Genes Dev* 2002; 16(2):165–170.

92. Taveggia C, Pizzagalli A, Fagiani E, et al. Characterization of a Schwann cell enhancer in the myelin basic protein gene. *J Neurochem* 2004; 91(4):813–824.

93. Trapp BD, Hauer P, Lemke G. Axonal regulation of myelin protein mRNA levels in actively myelinating Schwann cells. *J Neurosci* 1988;8(9):3515–3521.

94. Tumpel S, Maconochie M, Wiedemann LM, et al. Conservation and diversity in the cis-regulatory networks that integrate information controlling expression of Hoxa2 in hindbrain and cranial neural crest cells in vertebrates. *Dev Biol* 2002;246(1):45–56.

95. Valat J, Privat A, Fulcrand J. Experimental modifications of postnatal differentiation and fate of glial cells related to axo-glial relationships. *Int J Dev Neurosci* 1988;6(3):245–260.

96. Vallstedt A, Klos JM, Ericson, J. Multiple dorsoventral origins of oligodendrocyte generation in the spinal cord and hindbrain. *Neuron* 2005;45(1):55–67.

97. Vartanian T, Fischbach G, Miller R. Failure of spinal cord oligodendrocyte development in mice lacking neuregulin. *Proc Natl Acad Sci U S A* 1999;96(2): 731–735.

98. Vivian JL, Klein WH, Hasty P. Temporal, spatial and tissue-specific expression of a myogenin-lacZ transgene targeted to the Hprt locus in mice. *Biotechniques* 1999;27(1):154–162.

99. Wasserman WW, Palumbo M, Thompson W, et al. Human-mouse genome comparisons to locate regulatory sites. *Nat Genet* 2000;26(2):225–228.

100. Waterston RH, Lindblad-Toh K, Birney E, et al. Initial sequencing and comparative analysis of the mouse genome *Nature* 2002; 420(6915):520–562.

101. Wegner M. Expression of transcription factors during oligodendroglial development. *Microsc Res Tech* 2001;52(6):746–752.

102. Wei Q, Miskimins WK, Miskimins R. The Sp1 family of transcription factors is involved in p27(Kip1)-mediated activation of myelin basic protein gene expression. *Mol Cell Biol* 2003;23(12): 4035–4045.

103. Wei Q, Miskimins WK, Miskimins R. Stage-specific expression of myelin basic protein in oligodendrocytes involves Nkx2.2-mediated repression that is relieved by the Sp1 transcription factor. *J Biol Chem* 2005;280(16): 16284–16294.

104. Werner T. Models for prediction and recognition of eukaryotic promoters, *Mamm Genome* 1999;10(2): 168–175.

105. Wight PA, Duchala CS, Readhead C, et al. A myelin proteolipid protein-LacZ fusion protein is developmentally regulated and targeted to the myelin membrane in transgenic mice. *J Cell Biol* 1993;123(2): 443–454.

106. Wiktorowicz M, Roach A. Regulation of myelin basic protein gene transcription in normal and shiverer mutant mice, *Dev Neurosci* 1991;13(3):143–150.

107. Wingender E, Chen X, Fricke E, et al. The TRANS-FAC system on gene expression regulation. *Nucleic Acids Res* 2001;29(1):281-283.

108. Wolswijk G. Chronic stage multiple sclerosis lesions contain a relatively quiescent population of oligodendrocyte precursor cells. *J Neurosci* 1998a;18(2): 601–609.

109. Wolswijk G. Oligodendrocyte regeneration in the adult rodent CNS and the failure of this process in multiple sclerosis. *Prog Brain Res* 1998b;117:233–247.

110. Wood PM, Bunge RP. Evidence that axons are mitogenic for oligodendrocytes isolated from adult animals. *Nature* 1986;320(6064):756–758.

111. Woodruff RH, Franklin RJ. The expression of myelin protein mRNAs during remyelination of lysolecithin-induced demyelination. *Neuropathol Appl Neurobiol* 1999;25(3):226–235.

112. Wrabetz L, Taveggia C, Feltri ML, et al. A minimal human MBP promoter-lacZ transgene is appropriately regulated in developing brain and after optic enucleation, but not in shiverer mutant mice. *J Neurobiol* 1998;34(1):10–26.

113. Yuh CH, Bolouri H, Davidson EH. Genomic cis-regulatory logic: experimental and computational analysis of a sea urchin gene. *Science* 1998;279(5358): 1896-1902.

114. Yuh CH, Bolouri H, Davidson EH. Cis-regulatory logic in the endo16 gene: switching from a specification to a differentiation mode of control. *Development* 2001;128(5):617–629.

115. Zeller NK, Behar TN, Dubois-Dalcq ME, et al. The timely expression of myelin basic protein gene in cultured rat brain oligodendrocytes is independent of continuous neuronal influences. *J Neurosci* 1985;5(11): 2955–2962.

116. Zhang SC, Ge B, Duncan ID. Adult brain retains the potential to generate oligodendroglial progenitors with extensive myelination capacity. *Proc Natl Acad Sci USA* 1999;96(7):4089–4094.

6

Animal Models for Multiple Sclerosis

Trevor Owens

Department of Immunology, Montreal Neurological Institute, Montreal, Quebec, Canada

---

"The problem in MS is to understand the Disease itself,"
(*with apologies to Wilder Penfield, whose original quote I have modified*).

In seeking to understand the complexity of human disease, we are often frustrated by our inability to get inside the problem, to take it apart. For this reason we look to models of disease, which do allow such intervention. The history of using animals as models for human disease goes back to antiquity, although the necromancers and priests who pronounced on the basis of internal organ pathology in sacrificial animals may not have realized that this was what they were doing. Probably nowhere in modern clinical biology has the use of animal models had as much impact as in the study of autoimmune disease. The tissue-infiltrating pathology resulting from immune attack on self organs and tissues is remarkable for the simple message it conveys, and yet the very fact of autoimmune tissue destruction, coupled with the lengthy progression of most such diseases, severely limits our access to the disease as it initiates and establishes. We therefore turn to animal models.

Multiple sclerosis (MS) is among the more difficult of the organ-specific autoimmune diseases to model. Autopsy material is limited and usually represents long-established disease. Biopsy and autopsy examinations indicate that an autoimmune process had taken place but, since the disease process is located in the central nervous system (CNS), it is difficult to obtain or analyze biopsies or draining fluids that allow detailed monitoring of disease progression. It was relatively recently that imaging of live patients became possible and gave us new insights into previously inaccessible stages of disease. The purpose of this chapter is to review the animal models currently used in MS research, and to address the question of not whether they are "good" models for MS, but whether the tail has come to wag the dog—have animal models been overinterpreted in what they tell us about the disease, to the extent that we neglect what the disease itself tells us?

MS IS A DISEASE OF HETEROGENEOUS PATHOLOGY

First, we need to understand what it is we seek to model. MS is didactically taught to be an inflammatory demyelinating disease of probable autoimmune etiology. This description is usually inadequate and does not always hold up well to close examination. For many years, the most commonly used slides in introductions to lectures on MS have been drawings depicting multiple progressions. Most of them are variants on the theme of immune cell entry to the CNS preceding and roughly correlating with disease. In particular, most progressions include some degree of remission followed by relapse, with a satisfying correlation to waves of immune cell entry. (In the strictest sense, immune cell entry is not routinely shown for MS, but is inferred from magnetic resonance (MR) imaging. However, this is likely to be a reasonable inference, even though we await precise dissection of the cellular and molecular events that account for a gadolinium-enhancing MR lesion.) Many, if not most, patients show a general pattern of a relatively benign disease that shows occasional episodes or attacks, which increase in frequency and severity over an indefinite period of time [relapsing-remitting MS (RRMS)], and then progress to a disease where remission does not restore full functionality, with a progression to a more constant state of disability [secondary-progressive MS (SPMS)] (1,2). Described in this way, one gets the impression of a single disease that evolves in severity over time.

However, not all MS follows this pattern. For instance, primary progressive MS shows an inversion of the "usual" bias toward women and girls; shows considerably less axonal damage than SPMS (3); and doesn't fit the pattern of one stage of disease evolving into another (e.g., as RRMS does in its advance to SPMS disease (2). Primary progressive multiple sclerosis (PPMS) can therefore appear unrelated in its development to the other progressions. Other rapidly-progressing variants include acute or Marburg's MS, neuromyelitis optica (Devic's disease), and Balo's concentric sclerosis, and there are other rare but well-described, rapidly-progressing pathologies. Diagnoses of MS can also be extended to include disease patterns that are benign or even monoepisodic (2,4).

More recently, analyses of biopsy and autopsy material, principally by one multicenter collaborative group, have revealed heterogeneity of pathology underlying clinical MS (see Chapter 3 by Morales et al.). These analyses should be considered to be ongoing, but publications to date suggest there to be four distinct pathologies (5). The most common are two conventional immune-inflammatory pathologies, showing focal, perivascular lesions of T-cells + macrophages (Type I) and antibody + complement (Type II) associated to demyelination and axonal damage in white matter. Less common but convincingly established are pathologies reminiscent of viral- or toxin-induced damage, or those associated with ischemia, with diffuse white matter involvement (Type III), and what appears as a primary oligodendrocyte dystrophy (Type IV) (5,6). It remains contentious whether these pathologies can occur together in the same patient, and this will be resolved with further analyses (7,8). However, these studies have opened our eyes to the heterogeneity of pathology in MS. Furthermore, other work has shown that pathology in some forms of MS extends beyond the classical demyelinated plaque in white matter. The latter would seem to be a feature of acute and RRMS. By contrast, in chronic disease, cortical involvement becomes more evident, with widespread microglial activation and diffuse myelin and axonal loss (9,10). Cases of acute MS often do not show intrathecal immunoglobulin synthesis or oligoclonal immunoglobulin bands in cerebrospinal fluid (CSF), both of which are considered characteristic of MS and, indeed, formed the basis for diagnosis prior to the introduction of MRI. In many cases of SPMS, there is less evidence for immune involvement than in other forms of MS (e.g., reduced T-lymphocyte infiltration), although activated macrophages/microglia continue to feature (2).

INFLAMMATORY DEMYELINATION AS A TARGET FOR ANIMAL MODELS

MS is therefore not a monolithic disease. The challenge then is to decide which aspects best deserve to be featured in an animal model, which could then be studied to better understand the human disease, with the qualification that one should aim to keep the number of models as low as possible and not devise an animal model for each individual patient. A balance needs to be struck between narrow definitions for MS, making it easier to model, versus using a broad definition, so as to include as many of the sub-pathologies described above as possible. One aspect that is fairly consistent to most of the variants of MS is immune inflammation with demyelination, and almost all animal models involve inflammatory demyelination as a first requirement.

It is noteworthy that the three most common inflammatory diseases of the CNS, with varying degrees of demyelination and axonal damage, are MS, viral infection, and acute disseminated encephalomyelitis (ADEM). Etiological links between these diseases are suspected. There is much anecdotal and pathological evidence that viral infection acts as a trigger for MS, and ADEM often occurs as a postviral or postvaccination encephalomyelitis (11). It is perhaps not surprising, therefore, that the two most commonly studied genres of animal models for MS are infection with a neurotropic virus, and a broad spectrum of autoimmune diseases grouped together as experimental autoimmune encephalomyelitis (EAE). EAE is an autoimmune inflammatory demyelinating disease that was established by Thomas Rivers in 1933 as a model for ADEM (11a). Generically, though varying by strain and protocol, EAE and neurotropic viral models show inflammation, demyelination, and axonal damage (12–14). Use of such models has contributed to our understanding of MS, but may also have biased it.

INNATE IMMUNITY

To model inflammatory disease requires immune stimulation. Innate immunity is fundamental to initiation of immune responses. The term "innate immunity" refers to a broad array of preprogrammed responses to infection or ligands specific to infectious agents. An evolutionarily ancient recognition and signaling system forms the basis for pathogen recognition by innate components. The Toll-like receptors (TLRs), of which eleven have so far been described, are so-called because of their homology to Toll receptors, themselves first described as playing a role in development of the nervous system in Drosophila (15). TLRs specifically bind ligands that are uniquely expressed by microbes, fungi, and viruses. These pathogen-derived epitopes are termed pathogen-associated molecular patterns (PAMPs) (15). TLR signaling induces cytokine production, notably the Type I interferons, which are associated with early cellular responses to viral infection, and chemokines, which can induce leukocyte entry to the CNS (16,17). TLR-induced cytokines pave the way for the adaptive or antigen-specific lymphocyte response, and direct the quality of those responses. Thus, TLR-expressing cells in mucosae, epithelia, and endothelia are both located and equipped appropriately to serve as a frontline defense against pathogens. TLR-expressing cells are also found in the CNS and have been shown to mount early responses to PAMPs (18).

ADJUVANTS AND ADJUVANT EFFECTS

Initiation of T-cell immune responses, and thus of adaptive immune responses generally, is dependent on adequate provision of co-stimulatory signals. These are provided through ligation of signaling receptors on T-cells by co-stimulator ligands expressed on antigen-presenting cells (APC) (19). Expression of sufficient levels of co-stimulator ligands by APC is induced through TLR signals, as well as by other signals that include cytokines, many of which themselves are TLR-inducible (15). This is the immunological basis for use of adjuvants. Administration of a potential antigen with adjuvant facilitates its recognition in the context of a co-stimulator-adequate environment, and so ensures an immune response. It is important to recognize that adjuvants are essential for experimental initiation of immune responses, unless the immunogen is itself a TLR ligand (e.g., bacteria, viruses). Given that the quality of the immune response that is induced is influenced by the nature of the TLR ligand (20), then it becomes clear that an experimenter's choice of adjuvants directs the nature of the immune response. However, it is equally important to recognize that an experimenter's choices may themselves be limited by what works. This returns discussion to the issue of what aspect of MS one should wish to model. The focus on inflammatory pathology, coupled with the need for aggressive immunization in order to overcome self-tolerance, has driven rodent models toward use of complete Freund's adjuvant (CFA). The active ingredient in this oil-based emulsion is heat-killed *M. tuberculosis*. The debate as to how appropriate the delayed-type hypersensitivity (DTH) reaction that this provokes is to understanding MS continues to be unresolved (21).

Pertussis toxin (PT), or heat-killed *Bordetella pertussis*, is frequently used as a co-adjuvant, more so since the move toward gene-deficient "knockout" mice in EAE studies. The great majority of ESC lines used for the in vitro first step of homologous recombination in generation of a gene knockout are from mice of the 129/J background. Almost all knockouts are therefore initially 129/J, and are most frequently back-crossed to C57Bl/6 (22). Mice on the C57Bl/6 genetic background are relatively resistant to induction of EAE (23), and induction of EAE in C57Bl/6 mice almost always requires use of PT as well as CFA. This has become a popular model since the advent of gene-deficient mice.

Adjuvant remains a necessity for generation of a sufficiently potent T-cell response to produce CNS inflammation. It should be noted that neurotropic viruses serve as their own adjuvant, and similarities between the inflammatory response to virus and that in EAE are taken as support for physiological relevance of the adjuvant-induced EAE model. One might query the relevance of virus infection to MS in the first place, and this should always be kept in mind, although most commentators would agree that it is not unreasonable.

INFLAMMATORY VERSUS ANTIBODY-INDUCING IMMUNE RESPONSES

Adaptive immune responses are founded on activation of CD4+ T-lymphocytes. The CD4+ T-cell response can be very broadly categorized on the basis of cytokine production. The Th1 versus Th2 dichotomy is one of the enduring paradigms of modern immunology (24,25). Inflammatory CD4+ T-cells secrete Th1 cytokines, classically defined by interferon gamma (IFNγ) and tumor necrosis factor alpha (TNFα). Probably equally importantly, Th1 T-cells express profiles of adhesion ligands and chemokine receptors that direct migration to tissues (25), and together with their cytokine profile, this is likely why Th1 T-cells were originally defined as those that induced DTH responses (26). Both CFA and the commonly used neurotropic viruses such as Theiler's murine encephalitic virus (TMEV) bias the immune response toward a Th1 profile. With the exception of experimentally immunosuppressed or immunomodulated animals, Th2 responses (that lack IFNγ and TNFα, are dominated by interleukins 4, 5, and 10, and are associated with antibody responses) fail to induce MS-like disease in mice (27,28). It would be unwise to extrapolate from this information alone to suggest that MS is a Th1 disease (29). The fact that myelin-specific Th2 cells can induce CNS inflammation in mice that lack appropriate immunoregulatory systems (28) leaves open the possibility that MS may have a basis in immunoregulation deficiency, as has long been proposed (30). Antibodies most likely play a role in MS, whether or not a Th2 response would be required for them to be produced (2,31). Recent reports suggest that antibodies may influence the quality of disease in MS, rather than play an initiating role; this is broadly consistent with experimental demonstrations of synergy between antibodies against myelin oligodendrocyte glycoprotein (MOG) and myelin basic protein (MBP)-specific T-cells for induction of demyelinating EAE in rats (32–34). It is often overlooked that the CFA-based immunizations that are used to induce EAE can themselves induce antibody responses. Whether such antimyelin antibodies play a necessary role in EAE has been a contentious issue; most recent studies suggest that the nature of the myelin protein (peptide versus polypeptide, autologous versus xenogeneic) may influence their requirement (35,36).

CD4 VERSUS CD8 T-CELLS

Whereas the predominant infiltrating T-cell in most EAE models is the CD4[+] T-cell, there is evidence from MS that CD8[+] T-cells may play a greater role in human disease (37), and are particularly implicated as cytotoxic effectors. Earlier studies suggested that CD8[+] T-cells were either not necessary for or played an immunoregulatory role in EAE (38,39), whereas three recent papers show the ability of CD8[+] T-cells to induce EAE (40–41a). These represent a minority view to date, so that the CD4 versus CD8 dichotomy stands as one more discrepancy between MS and EAE. In this regard, viral models such as TMEV encephalomyelitis may be more faithful models of MS inflammation.

CHOICE OF SPECIES

The previous analysis develops the theme that in designing animal models for a disease with heterogeneous pathology, one must choose which aspect to model, and be aware that experimental variables such as adjuvants may constrain immunological models in ways that need careful consideration. A third consideration is whether the choice of animal species influences the behavior of the model.

The most commonly studied experimental animals are rodents, principally mice and rats. These two species have, by and large, supplanted guinea pigs, hamsters, rabbits, and other species that were once more commonly studied. There has recently been increased use of primates, which closes the circle from the early days when ADEM was first modeled in monkeys [see (42) for review]. Primates offer a number of advantages as models for MS, including the fact that primate colonies are outbred (like humans); their high degree of TCR and MHC homology allows prediction of peptide specificities; and the route to clinical application is shorter than from rodents. The primate model of MOGp14–36-induced EAE in the common marmoset *(Callithrix jacchus)* seems likely to supplant other primate models, such as Cynomolgus *(Macaca fascicularis)* and rhesus monkeys *(M. mulatta)*. The marmoset model shows 100% prevalence in a small animal that is nevertheless MR-imageable. It has a relapsing-remitting or primary-progressive clinical course; MS-like pathology including axonal pathology; evidence for B-cell/antibody involvement; and the possibility of adoptive transfer between chimeric twins. There is limited major histocompatibility complex (MHC) II polymorphism of DR- and DQ-equivalent regions and disease can also be induced by MBP or proteolipid protein (PLP). This EAE model is increasingly used in testing therapeutics (42a). That mouse models have come to dominate the MS field has much to do with the expense of working with primates, as well as the fact that mouse genetics outstripped any other species. The mouse is now the favorite species for generation of transgenic and gene-deficient animals, which have been critical for understanding the role of specific genes in many studies. Nevertheless, the current concentration of systems and questions through one species must be kept in mind when evaluating the information that comes from animal studies. Two specific instances where the variables discussed herein have influenced interpretation of animal studies for MS are studies on the role of IFNγ and of TNFα in EAE (discussed below). The strain of animal is also a significant influence. Depending on the strain of rat, EAE may be demyelinating or nondemyelinating, monophasic, or relapsing-remitting (23,32). Similarly, the same encephalitogenic peptide can induce either an RRMS-like or a PPMS-like EAE, depending on the strain of mouse and the choice of adjuvant (43).

TABLE 6-1 *Use of selected species of animal in studies of EAE since 1950*

Decade	Mouse	Rat	Rabbit	Guinea pig	Monkey
1950–1960	0	0	0	0	0
1960–1970	0	4	1	3	0
1970–1980	30	111	27	140	10
1980–1990	174	416	50	320	21
1990–2000	775	727	52	234	32
2000–	517 (1477)	274 (782)	24 (69)	54 (154)	38 (109)

Data are numbers of listings found in PubMed searching for Species (as per column headings) and EAE. Numbers in parentheses for 2000–2004 are projections for a 10-year period based on the approximately 3½ years already listed.

Since the first appearance of the term EAE in the PubMed service of the National Library of Medicine in 1962 (44), publications involving rat and guinea pig were neck-and-neck until the 1990s, when the mouse caught up and the guinea pig fell behind in popularity. In the first three and one-half years of this decade, publications identified using the search words "mouse + EAE" already outnumber all other "species + EAE" listings (Table 6-1, Fig. 6-1). It should also be noted that there was a three-fold decade-to-decade jump in "monkey + EAE" listings from the 1990s to this decade (projected), which points toward increased use of primates in the future.

THE INTERFERON-γ CONTROVERSY

Effects of IFNγ

As discussed above, IFNγ is the paradigmatic Th1 cytokine. This proinflammatory cytokine induces MHC, adhesion ligand, and co-stimulator ligand expression, as well as inducing expression of other cytokines such as TNFα. Levels of IFNγ protein and ribonucleic acid (RNA) were shown to increase in the target tissue of many autoimmune diseases, and in the CNS in MS and EAE (45). These levels correlated to severity of disease and fell in remission. It was logical to expect a causative

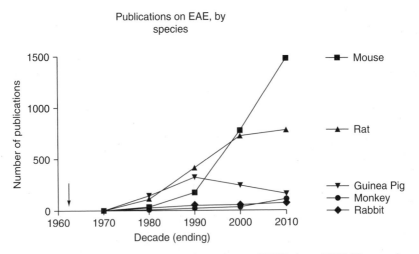

FIG. 6-1. Publications involving selected animal species and EAE since 1950. The number of listings in PubMed (*http://www.ncbi.nlm.nih.gov/entrez/query.fcgi?db=PubMed*) under "Species name" + "EAE" was obtained using decades (e.g., 1950–1960) as Limits. Numbers are plotted against the decade for the species shown. The arrow shows the date (1962) of the earliest listing identified using "EAE" as a search term.

relationship between IFNγ and CNS inflammatory disease. And, because IFNs are by definition antiviral mediators, and there was presumed to be a link between viral infection and MS, IFNγ was given by intravenous injection to RRMS patients with the expectation that the viral cause of disease would be targeted with benefit for the patients. Strikingly, there was an increase in the attack rate during the one month of weekly administration and the study was stopped for safety reasons (46). Notwithstanding some perceived deficiencies in study design [see commentary by Willenborg in same issue as (47)], it was evident that IFNγ promoted or exacerbated MS. A more recent study has involved administration of antibodies against the IFNγ-receptor to patients with SPMS. There was improvement in their progression, again consistent with a disease-exacerbating role for IFNγ in MS (48).

EFFECTS OF IFNγ IN EAE

Completely unexpectedly, analogous interventions in EAE models have had exactly opposite effects [see (45) for review of specific reports]. Some of these interventions have been more invasive than would be possible in clinical studies, involving use of viral vectors (49) or direct injection of antibodies to the CNS. It remains the case that the exact experimental design used in the MS study has never been replicated in animals, but the overall finding is that opposite results were obtained in MS and EAE. In MS, IFNγ makes the disease worse, whereas in EAE, IFNγ made the disease better or prevented its onset. The question arises whether the EAE model is the wrong one to use for MS, whether there are fundamental differences between animals and humans regarding the role of IFNγ, or something else.

CD8⁺ T-CELLS AND IFNγ

As to what that "something else" might be, three groups reported that EAE can be induced by CD8⁺ T-cells (40–41a). In one of those studies, anti-IFNγ antibodies prevented disease (41). This represents possibly the only instance

where IFNγ blockade has inhibited EAE, and so generated considerable interest (50). The suggestion was made that the discrepancy between EAE and MS regarding the effects of IFNγ blockade might reflect an artefactual predominance of CD4⁺ T-cells in EAE. However, as attractive as that seems, induction of EAE with CD8⁺ T-cells has not been repeated since the first publication and these two papers remain the only descriptions of CD8-induced EAE. An alternative perspective is offered by the demyelinating disease that occurs in mice overexpressing the co-stimulator ligand B7.2/CD86 on microglia. This disease is also mediated by CD8⁺ T-cells, which produce IFNγ, and its representation of an adjuvant-independent encephalomyelitis has been suggested as preferable to EAE as an animal model of inflammatory events in MS (51). It is not yet known whether IFNγ blockade inhibits this disease.

EFFECTS OF IFNγ IN VIRAL ENCEPHALOMYELITIS

One way to address these questions is to ask whether IFNγ plays analogous roles in viral inflammation in the CNS. The immune response to TMEV infection and subsequent demyelinating disease includes both CD4⁺ and CD8⁺ T-cells, and so offers an alternative system for evaluation of the role of IFNγ. The cytotoxic and humoral immune response to viral infection in the CNS is generally independent of IFNγ (52,53), though reduced expression of immune markers was noted in the CNS of IFNγ-deficient, TMEV-infected mice of susceptible background (14). Disease onset was accelerated by intracerebral administration of IFNγ (52). Motor dysfunction correlates to axonal damage (54), and both viral persistence and neuronal damage were increased by IFNγ blockade or deficiency (14,53). Interestingly, the demyelination that normally accompanies TMEV infection was not inhibited by IFNγ blockade or deficiency (14,53), which would indicate consistency between viral and autoimmune animal models. In IFNγ-deficient mice, demyelination was more severe, and IFNγ deficiency or blockade both overcame strain-dependent resistance to TMEV demyelination (14,53). In mice normally susceptible to TMEV encephalomyelitis, neuronal damage was exacerbated (14,53).

Such observations make an additional point, which is that intrastrain variation within a species can have effects as dramatic as intraspecies differences, in some cases. This is an important point to consider in interpreting findings (e.g., from EAE studies where, depending on the mouse strain, effects of a similar immunization may have very different results, ranging from no demyelination to severe loss of myelin).

EFFECTS OF TRANSGENIC OR "HYPODERMIC" IFNγ EXPRESSION IN CNS

Another approach to dissecting this controversy is to consider results from transgenic mice. All but one of the transgenic mice in which IFNγ is overexpressed in the CNS have used oligodendrocyte (OLG)-specific promoters, and all show proinflammatory effects, ranging from spontaneous demyelination and inflammation to a more severe disease when EAE was induced with myelin protein and adjuvant immunization (45,55,56). The effects of IFNγ seen in transgenic models thus differ from those observed following IFNγ or IFNγR blockade, or genetic deficiency of IFNγ. Interestingly, direct injection of IFNγ to the CNS (hypodermic administration) induced inflammation in rats (57,58) (so far this has not been reported in mice), so direct injection and transgenesis generate similar findings. One distinction between these experiments and those in which IFNγ played an immunoregulatory role is the absence of adjuvant in transgenic or hypodermic IFNγ models. Although this is an attractive target for criticism, it is not as clear-cut as might first appear. For instance, transgenic mice that expressed IFNγ in OLG showed greater severity of EAE induced by myelin basic protein with CFA (55).

All of these findings, from an ever-growing number of studies, provide plenty of material for discussion and debate. What can be distilled from them, however, is that both transgenic and

hypodermic administration of IFNγ to rodent CNS achieve effects consistent with those of two studies in which IFNγ was targeted in MS; IFNγ was revealed to be proinflammatory. By contrast, animal experiments in which IFNγ was targeted or administered during EAE showed an opposite, protective effect. IFNγ also showed a protective effect against virus infection and CNS damage in Theiler's virus encephalomyelitis (TMEV) (14,52). Two points deserve emphasis: the world of animal models is no more monolithic than MS, and the immunoregulatory effects of IFNγ on CNS inflammation have so far only been demonstrated in animals. So, depending on where one looks within the world of animal models for MS, one can find results that match or contradict the MS experience. The inflammatory role of IFNγ can indeed be modeled in rodents. Whether EAE is a good model for MS is, therefore, not the right question. The question should be whether one can obtain answers about specific questions regarding particular aspects of MS, by study of particular forms of EAE.

IS ADJUVANT A PROBLEM?

Finally, it remains true that effects of IFNγ differ in EAE versus MS. Despite imperfect correspondence, there do seem to be grounds for suspicion that adjuvant (or TLR signaling, as in the case of viral infection) may be a critical distinction between the MS-like and MS-unlike systems. This is reinforced by observation that immunosuppression in bacille Calmette-Guérin (BCG, *M. tuberculosis*)-infected mice was overcome in the absence of IFNγ (59), with attendant findings from the same and other groups showing an IFNγ-dependent nitric oxide (NO)–mediated T-cell suppressive mechanism (60,61). This kind of observation has tended to be made in CFA- or pathogen-involving experimental systems. At the same time, disease-ameliorating IFNγ was delivered to mice by a herpesvirus vector (49), and IFNγ deficiency revealed a protective role for this cytokine against TMEV encephalomyelitis in mice (14). Both viruses would be expected to act as TLR ligands. If there turns out to be a specific effect of bacterial PAMPs (e.g., from *M. tuberculosis*) in directing a protective role for IFNγ, then incidental infections might influence the course of MS. This suggests an interesting, though speculative, explanation for some reports of disparate pathologies of MS, and effects of antibiotics in some studies (62).

CHEMICAL VERSUS INFLAMMATORY ATTACK

Demyelinating pathology can also be obtained in animals through the use of myelin-specific toxins. The most commonly used toxins are the copper chelator cuprizone (63,64), the chromatin-disrupting agent ethidium bromide (EtBr) (65,66), and the lipid toxin lysolecithin/lysophosphatidylcholine (LPC) (67). These have been used to model aspects of demyelinating pathology, their advantage being that either local administration or intrinsic characteristics allow prediction of site of effect, unlike in EAE where lesion occurrence is always uncertain. Cuprizone and EtBr have been exploited for study of remyelination, and such studies have contributed to our understanding of oligodendrocyte precursor cells and their dynamics (64,66). It might be argued that toxin-induced demyelination is not a faithful model for MS; however, such models are not used with any expectation that these toxins cause disease, but, rather, to understand mechanism. In this way they contribute to our general understanding of demyelination and remyelination. There is a downstream, inflammatory component to toxin-induced demyelination, and study of cellular and cytokine/chemokine responses has contributed to better understanding of injury-reactive inflammation in the CNS, such as may indeed occur in MS (68,69). An analogous approach has been to transgenically promote demyelination through overexpression of the DM-20 myelin proteolipid (70). This generated a mouse (the ND4 transgenic) that myelinates normally but then develops spontaneous demyelination with attendant immune sequelae as it ages (71). This would seem to offer a useful model for Type IV MS pathology, as defined by Lucchinetti and colleagues (5).

HUMAN VERSUS MOUSE: SAME PRINCIPLES, DIFFERENT PLAYERS?

In general, one can learn from parallel situations in which the players differ but the principles are the same. Thus, if it should turn out that IFNγ-induced, NO-mediated immunoregulation is not a prominent feature of immunoregulation in humans, then one can expect that another cytokine-driven system will operate in its place. Whether human macrophages/microglia are an equivalent source of NO as their murine counterparts may be one critical species-specific difference (72). Reports of elevated iNOS expression and NO levels in MS tissue are interpreted as showing cytopathic effect for NO (73), but it should be kept in mind that exactly similar correlations were reported in EAE. It took a series of contradictory inhibitor studies, as well as unexpected findings for iNOS-deficient mice, to shift our thinking toward the possibility of a neuroprotective role for NO (72). There is some interest in IL-17 as a potential alternative inflammatory cytokine to IFNγ in promoting inflammatory responses in mice (74), and the parallels may become more obvious when this route is followed. We are already familiar with other species-specific differences, such as that there is no IL-8 in mice, and the preferential role of GM-CSF over IL-3 in hematopoietic stem cell growth in humans. Thus, we should not necessarily expect exact transspecies homology in mechanism of effect but, rather, look for the operation of analogous regulatory systems.

PERIPHERAL VERSUS CNS EFFECTS OF INTERVENTIONS

When working with animal models, it is possible to directly assess whether a reagent accesses the CNS. By contrast, in MS this is not possible, and very often the only thing one knows with certainty is that the drug or reagent accesses the periphery. The increased attack rate in the intravenous IFNγ study was suggested to reflect intra-CNS action of IFNγ, because of the likelihood of blood–brain barrier in these patients (46). However, it is equally possible that the cytokine, and the antireceptor antibody in a later study, acted purely on the peripheral immune response. Administration of IFNγ to mice or rats via viral infection of ependymal cells (49), or of cytokine or antibodies via the hypodermic route (57,58,75), places IFNγ or antibodies directly in the CNS, and it is possible that discrepant results between animals and MS patients reflect that difference in locale of action. This consideration may also help explain the discrepancy between effects of TNFα-targeting reagents in EAE versus in MS (76). Anti-TNFα antibodies inhibited EAE but drugs based on analogous principles did not improve MS. It would be important to know whether there was differential access to the CNS in MS patients versus in animals. The fact that some patients showed worsening of symptoms probably reflects differential effects of TNFα acting through either of the two receptors for this cytokine, one of which signals for oligodendrocyte precursor cell survival (77). Interestingly, the same drugs are effective against rheumatoid arthritis, but some patients showed evidence of neurological problems (78). It would be difficult to explain how this might occur if the anti-TNFα drugs did not access the CNS, although these are questions without answers for the moment.

CONCLUSIONS

Just as there is no one pathology that defines MS, there is no one animal model for MS. Choice of animal species is likely to be an overriding consideration and it may be useful to maintain studies of less-popular models to keep a broad perspective. The most commonly used animal model EAE shows some discrepancies in immune regulation and CNS pathology from MS, but remains a useful model for autoimmune inflammation (Table 6-2). Viral encephalomyelitis models show some of the same immunoregulatory distinctions as EAE, proba-

TABLE 6-2 *Comparison between MS and animal models*

MS disease characteristic	Whether faithfully modeled in:		
	EAE	TMEV	Transgenic or toxin models
Female:male ratio > 1 (except PPMS)	v	v	v B7.2/CD86 (51) X Toxins, not known for ND4 (70,71)
Demyelination	Varies with species/strain [see (22)]	v	v B7.2/CD86 (51) v ND4 (71) v Toxins
Macrophage infiltration	v	v	v B7.2/CD86 (51) v ND4 (71) v Toxins
Role for CD4 T-cells	v	v	X B7.2/CD86 (51) v ND4 (71) vLPC (68), X Cup, EtBr
Role for CD8 T-cells	v(2 reports)	v	v B7.2/CD86 (51) X Toxins, ND4 (71)
Relapsing/remitting progression	v	X	X B7.2/CD86 (51) X Toxins, ND4 (71)
Axonal damage	v (eg.(12))	v	v B7.2/CD86 (51) Not known for toxins, ND4
Oligodendrocyte-based dysmyelinating pathology	X	X	v ND4 (71) X B7.2/CD86 (51), toxins
Exacerbated by IFNγ	X (one report (41))	X	v MBP/IFNγ (55) Not known for toxins, ND4, B7.2/CD86

Note: This table has been assembled to highlight a range of characteristics of MS and how they are variously but not universally modeled by experimental and transgenic animal systems. Correspondence is indicated by a tick (v), lack of correspondence by an X. LPC, lysophosphatidylcholine/lysolecithin; Cup, cuprizone; EtBr, ethidium bromide.

bly because of being focused on mice. Transgenic models allow study to specific aspects of disease and its induction, although they are inevitably mouse models. Toxin-induced demyelination has been very useful for examination of regenerative processes, with the obvious caveat that there is little evidence for a role for toxins in MS. Finally, one has to choose whatever model works best for the question one wishes to address. The biggest risk is to overinterpret results from any one model as being representative of what is a globally heterogeneous disease.

ACKNOWLEDGMENTS

I thank the members of my lab for their continued inspiration, and the Canadian Institutes of Health Research, the Multiple Sclerosis Society of Canada, the National MS Society and the Wadsworth Foundation for their support for my research.

REFERENCES

1. Antel JP, Owens T. Immune regulation and CNS autoimmune disease. *J Neuroimmunol* 1999;100: 181–189.
2. Compston A, Coles A. Multiple sclerosis. *Lancet* 2002;359:1221–1231.
3. Bruck W, Lucchinetti C, Lassmann H. The pathology of primary progressive multiple sclerosis. *Mult Scler* 2002;8:93–97.
4. Lassmann H, Bruck W, Lucchinetti C. Heterogeneity of multiple sclerosis pathogenesis: implications for diagnosis and therapy. *Trends Mol Med* 2001;7:115–121.
5. Lucchinetti C, Bruck W, Parisi J, et al. Heterogeneity of multiple sclerosis lesions: implications for the pathogenesis of demyelination. *Ann Neurol* 2000;47: 707–717.
6. Barnett MH, Prineas JW. Relapsing and remitting multiple sclerosis: pathology of the newly forming lesion. *Ann Neurol* 2004;55:458–468.
7. Ludwin SK. The neuropathology of multiple sclerosis. *Neuroimaging Clin North Am* 2000;10:625–648 ,vii.
8. Trapp BD. Pathogenesis of multiple sclerosis: the eyes only see what the mind is prepared to comprehend. *Ann Neurol* 2004;55:455–457.
9. Kuhlmann T, Lingfeld G, Bitsch A, et al. Acute axonal damage in multiple sclerosis is most extensive in early disease stages and decreases over time. *Brain* 2002;125:2202–2212.
10. Bitsch A, Schuchardt J, Bunkowski S, et al. Acute axonal injury in multiple sclerosis: correlation with demyelination and inflammation. *Brain* 2000;123: 1174–1183.
11. Owens T. Overview of Immunology and Autoimmunity: EAE and ADEM. In: Ransohoff RM, ed. CONTINUUM Course on Neuroimmunology. St. Paul, MN: American Academy of Neurology; 2001.
11a.Available at www.nationalmssociety.org/Brochures-HistoryofMS1.asp.
12. Pitt D, Werner P, Raine CS. Glutamate excitotoxicity in a model of multiple sclerosis. *Nat Med* 2000;6:67–70.
13. Smith T, Groom A, Zhu B, et al. Autoimmune encephalomyelitis ameliorated by AMPA antagonists. *Nat Med* 2000;6:62–66.
14. Rodriguez M, Zoecklein LJ, Howe CL, et al. Gamma interferon is critical for neuronal viral clearance and protection in a susceptible mouse strain following early intracranial Theiler's murine encephalomyelitis virus infection. *J Virol* 2003;77:12252–12265.
15. Medzhitov R. Toll-like receptors and innate immunity. *Nat Rev Immunol* 2001;1:135–145.
16. Hertzog PJ, O'Neill LA, Hamilton JA. The interferon in TLR signaling: more than just antiviral. *Trends Immunol* 2003;24:534–539.
17. Yeh WC, Chen NJ. Immunology: another toll road. *Nature* 2003;424:736–737.
18. Rivest S, Lacroix S, Vallieres L, et al. How the blood talks to the brain parenchyma and the paraventricular nucleus of the hypothalamus during systemic inflammatory and infectious stimuli. *Proc Soc Exp Biol Med* 2000;223:22–38.
19. Chambers CA. The expanding world of co-stimulation: the two-signal model revisited. *Trends Immunol* 2001;22:217–223.
20. Jones BW, Means TK, Heldwein KA, et al. Different toll-like receptor agonists induce distinct macrophage responses. *J Leukoc Biol* 2001;69:1036–1044.
21. Matthys P, Vermeire K, Billiau A. Mac-1(+) myelopoiesis induced by CFA: a clue to the paradoxical effects of IFN-gamma in autoimmune disease models. *Trends Immunol* 2001;22:367–371.
22. Campbell IL, Owens T. Animal Models of Neurologic Disease. In: Antel J, Vincent A, Hartung H, eds. *Clinical Neuroimmunology*, 2nd ed. Malden, MA: Blackwell Science; 2004. In press.
23. Owens T, Sriram S. The immunology of multiple sclerosis and its animal model, experimental allergic encephalomyelitis. *Neurol Clin* 1995;13:51–73.
24. Mosmann TR, Coffman RL. TH1 and TH2 cells: different patterns of lymphokine secretion lead to different functional properties. *Annu Rev Immunol* 1989;7: 145–173.
25. Janeway C, Travers P, Walport M, Capra J. *Immunobiology: The Immune System in Health and Disease*. New York: Garland, 1999.
26. Mosmann TR, Cherwinski H, Bond MW, et al. Two types of murine helper T-cell clone. I. Definition according to profiles of lymphokine activities and secreted proteins. *J Immunol* 1986;136:2348–2357.
27. Martin R, McFarland HF, McFarlin DE. Immunological aspects of demyelinating diseases. *Annu Rev Immunol* 1992;10:153–187.
28. Lafaille JJ, Keere FV, Hsu AL, et al. Myelin basic protein-specific T helper 2 (Th2) cells cause experimental autoimmune encephalomyelitis in immunodeficient hosts rather than protect them from the disease. *J Exp Med* 1997;186:307–312.
29. Lassmann H, Ransohoff RM. The CD4-Th1 model for multiple sclerosis: a crucial reappraisal. *Trends Immunol* 2004;25:132–137.

30. Antel JP, Arnason BG, Medof ME. Suppressor cell function in multiple sclerosis: correlation with clinical disease activity. *Ann Neurol* 1979;5:338–342.

31. Genain CP, Cannella B, Hauser SL, et al. Identification of autoantibodies associated with myelin damage in multiple sclerosis. *Nat Med* 1999;5:170–175.

32. Linington C, Engelhardt B, Kapocs G, et al. Induction of persistently demyelinated lesions in the rat following the repeated adoptive transfer of encephalitogenic T-cells and demyelinating antibody. *J Neuroimmunol* 1992;40:219–224.

33. Berger T, Rubner P, Schautzer F, et al. Antimyelin antibodies as a predictor of clinically definite multiple sclerosis after a first demyelinating event. *N Engl J Med* 2003;349:139–145.

34. Antel JP, Bar-Or A. Do myelin-directed antibodies predict multiple sclerosis? *N Engl J Med* 2003;349: 107–109.

35. Lyons JA, Ramsbottom MJ, Cross AH. Critical role of antigen-specific antibody in experimental autoimmune encephalomyelitis induced by recombinant myelin oligodendrocyte glycoprotein. *Eur J Immunol* 2002;32:1905–1913.

36. Oliver AR, Lyon GM, Ruddle NH. Rat and human myelin oligodendrocyte glycoproteins induce experimental autoimmune encephalomyelitis by different mechanisms in C57BL/6 mice. *J Immunol* 2003;171: 462–468.

37. Babbe H, Roers A, Waisman A, et al. Clonal expansions of CD8(+) T-cells dominate the T-cell infiltrate in active multiple sclerosis lesions as shown by micromanipulation and single cell polymerase chain reaction. *J Exp Med* 2000;192:393–404.

38. Koh DR, Fung-Leung WP, Ho A, et al. Less mortality but more relapses in experimental allergic encephalomyelitis in CD8–/– mice. *Science* 1992;256:1210–1213.

39. Sriram S, Carroll L. In vivo depletion of Lyt-2 cells fails to alter acute and relapsing EAE. *J Neuroimmunol* 1988;17:147–157.

40. Sun D, Whitaker JN, Huang Z, et al. Myelin antigen-specific CD8+ T-cells are encephalitogenic and produce severe disease in C57BL/6 mice. *J Immunol* 2001;166: 7579–7587.

41. Huseby ES, Liggitt D, Brabb T, et al. A pathogenic role for myelin-specific cd8(+) T-cells in a model for multiple sclerosis. *J Exp Med* 2001;194:669–676.

41a. Ford ML, Evavold BD. Specificity, magnitude, and kinetics of MOG-specific CD8(+) T-cell responses during experimental autoimmune encephalomyelitis. *Eur J Immunol* 2005;35:76–85.

42. Johnson R, Griffin D, Gendleman H. Postinfectious encephalomyelitis. *Semin Neurol* 1985;5:180–190.

42a. Hart BA, Laman JD, Bauer J, et al. Modelling of multiple sclerosis: lessons learned in a non-human primate. *Lancet Neurol* 2004;3: 588–597.

43. Tsunoda I, Kuang LQ, Theil DJ, et al. Antibody association with a novel model for primary progressive multiple sclerosis: induction of relapsing-remitting and progressive forms of EAE in H2s mouse strains. *Brain Pathol* 2000;10:402–418.

44. Mueller PS, Kies MW, Alvord EC, Jr., et al. Prevention of experimental allergic encephalomyelitis (EAE) by vitamin C deprivation. *J Exp Med* 1962;115:329–338.

45. Owens T, Wekerle H, Antel J. Genetic models for CNS inflammation. *Nat Med* 2001;7:161–166.

46. Panitch HS, Hirsch RL, Haley AS, et al. Exacerbations of multiple sclerosis in patients treated with gamma interferon. *Lancet* 1987;1:893–895.

47. Owens T, Tran E, Hassan-Zahraee M, et al. Immune cell entry to the CNS—a focus for immunoregulation of EAE. *Res Immunol* 1998;149:781–789;[discussion] 844–846,855–860.

48. Skurkovich S, Boiko A, Beliaeva I, et al. Randomized study of antibodies to IFN-gamma and TNF-alpha in secondary progressive multiple sclerosis. *Mult Scler* 2001;7:277–284.

49. Furlan R, Brambilla E, Ruffini F, et al. Intrathecal delivery of IFN-gamma protects C57BL/6 mice from chronic-progressive experimental autoimmune encephalomyelitis by increasing apoptosis of central nervous system-infiltrating lymphocytes. *J Immunol* 2001;167:1821–1829.

50. Steinman L. Myelin-specific CD8 T-cells in the pathogenesis of experimental allergic encephalitis and multiple sclerosis. *J Exp Med* 2001;194:F27–F30.

51. Zehntner SP, Brisebois M, Tran E, et al. Constitutive expression of a costimulatory ligand on antigen-presenting cells in the nervous system drives demyelinating disease. *Faseb J* 2003;17:1910–1912.

52. Pullen LC, Miller SD, Dal Canto MC, et al. Alteration in the level of interferon-gamma results in acceleration of Theiler's virus-induced demyelinating disease. *J Neuroimmunol* 1994;55:143–152.

53. Rodriguez M, Pavelko K, Coffman RL. Gamma interferon is critical for resistance to Theiler's virus-induced demyelination. *J Virol* 1995;69:7286–7290.

54. Ure DR, Rodriguez M. Preservation of neurologic function during inflammatory demyelination correlates with axon sparing in a mouse model of multiple sclerosis. *Neuroscience* 2002;111:399–411.

55. Renno T, Taupin V, Bourbonniere L, et al. Interferon-gamma in progression to chronic demyelination and neurological deficit following acute EAE. *Mol Cell Neurosci* 1998;12:376–389.

56. LaFerla FM, Sugarman MC, Lane TE, et al. Regional hypomyelination and dysplasia in transgenic mice with astrocyte-directed expression of interferon-gamma. *J Mol Neurosci* 2000;15:45–59.

57. Simmons RD, Willenborg DO. Direct injection of cytokines into the spinal cord causes autoimmune encephalomyelitis-like inflammation. *J Neurol Sci* 1990;100:37–42.

58. Sethna MP, Lampson LA. Immune modulation within the brain: recruitment of inflammatory cells and increased major histocompatibility antigen expression following intracerebral injection of interferon-gamma. *Neuroimmunol* 1991;34:121–132.

59. Dalton DK, Haynes L, Chu CQ, et al. Interferon gamma eliminates responding CD4 T-cells during mycobacterial infection by inducing apoptosis of activated CD4 T-cells. *J Exp Med* 2000;192:117–122.

60. Willenborg DO, Fordham SA, Staykova MA, et al. IFN-gamma is critical to the control of murine autoimmune encephalomyelitis and regulates both in the periphery and in the target tissue: a possible role for nitric oxide. *J Immunol* 1999;163:5278–5286.

61. Cauley LS, Miller EE, Yen M, et al. Superantigen-induced CD4 T-cell tolerance mediated by myeloid cells and IFN-gamma. *J Immunol* 2000;165:6056–6066.

62. Sriram S, Stratton CW, Yao S, et al. Chlamydia pneumoniae infection of the central nervous system in multiple sclerosis. *Ann Neurol* 1999;46:6–14.

63. Ludwin SK. Central nervous system demyelination and remyelination in the mouse: an ultrastructural study of cuprizone toxicity. *Lab Invest* 1978;39:597–612.

64. Matsushima GK, Morell P. The neurotoxicant, cuprizone, as a model to study demyelination and remyelination in the central nervous system. *Brain Pathol* 2001;11:107–116.

65. Blakemore WF. Ethidium bromide induced demyelination in the spinal cord of the cat. *Neuropathol Appl Neurobiol* 1982;8:365–375.

66. Blakemore WF, Smith PM, Franklin RJ. Remyelinating the demyelinated CNS. *Novartis Found Symp* 2000; 231:289–298;[discussion]298–306.

67. Gensert JM, Goldman JE. Endogenous progenitors remyelinate demyelinated axons in the adult CNS. *Neuron* 1997;19:197–203.

68. Ousman SS, David S. Lysophosphatidylcholine induces rapid recruitment and activation of macrophages in the adult mouse spinal cord. *Glia* 2000;30:92–104.

69. Ousman SS, David S. MIP-1alpha, MCP-1, GM-CSF, and TNF-alpha control the immune cell response that mediates rapid phagocytosis of myelin from the adult mouse spinal cord. *J Neurosci* 2001;21: 4649–4656.

70. Johnson RS, Roder JC, Riordan JR. Over-expression of the DM-20 myelin proteolipid causes central nervous system demyelination in transgenic mice. *J Neurochem* 1995;64:967–976.

71. Mastronardi FG, Ackerley CA, Arsenault L, et al. Demyelination in a transgenic mouse: a model for multiple sclerosis. *J Neurosci Res* 1993;36:315–324.

72. Willenborg DO, Staykova MA, Cowden WB. Our shifting understanding of the role of nitric oxide in autoimmune encephalomyelitis: a review. *J Neuroimmunol* 1999;100:21–35.

73. Smith KJ, Lassmann H. The role of nitric oxide in multiple sclerosis. *Lancet Neurol* 2002;1:232–241.

74. Wheeler RD, Owens T. The Changing Face of Cytokines in the Brain: Perspectives from EAE. In: Hayley S, ed. *The Role of Cytokines in Neurodegenerative and Psychiatric Conditions: Multiple Mechanisms of Action.* Current Pharmaceutical Design; 2004.

75. Voorthuis JA, Uitdehaag BM, De Groot CJ, et al. Suppression of experimental allergic encephalomyelitis by intraventricular administration of interferon-gamma in Lewis rats. *Clin Exp Immunol* 1990;81:183–188.

76. The Lenercept Multiple Sclerosis Study Group and The University of British Columbia MS/MRI Analysis Group. TNF neutralization in MS: results of a randomized, placebo-controlled multicenter study. *Neurology* 1999;53:457–465.

77. Arnett HA, Mason J, Marino M, et al. TNF alpha promotes proliferation of oligodendrocyte progenitors and remyelination. *Nat Neurosci* 2001;4:1116–1122.

78. Feldmann M, Maini RN. Anti-TNF alpha therapy of rheumatoid arthritis: what have we learned? *Annu Rev Immunol* 2001;19:163–196.

7

Human Immune Studies in Multiple Sclerosis

Amit Bar-Or

Program in Experimental Therapeutics, Clinical Research Unit, Montreal Neurological Institute and McGill University, Montreal, Quebec Canada

The transition of multiple sclerosis (MS) into the category of treatable neurological illnesses has fueled an exponential growth in the MS literature. Particularly remarkable has been the surge in publications relating to the immunology of MS and its animal models. Here, we will focus on aspects of the human immune response that appear to be relevant to the pathophysiology of MS and to the rational development and application of current and future therapies. It should be kept in mind, however, that a more complete understanding of the MS process requires an appreciation of physiological aspects of central nervous system (CNS) immune-surveillance and neurobiology, as well as the intricacies of abnormal immune-neural interaction. These include dynamics at the level of the blood–brain barrier (BBB), the impact of immune mediators on neural responses and on CNS repair and, in turn, the effects of CNS

responses on the invading immune cells. A detailed review of such a broad literature is well beyond the scope of this chapter.

Much of what we believe we know about immune-pathophysiology in patients with MS has been based on studies in animal models of CNS inflammation. There is little doubt that animal studies continue to generate fundamental insights into mechanisms of immune–neural interaction. Indeed, the use of models such as experimental autoimmune encephalomyelitis (EAE) has become integral to the process of drug development for MS. There are, however, several examples of agents that were applied to MS clinical trials based on promising animal model data, and were found to be ineffective or, at times, even harmful. A corollary is that some potentially useful MS therapies may never be pursued because of a lack of measured benefit in preclinical models. Directly translating animal model-based observations to human disease mechanisms and putative therapeutic targets therefore remains problematic. More and more studies are emerging on human immune cells in vitro, as well as on human immune responses that are modulated in vivo. The practicing clinician is thus confronted with a daunting body of animal and human studies that may, at times, appear to be in conflict. Part of the challenge is to somehow distinguish between results that are plausible based on animal or in vitro studies, and those that are drawn from direct observations of the natural history of patients, or of patients subjected to a given therapy. Even the latter observations are not foolproof, however, since one might measure a real biological response or effect of therapy in patients, which may or may not be relevant to the disease itself. The true involvement of immune responses in MS is bound to be multifaceted, and our current understanding of the disease process remains largely speculative.

This chapter strives to examine our more established assumptions regarding immune contributions to the distinct phases of MS, and should provide a useful background for considering how to approach new immune therapeutic strategies. We will highlight studies in humans, including patients with MS, occasionally drawing from animal model findings to underscore principles of CNS inflammatory responses that are likely to be relevant to the human condition. We will consider how well MS meets the definition and requirements of an autoimmune disease. A simplified model of MS immunepathophysiology will illustrate the basic principles by which peripheral immune activation is thought to impact upon the CNS compartment, and identify the putative sites of action of current and future MS treatments.

IS MS INITIATED AS AN AUTOIMMUNE DISEASE?

An ongoing challenge for the normal immune system is the ability to efficiently discriminate between foreign antigens, and components of self (self-antigens). Of the immune cell repertoire, T-cells and B-cells have the capacity to recognize and develop so-called memory to spe-

cific antigenic targets. As such, these cells contribute to the adaptive immune response that can more efficiently respond to the same target in the future. Within the normal T-cell and B-cell repertoire, there are cells that can recognize and react to self-antigens. These autoreactive cells normally do not mount vigorous immune responses that could be harmful to the host. Instead, autoreactive cells are kept in check as part of the state of tolerance to self-antigens. This normal state of autoimmunity is likely to serve important homeostatic functions.

Immune responses can cause damage by targeting a person's own tissue when the normal state of autoimmunity becomes dysregulated and tolerance to particular self-antigens is broken. This is referred to as autoimmune disease (1). Why some individuals develop autoimmune disease, and why there is selectivity toward particular target organs, remains unclear. The prevailing thought is that these conditions manifest when immune dysregulation is triggered by environmental exposures (such as one or more common viruses), in genetically susceptible hosts (likely reflecting involvement of multiple risk-conferring and protective genes, each contributing relatively little to the overall susceptibility).

The observation of immune cells infiltrating sites of CNS injury, as a hallmark of MS pathology, has long supported the contention that MS is an autoimmune disease. However, since one of the main roles of the normal immune system is to respond to all forms of tissue injury, the mere presence of immune mediators in MS lesions does not necessarily mean that the immune system initiated the disease process. For a disease to have a frank autoimmune etiology, several criteria must be met. These include observations that (a) immune mediators are present within the sites of pathology in patients with the illness; (b) the same mediators are not present in persons or tissues without the illness; (c) the putative immune mediators can adoptively transfer the disease; and (d) removal of these mediators has beneficial effects on the host. While MS fulfills the first requirement reasonably well, relatively few features of MS lesions have been established as specific to the MS pathologic state. Unlike passive transfer experiments in myasthenia gravis in which patient serum can induce disease in recipient animals, similar findings with MS serum or cells have not been established. The exception may be the very unique circumstances where transgenic mice are engineered to have all their T-cells respond to a specific myelin antigen, resulting in spontaneous CNS inflammatory demyelination (2). The ongoing clinical progression of patients in the face of the approved immune-modulating therapies and a variety of immune-suppressing agents remains troubling. At the very least, it invokes processes in the CNS that may be relatively independent of the classical concept of immune responses.

Whether immune dysregulation is a primary initiating event or a secondary response in MS, the presence of activated immune cells and mediators at the site of CNS pathology and observations that manipulating immune responses in patients can both aggravate or diminish disease activity argues that immune responses are not merely epiphenomena of CNS tissue injury, but, rather, play an important role in the pathophysiology of MS. The following sections examine

how immune mediators are thought to contribute to MS relapses, remissions, and disease progression.

THE PRESUMED TRIGGER OF MS RELAPSES: PERIPHERAL IMMUNE ACTIVATION

In MS, the immune system is separated from the CNS target by the BBB (Fig. 7-1), representing the typical three-compartment model of immune-mediated disease. A key event in the triggering of an MS relapse is thought to be the activation outside the target organ (Step 1) of T-cells that can recognize antigens in the CNS. Through a sequence of subsequent events, these activated immune cells then undergo adhesion to the endothelial barrier (Step 2), attraction (Step 3), and active invasion (Step 4) into the target organ, where they may become reactivated (Step 5) and subsequently participate in the disease process (Step 6). The differentiation state of the invading cells determines whether they contribute to injury or, possibly, counter the injury process. This model will be used as a framework to discuss

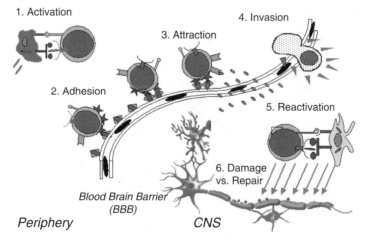

FIG. 7-1. A simplified model of MS immunopathogenesis. Immune cells activated in the periphery (Step 1) up-regulate surface molecules that enable them to more efficiently adhere (Step 2) to the endothelial cells of the blood–brain barrier (BBB) and respond to local chemokine gradients (Step 3). Active secretion of matrix proteases (Step 4) facilitates immune cell invasion into the CNS where they may become reactivated (Step 5) and impact on the biology of CNS elements (Step 6). These steps represent potential therapeutic targets for MS therapies.

how abnormalities at each of these steps may contribute to the MS process and how targeting one or more of these steps may be of therapeutic benefit.

It was Pasteur's introduction of a neural tissue containing vaccine as a therapy for rabies, resulting in episodes of acute disseminated encephalomyelitis (postvaccination ADEM), that first led to the consideration that triggering an autoreactive immune response in the periphery could translate into a CNS inflammatory attack in humans (3). This sparked the development of the commonly used EAE model of MS in which peripheral immunization with components of myelin [including myelin basic protein (MBP), myelin oligodendrocyte glycoprotein (MOG), and myelin oligodendrocyte glycoprotein (PLP)] can induce inflammatory CNS demyelination (4–6). EAE can also be induced in naïve animals by means of adoptive transfer of activated (but not resting) myelin reactive CD4+ T-cells from animals with established disease (7). The choice of animal strain, the spe-

cific antigen selected, and the immunization regimen can result in distinct phenotypes of EAE, with particular anatomical predilection such as spinal cord or optic nerve, or characteristic clinical patterns, including relapsing and chronic disease forms (6). This and other animal models (see Chapter 6 dedicated to animal models of MS, by Owens) establish that peripheral activation of T-cells that recognize CNS antigens can result in a CNS inflammatory disease.

By analogy with EAE, initiation of MS (or at least an MS relapse) is thought to be triggered by peripheral activation of autoaggressive, CNS-directed T-cells. T-cells recognize antigens that bind with sufficient affinity and avidity to their T-cell receptor (TCR). The appropriate antigen fragment must be presented to the TCR within the pocket of the major histocompatibility molecule (MHC), expressed on the surface of antigen-presenting cells (APCs) (Fig. 7-2). Effective APCs include dendritic cells, monocyte/macrophage, B-cells, and CNS microglial cells. Successful binding of the antigen–MHC

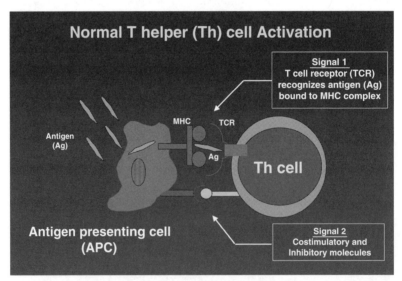

FIG. 7-2. T-cell activation: interaction with antigen-presenting cell (APC). The APC processes antigen (Ag) and presents to the T-cell in the context of the major histocompatibility molecule (MHC). A T-cell bearing an appropriate T-cell receptor capable of binding the Ag–MHC complex receives "Signal 1." Productive activation of T-cells (particularly naïve T-cells) requires additional co-stimulatory signals that can be provided by the APC or by other mediators in the local environment. The integration of the signal through the TCR (Signal 1) and additional co-stimulatory as well as inhibitory signals (collectively referred to as Signal 2), influences whether the T-cell becomes activated and may also impact on the functional response profile of the activated T-cell.

complex to the TCR delivers a T-cell-activating signal. However, this signal alone is not usually sufficient for full T-cell activation. Co-stimulatory signals are also required and may be delivered by APCs that express co-stimulatory molecules on their surfaces. A T-cell stimulated only via its TCR (in the absence of co-stimulation) may become anergic, and no longer react to its antigen. In contrast, a T-cell receiving both a TCR-mediated signal, and co-stimulation can become fully activated, proliferate, and release a range of cytokines and other effector molecules. These may, in turn, impact the target organ directly or through modulation of the functions of other immune cells. When APCs are exposed to factors such as infectious particles [for example, through Toll-like receptors (TLRs)], various other inflammatory mediators, or to injured tissue, they become activated and up-regulate their surface expression of co-stimulatory molecules (8). Several families of co-stimulatory molecules and their receptors are thought to play key roles in regulating immune responses in both health and disease states in humans. One important co-stimulatory pathway is represented by the CD28 or CTLA-4 molecules on T-cells, being engaged by the CD80 (B7.1) or CD86 (B7.2) co-stimulatory molecules expressed on APCs. Engagement of CD28 by B7 molecules stimulates the T-cell, while the same B7 molecules engaging CTLA-4 mediates an inhibitory signal. Whether a T-cell becomes productively activated thus depends on the integration of signals mediated by the TCR, and on the profile of co-stimulatory molecules available in the particular microenvironment (9,10). Modulating T-cell responses by targeting the B7 co-stimulatory pathway, as well as more recently described co-stimulatory molecules and their ligands (11–15), provides an attractive therapeutic approach for immune-mediated diseases, including MS.

As part of the normal immune system's capacity to generate effector T-cells that can respond in different ways depending on the circumstance, the same naïve T-cells can differentiate into functionally distinct subsets that are distinguishable based on their cytokine production profiles (16,17). The microenvironment during initial activation critically determines how the T-cells differentiate. In addition to the strength of activation (including signals mediated by the TCR and the available profile of co-stimulation), cytokines represent important contextual cues that can influence T-cell differentiation. Certain cytokines released by APCs can critically define subsequent T-cell responses. For example, interleukin (IL)-12 or IL-23 can preferentially generate T-cells that subsequently secrete interferon-gamma (IFNγ and tumor necrosis factor alpha (TNFα) (18). These T-cells have been arbitrarily referred to as T-helper type-1 (Th1) cells, and are effective as part of the normal anti-viral response (19). In contrast, T-cells that initially become activated in the presence of IL-4 and in the absence if IL-12 subsequently produce cytokines including IL-4, IL-5, IL-13, and possibly IL-10. These Th2 cells are important in responses against parasitic infections. Normal humans must therefore be able to mount both Th1 and Th2 responses, depending on the circumstance. A dysregulation in the body's normal balance between Th1 and Th2 responses can result in disease states. Unchecked Th2 responses may contribute to asthma or atopic conditions, and too much of a Th1 response has been implicated in certain target-directed autoimmune diseases.

In the EAE model of MS, CNS-autoreactive Th1 T-cells can adoptively induce disease, whereas transfer of Th2 cells that recognize the same CNS antigens does not usually induce disease. Moreover, the Th2 cells may protect the animal from getting the Th1-mediated disease. By extension, it has been suggested that in MS, CNS-directed Th1 responses may be proinflammatory and cause damage, whereas Th2 responses may be anti-inflammatory and possibly protective (20–23). Additional T-cell subsets have been identified that likely play important roles in the regulation of human immune responses (23), and are further discussed in subsequent sections. It must be emphasized that the Th1/Th2 paradigm does not adequately capture the true complexity of immune regulation, and should not be taken as dogma. For example, driving Th2 responses too far can result in a form of EAE caused by the Th2 cells (24,25).

Nonetheless, the appreciation that T-cells can adopt distinct effector profiles and that dysregulation among different subsets of T-cells may contribute to pathologic states is relevant.

What is the evidence that human T-cells reactive to specific CNS antigens are involved in the MS disease process? To date, no single CNS antigen has been established as the major MS target. In all likelihood, the predominant target during MS relapses is different across patients and may, indeed, change within the same individual over time (epitope spread). Hence, multiple T-cell targets are likely involved in MS (26–31), though studies have tended to focus on reactivity to MBP, in part because human MBP is easier to isolate for in vitro studies than the much less-water-soluble PLP, or MOG that is present in very small amounts. All individuals (including those without MS) have circulating T-cells that can react to CNS antigens, including MBP (32–34). Thus, the mere presence of such CNS-reactive T-cells is not sufficient to cause disease. Studies that compare MS patients to controls have suggested that MBP-reactive T-cells from patients are in a higher state of activation (35,36), require less costimulation (37,38), tend to be of higher avidity (36), and preferentially belong to the memory T-cell pool (39–41). There is also some evidence that MBP-reactive T-cells isolated from MS patients are more likely to produce proinflammatory (Th1), rather than anti-inflammatory mediators (42,43). In immunohistochemical studies, using an antibody that identifies the encephalitogenic fragment $MBP_{(85-99)}$ (only when it is bound within the DR2 (MHC Class II) molecule), it has been shown that the DR2–MBP complex is presented by APCs within MS lesions at a higher frequency than in brains from normal DR2+ individuals (44).

Much of the focus has centered on the roles of CNS autoreceptive CD4 helper T-cells, in part because of technical difficulties in maintaining CD8 cytotoxic T-cells in culture. There is now good evidence in studies of MS patients that points to an important contribution of CD8 T-cells. A prominence of CD8 over CD4 T-cell responses is observed within MS lesions (45,46) and molecular studies demonstrate that specific CD8 (rather than CD4) T-cells are expanded and

persist long-term within the CNS compartment of patients (45,47). A higher prevalence of CNS autoreactive CD8 T-cells is confirmed in the circulation of MS patients compared to controls (48–50). The roles of natural killer (NK) cells, NK T-cells, and γ/δ T-cells in MS are also under investigation (51,52).

The most compelling evidence to date that peripherally activated, CNS-autoreactive T-cells indeed participate in the MS disease process stems from careful immune studies of patients treated with an altered peptide ligand (APL) of MBP. An altered peptide ligand refers to a peptide antigen that is altered by replacing one or more of its amino acids. T-cells that recognize a particular antigen may still recognize an APL of that antigen, though the T-cell response to this APL may be considerably different. Studies initiated in EAE found that an APL of an encephalitogenic epitope of MBP led to a Th2 shift in MBP reactivity, associated with improved clinical outcomes (53,54). The same APL was subsequently introduced into early-phase MS clinical trials. At relatively low doses, subcutaneous injection of the APL was found to induce the anticipated Th2 responses to MBP in MS patients, and suggested possible benefit on MRI outcomes (55). However, in another trial, a higher dose of the same APL was associated with significant increases in MRI activity in several patients, with or without clinical correlates (56). In these patients, elegant immune monitoring identified a strong induction of MBP-reactive CD4 T-cells both in the periphery and in the CSF. These MBP-reactive T-cells were notable for their production of high levels of the Th1 cytokine, IFNγ. Based on the above studies, MS therapeutics are often considered in terms of their capacity to inhibit the activation of Th1 CNS autoreactive cells or promote Th2 responses to CNS targets. It should be emphasized that the relationship between Th1 and Th2 responses (loosely designated as proinflammatory and anti-inflammatory, respectively) and tissue damage or protection in MS remains only partially understood, as recent studies have suggested that Th1 responses may not always be detrimental (57,58). Indeed, immune system cells are not all "bad" or all "good." The challenge is to elucidate which immune responses may be injurious, and when, so that appropriate therapies can be most appropriately developed and applied.

Is there evidence to suggest where and how CNS-reactive T-cells become activated in patients with MS? It is now accepted that lymphocyte trafficking into the CNS occurs under normal physiologic conditions (59–61), and that resident CNS microglial cells (both peri-vascular and parenchymal) can serve as competent antigen-presenting cells (6,23). In this context, abnormal profiles of co-stimulatory molecule expression may contribute to the activation of CNS autoreactive T-cells, both within and outside of the CNS. Expression of CD80 (B7.1) is reported to be selectively up-regulated in MS plaques (62,63), and CD80 (but not CD86) was found to be up-regulated on immune cells in cerebrospinal fluid (CSF) and peripheral blood of MS patients compared to controls (64). Blockade of CD80 signaling in EAE inhibits the induction phase of the disease (65–67). Another potential source of APCs capable of presenting antigens to T-cells within the CNS may be found in the CSF and meninges. Studies of these sites in patients with MS have revealed chronically activated B-cells/plasma cells, organized in structures resembling germinal centers, and expressing high levels of co-stimulatory molecules (68).

CNS autoreactive cells may also become activated outside the CNS, for example, by encountering fragments of CNS self-antigens that are released, or carried by APCs, into cervical lymph nodes that drain the brain (69–71). Molecular mimicry represents another mechanism by which autoreactive T-cells might become activated and contribute to autoimmune responses. In the context of MS, this could occur when T-cells that can recognize particular CNS antigens become activated upon encounter with fragments of foreign (nonself) antigens that are sufficiently similar to the CNS self-antigen. In support of this mechanism are observations that some human MBP-reactive T-cells can become activated by antigenic fragments derived from common viruses (including herpes simplex, Epstein–Barr, or influenza viruses) presented by the same MHC molecules (72,73). Extending this further is the elegant concept of structural equivalence, wherein two different MHC molecules (encoded by the individual's two MHC alleles), loaded with two distinct antigens, create two antigen–MHC complexes that may be sufficiently similar in structure, that they are both recognized by the same CNS-reactive T-cell (73).

IMMUNE CELL INTERACTION WITH THE BLOOD–BRAIN BARRIER: ADHESION, ATTRACTION, AND INVASION

When immune cells become activated, they up-regulate the expression of several families of molecules that facilitate their migration across endothelial barriers and into the target organ (Fig. 7-1). The process of transmigration involves a tightly regulated sequence of events (74,75). Up-regulated selectins and integrins on the activated immune cells interact with ligands expressed on the endothelial cells of the BBB, resulting in immune cell "rolling" and "tethering/arresting," respectively (Step 2). Chemokines secreted by endothelial cells, injured tissue, or immune cells themselves can promote integrin activation and further contribute to cell arrest (76). Chemokines also drive the migration of cells expressing the corresponding chemokine receptors toward the source of the chemical gradient (Step 3). Production of enzymes (Step 4), such as the matrix metalloproteinases (MMP), results in breakdown of the basement membrane and facilitates tissue infiltration (77). Selected evidence implicating these molecular steps in disease pathogenesis is provided below and identifies potential therapeutic targets for MS.

Implicating Adhesion Molecules in MS

Endothelial cells within MS lesions have been shown to express abnormally elevated levels of adhesion molecules including ICAM-1 and VCAM-1, which correlate with the extent of leukocyte infiltration (75,78–80). Their ligands (LFA-1 and VLA-4, respectively) have been identified on the perivascular inflammatory cells within MS lesions (81). These, and related animal model studies, provide the foundation for therapeutic targeting of cell migration in patients with MS with agents such as natalizumab. It is interesting to note that adhesion molecules such as VCAM-1 and LFA-1 are also expressed on glial cells within MS lesions (82), possibly pointing to additional roles for these molecules in antigen presentation and T-cell co-stimulation (81,83,84).

Selective Expression of Chemokines and Chemokine Receptors in MS

The normal immune system utilizes a complex network of chemokines and chemokine receptors to regulate movement of immune cells within and between tissues. Such chemokine–chemokine receptor interactions are also involved in the trafficking of immune cells into the CNS of patients with MS (Fig. 7-1, Step 3). The majority of cells in the CSF of MS patients are memory T-cells that express CCR7, consistent with a so-called central memory phenotype of cells that participate in immune-surveillance. With the MS lesions themselves, essentially all T-cells do not express CCR7, consistent with the so-called effector memory phenotype. Cells expressing MHC Class II, CD68, CD86, and the chemokine receptor CCR7, consistent with maturing dendritic cells, are abundant both within the CSF and the lesions of MS patients (71). These observations support a model in which the afferent limb of CNS-directed immune responses involves entry of dendritic cells that undergo maturation when they capture CNS antigens within the MS lesions. The maturing dendritic cells then migrate via the CSF into the deep cervical lymph nodes, where they may present CNS antigens to T-cells. The T-cells turn into central memory (CCR7+) cells, which participate in the efferent limb of CNS immune responses by entering the CSF and subsequently down-regulating CCR7 (becoming CCR7-effector memory T-cells) upon restimulation by antigen within the CNS compartment. The effector memory T-cells are retained within the MS lesions, where they contribute to the disease process (71).

Studies in both EAE and MS implicate certain chemokines in the selective recruitment of T-cells and monocytes/dendritic cells into the inflamed CNS (85). For example, RANTES (CCL5) that is chemotactic for lymphocytes and monocytes expressing CCR5, is up-regulated at the edge of active MS lesions (86), and MCP-1 (CCL2), a chemokine that attracts monocytes expressing CCR2, is expressed by local astrocytes (87). Compared to neurological controls, CSF from MS patients was observed to contain elevated levels of both IP-10 (CXCL10), as well as CCL5, both chemotactic for activated T-cells expressing the chemokine receptor CXCR3 (88). An increased frequency of CD4+ and CD8+ T-cells from the CSF of MS patients were seen to express CXCR3. Immunohistochemistry confirmed an increased perivascular expression of CXCR3 as well as CCR5 on immune cells infiltrating MS lesions. Thus, the data suggest that CCL2/CCR2, CXCL10/CXCR3, and CCL5/CCR5 interactions may be selectively involved in MS pathogenesis. Certain chemokine–chemokine receptor interactions may preferentially contribute to the trafficking of proinflammatory Th1 T-cell populations (86,88–91), though this may not always be the case for individual T-cells (92).

Selective Expression of Matrix Proteinases (MPs) in MS

The family of MPs is composed of tightly regulated proteolytic enzymes, including the matrix metalloproteinases (MMPs), that contribute to diverse biological processes such as normal organ development, tissue remodeling, and immune responses. The ability of activated immune cells to migrate across barriers such as the BBB and infiltrate the extracellular matrix of the target tissue is predicated, in part, on the local production of such lytic enzymes (Fig. 7-1, Step 4). Dysregulation of MMP and the related ADAM (a disintegrin and metalloproteinase) family of molecules may contribute to abnormal tissue invasion by immune cells (77,93–95). MMPs and ADAMs are typically produced as proenzymes requiring proteolytic cleavage to become activated. Tissue inhibitors of matrix proteinases (TIMPs) function to down-regulate the matrix protease effects (96). Expression of matrix proteases is not restricted to activated immune cells; it is also seen in CNS glial cells such as astrocytes and microglia (97–99). The potential contribution of matrix protease family molecules to the MS process may thus include (a) disruption of the BBB basement membrane and extracellular matrix (96), thereby facilitating parenchymal infiltration of immune cells (97); (b) facilitating the action of membrane-bound proinflammatory cytokines, such as TNFα, by cleaving them off the cell surface (100,101); and (c) directly damaging elements of the CNS (102). It should be kept in mind that certain matrix proteases may also be required during processes of repair and regeneration within the CNS (77). In MS patients, increased activity of several CSF MMPs has been reported, compared to individuals without MS (103,104). For example, gelatinase B (MMP-9) levels are abnormally elevated in both the serum and CSF of MS patients, particularly during acute relapses. These elevated levels correlate with the degree of BBB disruption measured as the number of gadolinium-enhancing MRI lesions (105,106). Analysis of MMP, ADAM, and TIMP levels in different immune cell subsets reveals distinct expression profiles in T-cells, B-cells, and monocytes in both normals and in patients with MS (107,108). Of interest, monocytes express a broader range and often higher amounts of different proteolytic enzymes compared to T-cells and B-cells (107), which is consistent with the observation that invading monocyte/macrophage are a major contributor to the MS inflammatory lesions.

It is important to keep in mind that the multi-step molecular machinery described above (involving adhesion molecules, chemokines, and matrix proteases) is fundamental to normal processes of immune surveillance and adaptive immunity, in which cells migrate across different endothelial barriers, including the BBB (59–61,109). However, dysregulated expression or function of these families of molecules is likely to contribute to the pathology of immune-mediated diseases. Ongoing efforts are aimed at elucidating how these molecular interactions may be involved in the MS pathophysiology, and how distinct steps of cell trafficking may be targeted therapeutically, while minimizing the impact on normal immune functions.

INVOLVEMENT OF B-CELL AND ANTIBODY RESPONSES IN MS

Like T-cells, B-cells have the capacity to recognize particular antigens, which they do through their B-cell receptor (BCR) expressed on the cell surface. B-cells typically become activated when they are first stimulated upon encounter with an antigen that binds the BCR, and subsequently receive "help" from T-cells. The B-cells may then proliferate and differentiate into memory B-cells as well as plasma cells that secrete antibodies (immunoglobulins, Ig), and contribute to the humoral immune response against the stimulating antigen. The potential role of B-cells in MS pathophysiology has generally been considered in terms of their ability to react to CNS antigens and the subsequent production of CNS-directed autoantibodies. It has long been appreciated that the CSF of MS patients frequently contains elevated levels of Ig, which typically displays an oligoclonal pattern when run on an electrophoretic gel. Though the actual target(s) of these antibodies remains unknown, molecular biology studies (somatic hypermutation analysis) of B-cells found within MS lesions and CSF indicates that certain B-cells are expanded in response to antigenic encounter within the CNS compartment. The presence of deposited Ig and complement molecules is reportedly a common occurrence in MS lesions and, in both MS and EAE, antibodies bound to fragments of myelin are found within phagocytic cells at sites of demyelination (110,111). Together, these findings point to possible contribution of complement-mediated injury and antibody-directed cytotoxicity (ADCC), to the MS disease process (112,113). However, in contrast to antibodies against pancreatic antigens (e.g., GAD) that can be detected in patients with *Diabetes mellitus*, antibodies against CNS myelin components (such as MBP and MOG) appear to be of relatively low affinity, raising questions as to their actual involvement in MS pathology (114). Another possibility is that anti-CNS antibodies do not directly contribute to injury, but represent part of the immune system's response to injury. As such, the presence of anti-CNS antibodies may provide a marker of how aggressive the inflammatory process is (115,116). It has also been suggested that certain antibodies to CNS elements may actually be beneficial, such as anti-myelin antibodies that may support remyelination (117,118), or others that could function to remove debris, including growth inhibitory molecules (119), thereby contributing to an environment that is more permissive to axonal regeneration.

B-cell contribution to MS has also been considered beyond their capacity to become antibody-producing cells. For example, B-cell subsets have been identified that can function as effective APCs to T-cells (120) and the meninges and CSF of patients with MS are found to contain chronically activated B-cells (31) in structures reminiscent of germinal centers, that may promote ongoing T-cell activation and propagation of the MS disease activity (68,121,122).

Furthermore, normal human B-cells are now thought to actively contribute to the regulation of immune responses through secretion of distinct effector cytokine profiles in a context-dependent fashion (123,124). Abnormalities in this regulatory function may be relevant to autoimmune diseases, including MS (123,125). Targeting certain B-cell subsets may emerge as a useful therapeutic approach for subsets of patients. In this context it is noteworthy that the molecular interactions that underlie human B-cell entry into the CNS (involving adhesion molecules, chemokines, and MMP) partially overlap, but are not identical to those employed by T-cells (107,108). This becomes relevant when considering the impact of T-cell-directed therapies on B-cell physiology, as well as the optimal approach to the development of B-cell-directed therapies.

REACTIVATION OF IMMUNE CELLS WITHIN THE CNS

Following infiltration into the CNS, T-cells and B-cells may become reactivated (Fig. 7-1, Step 5). Antigen presentation could be accomplished by resident cells such as CNS microglia, or by invading monocyte/macrophage, and dendritic cells (126–129). The presence of inflammatory factors produced within the CNS, including cytokines, chemokines, and matrix proteases, can stimulate invading APC, as well as primed T-cells and B-cells, in the process of so-called bystander activation. Tissue damage may expose additional myelin components that can become targets of subsequent immune attack (epitope spread), possibly contributing to clinical relapses (130).

Active immune responses could impact the integrity of CNS myelin, oligodendrocytes, and neural elements by several distinct mechanisms (Fig. 7-1, Step 6, and Tables 7-1 and 7-2). CD4 and CD8 T-cells can mediate antigen-specific injury to targets that they recognize. Autoreactive antibodies may contribute to antigen-specific injury through complement fixation or ADCC. In vitro studies suggest that CD4 and CD8 T-cells may also impact the health of neurons by nonspecific cytotoxic mechanisms (131,132). A variety of soluble factors, including proinflammatory cytokines, glutamate, matrix proteases, nitric oxide, oxygen radicals,

TABLE 7-1 *Immune mechanisms that could contribute to CNS injury*

Cytotoxicity mediated by immune cells, including:
 (i) Antigen-specific, CNS-reactive CD8 T-cells and CD4 T-cells
 (ii) Nonantigen-specific CD8 and CD4 T-cells (bystander injury)
 (iii) Macrophage; reactive microglia
 (iv) Natural killer (NK) cells; NK T-cells; γ/δ T-cells
 (v) Failure to down-regulate the immune response (prolonged retention, and/or limited apoptosis of proinflammatory cells)
 (vi) Apoptotic signals (leading to neural cell death)

Injury by soluble (humoral) immune mediators, including:
 (i) Antigen-specific, CNS-reactive antibodies: injury through complement fixation and/or antibody-dependent cytotoxicity (ADCC)
 (ii) Proinflammatory cytokines (including Th1 cytokines, osteopontin, TNFα, IL-1β)
 (iii) Nitric oxide and reactive oxygen species
 (iv) Leukotrienes, plasminogen activators
 (v) Matrix metalloproteinases (MMPs)
 (vi) Glutamate-mediated cytotoxicity

TABLE 7-2 *Immune mechanisms that could contribute to CNS recovery, protection, and repair*

Mediators that could serve to decrease proinflammatory responses, including:
 (i) Anti-inflammatory cytokines (including Th2 cytokines, IL-10, TGFβ)
 (ii) Anti-inflammatory, antigen-presenting cells
 (iii) Regulatory/suppressive T-cell subsets (Tr1, Th2, Th3, CD4+CD25hi; CD8 HLA-E)
 (iv) Proapoptotic signals (leading to death of proinflammatory immune cells)
 (v) Tissue inhibitors of matrix metalloproteinases (TIMPs)

Mechanisms that could promote CNS protection and repair, including:
 (i) Release of neurotrophic factors (BDNF, NGF, others)
 (ii) Clearance of inhibitory myelin molecules (Nogo, MAG) by macrophage/microglia
 (iii) Cytokines promoting CNS progenitor cells (e.g., TNFα via TNFR2) and remyelination (IL-1β inducing IGF-1)
 (iv) Protective autoimmunity
 (v) Promyelinating antibodies
 (vi) Some prostaglandins, lipoxins, antithrombin

and proapoptotic signals may also mediate injury in a nonantigen-dependent way (23,41, 57,133).

CONTRIBUTION OF IMMUNE RESPONSES TO REMISSIONS

Recovery from an MS relapse involves both immune and nonimmune mechanisms. Examples of nonimmune mechanisms include early redistribution of sodium channels on demyelinated nerve segments (134), remyelination (135), axonal regeneration, and reorganization of networks (136). Immune mechanisms contributing to recovery include active resolution and/or suppression of the damaging inflammatory processes, as well as promotion of immune responses that support protection and repair. Resolution of active inflammation requires clearance of infiltrating immune cells through migration out of the CNS or through apoptosis in situ. This limits further injury and enables reversal of acute edema. It is the balance between locally expressed proinflammatory cytokines and proretention chemokines,

as well as the profile of proapoptotic and anti-apoptotic molecules, which together determine whether activated immune cells persist within MS lesions and impact upon recovery (57).

In keeping with the theme that active immune responses are not necessarily detrimental during CNS inflammation, Table 7-2 identifies several ways in which immune mediators may be beneficial in MS. One general theme relates to how particular immune responses can suppress or downregulate others. Th2 cytokines are known to inhibit Th1 differentiation, such that activated Th2 cells within the CNS could limit proinflammatory Th1 responses through a process termed bystander suppression. Modulation of infiltrating monocyte/macrophage as well as resident microglia toward a Type 2 APC phenotype could promote anti-inflammatory Th2 responses within the CNS (129,137). Importantly, overly aggressive shifts toward Th2 responses may be harmful (24,25) and, in some settings, Th1 responses have been identified as potentially beneficial, pointing to a possible role for protective autoimmunity (138). Several subsets of T-cells may have potential immune-regulatory properties (139–141). The roles of CD25[hi] CD4 cells, IL-10-producing Tr1 cells, or TGFβ-producing Th3 cells (142–144), as well as distinct CD8 T-cell subsets (such as HLA-E restricted CD8 suppressors) (145,146) are of considerable interest.

In addition to the provision of down-regulatory or anti-inflammatory signals, further mechanisms by which immune responses may be beneficial in the CNS of MS patients include active contributions to survival and repair of neural elements through release of neurotrophic factors (147,148), release of cytokines that may induce proliferation of oligodendrocyte progenitor cells (e.g., TNFα) (149), and production of myelin-directed antibodies that may actually support remyelination (117,119,150,151). Immune responses may also contribute to repair by promoting a more permissive CNS environment, through the removal of molecules that otherwise inhibit axonal regeneration such as Nogo and MAG (152). It is noteworthy (Tables 7-1 and 7-2) that certain immune mediators (such as IL-1β, TNFα, apoptotic molecules) may have both detrimental and beneficial effects during CNS inflammation. For example, IL-1β can contribute to CNS injury by promoting the action of certain MMP and by exacerbating glutamate cytotoxicity, but is also required for the production of the nerve growth factor CNTF (153), and is able to promote remyelination by inducing the growth factor IGF-1 (154). Similarly, TNFα is considered a Th1 proinflammatory cytokine that may be directly cytotoxic when acting via TNFR1, but can be supportive of remyelination when acting via TNFR2. This poses particular therapeutic challenges and may explain why anti-TNFα therapies (which work well for patients with rheumatoid arthritis) have been unsuccessful and, indeed, detrimental in MS.

IMMUNE MECHANISMS OF DISEASE PROGRESSION

The contribution of inflammatory mechanisms to progressive and persistent neurological disability in MS patients remains to be fully defined. Failure of the resolution phase of acute relapses, due to persistence of proretention and prosurvival cues (Table 7-1), may play a role in prolonging the injurious impact of infiltrating immune cells. Chronic activation of resident CNS glial cells, such as microglia and astrocytes, may provide the basis for the generation or maintenance of progressive pathologic responses, even in the absence of acute waves of infiltrating inflammatory cells from the periphery. CNS resident cells may become activated through TLR or by scavenging the CNS debris itself. There is speculation that germinal center-like structures develop within the CNS providing the nidus for chronic activation (68,121, 122). Collectively, the activated cells residing within the CNS could be sources of potential effector molecules that contribute to smoldering tissue injury.

A so-called multi-hit model is likely relevant to the gradual loss of neural elements and neurological function over the lifelong course of MS. Sublethal injury may render oligodendrocytes (OLG) and neurons more vulnerable to accumulating insults. For example, OLG chronically exposed to an inflammatory environment up-regulate intracellular p53, leading to surface up-regulation of death receptors which now make the cell more susceptible to apoptosis mediated by Fas-ligand and tumor necrosis factor–related apoptosis-inducing ligand (TRAIL) (155). Injury of OLG progenitor cells early in the disease course may lead to their eventual depletion and a progressively limited capacity of the CNS to remyelinate (156). Axons, in turn, rely on support from OLG. In their absence, the axons likely become more vulnerable to insults that would otherwise have a lesser impact. A combination of sublethal insults is thus likely to contribute to the chronic loss of CNS elements (157). Though the clinical manifestations of the above processes may not be apparent early in the disease course, it is likely that these mechanisms contribute to CNS tissue injury from the earliest stages of MS. This is borne out in EAE, where features of acute and more chronic disease patterns overlap, implying the coexistence of distinct pathogenic mechanisms through much of the disease course. It is not known whether the mechanisms underlying chronic progression in patients with the primary progressive form of MS (PPMS) are identical to those which account for the more common secondary progression (SPMS) form of disease.

IMMUNE MODULATORS IN MS: PROPOSED MECHANISMS OF ACTION

Studying the in vivo mode of action of MS treatments is essential to the generation of novel therapies. The thoughtful development of biological assays and their implementation into well-designed clinical trials of experimental therapies for MS are paramount. These mechanistic studies not only provide proof of biologic concept and insights into the relevant mode of action of the therapy in question, but also provide critical windows into the disease itself. Combining clinical, imaging and biological outcome measures enables more comprehensive prospective monitoring of patients in trials, as well as the development and validation of biomarkers of disease activity, treatment response, and prognosis. The simplified model presented above (Fig. 7-1) identifies potential targets for intervention in MS. In

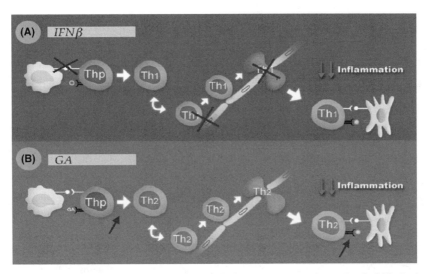

FIG. 7-3. Presumed modes of action of IFNβ and glatiramer acetate therapies in MS. **A.** As a family, interferon-beta (IFNβ) therapies likely to mediate their therapeutic effects by suppressing immune cell activation and by inhibiting expression of adhesion molecules and matrix proteases, resulting in diminished adhesion and invasion of activated immune cells into the CNS. This would translate into less CNS inflammation and damage. **B.** Glatiramer acetate (GA) is thought to act by modulating the activated immune cells that adopt an anti-inflammatory cytokine profile and migrate into the CNS. There, these cells are thought to counter the local inflammation and decrease damage.

general terms, treatments that can prevent CNS-reactive cells from becoming abnormally activated or from entering their target are considered beneficial in MS; this also applies to treatments that can shift the immune response from a proinflammatory to an anti-inflammatory profile, and treatments that can promote CNS protection and repair. Therapies can thus be considered in terms of their potential to (a) inhibit co-stimulation and peripheral immune activation of proinflammatory cells, or promote the same for anti-inflammatory cells (Fig. 7-1, Step 1); (b) modulate CNS infiltration through inhibition or promotion of selected molecules involved in adhesion (Step 2), attraction (Step 3), or trans-migration (Step 4); (c) impact immune reactivation within the CNS or the capacity to suppress or regulate immune effector profiles (Step 5); and (d) contribute to local tissue protection and repair (Step 6).

Converging studies suggest that the IFNβ medications share the same therapeutic mechanisms of action in MS, which are thought to include (a) inhibiting co-stimulatory molecule expression resulting in decreased T-cell activation (64); (b) inducing immune suppressive cytokine production such as IL-10 (158); and (c) reducing the capacity of immune cell migration into the CNS by inhibiting their expression of adhesion molecules (159) and matrix proteases (Fig. 7-3A) (160–162). In contrast, studies of the therapeutic mode of action of glatiramer acetate in MS (a) initially considered its capacity to inhibit myelin-reactive T-cells (163) and subsequently focused on (b) its ability to promote anti-inflammatory T-cells (20,164–171) and Type 2 (anti-inflammatory) APCs (129,137) that migrate into the CNS where they may counter inflammatory responses, and (c) possibly contribute to protection of CNS elements through the release of neurotrophic factors (Fig. 7-3B) (172,173). More detailed discussion of the currently used immune modulators and immune suppressants, as well as future therapies of MS, can be found in the subsequent chapters.

REFERENCES

1. Ermann J, Fathman CG. Autoimmune diseases: genes, bugs and failed regulation. *Nat Immunol* 2001;2(9):759–761.

2. Bettelli E, Pagany M, Weiner HL, et al. Myelin oligo-dendrocyte glycoprotein-specific T-cell receptor transgenic mice develop spontaneous autoimmune optic neuritis. *J Exp Med* 2003;197(9):1073–1081.

3. Stuart G, Krikorian KS. The neuro-paralytic accidents of anti-rabies treatment. *Ann Trop Med Parasitol* 1928;22:327–377.

4. Rivers TM, Schwentker FF. Encephalomyelitis accompanied by myelin destruction experimentally produced in monkeys. *J Exp Med* 1935;61:689–702.

5. Kabat EA, Wolf A, Bezer AE. The rapid production of acute disseminated encephalomyelitis in rhesus monkeys by injection of heterologous and homologous brain tissue with adjuvants. *J Exp Med* 1947;85:117–130.

6. Wekerle H. Antigen Presentation by CNS Glia. In: Kettenmann H, Ranson B, eds. *Neuroglia*. Oxford: Oxford University Press, 1994.

7. Paterson PY. Transfer of allergic encephalomyelitis in rats by means of lymph node cells. *J Exp Med* 1960;111:119–136.

8. Cook DN, Pisetsky DS, Schwartz DA. Toll-like receptors in the pathogenesis of human disease. *Nat Immunol* 2004;5(10):975–979.

9. Anderson DE, Bieganowska KD, Bar-Or A, et al. Paradoxical inhibition of T-cell function in response to CTLA-4 blockade; heterogeneity within the human T-cell population. *Nat Med* 2000;6(2):211–214.

10. Vijayakrishnan L, Slavik JM, Illes Z, et al. An autoimmune disease-associated CTLA-4 splice variant lacking the B7 binding domain signals negatively in T-cells. *Immunity* 2004;20(5):563–575.

11. Chitnis T, Khoury SJ. Role of costimulatory pathways in the pathogenesis of multiple sclerosis and experimental autoimmune encephalomyelitis. *J Allergy Clin Immunol* 2003;112(5):837–849;[quiz]850.

12. Dong C, Juedes AE, Temann UA, et al. ICOS co-stimulatory receptor is essential for T-cell activation and function. *Nature* 2001;409(6816):97–101.

13. Okazaki T, Iwai Y, Honjo T. New regulatory co-receptors: inducible co-stimulator and PD-1. *Curr Opin Immunol* 2002;14(6):779–782.

14. Salama AD, Chitnis T, Imitola J, et al. Critical role of the programmed death-1 (PD-1) pathway in regulation of experimental autoimmune encephalomyelitis. *J Exp Med* 2003;198(1):71–78.

15. Schreiner B, Mitsdoerffer M, Kieseier BC, et al. Interferon-beta enhances monocyte and dendritic cell expression of B7-H1 (PD-L1), a strong inhibitor of autologous T-cell activation: relevance for the immune modulatory effect in multiple sclerosis. *J Neuroimmunol* 2004;155(1–2):172–182.

16. Abbas AK, Murphy KM, Sher A. Functional diversity of helper T lymphocytes. *Nature* 1996;383(6603):787–793.

17. O'Garra A. Cytokines induce the development of functionally heterogeneous T helper cell subsets. *Immunity* 1998;8(3):275–283.

18. Murphy CA, Langrish CL, Chen Y, et al. Divergent pro- and antiinflammatory roles for IL-23 and IL-12 in joint autoimmune inflammation. *J Exp Med* 2003;198(12):1951–1957.

19. Mosmann TR, Coffman RL. Heterogeneity of cytokine secretion patterns and functions of helper T-cells. *Adv Immunol* 1989;46:111–147.

20. Farina C, Then Bergh F, Albrecht H, et al. Treatment of multiple sclerosis with Copaxone (COP): Elispot assay detects COP-induced interleukin-4 and interferon-gamma response in blood cells. *Brain* 2001;124(Pt 4):705–719.

21. Hemmer B, Archelos JJ, Hartung HP. New concepts in the immunopathogenesis of multiple sclerosis. *Nat Rev Neurosci* 2002;3(4):291–301.

22. Steinman L, Martin R, Bernard C, et al. Multiple sclerosis: deeper understanding of its pathogenesis reveals new targets for therapy. *Annu Rev Neurosci* 2002;25:491–505.

23. Antel J, Owens T. Multiple sclerosis and immune regulatory cells. *Brain* 2004;127(Pt 9):1915–1916.

24. Genain CP, Abel K, Belmar N, et al. Late complications of immune deviation therapy in a nonhuman primate. *Science* 1996;274(5295):2054–2057.

25. Pedotti R, Mitchell D, Wedemeyer J, et al. An unexpected version of horror autotoxicus: anaphylactic shock to a self-peptide. *Nat Immunol* 2001;2(3):216–222.

26. Ota K, Matsui M, Milford EL, et al. T-cell recognition of an immunodominant myelin basic protein epitope in multiple sclerosis. *Nature* 1990;346(6280):183–187.

27. Sun JB, Olsson T, Wang WZ, et al. Autoreactive T- and B-cells responding to myelin proteolipid protein in multiple sclerosis and controls. *Eur J Immunol* 1991;21(6):1461–1468.

28. Markovic-Plese S, Fukaura H, Zhang J, et al. T-cell recognition of immunodominant and cryptic proteolipid protein epitopes in humans. *J Immunol* 1995;155(2):982–992.

29. Kerlero de Rosbo N, Hoffman M, Mendel I, et al. Predominance of the autoimmune response to myelin oligodendrocyte glycoprotein (MOG) in multiple sclerosis: reactivity to the extracellular domain of MOG is directed against three main regions. *Eur J Immunol* 1997;27(11):3059–3069.

30. Allegretta M, Nicklas JA, Sriram S, et al. T-cells responsive to myelin basic protein in patients with multiple sclerosis. *Science* 1990;247(4943):718–721.

31. Pender MP. Infection of autoreactive B lymphocytes with EBV, causing chronic autoimmune diseases. *Trends Immunol* 2003;24(11):584–588.

32. Martin R, Jaraquemada D, Flerlage M, et al. Fine specificity and HLA restriction of myelin basic protein-specific cytotoxic T-cell lines from multiple sclerosis patients and healthy individuals. *J Immunol* 1990;145(2):540–548.

33. Pender MP, Csurhes PA, Greer JM, et al. Surges of increased T-cell reactivity to an encephalitogenic region of myelin proteolipid protein occur more often in patients with multiple sclerosis than in healthy subjects. *J Immunol* 2000;165(9):5322–5331.

34. Pette M, Fujita K, Kitze B, et al. Myelin basic protein-specific T lymphocyte lines from MS patients and healthy individuals. *Neurology* 1990;40(11):1770–1776.

35. Zhang J, Markovic-Plese S, Lacet B, et al. Increased frequency of interleukin 2-responsive T-cells specific for myelin basic protein and proteolipid protein in peripheral blood and cerebrospinal fluid of patients with multiple sclerosis. *J Exp Med* 1994;179(3):973–984.

36. Bielekova B, Sung MH, Kadom N, et al. Expansion and functional relevance of high-avidity myelin-specific CD4+ T-cells in multiple sclerosis. *J Immunol* 2004;172(6):3893–3904.

37. Scholz C, Patton KT, Anderson DE, et al. Expansion of autoreactive T-cells in multiple sclerosis is independent of exogenous B7 costimulation. *J Immunol* 1998; 160(3):1532–1538.

38. Lovett-Racke AE, Trotter JL, Lauber J, et al. Decreased dependence of myelin basic protein-reactive T-cells on CD28-mediated costimulation in multiple sclerosis patients. A marker of activated/memory T-cells. *J Clin Invest* 1998;101(4):725–730.

39. Burns J, Bartholomew B, Lobo S. Isolation of myelin basic protein-specific T-cells predominantly from the memory T-cell compartment in multiple sclerosis. *Ann Neurol* 1999;45(1):33–39.

40. Bielekova B, Muraro PA, Golestaneh L, et al. Preferential expansion of autoreactive T lymphocytes from the memory T-cell pool by IL-7. *J Neuroimmunol* 1999;100(1–2):115–123.

41. Bar-Or A, O'Connor K, Hafler DA. Multiple Sclerosis. In: Austen KF, Frank MM, Atkinson JP, Cantor H, eds. *Samter's Immunologic Diseases*. 6th ed. Philadephia: Lippincott Williams & Wilkins, 2001: 711–737.

42. Becher B, Giacomini PS, Pelletier D, et al. Interferon-gamma secretion by peripheral blood T-cell subsets in multiple sclerosis: correlation with disease phase and interferon-beta therapy. *Ann Neurol* 1999;45(2): 247–250.

43. Biddison WE, Cruikshank WW, Center DM, et al. CD8+ myelin peptide-specific T-cells can chemoattract CD4+ myelin peptide-specific T-cells: importance of IFN-inducible protein 10. *J Immunol* 1998;160(1): 444–448.

44. Krogsgaard M, Wucherpfennig KW, Cannella B, et al. Visualization of myelin basic protein (MBP) T-cell epitopes in multiple sclerosis lesions using a monoclonal antibody specific for the human histocompatibility leukocyte antigen (HLA)-DR2-MBP 85–99 complex. *J Exp Med* 2000;191(8):1395–1412.

45. Babbe H, Roers A, Waisman A, Lassmann H, et al. Clonal expansions of CD8(+) T-cells dominate the T-cell infiltrate in active multiple sclerosis lesions as shown by micromanipulation and single cell polymerase chain reaction. *J Exp Med* 2000;192(3): 393–404.

46. Hoftberger R, Aboul-Enein F, Brueck W, et al. Expression of major histocompatibility complex class I molecules on the different cell types in multiple sclerosis lesions. *Brain Pathol* 2004;14(1):43–50.

47. Skulina C, Schmidt S, Dornmair K, et al. Multiple sclerosis: brain-infiltrating CD8+ T-cells persist as clonal expansions in the cerebrospinal fluid and blood. *Proc Natl Acad Sci USA* 2004;101(8):2428–2433.

48. Tsuchida T, Parker KC, Turner RV, et al. Autoreactive CD8+ T-cell responses to human myelin protein-derived peptides. *Proc Natl Acad Sci USA* 1994;91(23): 10859–10863.

49. Buckle GJ, Hollsberg P, Hafler DA. Activated CD8+ T-cells in secondary progressive MS secrete lymphotoxin. *Neurology* 2003;60(4):702–705.

50. Crawford MP, Yan SX, Ortega SB, et al. High prevalence of autoreactive, neuroantigen-specific CD8+ T-cells in multiple sclerosis revealed by novel flow cytometric assay. *Blood* 2004;103(11):4222–4231.

51. Illes Z, Kondo T, Newcombe J, et al. Differential expression of NK T-cell V alpha 24J alpha Q invariant TCR chain in the lesions of multiple sclerosis and chronic inflammatory demyelinating polyneuropathy. *J Immunol* 2000;164(8):4375–4381.

52. Murzenok PP, Matusevicius D, Freedman MS. Gamma/delta T-cells in multiple sclerosis: chemokine and chemokine receptor expression. *Clin Immunol* 2002;103(3 Pt 1):309–316.

53. Karin N, Mitchell DJ, Brocke S, et al. Reversal of experimental autoimmune encephalomyelitis by a soluble peptide variant of a myelin basic protein epitope: T-cell receptor antagonism and reduction of interferon gamma and tumor necrosis factor alpha production. *J Exp Med* 1994;180(6):2227–2237.

54. Young DA, Lowe LD, Booth SS, et al. IL-4, IL-10, IL-13, and TGF-beta from an altered peptide ligand-specific Th2 cell clone down-regulate adoptive transfer of experimental autoimmune encephalomyelitis. *J Immunol* 2000;164(7):3563–3572.

55. Kappos L, Comi G, Panitch H, et al. Induction of a non-encephalitogenic type 2 T helper-cell autoimmune response in multiple sclerosis after administration of an altered peptide ligand in a placebo-controlled, randomized phase II trial. The Altered Peptide Ligand in Relapsing MS Study Group. *Nat Med* 2000;6(10): 1176–1182.

56. Bielekova B, Goodwin B, Richert N, et al. Encephalitogenic potential of the myelin basic protein peptide (amino acids 83–99) in multiple sclerosis: results of a phase II clinical trial with an altered peptide ligand. *Nat Med* 2000;6(10):1167–1175.

57. Martino G, Adorini L, Rieckmann P, et al. Inflammation in multiple sclerosis: the good, the bad, and the complex. *Lancet Neurol* 2002;1(8):499–509.

58. Moalem G, Leibowitz-Amit R, Yoles E, et al. Autoimmune T-cells protect neurons from secondary degeneration after central nervous system axotomy. *Nat Med* 1999;5(1):49–55.

59. Wekerle H, Linington C, Lassmann H.. Cellular immune reactivity within the CNS. *Trends Neurosci* 1986;9:271–277.

60. Hickey WF. Migration of hematogenous cells through the blood-brain barrier and the initiation of CNS inflammation. *Brain Pathol* 1991;1(2):97–105.

61. Kivisäkk P, Mahad DJ, Callahan MK, et al. Human cerebrospinal fluid central memory CD4+ T-cells: evidence for trafficking through choroid plexus and meninges via P-selectin. *Proc Natl Acad Sci USA* 2003;100(14):8389–8394.

62. Williams K, Ulvestad E, Antel JP. B7/BB-1 antigen expression on adult human microglia studied in vitro and in situ. *Eur J Immunol* 1994;24(12):3031–3037.

63. Windhagen A, Newcombe J, Dangond F, et al. Expression of costimulatory molecules B7–1 (CD80), B7–2 (CD86), and interleukin 12 cytokine in multiple sclerosis lesions. *J Exp Med* 1995;182(6):1985–1996.

64. Genc K, Dona DL, Reder AT. Increased CD80(+) B-cells in active multiple sclerosis and reversal by interferon beta-1b therapy. *J Clin Invest* 1997;99(11):2664–2671.

65. Kuchroo VK, Das MP, Brown JA, et al. B7-1 and B7-2 costimulatory molecules activate differentially the Th1/Th2 developmental pathways: application to autoimmune disease therapy. *Cell* 1995;80(5):707–718.

66. Racke MK, Scott DE, Quigley L, et al. Distinct roles for B7-1 (CD-80) and B7-2 (CD-86) in the initiation of

experimental allergic encephalomyelitis. *J Clin Invest* 1995;96(5):2195–2203.

67. Miller SD, Vanderlugt CL, Lenschow DJ, et al. Blockade of CD28/B7–1 interaction prevents epitope spreading and clinical relapses of murine EAE. *Immunity* 1995;3(6):739–745.

68. Corcione A, Casazza S, Ferretti E, et al. Recapitulation of B-cell differentiation in the central nervous system of patients with multiple sclerosis. *Proc Natl Acad Sci USA* 2004;101(30):11064–11069.

69. Cserr HF, Harling-Berg CJ, Knopf PM. Drainage of brain extracellular fluid into blood and deep cervical lymph and its immunological significance. *Brain Pathol* 1992;2(4):269–276.

70. de Vos AF, van Meurs M, Brok HP, et al. Transfer of central nervous system autoantigens and presentation in secondary lymphoid organs. *J Immunol* 2002; 169(10):5415–5423.

71. Kivisäkk P, Mahad DJ, Callahan MK, et al. Expression of CCR7 in multiple sclerosis: implications for CNS immunity. *Ann Neurol* 2004;55(5):627–638.

72. Wucherpfennig KW, Strominger JL. Molecular mimicry in T-cell-mediated autoimmunity: viral peptides activate human T-cell clones specific for myelin basic protein. *Cell* 1999;80:695–705.

73. Lang HL, Jacobsen H, Ikemizu S, et al. A functional and structural basis for TCR cross-reactivity in multiple sclerosis. *Nat Immunol* 2002;3(10):940–943.

74. Springer TA. Traffic signals for lymphocyte recirculation and leukocyte emigration: the multistep paradigm. *Cell* 1994;76(2):301–314.

75. Ransohoff RM. Mechanisms of inflammation in MS tissue: adhesion molecules and chemokines. *J Neuroimmunol* 1999;98(1):57–68.

76. Campbell JJ, Hedrick J, Zlotnik A, et al. Chemokines and the arrest of lymphocytes rolling under flow conditions. *Science* 1998;279(5349):381–384.

77. Yong VW, Power C, Forsyth P, et al. Metalloproteinases in biology and pathology of the nervous system. *Nat Rev Neurosci* 2001;2(7):502–511.

78. Sobel RA, Mitchell ME, Fondren G. Intercellular adhesion molecule-1 (ICAM-1) in cellular immune reactions in the human central nervous system. *Am J Pathol* 1990;136(6):1309–1316.

79. Washington R, Burton J, Todd RF, 3rd, et al. Expression of immunologically relevant endothelial cell activation antigens on isolated central nervous system microvessels from patients with multiple sclerosis. *Ann Neurol* 1994;35(1):89–97.

80. Cannella B, Raine CS. The adhesion molecule and cytokine profile of multiple sclerosis lesions. *Ann Neurol* 1995;37(4):424–435.

81. Bo L, Peterson JW, Mork S, et al. Distribution of immunoglobulin superfamily members ICAM-1, -2, -3, and the beta 2 integrin LFA-1 in multiple sclerosis lesions. *J Neuropathol Exp Neurol* 1996;55(10): 1060–1072.

82. Brosnan CF, Cannella B, Battistini L, et al. Cytokine localization in multiple sclerosis lesions: correlation with adhesion molecule expression and reactive nitrogen species. *Neurology* 1995;45[Suppl 6]S16–S21.

83. Damle NK, Klussman K, Leytze G, et al. Costimulation with integrin ligands intercellular adhesion molecule-1 or vascular cell adhesion molecule-1

augments activation-induced death of antigen-specific CD4+ T lymphocytes. *J Immunol* 1993;151(5): 2368–2379.

84. Moingeon P, Chang HC, Wallner BP, et al. CD2-mediated adhesion facilitates T lymphocyte antigen recognition function. *Nature* 1989;339(6222):312–314.

85. Karpus WJ, Ransohoff RM. Chemokine regulation of experimental autoimmune encephalomyelitis: temporal and spatial expression patterns govern disease pathogenesis. *J Immunol* 1998;161(6):2667–2671.

86. Hvas J, McLean C, Justesen J, et al. Perivascular T-cells express the pro-inflammatory chemokine RANTES mRNA in multiple sclerosis lesions. *Scand J Immunol* 1997;46(2):195–203.

87. Van Der Voorn P, Tekstra J, Beelen RH, et al. Expression of MCP-1 by reactive astrocytes in demyelinating multiple sclerosis lesions. *Am J Pathol* 1999;154(1): 45–51.

88. Sorensen TL, Tani M, Jensen J, et al. Expression of specific chemokines and chemokine receptors in the central nervous system of multiple sclerosis patients. *J Clin Invest* 1999;103(6):807–815.

89. Siveke JT, Hamann A. T helper 1 and T helper 2 cells respond differentially to chemokines. *J Immunol* 1998;160(2):550–554.

90. Balashov KE, Rottman JB, Weiner HL, et al. CCR5(+) and CXCR3(+) T-cells are increased in multiple sclerosis and their ligands MIP-1alpha and IP-10 are expressed in demyelinating brain lesions. *Proc Natl Acad Sci USA* 1999;96(12):6873–6878.

91. Misu T, Onodera H, Fujihara K, et al. Chemokine receptor expression on T-cells in blood and cerebrospinal fluid at relapse and remission of multiple sclerosis: imbalance of Th1/Th2-associated chemokine signaling. *J Neuroimmunol* 2001;114(1–2):207–212.

92. Nanki T, Lipsky PE. Lack of correlation between chemokine receptor and T(h)1/T(h)2 cytokine expression by individual memory T-cells. *Int Immunol* 2000;12(12):1659–1667.

93. Yong VW, Krekoski CA, Forsyth PA, et al. Matrix metalloproteinases and diseases of the CNS. *Trends Neurosci* 1998;21(2):75–80.

94. Kieseier BC, Seifert T, Giovannoni G, et al. Matrix metalloproteinases in inflammatory demyelination: targets for treatment. *Neurology* 1999;53(1):20–25.

95. Kieseier BC, Pischel H, Neuen-Jacob E, et al. ADAM-10 and ADAM-17 in the inflamed human CNS. *Glia* 2003;42(4):398–405.

96. Rosenberg GA, Kornfeld M, Estrada E, et al. TIMP-2 reduces proteolytic opening of blood-brain barrier by type IV collagenase. *Brain Res* 1992;576(2):203–207.

97. Leppert D, Waubant E, Galardy R, et al. T-cell gelatinases mediate basement membrane transmigration in vitro. *J Immunol* 1995;154(9):4379–4389.

98. Cuzner ML, Gveric D, Strand C, et al. The expression of tissue-type plasminogen activator, matrix metalloproteases and endogenous inhibitors in the central nervous system in multiple sclerosis: comparison of stages in lesion evolution. *J Neuropathol Exp Neurol* 1996;55(12):1194–1204.

99. Maeda A, Sobel RA. Matrix metalloproteinases in the normal human central nervous system, microglial nodules, and multiple sclerosis lesions. *J Neuropathol Exp Neurol* 1996;55(3):300–309.

100. Hartung HP, Jung S, Stoll G, et al. Inflammatory mediators in demyelinating disorders of the CNS and PNS. *J Neuroimmunol* 1992;40(2–3):197–210.

101. Black RA, Rauch CT, Kozlosky CJ, et al. A metalloproteinase disintegrin that releases tumour-necrosis factor-alpha from cells. *Nature* 1997;385(6618): 729–733.

102. Proost P, Van Damme J, Opdenakker G. Leukocyte gelatinase B cleavage releases encephalitogens from human myelin basic protein. *Biochem Biophys Res Commun* 1993;192(3):1175–1181.

103. Cuzner ML, Davison AN, Rudge P. Proteolytic enzyme activity of blood leukocytes and cerebrospinal fluid in multiple sclerosis. *Ann Neurol* 1978;4(4): 337–344.

104. Gijbels K, Masure S, Carton H, et al. Gelatinase in the cerebrospinal fluid of patients with multiple sclerosis and other inflammatory neurological disorders. *J Neuroimmunol* 1992;41(1):29–34.

105. Leppert D, Ford J, Stabler G, et al. Matrix metalloproteinase-9 (gelatinase B) is selectively elevated in CSF during relapses and stable phases of multiple sclerosis. *Brain* 1998;121 (Pt 12):2327–2334.

106. Lee MA, Palace J, Stabler G, et al. Serum gelatinase B, TIMP-1 and TIMP-2 levels in multiple sclerosis. A longitudinal clinical and MRI study. *Brain* 1999;122 (Pt 2):191–197.

107. Bar-Or A, Nuttall RK, Duddy M, et al. Analyses of all matrix metalloproteinase members in leukocytes emphasize monocytes as major inflammatory mediators in multiple sclerosis. *Brain* 2003;126(Pt 12):2738–2749.

108. Alter A, Duddy M, Hebert S, et al. Determinants of human B-cell migration across brain endothelial cells. *J Immunol* 2003;170(9):4497–4505.

109. Hickey WF, Hsu BL, Kimura H. T-lymphocyte entry into the central nervous system. *J Neurosci Res* 1991;28(2):254–260.

110. Genain CP, Cannella B, Hauser SL, et al. Identification of autoantibodies associated with myelin damage in multiple sclerosis. *Nat Med* 1999;5(2):170–175.

111. Raine CS, Cannella B, Hauser SL, et al. Demyelination in primate autoimmune encephalomyelitis and acute multiple sclerosis lesions: a case for antigen-specific antibody mediation. *Ann Neurol* 1999;46(2):144–160.

112. Piddlesden SJ, Lassmann H, Zimprich F, et al. The demyelinating potential of antibodies to myelin oligodendrocyte glycoprotein is related to their ability to fix complement. *Am J Pathol* 1993;143(2):555–564.

113. Pender MP. The pathogenesis of primary progressive multiple sclerosis: antibody-mediated attack and no repair? *J Clin Neurosci* 2004;11(7):689–692.

114. O'Connor KC, Chitnis T, Griffin DE, et al. Myelin basic protein-reactive autoantibodies in the serum and cerebrospinal fluid of multiple sclerosis patients are characterized by low-affinity interactions. *J Neuroimmunol* 2003;136(1–2):140–148.

115. Berger T, Rubner P, Schautzer F, et al. Antimyelin antibodies as a predictor of clinically definite multiple sclerosis after a first demyelinating event. *N Engl J Med* 2003;349(2):139–145.

116. Antel JP, Bar-Or A. Do myelin-directed antibodies predict multiple sclerosis? *N Engl J Med* 2003;349(2): 107–109.

117. Miller DJ, Asakura K, Rodriguez M. Experimental strategies to promote central nervous system remyelination in multiple sclerosis: insights gained from the Theiler's virus model system. *J Neurosci Res* 1995;41(3):291–296.

118. Miller DJ, Njenga MK, Murray PD, et al. A monoclonal natural autoantibody that promotes remyelination suppresses central nervous system inflammation and increases virus expression after Theiler's virus-induced demyelination. *Int Immunol* 1996;8(1): 131–141.

119. Li W, Walus L, Rabacchi SA, et al. A neutralizing anti-Nogo66 receptor monoclonal antibody reverses inhibition of neurite outgrowth by central nervous system myelin. *J Biol Chem* 2004;279(42): 43780–43788.

120. Bar-Or A, Oliveira EM, Anderson DE, et al. Immunological memory: contribution of memory B-cells expressing costimulatory molecules in the resting state. *J Immunol* 2001;167(10):5669–5677.

121. Prineas JW. Multiple sclerosis: presence of lymphatic capillaries and lymphoid tissue in the brain and spinal cord. *Science* 1979;203(4385):1123–1125.

122. Serafini B, Rosicarelli B, Magliozzi R, et al. Detection of ectopic B-cell follicles with germinal centers in the meninges of patients with secondary progressive multiple sclerosis. *Brain Pathol* 2004;14(2):164–174.

123. Duddy ME, Alter A, Bar-Or A. Distinct profiles of human B-cell effector cytokines: a role in immune regulation? *J Immunol* 2004;172(6):3422–3427.

124. Anderson AC, Reddy J, Nazareno R, et al. IL-10 plays an important role in the homeostatic regulation of the autoreactive repertoire in naive mice. *J Immunol* 2004;173(2):828–834.

125. Fillatreau S, Sweenie CH, McGeachy MJ, et al. B-cells regulate autoimmunity by provision of IL-10. *Nat Immunol* 2002;3(10):944–950.

126. Aloisi F, Ria F, Penna G, et al. Microglia are more efficient than astrocytes in antigen processing and in Th1 but not Th2 cell activation. *J Immunol* 1998;160(10): 4671–4680.

127. Williams K, Ulvestad E, Antel J. Immune regulatory and effector properties of human adult microglia studies in vitro and in situ. *Adv Neuroimmunol* 1994; 4(3):273–281.

128. Ulvestad E, Williams K, Bjerkvig R, et al. Human microglial cells have phenotypic and functional characteristics in common with both macrophages and dendritic antigen-presenting cells. *J Leukoc Biol* 1994;56(6):732–740.

129. Kim HJ, Ifergan I, Antel JP, et al. Type 2 monocyte and microglia differentiation mediated by glatiramer acetate therapy in patients with multiple sclerosis. *J Immunol* 2004;172(11):7144–7153.

130. Tuohy VK, Yu M, Yin L, et al. The epitope spreading cascade during progression of experimental autoimmune encephalomyelitis and multiple sclerosis. *Immunol Rev* 1998;164:93–100.

131. Giuliani F, Goodyer CG, Antel JP, et al. Vulnerability of human neurons to T-cell-mediated cytotoxicity. *J Immunol* 2003;171(1):368–379.

132. Neumann H, Medana IM, Bauer J, et al. Cytotoxic T lymphocytes in autoimmune and degenerative CNS diseases. *Trends Neurosci* 2002;25(6):313–319.

133. Waxman SG. Nitric oxide and the axonal death cascade. *Ann Neurol* 2003;53(2):150–153.

134. Waxman SG. Acquired channelopathies in nerve injury and MS. *Neurology* 2001;56(12):1621–1627.

135. Chari DM, Blakemore WF. New insights into remyelination failure in multiple sclerosis: implications for glial cell transplantation. *Mult Scler* 2002;8(4):271–277.

136. Reddy H, Narayanan S, Matthews PM, et al. Relating axonal injury to functional recovery in MS. *Neurology* 2000;54(1):236–239.

137. Weber MS, Starck M, Wagenpfeil S, et al. Multiple sclerosis: glatiramer acetate inhibits monocyte reactivity in vitro and in vivo. *Brain* 2004;127(Pt 6):1370–1378.

138. Schwartz M. Protective autoimmunity as a T-cell response to central nervous system trauma: prospects for therapeutic vaccines. *Prog Neurobiol* 2001;65(5):489–496.

139. Sakaguchi S, Sakaguchi N, Asano M, et al. Immunologic self-tolerance maintained by activated T-cells expressing IL-2 receptor alpha-chains (CD25). Breakdown of a single mechanism of self-tolerance causes various autoimmune diseases. *J Immunol* 1995;155(3):1151–1164.

140. Anderton S, Burkhart C, Metzler B, et al. Mechanisms of central and peripheral T-cell tolerance: lessons from experimental models of multiple sclerosis. *Immunol Rev* 1999;169:123–137.

141. Kohm AP, Carpentier PA, Anger HA, et al. Cutting edge: CD4+CD25+ regulatory T-cells suppress antigen-specific autoreactive immune responses and central nervous system inflammation during active experimental autoimmune encephalomyelitis. *J Immunol* 2002;169(9):4712–4716.

142. Baecher-Allan C, Viglietta V, Hafler DA. Human CD4+CD25+ regulatory T-cells. *Semin Immunol* 2004;16(2):89–98.

143. Viglietta V, Baecher-Allan C, Weiner HL, et al. Loss of functional suppression by CD4+CD25+ regulatory T-cells in patients with multiple sclerosis. *J Exp Med* 2004;199(7):971–979.

144. Cottrez F, Groux H. Specialization in tolerance: innate CD(4+)CD(25+) versus acquired TR1 and TH3 regulatory T-cells. *Transplantation* 2004;77[1 Suppl]S12–S15.

145. Hu D, Ikizawa K, Lu L, et al. Analysis of regulatory CD8 T-cells in Qa-1-deficient mice. *Nat Immunol* 2004;5(5):516–523.

146. Chess L, Jiang H. Resurrecting CD8+ suppressor T-cells. *Nat Immunol* 2004;5(5):469–471.

147. Kerschensteiner M, Gallmeier E, Behrens L, et al. Activated human T-cells, B-cells, and monocytes produce brain-derived neurotrophic factor in vitro and in inflammatory brain lesions: a neuroprotective role of inflammation? *J Exp Med* 1999;189(5):865–870.

148. Stadelmann C, Kerschensteiner M, Misgeld T, et al. BDNF and gp145trkB in multiple sclerosis brain lesions: neuroprotective interactions between immune and neuronal cells? *Brain* 2002;125(Pt 1):75–85.

149. Arnett HA, Mason J, Marino M, et al. TNF alpha promotes proliferation of oligodendrocyte progenitors and remyelination. *Nat Neurosci* 2001;4(11):1116–1122.

150. Miller DJ, Rodriguez M. A monoclonal autoantibody that promotes central nervous system remyelination in a model of multiple sclerosis is a natural autoantibody encoded by germline immunoglobulin genes. *J Immunol* 1995;154(5):2460–2469.

151. Reindl M, Khantane S, Ehling R, et al. Serum and cerebrospinal fluid antibodies to Nogo-A in patients with multiple sclerosis and acute neurological disorders. *J Neuroimmunol* 2003;145(1–2):139–147.

152. Schwab ME. Nogo and axon regeneration. *Curr Opin Neurobiol* 2004;14(1):118–124.

153. Herx LM, Rivest S, Yong VW. Central nervous system-initiated inflammation and neurotrophism in trauma: IL-1 beta is required for the production of ciliary neurotrophic factor. *J Immunol* 2000;165(4):2232–2239.

154. Mason JL, Suzuki K, Chaplin DD, et al. Interleukin-1beta promotes repair of the CNS. *J Neurosci* 2001;21(18):7046–7052.

155. Wosik K, Antel J, Kuhlmann T, et al. Oligodendrocyte injury in multiple sclerosis: a role for p53. *J Neurochem* 2003;85(3):635–644.

156. Niehaus A, Shi J, Grzenkowski M, et al. Patients with active relapsing-remitting multiple sclerosis synthesize antibodies recognizing oligodendrocyte progenitor cell surface protein: implications for remyelination. *Ann Neurol* 2000;48(3):362–371.

157. Antel JP, Bar-Or A. Multiple Sclerosis: Therapy. In: Lazzarini R, ed. *Myelin Biology and Disorders*: Boston: Elsevier Academic Press, 2004: 791–806.

158. Rudick RA, Ransohoff RM, Peppler R, et al. Interferon beta induces interleukin-10 expression: relevance to multiple sclerosis. *Ann Neurol* 1996;40(4):618–627.

159. Kilinc M, Saatci-Cekirge I, Karabudak R. Serial analysis of soluble intercellular adhesion molecule-1 level in relapsing-remitting multiple sclerosis patients during IFN-beta1b treatment. *J Interferon Cytokine Res* 2003;23(3):127–133.

160. Karabudak R, Kurne A, Guc D, et al. Effect of interferon beta-1a on serum matrix metalloproteinase-9 (MMP-9) and tissue inhibitor of matrix metalloproteinase (TIMP-1) in relapsing remitting multiple sclerosis patients. One year follow-up results. *J Neurol* 2004;251(3):279–283.

161. Galboiz Y, Shapiro S, Lahat N, et al. Matrix metalloproteinases and their tissue inhibitors as markers of disease subtype and response to interferon-beta therapy in relapsing and secondary-progressive multiple sclerosis patients. *Ann Neurol* 2001;50(4):443–451.

162. Yong VW. Differential mechanisms of action of interferon-beta and glatiramer aetate in MS. *Neurology* 2002;59(6):802–808.

163. Teitelbaum D, Meshorer A, Hirshfeld T, et al. Suppression of experimental allergic encephalomyelitis by a synthetic polypeptide. *Eur J Immunol* 1971;1(4):242–248.

164. Miller A, Shapiro S, Gershtein R, et al. Treatment of multiple sclerosis with copolymer-1 (Copaxone): implicating mechanisms of Th1 to Th2/Th3 immune-deviation. *J Neuroimmunol* 1998;92(1–2):113–121.

165. Qin Y, Zhang DQ, Prat A, et al. Characterization of T-cell lines derived from glatiramer-acetate-treated multiple sclerosis patients. *J Neuroimmunol* 2000;108(1–2):201–206.

166. Neuhaus O, Farina C, Yassouridis A, et al. Multiple sclerosis: comparison of copolymer-1-reactive T-cell lines from treated and untreated subjects reveals cytokine shift from T helper 1 to T helper 2 cells. *Proc Natl Acad Sci USA* 2000;97(13):7452–7457.

167. Karandikar NJ, Crawford MP, Yan X. Glatiramer acetate (Copaxone) therapy induces CD8(+) T-cell responses in patients with multiple sclerosis. *J Clin Invest* 2002;109:641–649.

168. Schmied M, Duda PW, Krieger JI, et al. In vitro evidence that subcutaneous administration of glatiramer acetate induces hyporesponsive T-cells in patients with multiple sclerosis. *Clin Immunol* 2003;106(3): 163–174.

169. Hafler DA. Degeneracy, as opposed to specificity, in immunotherapy. *J Clin Invest* 2002;109(5):581–584.

170. Duda PW, Schmied MC, Cook SL, et al. Glatiramer acetate (Copaxone) induces degenerate, Th2-polarized immune responses in patients with multiple sclerosis. *J Clin Invest* 2000;105(7):967–976.

171. Kim HJ, Biernacki K, Prat A, et al. Inflammatory potential and migratory capacities across human brain endothelial cells of distinct glatiramer acetate-reactive T-cells generated in treated multiple sclerosis patients. *Clin Immunol* 2004;111(1):38–46.

172. Ziemssen T, Kumpfel T, Klinkert WE, et al. Glatiramer acetate-specific T-helper 1- and 2-type cell lines produce BDNF: implications for multiple sclerosis therapy. Brain-derived neurotrophic factor. *Brain* 2002;125(Pt 11):2381–2391.

173. Chen M, Valenzuela RM, Dhib-Jalbut S. Glatiramer acetate-reactive T-cells produce brain-derived neurotrophic factor. *J Neurol Sci* 2003;215(1–2):37–44.

8

Making the Diagnosis of Multiple Sclerosis

Gary Birnbaum

MS Treatment and Research Center, Minneapolis Clinic of Neurology, Golden Valley, Minnesota

"I don't need any tests to diagnose MS. I can smell it."

A well-known MS specialist

For those of us who do not have the olfactory perspicacity of our colleague, the diagnosis of MS remains a challenge. New techniques and criteria have increased our ability to diagnosis the progressive, inflammatory, central nervous system disease that is MS, but at the same time have allowed us to detect pathologic and nonpathologic changes that can mimic MS in ways that increase the difficulty of diagnosis. In the final analysis, MS remains a clinical diagnosis with laboratory parameters that are of value in supporting the diagnosis and in excluding MS "look-alikes."

More experienced readers of this chapter will almost certainly recall individuals presenting with a variety of unusual symptoms and signs not mentioned by me. My intent in this chapter is not to be encyclopedic and list all permutations of this enormously pleomorphic disease, but to pro-vide a fundamental foundation for assessment, utilizing the most common features of this illness.

PATTERNS OF DISEASE PRESENTATION

Before proceeding to a discussion of the particular clinical signs and symptoms of MS, one must understand the different patterns of disease progression and how initial clinical presentations will vary depending on the pattern of an individual's MS. Four general patterns of disease progression are described (1).

The most common pattern, noted in about 85% of persons with MS, is one of relapsing and remitting neurologic symptoms. Neurologic symptoms may appear over minutes to hours and remit, either partially or completely, over days to months. Intervals between relapses vary greatly. The next most common is a pattern of onset characterized by the insidious development of neurologic symptoms over weeks to months. Symptoms slowly progress with no true remission but with intermittent periods of disease stability. This pattern is called primary progressive MS and diagnostic criteria for this pattern of disease differ from those of relapsing-remitting MS (2). Primary progressive MS must be differentiated from secondary progressive MS, discussed below. Least common and noted, at most, in only 5% of persons with MS, is a pattern of disease characterized by insidious onset of neurologic difficulties with occasional, superimposed relapses and remissions. This pattern is called, appropriately, progressive relapsing MS. A large proportion of persons with relapsing-remitting MS will change their pattern of disease over time to one of gradual progression of neurologic difficulty with no superimposed relapses. In this pattern, individuals with an initial disease presentation of relapses and remissions note a gradual decrease in relapse frequency (a phase called transitional MS), followed by a gradually progressive increase in neurologic difficulties. This pattern is called secondary progressive MS and can manifest itself many years after an antecedent relapse. This is important for the diagnostician, since recall of one or two minor relapses decades earlier may be difficult and progression of symptoms may be comparable to those noted with primary progressive MS. However, the pathogenesis and treatments of these two patterns of MS may be different (3,4) so every effort should be made to identify any prior, acute neurologic episodes in persons with gradually increasing neurologic dysfunction before making a diagnosis of primary progressive MS.

Demographics of the Different Forms of MS

While not essential for making a diagnosis of MS, understanding the demographics of the different patterns of MS is of value. Relapsing-remitting MS is a disease of young adults, usually presenting between the ages of 15 and 50. While individuals outside these age limits are described, they are relatively uncommon. Women predominate at ratios of 2–3:1 over men. In contrast, primary progressive MS is most common in adults in their middle years, between ages 30 and 60, with equal ratios of men and women. Patients with progressive relapsing MS are similar to those with primary progressive MS.

THE GENETICS OF MS

While the multitude of genes involved in the pathogenesis of MS are not known, they most likely first segregated in northern Europe (5). As a result, most persons with MS are either of northern European origin or have ancestors from that region. As a corollary, while there may be only six degrees of separation between all of us, MS is very rare in certain racial populations. These are well described (6), and include American Indians, African blacks, Hutterites (7), and Asians. While demyelinating diseases can occur in Asians, their patterns of presentation are different than those of MS, as are their laboratory findings (8,9). Further details will be discussed in the section on the differential diagnosis of MS (Excluding MS "Look-alikes"). The genes most associated with susceptibility to MS are those of the major histocompatibility complex (10), especially the HLA-DR2 genes, but there is sufficient heterogeneity of these genes in persons with MS that they are of no value in terms of diagnosis.

Initial Clinical Symptoms in Persons with Relapsing-Remitting MS

The initial symptoms of relapsing-remitting MS are as varied as the functions of the central nervous system. None are specific for MS and, as will be repeated throughout this chapter, other illnesses causing similar symptoms must be excluded. However, certain symptoms are much more common in MS and can suggest the possibility of an inflammatory central nervous system process.

Presenting symptoms often are described both in neurologic terms (numbness, weakness, tremors), and in changes of function, such as increased difficulty with handwriting or doing up buttons, increased difficulty with walking, running, or leg coordination, or difficulty tracking with reading, Such symptoms are diverse in their possible etiologies, and the diagnostician may need to rely on physical signs for greater clarification. However, it is essential to remember that, in the absence of objective data indicating the presence of central nervous system dysfunction, one cannot make a diagnosis of MS. In other words, symptoms alone are insufficient to diagnose MS (11).

Among the most common presenting symptoms are changes in visual function. These can take the form of monocular (rarely binocular) decreased visual acuity or blurred vision, described as "looking through a fogged window or smudged eyeglasses," often involving central vision more than peripheral vision. Less common is a loss of color intensity, with everything appearing "bleached" or lighter. In severe instances, vision is lost entirely. If the visual loss results from inflammation of the optic nerve, as opposed to an optic chiasmal lesion, there may be sharp or dull pain behind and over the eye, worse with eye movement, and at times preceding the onset of visual difficulty by days to weeks. In MS, these visual difficulties are most likely the result of an inflammation of the optic nerve (optic neuritis) and can occur over a matter of hours to days, often subsiding completely without treatment, over weeks to months.

Sensory symptoms as presenting features in MS are also very frequent. Their onset, in contrast to sensory changes of compressive neuropathies or radiculopathies, is usually painless, with some exceptions (12). Patterns of sensory change vary widely, at times involving particular dermatomes, such as the C7–T2 dermatomes, hands, feet, and legs. Gradually ascending sensory symptoms are common, often involving tightness in the abdomen or thorax ("like a girdle or rope"). Less commonly, facial and tongue numbness and tingling are noted. Symptoms may be unilateral or bilateral and can be worsened with fatigue or increased body temperature. The nature of the sensory changes varies, ranging from numbness, to numbness and tingling, to a dysesthetic, uncomfortable, prickling, and often burning sensation (causalgia). None of these sensory changes is unique to MS but, if present bilaterally and associated with a buzzing, electric, shock-like sensation into the back and/or limbs upon neck flexion (L'hermitte sign), strongly suggests the presence of spinal cord dysfunction. As with visual diffi-

culties, symptoms may spontaneously resolve partially or completely over days to weeks.

Vertigo or feelings of imbalance or dizziness are among the most common symptoms in any clinical practice of neurology and can be related to medication, changes in blood pressure, inner ear (vestibular) dysfunction, musculo-skeletal abnormalities of the neck (cervical vertigo), and, of course, brainstem dysfunction in MS. The dizziness and vertigo of central nervous system origin can be positional and worsened with rapid eye movements, but it is unusual for tinnitus and decreased hearing to be part of that symptom complex. Since inflammation of the brain stem in MS often involves other nuclei, the vertigo associated with MS is often associated with other symptoms such as diplopia, oscillopsia, dysarthria, and/or numbness. Isolated vertigo in persons with MS is most often due to inner ear dysfunction rather than central nervous system inflammation (13), and deciding whether an antecedent episode of vertigo was of central or peripheral origin can be difficult.

Double vision with or without oscillopsia (the symptom of nystagmus, with bouncing or jumping vision) can be a presenting symptom in MS. Again, other conditions such as diabetes, vascular disease of the central nervous system (either ischemic or aneurysmal), myasthenia gravis, and neoplastic processes can cause identical symptoms. In MS the diplopia is usually not associated with any pupillary or eyelid changes, and is often present on gaze to either side and vertically. The presence of skew diplopia, or dislocation of objects in the vertical as opposed to horizontal plane, is very suggestive of a central nervous system origin of the diplopia.

Weakness is a common presenting symptom in MS. Often symptoms of weakness will only be noted in a context of prolonged exertion ("My right leg begins to drag only after I've walked five miles"), or with elevations of core body temperature, such as with infections or hot weather. Weakness may involve any part of body but most commonly affects the lower extremities, either proximally or distally. Bilateral lower extremity weakness is most suggestive of spinal cord dysfunction and often is associated with changes in bowel or bladder function as well as changes in tone, with onset of muscle cramping or the appearance of myoclonic jerks, often when lying down at night.

One of the most common symptoms of MS is fatigue, not the kind of fatigue one has from insufficient rest or sleep—that is quickly eased with a nap or a good night's rest. Rather, it is the kind of fatigue one feels after a bout of the flu or other viral infection, namely, a more permeating fatigability that is not eased with rest alone and verges on a generalized feeling of weakness. It can vary in degree from mild to severe, and can be a major component of the initial presentation of MS. A change in energy levels at the time of presentation with any of the above symptoms should make one consider a central nervous system inflammatory process such as MS as a potential cause. However, fatigue can have a multitude of causes ranging from hematologic, metabolic, endocrine, and psychologic (14), and these must all be considered first.

Changes in bowel, bladder, and sexual function, occurring in isolation, are unusual in MS, but frequently occur in association with sensory and motor changes, especially those of the lower extremities, suggesting spinal cord dysfunction. Most common are changes in pattern, with more bladder urgency frequency, more constipation or alternating constipation and diarrhea, and more difficulty with arousal and orgasm. Onset of symptoms of MS may be precipitous, occurring over minutes to hours, or insidious, occurring over days, weeks, and months. Most symptoms of MS persist for more than 48 hours, though fluctuations may be considerable, especially when fatigue or elevations of ambient or core temperature are present, such as with fever, exercise, or hot baths. Worsening of symptoms with elevations of core temperature is called the Uhthoff phenomenon and results from increased conduction block of nerve impulses along already damaged and compromised pathways. Occasionally, presenting MS symptoms may be paroxysmal, such as those occurring with trigeminal neuralgia due to an inflammatory nidus in the region of the Vth cranial nerve. Ten percent of persons with MS will have seizures as a result of cortical inflammation, but seizures as a presenting symptom are unusual and should provoke a search for other causes. Even less

frequent are paroxysmal, dystonic hemicorporeal episodes, lasting for seconds to minutes, and provoked by movement. These are believed to be of spinal origin and are usually seen in individuals with antecedent spinal cord dysfunction. It is unusual for a L'hermitte sign to be a presenting symptom of MS, but it almost always indicates cervical spinal cord dysfunction, either from structural impingement due to cervical spine disease, or to intrinsic cervical spinal cord disease. It is important, though at times very difficult, to distinguish the common neck pain, with neck "crunching and crackling," and radiating muscle spasms, from the painless, electrical "buzzing" of the L'hermitte sign precipitated by neck flexion.

Presenting Symptoms of Primary Progressive MS

In contrast to the often precipitous onset of symptoms in persons with relapsing-remitting MS, the onset of symptoms in persons with primary progressive MS may be so insidious as to preclude determining a time of onset with precision greater than months or years. In addition, visual or cranial nerve symptoms at onset of primary progressive MS are most unusual, in keeping with the pathophysiology of the disease, which mainly involves the spinal cord. Most common symptoms are those of gradually increasing imbalance, extremity weakness, limb tightness, numbness and tingling of either a limb or limbs (usually the legs), and often the lower trunk, with changes in bowel, bladder, and sexual function, similar to those noted with relapsing-remitting MS. Needless to say, this pattern of neurologic change is not unique to persons with primary progressive MS.

PRESENTING SIGNS IN MULTIPLE SCLEROSIS

In general, the findings on neurologic exam are appropriate to the presenting symptoms of an individual. Thus, in persons presenting with the visual difficulties of an optic neuritis, there almost always is decreased visual acuity that is noncorrectable with glasses, visual field defects (usually in the form of central or paracentral scotomata, loss or decrease of color intensity, especially to red), an afferent papillary defect, and, less commonly, edema of the optic nerve. Since demyelination of optic nerves can occur subclinically, the presence of optic atrophy or an afferent papillary defect on neurologic exam, even in the absence of an antecedent history of visual symptoms, can be of great value in identifying the presence of multifocal neurologic dysfunction ("dissemination of neurologic signs in space"). Sensory changes in MS often will not be sharply defined, as they are with peripheral nervous system abnormalities, except for those associated with transverse spinal cord dysfunction where sensory levels on the abdomen or thorax can be very sharply demarcated.

The signs in persons presenting with diplopia are most often those of an internuclear ophthalmoplegia (INO), or an abducens weakness. The INO is usually bilateral; the abducens weakness is usually unilateral. Nystagmus is a feature of an INO yet, in my experience, it usually is not associated with oscillopsia. Rather, persons describe visual blurring with lateral gaze, trouble with tracking when reading, or a discomfort on lateral gaze that cannot be clearly defined.

Persons with symptoms of limb weakness may have demonstrable weakness on formal testing, with or without associated changes in tone. Muscle tone may be normal or diffuse increased with or without spasticity. Reflexes are usually increased and Babinski responses are common.

It is common for the biologic onset of MS to precede the initial clinical presentation. The MRI typically demonstrates much more silent disease than is associated with clear clinical symptoms and signs, so much so that less than 1 in 10 new T2 or contrast-enhancing lesions is associated with the appearance or worsening of a symptom. As a result, there may be findings on neurologic exam that were not noted by the individual and were not associated with any symptom. As noted above, this is commonly seen with abnormalities of the optic nerve where the presence of temporal disc pallor may indicate the presence of a subclinical episode of optic neuritis. Equally common are findings of deep

tendon reflex asymmetry, usually with disproportionately active reflexes of the lower extremities. At times, especially in individuals with symptoms suggestive of spinal cord dysfunction, Babinski responses will be found, with or without associated hyperreflexia and increased lower extremity (LE) tone. Imbalance or gait ataxia may not be noted by the individual but can be seen when attempting to do tandem gait. The causes of such imbalance are multiple, ranging from poor vision, sensory loss, cerebellar dysfunction, or weakness, and this finding must be interpreted in these contexts.

Just as the presence of particular symptoms and signs may suggest a diagnosis of MS, their absence can cast the diagnosis in doubt. Rudick et al. (15) suggested a series of so-called red flag negatives that should cause a diagnostician pause. These include the absence of objective optic nerve or oculomotor findings, the absence of clinical remissions, the absence of sensory findings, the absence of bowel or bladder difficulties, and normal or atypical MRI and CSF findings. None of these is totally exclusionary, especially early in the course of MS or in persons with variants of MS, such as those with primary progressive MS. However, in persons with long neurologic histories and many of the above negatives, a history of diseases other than MS should be considered.

Magnetic Resonance Imaging (MRI)

The advent of MRI has both simplified and complicated making a diagnosis of MS. Since MS is a multifocal, progressive, inflammatory disease of the central nervous system, MRIs are able to demonstrate these changes. However, the changes seen on MRI are based on changes in proton density (water content) and thus are intrinsically nonspecific. "Spots" on MRI thus can occur with any condition that results in changes of brain water content. These can range from normal aging, to migraine, high blood pressure, head injury, infection, or vasculitis. Thus, changes on MRI should never be used in isolation to make a diagnosis of MS, regardless of what the radiology report may state. That said, there are changes on MRI that are very suggestive of the diagnosis of MS.

The changes on MRI seen in persons with MS correlate with the gross and histologic pathology of the disease (16,17). While lesions of MS can occur anywhere, they are most often periventricular and subcortical. Lesions in the corpus callosum and corona radiata are equally common. Less common are lesions in the posterior fossa, but their presence in this region is atypical for many of the other causes of supratentorial "spots," such as hypertension and migraine, and thus reduce the list of possible disease processes. Spinal cord lesions are also common in MS and uncommon in many of the other diseases causing supratentorial changes (18). Their presence again reduces the list of diagnostic possibilities. Pathologically, changes of MS are common in cortical gray matter, and can be very extensive (19). While I have seen changes on MRI in the gray matter, they are uncommon.

In addition to the location of lesions in MS, their configuration, especially on T2/FLAIR (fluid-attenuated inversion-recovery) imaging, can be of value. Again, the MRI changes reflect the pathology of the disease. The inflammation of MS is often perivenular and, as a result, the lesions of MS may have an elongated or oval appearance. When present in rows along the ventricular edge, they have been called Dawson's Fingers. Many lesions are round, and when present subcortically have a curved appearance, reflecting the configuration of the subcortical "U fibers." Criteria for the shape and distribution of MRI lesions suggestive of MS are published. As expected, given the relative nonspecificity of the changes seen on MRI, the sensitivity and specificity of such changes for MS is not 100%. Among the more stringent criteria being used are those promulgated by Barkhoff et al. (20). These are utilized in the diagnostic algorithm proposed by McDonald et al. (21), discussed below. Table 8-1 lists the Barkhoff et al. criteria. While their specificity for MS is high, their sensitivity is of necessity lower, resulting in more false negative assessments.

The MRI can be configured in multiple ways to give different images of lesions. In MS, most lesions are seen with T2/FLAIR imaging. However, other MRI configurations also provide valuable information on the nature of the spots seen. With T1 imaging, the lesions of MS may appear hypointense, giving rise to so-called black holes. There are two kinds of black holes; those that appear transiently (in areas of acute inflammation—these most probably represent focal edema), and those that are permanent (22). Several studies have shown that permanent black holes represent areas of focal axonal loss (23,24). The presence of such black holes in the MRIs of persons with MS suggests a more destructive pattern of disease, one that can lead to another change in MRI, namely, atrophy (25,26).

Recent data show that brain atrophy is an early feature of MS (19,27,28). Measures of atrophy are not standardized (25) and assessing atrophy on MRI can be difficult, using only one's eyeballs. However, in some individuals atrophy, in the form of ventricular enlargement, callosal thinning, and sulcal widening, can be seen at onset of the disease, to an extent disproportionate to the numbers of T2/FLAIR and T1 lesions present (19,27,28). Such observations have led to the hypothesis that pathophysiology of MS may consist of two linked but separable processes—inflammation and primary degeneration (29).

The acute inflammatory lesions of MS are associated with a breakdown of the blood–brain barrier (30). Thus, when a compound such as gadolinium is injected into the veins of a person with MS, the material can leak into such active lesions and be visible on MRI (31–34). Enhancement can persist for periods of up to four to six weeks (35). Such lesions are called contrast-enhancing, and have been used as an assessment of therapeutic efficacy in multiple clinical trials (36–39). Contrast-enhancing lesions are not unique to MS, and can be seen in any condition associated with a breakdown of the blood–brain barrier. However, the presence of contrast-enhancing lesions in association with multiple

TABLE 8-1 *MRI criteria for aiding in the diagnosis of MS (Barkhoff et al.)*

At least three of the four following changes must be noted:
1. At least one gadolinium-enhancing lesion or nine T2 hyperintense lesions
2. At least one infratentorial (or spinal cord) lesion
3. At least one subcortical lesion
4. At least three periventricular lesions

T2/FLAIR lesions, in the appropriate distribution and of the appropriate shape, would be very supportive of a diagnosis of MS (20). However, there are many caveats to the use of this technique in both making a diagnosis of MS and in establishing the efficacy of treatment. First is the fact that some persons with MS tend to have large numbers of contrast-enhancing lesions, while others do not. This pattern of response holds true for extended periods of time (40,41). Second, visualization of enhancement is very technique-dependent (42). If the amount of gadolinium is increased, or the time between injection and scanning is increased, the numbers of contrast-enhancing lesions will be increased. Thus, to an extent, the presence or absence of such lesions is an artifact of the technique used. It is clear that inflammation and disease progression can occur in the complete absence of contrast enhancement, so the absence of this phenomenon should not dissuade one from a diagnosis of MS.

The MRI is also of great value in predicting which individuals presenting with their first episode of neurologic dysfunction [a clinically isolated syndrome (CIS)] will go on to develop clinically definite MS. Several studies (43,44) have demonstrated that persons with CIS who have lesions on their brain MRIs compatible with the presence of a central nervous system inflammatory process like MS have a greatly increased risk of developing clinically definite MS, and this risk increases with the numbers of lesions present, being almost 100% if more than 10 lesions are present. In addition, the numbers of lesions seen on MRI at initial presentation is a predictor of the rate of disease progression. Persons with more than 10 lesions on MRI have a greatly increased risk of having a significant disability within 15 years of onset (43,44).

EVOKED RESPONSES

Disease activity in MS occurs subclinically, resulting in physiologic changes in visual, auditory, and sensory pathways without a history of symptoms referable to these pathways. Additionally, both peripheral and central nervous system diseases can cause similar symptoms, and differentiating these two possibilities can be important in making a diagnosis of MS. It is in these contexts that evoked-response testing can be useful. Multiple types of evoked responses are possible. The most common are patterned, visual evoked responses (PVERs), measuring latencies of nerve conduction in prechiasmatic visual pathways; brainstem auditory evoked responses (BAERs), measuring latencies in brainstem auditory pathways; and somatosensory evoked responses (SSERs), measuring latencies in central somatosensory pathways. Multiple studies have been done assessing the usefulness of these tests in terms of sensitivity and specificity. The most reliable of these is the patterned visual evoked response test (45,46). If retinal abnormalities are excluded, delays in P100 latencies, or significant interocular differences in P100 latencies, would be indicative of abnormalities in one or both optic nerves. Changes may also be noted in wave amplitudes and configuration. In isolation, such changes are less specific in terms of defining demyelinating abnormalities of optic nerves. BAERs and SSERs are technically more difficult and more susceptible to artifact with less specificity for demyelinating processes. In an individual presenting with a clinically isolated syndrome and a paucity of findings on neurologic exam and MRI, findings evidence for subclinical dysfunction of central nervous system pathways can help in the diagnosis of MS. Similarly, if there is uncertainty as to the anatomic location of visual, auditory, or sensory symptoms, evoked-response testing can be of value.

CEREBROSPINAL FLUID (CSF) ANALYSIS

In up to 90% of individuals with clinically definite MS, the spinal fluid will show changes of low-grade inflammation. These changes are both measured directly in CSF, such as the immunoglobulin G (IgG) concentration and oligoclonal bandings, and are calculated from measurements of CSF and serum IgG, and albumin. Calculated values, using standard formulae, include the IgG index and IgG synthesis rate. This presence of these changes is a function of both the extent of disease and the anatomic location of the inflammatory lesions. Those near ventricular surfaces will result in abnormalities of spinal fluid. However, with more extensive involvement of the blood–brain barrier, the specificity of the calculated changes seen in MS CSF (such as the IgG synthesis rate) decreases (47). A corollary of these facts is that early in the course of disease, when changes in spinal fluid are of greatest value in supporting a diagnosis of MS, the spinal fluid is often normal (48) but can become abnormal over time (49). In up to almost 20% of patients with clinically definite MS, the spinal fluid remains normal (50), perhaps related to differences in the pathogenesis of disease in these individuals (51). Nevertheless, the presence of a low-grade inflammation in CSF, in the absence of other diseases that could cause similar changes, would support a diagnosis of MS.

The inflammatory changes seen in the CSF of persons with MS are several, and none are specific for MS since similar changes can be seen in a large number of other diseases (52). In addition, these changes must be interpreted in the context that several of the values are calculated rather than measured directly. Their sensitivity and specificity for MS is greatest when blood–brain barrier breakdown is low and total spinal fluid protein is normal. The presence of significantly elevated total of spinal fluid protein (relatively uncommon in MS) will give rise to elevated values of the calculated parameters.

The changes most commonly seen in the spinal fluids of persons with MS are shown in Table 8-2. As noted above, mild elevations in numbers of mononuclear cells are fairly common in persons with relapsing-remitting MS, and much less common in the less inflammatory stages of MS such as primary progressive MS or secondary progressive MS. Numbers are almost always under 20 per cubic mm and numbers of cells above 50 per cubic mm should prompt a reconsideration of the diagnosis of MS. The majority of cells are lymphocytes or mononuclear cells. In very acute phases of MS, some polymorphonuclear neutrophils (PMNs) can be present.

Increased amounts of IgG in the CSF, in the presence of a normal total protein concentration, are characteristic of any low-grade central nervous system inflammatory response. Calculated values, based on serum and CSF IgG and total protein, are used to calculate the IgG index and the IgG synthesis rate. Again, in the presence of a normal CSF total protein they suggest the presence of an in situ inflammatory response in the central nervous system. The increased concentrations of IgG in MS CSF result from increases in particular subpopulations of IgG rather than a general increase in all antibodies. When tested in an appropriate fashion, the presence of these increased subpopulations of antibodies is demonstrated by the presence of oligoclonal bands, present in CSF but not in serum. Proper

TABLE 8-2   *Spinal fluid findings in persons with multiple sclerosis*

Finding	Description	Usefulness
Mononuclear pleocytosis	< 50 cells with some PMNs if very acute disease	Not very common but useful when present. If > 50 cells/mm³, consider another diagnosis than MS.
Increased IgG concentration	Measures total CSF IgG	Very useful in the presence of a normal total CSF protein
Increased IgG index	A calculated value based on the concentrations of IgG in serum and CSF	Very useful in the presence of a normal total CSF protein
Increased IgG synthesis rate	A calculated value based on the concentrations of IgG in serum and CSF	Very useful in the presence of a normal total CSF protein
Oligoclonal banding	Bands of proteins in the IgG portion of the gel, not seen in serum	Very useful when present but serum must always be used as a comparison. Also, a high incidence of false negative results if proper assay techniques not utilized
Myelin basic protein (MBP) elevations	Increased concentrations of an important structural myelin protein	Not very useful since results usually are normal. Will usually be elevated in cases with more acute, widespread disease. Also, not specific for inflammatory states since any destructive myelin process will result in MBP elevations.

technique is essential to maximize the sensitivity of detecting such bands. At present, the standard assay should consist of isoelectric focusing of the proteins, followed by immunofixation to demonstrate the bands in the IgG region (53) (see also Chapter 10 by Thompson and Freedman).

RULING OUT "MS LOOK-ALIKES"

As noted initially, none of the historical, physical, or laboratory changes of MS are unique to that disease and every effort must be made to exclude diseases that can mimic the symptoms, signs, and laboratory changes of MS. Most can be excluded by simple blood or CSF tests. Others, especially those involving genetic mutations, require more sophisticated and expensive testing. In addition, there are demyelinating diseases that have a different clinical course than does MS and probably have a different pathogenesis, too.

Most common of the non-MS demyelinating diseases is acute disseminated encephalomyelitis (ADEM). While usually a disease of children, occurring after a viral infection, the disease can occur in adults and is associated with multifocal neurologic signs and symptoms, very similar to those noted above in persons with MS. In addition, the MRIs of persons with ADEM look similar to those of persons with MS. However, in addition to the neurologic findings, persons with ADEM can have systemic signs of inflammation, with fever, altered levels of consciousness, and leukocytosis. The spinal fluid in ADEM often is more intensely inflammatory than that seen in MS. Most importantly, ADEM is a monophasic illness. Once the disease has run its course there should be no new physical signs and the MRI should remain stable. Differentiating acute MS from ADEM can be difficult and follow-up over time may be the only way to separate the two illnesses.

Devic's disease (neuromyelitis optica) is, as the name suggests, a demyelinating/necrotizing disease of the optic nerves and the spinal cord. The pattern of disease is very variable, with either optic nerve or spinal cord presentations predominating, and with different temporal patterns. Some persons present with recurrent bouts of transverse myelopathy of varying severity. Others have predominantly visual diffi-culties, either unilateral or bilateral. Degrees of recovery vary widely, but with the more acute, necrotizing form of the disease, severe neurological deficits can persist. The pathology of Devic's disease differs from that of MS. Cerebral signs and symptoms are absent and the brain MRI will be normal. The CSF often is more inflammatory than that seen in MS, in terms of numbers of WBCs (> 50 per mm³) and with breakdown of the blood–brain barrier, with or without oligoclonal banding (OCBs) (54). Pathologically, there is an inflammatory vasculitis, associated with the presence of antibodies and complement (55). Recently, an antibody has been described that is both sensitive to and specific for Devic's disease (55a). If corroborated by other labs, presence of this antibody could serve as a useful diagnostic tool. (See also Chapters 19 and 20, by Wingerchuk.)

Other uncommon demyelinating diseases are described, such as Baló's concentric sclerosis (56,57) and Marburg's disease (58,59), but these are probably variations of MS, differentiated mainly on the basis of the MRI findings (MRIs in persons with Baló's concentric sclerosis show concentric circles of T2 lesions (60,61)) and the acuteness of the clinical course (very acute in Marburg's disease). No data to at this time allow one to separate these illnesses on the basis of differences in pathophysiology.

A partial list of infectious, inflammatory, genetic, and neoplastic diseases that can mimic MS and that should be considered prior to making a diagnosis of MS are listed in Table 8-3. This list is by no means inclusive, since more than 100 look-alikes are described. Rather, it lists the most common look-alikes, though none are truly common. Indeed, in the case of Lyme disease, one series from a geographic area endemic for this illness failed to show infection with *Borrelia burgdorferi* in any patient originally believed to have MS (62,63). (See also Chapter 11, by Herndon.)

Up to 25% of patients presenting to an MS specialty clinic with a multitude of symptoms suggestive of multifocal central nervous system dysfunction are found not to have either MS or any other pathologic process, with normal or functional neurologic exams, normal MRIs, blood tests, and CSF analyses (personal observations).

TABLE 8-3 *Diseases that can mimic multiple sclerosis*

Disease	Description	Diagnostic testing required
Lyme disease	Central nervous system involvement is seen in the tertiary form of this disease, with multifocal central nervous system and peripheral nervous system findings, and with inflammatory changes on MRI and in CSF	Testing for the presence of antibodies in CSF and serum. Since false positives can occur in response to other spirochetes, if antibodies are present, Western blots should be obtained to look for patterns of antibody banding specific for infection with *Borrelia burgdorferi*
Sjögren's Syndrome	A systemic autoimmune disease with ocular, buccal, and joint abnormalities	Dry eyes and mouth are prominent. Diagnosis is made with either salivary gland biopsy or testing for SSA and SSB antibodies
Sarcoid	A systemic inflammatory disease of the lungs, skin, joints, and other organs	Causes an inflammatory meningitis, often basilar, affecting cranial nerves and spinal cord. MRIs show meningeal involvement. Diagnosis is made with biopsy of affected non-CNS organs and by the presence of elevated levels of ACE.
Primary central nervous system vasculitis	An autoimmune vasculitis affecting only the central nervous system	Can cause relapsing, multifocal, central nervous system signs and symptoms, often stroke-like in nature, affecting both grey and white matter. Can be diagnosed with cerebral angiography and the presence of various autoantibodies.
CNS syphilis	Caused by chronic central nervous system infection with *Treponema pallidum*	Can cause optic nerve and spinal cord injury, usually chronically progressive but with the vascular form of infection, more rapid in onset. Diagnosed by the presence of serum and CSF FTA-antibodies.
B_{12} deficiency	Caused by a deficiency of either B_{12} absorption or of a deficiency of a cyanocobalamin carrier protein	Can cause both optic nerve and spinal cord dysfunction. Usually a subacute disease with normal MRI and a noninflammatory CSF with low B_{12} levels
CADASIL (Cerebral autosomal dominant arteriopathy with subcortical infarcts and leukoence-phalopathy)	Results from an autosomal dominant mutation in the Notch 3 gene, causing a microangiopathy with associated migraines and often cognitive impairment. Involves both grey and white matter	MRIs can look very similar to MS but CSF is usually noninflammatory and headaches are a prominent feature of the illness. Diagnosed with genetic testing for the Notch 3 gene mutation
Central nervous system lymphoma	Multifocal infiltrating tumor of the brain can cause progressive multifocal neurologic difficulties; responsive to steroids	Usually older individuals without a relapsing-remitting course, and a CSF that is noninflammatory but has malignant cells. Brain biopsy may be needed at times

Such individuals are usually categorized as having a somatization disorder, hypochondriasis, or conversion reaction, with a large number of such individuals also being clinically depressed. Despite the complexity and severity of their symptoms, a diagnosis of MS on symptoms alone cannot be made.

The importance of early, accurate diagnosis of MS is not only to exclude diseases that may be amenable to treatments, but to consider initiating treatment with immune-modulating therapies as early as the possible. As is described in other chapters in this book, MS is a complex illness with different pathogenic processes probably occurring concomitantly. Since the inflammatory component of MS predominates early in the course of the disease in most individuals with relapsing-remitting MS, treatment with anti-inflammatory, immune-modulating therapy, early in the course of the disease, is most effective.

ALGORITHMS FOR THE DIAGNOSIS OF MS

Several algorithms are published to assist in establishing the diagnosis of MS. Their intent is to provide uniformity to the diagnosis of a disease as pleomorphic as MS and to allow the diagnosis to be made with accuracy as early in the course of disease as possible. This is especially true for those individuals who present with their first episode of neurologic dysfunction, that is, those with a clinically isolated syndrome (CIS). A high percentage of such individuals will progress to clinically definite MS and identifying them early, to start immune-modulating therapy, is important.

The most utilized algorithms are those published by Poser et al. (64) and McDonald et al. (21). The former utilizes clinical, laboratory, and imaging criteria to establish the presence of an inflammatory disease of the central nervous system that is disseminated in time and space. The latter utilizes the same clinical, laboratory, and imaging criteria, but utilizes imaging data subsequent to the first neurologic episode to establish dissemination of disease in time and space. Both sets of criteria make it essential to first exclude other possible causes of neurologic illness. The Poser Committee's criteria categorize diagnostic certainty into four groups, listed below. The McDonald Committee's criteria utilize three categories of diagnosis (definite MS, possible MS, and not MS). Details of the criteria for each of the algorithms can be obtained from the articles. A summary of the Poser et al. and the McDonald et al. criteria are listed in Tables 8-4 and 8-5.

TABLE 8-4 *Summary of the Poser Committee's criteria for the diagnosis of MS*

Diagnosis	Clinical episodes	Neurologic exam	Imaging data	CSF analyses
Clinically definite MS	2	Two anatomic sites of neurologic dysfunction		
	2	One anatomic site of neurologic dysfunction	More than one separate lesion not explaining the site of neurologic dysfunction	
Laboratory supported definite MS	2	One anatomic site of neurologic dysfunction or more than one separate lesion not explaining the site of neurologic dysfunction		Immunologic abnormalities compatible with MS
	1	Two anatomic sites of neurologic dysfunction		Immunologic abnormalities compatible with MS
	1	One anatomic site of neurologic dysfunction or more than one separate lesion not explaining the site of neurologic dysfunction		Immunologic abnormalities compatible with MS
Clinically probable MS	2	One anatomic site of neurologic dysfunction		
	1	Two anatomic sites of neurologic dysfunction		
	1	One anatomic site of neurologic dysfunction or more than one separate lesion not explaining the site of neurologic dysfunction		
Laboratory supported probable MS	2			Immunologic abnormalities compatible with MS

TABLE 8-5 *Summary of the McDonald Committee's criteria for the diagnosis of MS*

Clinical evidence at presentation				Additional clinical or laboratory evidence required if clinical evidence is insufficient	
Clinical settings/ conditions	Attacks	Lesions suggestive of MS (see above criteria)	Criteria proven	Dissemination in space	Dissemination in time
1 Definite MS on clinical grounds	=2	=2	Dissemination in time and space	Proven	Proven
2 Localized disease	=2	1	Dissemination in time	New T2 or enhancing lesion suggestive of MS, at least three months later, or new T2 lesion and (+) CSF	Proven
3 Multifocal attack (can be initial presenting attack or CIS, too)	1	=2	Dissemination in space	Proven	New T2 or enhancing lesion suggestive of MS or a second attack
4 First, mono-symptomatic episode (CIS)	1	1	Neither	New T2 or enhancing lesion suggestive of MS, at least three months later, or new T2 lesion and (+) CSF	New T2 or enhancing lesion suggestive of MS or a second attack
5 Primary progressive MS	Insidious onset with gradual progression of neurological deficits			Multiple T2 lesions with (+) CSF and abnormal PVERs	New T2 or enhancing lesion suggestive of MS, at least three months later, or clinical progression for longer than one year

As expected, the correlation between the Poser Committee's criteria and those of the McDonald Committee is not 100% in terms of establishing the diagnosis of clinically definite MS. Several recent prospective studies (65–67) addressed this question and compared the sensitivity of the two criteria, following CIS patients for up to three years. In the Dalton et al. study (65), which looked at individuals with a CIS, the rate of conversion from CIS to clinically definite MS was 2.4 times higher at the end of one year using McDonald Committee criteria compared to Poser Committee criteria, indicating that utilization of subclinical changes on MRI were more sensitive than clinical changes in detecting disease progression. Similar findings were noted in the study by Tintore et al. (66). Thus, the McDonald et al. guidelines could allow the earlier institution of disease-modifying therapy. However, in the Dalton et al. study, after three years of follow-up there were still 28% of patients diagnosed with clinically definite MS by McDonald Committee criteria that had not met Poser Committee criteria. These individuals could still develop additional clinical episodes at a later date, thus fulfilling the Poser Committee criteria, but their rate of clinical (as opposed to MRI) progression was not known. An important caveat of this study was that CSF findings were not utilized in either of the diagnostic algorithms. In the study by Fangerau et al. (67), clinically definite MS was diagnosed more often using the McDonald Committee criteria compared to utilization of the "clinically definite" criteria defined by Poser et al. However, when both clinically definite and "laboratory supported definite" criteria were used, the Poser Committee's guidelines yielded a higher percentage of definite MS. In summary, what can be said is that, using both clinical and laboratory assessments, the McDonald Committee's criteria allow the diagnosis of clinically definite MS to be made earlier, thus allowing the earlier initiation of disease-modifying drugs and, hopefully, having a more salubrious effect on the disease.

REFERENCES

1. Lublin FD, Reingold SC. Defining the clinical course of multiple sclerosis: results of an international survey. National Multiple Sclerosis Society (USA) Advisory Committee on Clinical Trials of New Agents in Multiple Sclerosis. *Neurology* 1996;46(4):907–911.
2. Thompson AJ, et al. Diagnostic criteria for primary progressive multiple sclerosis: a position paper. *Ann Neurol* 2000;47(6):831–835.
3. Lucchinetti C, et al. Heterogeneity of multiple sclerosis lesions: implications for the pathogenesis of demyelination. *Ann Neurol* 2000;47(6):707–717.
4. Bruck W, Lucchinetti C, Lassmann H. The pathology of primary progressive multiple sclerosis. *Mult Scler* 2002; 8(2):93–97.
5. Poser CM. The dissemination of multiple sclerosis: a Viking saga? A historical essay. *Ann Neurol* 1994;36 [Suppl 2]S231–S243.
6. Rosati G. The prevalence of multiple sclerosis in the world: an update. *Neurol Sci* 2001;22(2):117–139..
7. Hader WJ, et al. The occurrence of multiple sclerosis in the Hutterites of North America. *Can J Neurol Sci* 1996;23(4):291–295.
8. Kira J. Multiple sclerosis in the Japanese population. *Lancet Neurol* 2003;2(2):117–127.
9. Misu T, et al. Pure optic-spinal form of multiple sclerosis in Japan. *Brain* 2002;125(Pt 11):2460–2468.
10. Kenealy SJ, Pericak-Vance MA, Haines JL. The genetic epidemiology of multiple sclerosis. *J Neuroimmunol* 2003;143(1–2):7–12.
11. Levy DE. Transient CNS deficits: a common benign syndrome in young adults. *Neurology* 1988;38(6):831–836.
12. Ramirez-Lassepas M, et al. Acute radicular pain as a presenting symptom in multiple sclerosis. *Arch Neurol* 1992;49(3):255–258.
13. Frohman EM, et al. Benign paroxysmal positioning vertigo in multiple sclerosis: diagnosis pathophysiology and therapeutic techniques. *Mult Scler* 2003;9(3): 250–255.
14. Schwid SR, et al. Fatigue in multiple sclerosis: current understanding and future directions. *J Rehabil Res Dev* 2002;39(2):211–224.
15. Rudick RA, et al. Multiple sclerosis. The problem of incorrect diagnosis. *Arch Neurol* 1986;43(6):578–583.
16. Bo L, et al. Magnetic resonance imaging as a tool to examine the neuropathology of multiple sclerosis. *Neuropathol Appl Neurobiol* 2004;30(2):106–117.
17. De Groot CJ, et al. Post-mortem MRI-guided sampling of multiple sclerosis brain lesions: increased yield of active demyelinating and (p) reactive lesions. *Brain* 2001;124(Pt 8):1635–1645.
18. Lycklama G, et al. Spinal-cord MRI in multiple sclerosis. *Lancet Neurol* 2003;2(9):555–562.
19. Dalton CM, et al. Early development of multiple sclerosis is associated with progressive grey matter atrophy in patients presenting with clinically isolated syndromes. *Brain* 2004;127(Pt 5):1101–1107.
20. Barkhof F, et al. Comparison of MRI criteria at first presentation to predict conversion to clinically definite multiple sclerosis. *Brain* 1997;120 (Pt 11):2059–2069.
21. McDonald WI, et al. Recommended diagnostic criteria for multiple sclerosis: guidelines from the International Panel on the diagnosis of multiple sclerosis. *Ann Neurol* 2001;50(1):121–127.
22. Bagnato F, et al. Evolution of T1 black holes in patients with multiple sclerosis imaged monthly for 4 years. *Brain* 2003 126(Pt 8):1782–1789.
23. van Waesberghe JH, et al. Axonal loss in multiple sclerosis lesions: magnetic resonance imaging insights into substrates of disability. *Ann Neurol* 1999;46(5): 747–754.
24. Bitsch A, et al. A longitudinal MRI study of histopathologically defined hypointense multiple sclerosis lesions. *Ann Neurol* 2001;49(6):793–796.
25. Miller DH, et al. Measurement of atrophy in multiple sclerosis: pathological basis methodological aspectsand clinical relevance. *Brain* 2002;125(Pt 8):1676–1695.
26. Turner B, et al. Cerebral atrophy and disability in relapsing-remitting and secondary progressive multiple sclerosis over four years. *Mult Scler* 2003;9(1):21–27.
27. Brex PA, et al. Detection of ventricular enlargement in patients at the earliest clinical stage of MS. *Neurology* 2000;54(8):1689–1691.
28. Dalton CM, et al. Progressive ventricular enlargement in patients with clinically isolated syndromes is associated with the early development of multiple sclerosis. *J Neurol Neurosurg Psychiatry* 2002;73(2):141–147.
29. Ge Y, et al. Neuronal cell injury precedes brain atrophy in multiple sclerosis. *Neurology* 2004;62(4):624–627.
30. Sobel RA. The pathology of multiple sclerosis. *Neurol Clin* 1995;13(1):1–21.
31. Larsson HB, et al. Quantitation of blood-brain barrier defect by magnetic resonance imaging and gadolinium-DTPA in patients with multiple sclerosis and brain tumors *Magn Reson Med* 1990;16(1):117–131.
32. Grossman RI, et al. Multiple sclerosis: serial study of gadolinium-enhanced MR imaging. *Radiology* 1988;169(1):117–122.
33. Kermode AG, et al. Heterogeneity of blood-brain barrier changes in multiple sclerosis: an MRI study with gadolinium-DTPA enhancement. *Neurology* 1990;40 (2):229–235.

34. Katz D, et al. Correlation between magnetic resonance imaging findings and lesion development in chronic active multiple sclerosis. *Ann Neurol* 1993;34(5): 661–669.

35. Cotton F, et al. MRI contrast uptake in new lesions in relapsing-remitting MS followed at weekly intervals. *Neurology* 2003;60(4):640–646.

36. Li DK, Paty DW. Magnetic resonance imaging results of the PRISMS trial: a randomized double-blind placebo-controlled study of interferon-beta1a in relapsing-remitting multiple sclerosis Prevention of relapses and disability by interferon-beta1a subcutaneously in multiple sclerosis. *Ann Neurol* 1999;46(2):197–206.

37. Ge Y, et al. Glatiramer acetate (Copaxone): treatment in relapsing-remitting MS: quantitative MR assessment. *Neurology* 2000;54(4):813–817.

38. Paty DW, Li DK. Interferon beta-1b is effective in relapsing-remitting multiple sclerosis. II. MRI analysis results of a multicenter randomized double-blind placebo-controlled trial. UBC MS/MRI Study Group and the IFNB Multiple Sclerosis Study Group. *Neurology* 1993;43(4):662–667.

39. Simon JH, et al. Magnetic resonance studies of intra-muscular interferon beta-1a for relapsing multiple sclerosis. The Multiple Sclerosis Collaborative Research Group. *Ann Neurol* 1998;43(1):79–87.

40. McFarland HF, et al. Using gadolinium-enhanced magnetic resonance imaging lesions to monitor disease activity in multiple sclerosis. *Ann Neurol* 1992;32(6): 758–766.

41. Frank JA, et al. Serial contrast-enhanced magnetic resonance imaging in patients with early relapsing-remitting multiple sclerosis: implications for treatment trials. *Ann Neurol* 1994;36[Suppl]:S86–S90.

42. Rovaris M, et al. MRI evolution of new MS lesions enhancing after different doses of gadolinium. *Acta Neurol Scand* 1998;98(2):90–93.

43. Brex PA, et al. A longitudinal study of abnormalities on MRI and disability from multiple sclerosis. *N Engl J Med* 2002;346(3):158–164.

44. O'Riordan JI, et al. The prognostic value of brain MRI in clinically isolated syndromes of the CNS. A 10-year follow-up. *Brain* 1998;121(Pt 3):495–503.

45. Fischer C, et al. [Visual early auditory and somatosensory evoked potentials in multiple sclerosis (917 cases). *Rev Neurol (Paris)* 1986;142(5):517–523.

46. Sanders EA, et al. Electrophysiological disorders in multiple sclerosis and optic neuritis. *Can J Neurol Sci* 1985;12(4):308–313.

47. Blennow K, et al. Formulas for the quantitation of intrathecal IgG production Their validity in the presence of blood-brain barrier damage and their utility in multiple sclerosis. *J Neurol Sci* 1994;121(1):90–96.

48. Moulin D, Paty DW, Ebers GC. The predictive value of cerebrospinal fluid electrophoresis in `possible' multiple sclerosis. *Brain* 1983;106(Pt 4):809–816.

49. Zeman AZ, et al. A study of oligoclonal band negative multiple sclerosis. *J Neurol Neurosurg Psychiatry* 1996;60(1):27–30.

50. Rocchelli B, et al. Clinical and CSF findings in multiple sclerosis patients with or without IgG oligoclonal bands at isoelectric focusing examination of CSF and serum proteins. *Eur Neurol* 1983;22(1):35–42.

51. Farrell MA, et al. Oligoclonal bands in multiple sclerosis: clinical-pathologic correlation. *Neurology* 1985;35(2):212–218.

52. Strony LP, Wagner K, Keshgegian AA. Demonstration of cerebrospinal fluid oligoclonal banding in neurologic diseases by agarose gel electrophoresis and immunofixation. *Clin Chim Acta* 1982;122(2):203–212.

53. Marchetti P, et al. Identification of IgG-specific oligoclonal banding in serumand cerebrospinal fluid by isoelectric focusing: description of a simplified method for the diagnosis of neurological disorders. *Clin Chem Lab Med* 1999;37(7):735–738.

54. Ghezzi A, et al. Clinical characteristics course and prognosis of relapsing Devic's neuromyelitis optica. *J Neurol* 2004;251(1):47–52.

55. Lucchinetti CF, et al. A role for humoral mechanisms in the pathogenesis of Devic's neuromyelitis optica. *Brain* 2002;125(Pt 7):1450–1461.

55a. Lennon V, et al. A serum antibody marker of neuromyelitis optica:distinction from multiple sclerosis. *Lancet* 2004;364(9451):2106–2112.

56. Morioka C, et al. The evolution of the concentric lesions of atypical multiple sclerosis on MRI. *Radiat Med* 1994;12(3):129–133.

57. Moore GR, et al. Balo's concentric sclerosis: new observations on lesion development. *Ann Neurol* 1985;17(6): 604–611.

58. Johnson MD, Lavin P, Whetsell Jr WO. Fulminant monophasic multiple sclerosis Marburg's type. *J Neurol Neurosurg Psychiatry* 1990;53(10):918–921.

59. Mendez MF, Pogacar S. Malignant monophasic multiple sclerosis or "Marburg's disease." *Neurology* 1988;38(7):1153–1155.

60. Revel MP, et al. Concentric MR patterns in multiple sclerosis. Report of two cases. *J Neuroradiol* 1993;20(4):252–257.

61. Bolay H, et al. Balo's concentric sclerosis. Report of two patients with magnetic resonance imaging follow-up. *J Neuroimaging* 1996;6(2):98–103.

62. Coyle PK, Krupp LB, Doscher C. Significance of reactive Lyme serology in multiple sclerosis. *Ann Neurol* 1993;34(5):745–747.

63. Coyle PK *Borrelia burgdorferi* antibodies in multiple sclerosis patients. *Neurology* 1989;39(6):760–761.

64. Poser CM, Brinar VV. Diagnostic criteria for multiple sclerosis: an historical review. *Clin Neurol Neurosurg* 2004;106(3):147–158.

65. Dalton CM, et al. Application of the new McDonald criteria to patients with clinically isolated syndromes suggestive of multiple sclerosis. *Ann Neurol* 2002;52(1): 47–53.

66. Tintore M, et al. New diagnostic criteria for multiple sclerosis: application in first demyelinating episode. *Neurology* 2003;60(1):27–30.

67. Fangerau T, et al. Diagnosis of multiple sclerosis: comparison of the Poser criteria and the new McDonald criteria. *Acta Neurol Scand* 2004;109(6):385–389.

9

The Role of MRI in the Diagnosis of Multiple Sclerosis

Anthony L. Traboulsee[1] and David K.B. Li[2]

[1]*Division of Neurology, Department of Medicine, The University of British Columbia, Vancouver, British Columbia, Canada;* [2]*Department of Radiology, The University of British Columbia, Vancouver, British Columbia, Canada.*

INTRODUCTION

Magnetic resonance imaging (MRI) is the most important paraclinical test for the diagnosis of multiple sclerosis. The hallmark pathologic features of MS are multiple plaques or lesions throughout the central nervous system affecting the brain, optic nerves, and spinal cord. These lesions can be readily seen with conventional MRI techniques (Fig. 9-1) early in the disease course, even before the diagnosis is established clinically. MRI is the most sensitive neuroimaging method for detecting these lesions for dissemination in both space and in time. MRI is safe, provides full coverage of the brain in minutes, and is increasingly more available throughout the world. There is no single test that is diagnostic for MS, and the lesions detected with brain MRI are not specific to MS. Other diseases may have a similar appearance, and the diagnosis

of MS must rely on the presence of the appropriate clinical features. For most patients, brain MRI is not required to establish the diagnosis of MS. However, it is strongly recommended that a brain MRI be performed when the technology is available, in part to rule out alternative diagnosis. The International Panel Diagnostic Criteria formally incorporate the common MRI abnormalities found in MS patients. This allows for an earlier diagnosis of MS for patients who have had only a single clinical event consistent with demyelination (clinically isolated syndrome or CIS) and do not fulfill clinical criteria for MS. The required abnormalities for a diagnostic MRI increase as the clinical evidence weakens. It is common to encounter situations where the clinical story is incomplete because of poor recall or other reasons, and the neurological exam can be essentially normal. Care is required in these situations to not assume that MRI lesions alone are

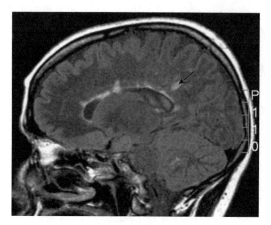

FIG. 9-1. Sagittal FLAIR brain image showing typical multiple sclerosis "T2" lesions. Classic MS lesions include ovoid-shaped, corpus callosum (incidence 51% CIS, 93% MS, 2% other neurological diseases) and flame-shaped Dawson Fingers (*arrow*). Other common lesions include juxtacortical, infratentorial (brainstem and cerebellum), and T1W gadolinium-enhancing lesions (Fig. 9-2). Corpus callosum lesions are best appreciated on sagittal FLAIR or proton density (PD) images.

MRI Protocol for Brain and Spinal Cord Imaging in Suspected MS

Terminology

MRI does not use radiation and is extremely safe for repeated use. In a fluctuating magnetic field, water molecules change energy states. The resultant signal that provides the characteristic images reflects a "water signature" for each tissue type, such as cerebrospinal fluid (CSF) and grey and white matter. Clinically, two basic sets of images are used: T2-weighted and T1-weighted images. T1 and T2 refer to the time it takes for the spin of protons to return to normal after application of a magnetic field. T1-weighted (T1W) images give a brighter signal in matter composed mainly of fat and the lesions appear dark, while proton density (PD), T2-weighted (T2W), and fluid-attenuated inversion-recovery (FLAIR) images give a brighter water signal for lesions (Fig. 9-2). Gadolinium, a nonradioactive dye injected into venous blood, normally does not cross the blood–brain barrier to appear in the brain parenchyma unless there is blood vessel disruption, in which case it would show as a bright lesion on T1W imaging. Gadolinium enhancement would be difficult to detect on T2W imaging since most lesions also appear bright. By convention, lesions that appear hyperintense (bright) on T2-weighted, PD-weighted, and FLAIR imaging are collectively called T2 lesions throughout this chapter.

Brain MRI Protocol

The lack of standardization of clinical MRI protocols and reporting can undermine its effectiveness (refer to Table 9-1). A standardized clinical protocol for MRI in MS or suspected MS has been recommended by an expert panel convened by the Consortium of MS Centers (1). The MRI techniques used in the diagnostic workup of suspected MS are the sequences that are routinely available on a standard clinical MRI scanner. Commonly used protocols range from 5-mm thick slices with 2.5-mm interslice gaps to 3-mm contiguous slices. There is better reproducibility and slightly higher lesion volume detection using 3-mm rather than 5-mm slice thickness

sufficient to diagnose MS. There are no routine indications for advanced MRI techniques including MR spectroscopy, magnetization transfer imaging, diffusion weighted imaging, and functional MRI in establishing the diagnosis of MS. These techniques are used at the discretion of local expertise.

This chapter includes standardized MRI protocols for the brain and spinal cord that are relatively thorough for the investigation of suspected MS and are essential for comparing serial, clinical MRI studies. When a practitioner is faced with diagnostic challenges, an understanding of the characteristic MRI abnormalities of MS, the natural history of their evolution, and of the role gadolinium and spinal cord imaging play can partially overcome the lack of pathologic specificity of MRI lesions. The role of MRI as evidence for dissemination in space and time in the International Panel Diagnostic Criteria for MS applies to patients who have had a documented clinical event consistent with demyelination, and emphasizes specificity over sensitivity.

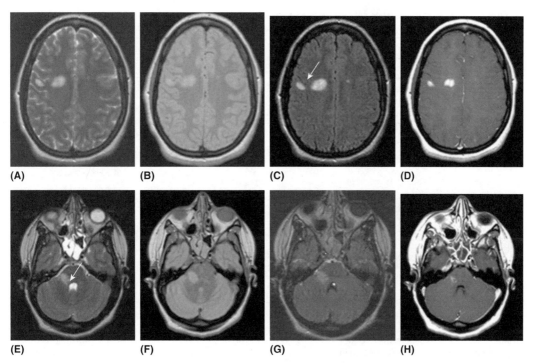

FIG. 9-2. Axial images from two levels in the same patient. MS lesions appear bright (hyperintense) on T2-weighted (**A** and **E**), proton density (**B** and **F**) and FLAIR imaging (**C** and **G**). FLAIR is preferable for juxtacortical lesions closed (*arrow*). T2 is more sensitive for infratentorial lesions (*open arrow*). Most T2 lesions are not seen on T1-weighted imaging (**D** and **H**) unless there is active inflammation with leakage of the blood–brain barrier. Active lesions appear as transient, gadolinium-enhancing on T1W postcontrast images (**D** and **H**) and as permanent, new, or enlarging T2 lesions on routine follow-up studies. This patient fulfills the modified Barkhof criteria for dissemination in space with a juxtacortical lesion, an infratentorial lesion, and at least one gadolinium-enhancing lesion.

(2,3). The Consortium of MS Centers MRI Working Group recommends contiguous 3-mm thick slices with no gap at a field strength of 1 Tesla or greater. A standardized protocol is invaluable for comparing across studies and for detecting longitudinal changes that may improve the diagnostic accuracy of the test. In clinical practice, the standardized MS protocol will provide a relatively thorough initial evaluation for most patients, even if the clinical scenario is not straightforward. Additional sequences such as diffusion-weighted imaging or MR angiography may be required in those cases where the clinical syndrome is atypical and the differential diagnosis includes a broad range of etiologies; this should be discussed with the radiologist.

The basic sequences that are recommended for lesion identification include: (a) an axial PD/T2W spin echo and a FLAIR sequence, and (b) a sagittal FLAIR sequence that covers the corpus callosum. Conventional spin echo (SE) techniques simultaneously acquire the PD and T2W images (double echo). Repetition times (TR) are long (2,500 to 3,000 msec), and lesion intensity increases with the longer echo time (TE) of the T2W (TE = 80 to 120 msec) compared to PD (TE = 15 to 40 msec) sequences. Posterior fossa lesions are best seen on T2W images and periventricular lesions are best seen with PD or FLAIR images (Fig. 9-2). Faster acquisition sequences ("fast" or "turbo spin echo") that allow additional signal averaging may miss smaller lesions due to the edge blur-

TABLE 9-1. *Consortium of MS centers standardized protocols for brain and spinal cord MRI in suspected MS*

Brain MRI protocol[1]		Spinal cord protocol[1]	
Sequence	Comment	Sequence	Comment
Scout localizer	Set up axial slices through subcallosal line[2]	Scout localizer	Use phased array coil if available
Sagittal Fast FLAIR	Convenient for identifying corpus colossal lesions	Sagittal T1 (precontrast)	Substitute with the postcontrast sagittal sequence if the spinal cord study immediately follows a contrast brain MRI
Axial FSE PD/T2	Sensitive for infratentorial lesions	Sagittal FSE PD/T2	PD optimally sensitive when the normal cord is isointense to CSF
Axial Fast FLAIR	Sensitive for juxtacortical and periventricular lesions	Axial FSE PD/T2	Through suspicious lesions
Axial T1 (precontrast)	Used to assess for T1 black holes	3D T1	Optional
3D T1	Optional	Sagittal T1 (postcontrast)	Same dose of gadolinium as for brain MRI No additional gadolinium is required if the spinal cord study immediately follows the contrast brain MRI
Axial T1 (postcontrast)[3]	Standard IV dose of 0.1 mmole/kg injected over 30 seconds Scan starting minimum 5 minutes after start of injection.	Axial T1 (postcontrast)	Through suspicious lesions to confirm findings on sagittal series and appearance

[1]Recommended field strength ≥ 1 Tesla.
[2]Subcallosal line is the line joining the undersurface of the front and back of the corpus callosum.
Contiguous 3-mm thick slices.
In-plane resolution = 1mm × 1mm.
FSE, fast spin echo or turbo spin echo. TE_1 minimum = 30 msec, TE_2 = 80 msec.
[3]Gadolinium may not be necessary if there are no lesions on the PD/T2 or FLAIR images.

ring associated with the shorter effective TE. This should not be of significant concern when contiguous, thin (≤ 3-mm) slices are obtained. Fast FLAIR is popular for periventricular and juxtacortical lesion identification because of the excellent suppression of cerebrospinal fluid partial volume effects (4). FLAIR may be less sensitive for some brainstem and spinal cord lesions (5,6), and PD/T2W are preferred.

Gadolinium

Inclusion of a gadolinium-enhanced, T1-weighted imaging is extremely useful for identifying new lesion activity. Higher (double or triple) doses of gadolinium, longer delays between injecting the gadolinium and acquiring the postcontrast T1W images, using thinner slices, and incorporating a magnetization transfer sequence have each been shown to increase the number of enhancing MS lesions as well as the intensity of some lesions (7,8). For routine diagnostic or clinical MRI scans, the recommended standard dose of gadolinium is 0.1 mmol/kg, with a minimum delay of 5 minutes after injection before acquiring the postcontrast T1W images. If a spinal MRI is also being obtained at the same visit, no further gadolinium is required.

Spinal Cord Protocol

The Consortium of MS Centers MRI Working Group recommends using a phase array coil for

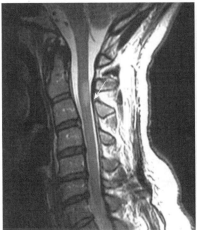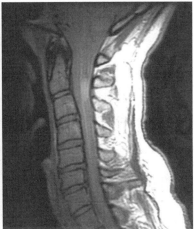

FIG. 9-3. Sagittal T2-weighted and proton density (PD) images of an MS lesion in the cervical spinal cord (*arrow*). Spinal cord imaging is useful when the symptoms are localized to the spinal cord and have not resolved to rule out alternative diagnosis, including spinal stenosis and tumor, or when the brain MRI is equivocal in suspected MS.

spinal cord imaging, if available. The spinal cord region to be covered will depend on the clinical findings, but often includes cervical and thoracic. The sequences should include pre- and postgadolinium-enhanced sagittal T1W, sagittal fast spin echo PD/T2 (Fig. 9-3), and axial PD/T2, as well as axial postcontrast T1W through suspicious lesions. Slice thickness should be ≤ 3 mm and there should be no gap between slices. As for brain MRI, the dose of gadolinium used is 0.1 mmol/kg injected over 30 seconds. Additional gadolinium is not required if the spinal MRI immediately follows a contrast brain MRI. In this case, the precontrast sagittal T1W images are excluded.

T2 Lesion Characteristics

Prevalence of T2 Lesions

Up to 100% of clinically definite MS patients have T2 lesions on brain MRI (9,10–17). However, early in the disease course, after a single attack of demyelination (CIS), approximately 20% of patients who eventually develop MS have a normal brain MRI (18). It would be extremely unusual for a patient with well-established MS not to have brain MRI lesions at some stage in the disease course; for those individuals,

further investigations along with careful consideration of alternative diagnoses are recommended.

Lesion Morphology and Distribution

The common MRI appearance is multiple white matter lesions with periventricular predominance; it would be unusual if this region was spared in MS. Lesions can occur in any central nervous system (CNS) tissue where there is myelin, including the cortex. However, most of these lesions are missed with conventional MRI due to similarities in signal intensities of MS lesions and grey matter, and the partial volume effects of CSF within the adjacent sulci (19). FLAIR sequences currently are preferred for the detection of cortical lesions (20). Dawson Fingers refer to the oval, elongated lesions in the corona radiata and the centrum semiovale (Fig. 9-1). These lesions are oriented along subependymal veins that are perpendicular to the walls of the ventricles, representing perivenular inflammation that is a unique pathologic feature of MS (21). These are best seen on the sagittal PD/T2W or FLAIR images. Lesions are also often seen in the temporal lobes, at the grey–white matter junction (juxtacortical), brainstem, cerebellum, optic nerves, and spinal cord.

The sagittal image is also useful for demonstrating lesions within the corpus callosum (Fig. 9-1) (22,23). Corpus callosal lesions were seen in 93% of 42 patients with established MS and only in 2% of 127 patients with white matter disease due to other causes (24). Since these early studies, there have been several reports of other disorders with involvement of the corpus callosum, including stroke (25), cerebral autosomal dominant arteriopathy subcortical infarctions and leukoencephalopathy (CADASIL) (26), lymphoma (27), Sjögren's disease (28), and progressive multifocal leukoencephalopathy (29), as some of the more common examples. The presence of corpus callosal lesions in CIS, though common (51% of patients), did not improve the final statistical model used by Barkhof et al. (30) for predicting which CIS patients would develop MS within three years of follow-up.

Optic nerve imaging is not routinely required in the diagnostic work-up of suspected MS unless there are atypical clinical features that are suspicious for an alternative diagnosis affecting the optic nerve or chiasm, such as a compressive or invasive lesion. A fat-suppression technique improves the sensitivity to detect lesions within the optic nerves (31). Asymptomatic optic nerve involvement was detected on MRI in 76% of 25 patients investigated, only four of whom had a history of optic neuritis (32).

Lesion Specificity

Postmortem studies have validated that the T2 lesions seen on MRI correlate with the typical plaques of MS seen on gross pathology (33). MS plaques appear as bright T2 lesions because of the longer T2 relaxation times. However, the T2 lesions are not specific for plaque age, degree of myelin loss, amount of inflammation and edema, or the degree of axonal loss (34). Most lesions have an expanded extracellular space, in part due to the edema, particularly with new inflammation (35). Lipids are effectively invisible on conventional MRI because of their short T2 relaxation time. Therefore, the lipid loss due to myelin sheath breakdown in demyelination does not directly contribute to the lesions seen

on conventional MRI. However, the loss of myelin lipid does create a more hydrophilic environment and the increased water content will lead to proton density increase and prolonged T1 and T2 relaxation times (bright lesions on PD/T2W and dark lesions on T1W sequences). Thus, other pathologies such as infarcts, infection, tumors, and inflammation can produce similar MRI signal changes due to abnormal water content that appears bright on PD/T2W and FLAIR images.

With increasing age, nonspecific MRI abnormalities (unidentified bright objects or UBOs) become increasingly common (36). UBOs are more frequent in women and a few small UBOs are common by the early to mid-forties (37). Patients with hypertension can also have confluent white matter lesions that are, indistinguishable from MS (38). Additional false positive lesion-like abnormalities on MRI due to normal structures include enlarged perivascular (Virchow–Robin) spaces, flow artifact, and volume averaging between adjacent slices. Perivascular spaces appear as punctate white matter lesions and commonly occur in the lower third of the corpus striatum, the midbrain, and the lenticular nucleus (39,40,41). Four percent of healthy controls of all ages can have periventricular changes that cannot be distinguished from MS (16). Table 9-2 lists some of the many diseases that can cause MRI lesions which at times mimic the appearance of MS.

Gadolinium-Enhancing, T1-Weighted Lesions

New disease activity (inflammation) can be detected by conventional MRI as gadolinium enhancement on the postcontrast T1W image (Fig. 9-2), and as new and enlarging T2 lesions on serial studies (see below). T2-weighted imaging techniques (i.e., T2W, PD, or FLAIR) are the most sensitive conventional MRI technique for detecting MS plaques but do not distinguish between acute and chronic lesions. T1-weighted imaging will only detect approximately one-third of the total number of T2 lesions; they will show up as hypointense (black) lesions on a pregadolinium (unen-

TABLE 9-2 *Differential diagnosis for multiple white matter lesions seen on brain MRI*

Common structures	Virchow–Robin spaces
	Flow artifact
	Partial volume
	Blood vessel or vascular malformation on gadolinium-enhanced scan
Unknown significance	Age-related changes
	UBOs (any age)
	Chronic hypertension
	Migraine
	Epilepsy (transient)
Inflammatory disorders	Acute disseminated encephalomyelitis (ADEM)
	Systemic lupus and connective tissue disorders
	Sjögren's syndrome
	Sarcoidosis
	Baló's concentric sclerosis
	Marburg's disease
	Chronic inflammatory demyelinating polyneuropathy
Infectious disorders	Neuroborreliosis (Lyme disease) and syphilis
	Progressive multifocal leukoencephalopathy (PML)
	Toxoplasmosis
	Abcess and tuberculomas
	Human immunodeficiency virus (HIV)
	Human T-cell lymphotropic virus (HTLV I/II)
	Encephalitis
	Cysticercosis
Vascular disorders	CNS vasculitis and antiphospholipid syndrome
	Behçet's disease
	Susac syndrome
	Lacunar stroke
	Multiple embolic strokes
	Degos disease
	Cerebral autosomal dominant arteriopathy with strokes and leukoencephalopathy (CADASIL)
Multifocal Tumor	Lymphoma
	Gliomatosis cerebri
	Metastases
Iatrogenic	Trauma (diffuse axonal injury)
	Central pontine myelinolysis (CPM)
	Radiation therapy
Toxic	Chemotherapy (e.g., 5 fluorouracil)
	Machiafava–Bignami disease
Metabolic	Wilson disease, porphyria, phenylketonuria (PKU)
	Mitochondrial disorders
Leukodystrophies	Globoid cell, adrenomyeloneuropathy, metachromatic

hanced) T1W scan. Pathologically, some of these will represent acute edema associated with a new or active lesion and these will often enhance with gadolinium. Gadolinium does not normally cross the intact blood–brain barrier (BBB). New MS lesions pathologically coincide with disruption of the BBB and inflammation, and appear on T1W imaging as gadolinium-enhancing lesions. Weekly MRI studies demonstrate that gadolinium enhancement always occurs before or during the development of all new T2 lesions (42,43) and represents breakdown of the blood–brain bar-

rier as proinflammatory T-cells infiltrate into the brain parenchyma (44). However, weekly imaging is not feasible for routine clinical practice, and only approximately 30% of clinical scans will have evidence of gadolinium-enhancing lesions during a routine MRI study because of the transient enhancement that is characteristic of active MS lesions and the random occurrence of new lesions.

The majority of new T2 lesions will enhance with gadolinium. Also, pre-existing T2 lesions can re-enhance, indicating new activity; in monthly MRI studies T1W gadolinium-enhancing lesions are seen twice as often as new T2 activity (new or enlarging T2 lesions). However, in clinical practice, the most common evidence of previous MS lesion activity is the accumulation of new T2 and enlarging T2 lesions since the last clinical scan.

The enhancement pattern can change with evolution and resolution of inflammation. The pattern ranges from diffuse to nodular and ring-like. The enhancement is more often solid and homogeneous with fresh lesions, particularly when they are small, and may appear ring-like with lesions that are larger and several weeks old. In rare cases where extremely large MS lesions appear tumor-like, the "open ring" sign favors demyelination over tumor or abscess (45).

Gadolinium Enhancement Is Transient

Enhancement usually lasts 4 weeks (range 1 to 16 weeks) with a gradual decline over the next 2 to 4 weeks (46,47). Gadolinium enhancement is sensitive to steroids and other anti-inflammatory treatments used in MS. It is extremely unusual for an MS lesion to have gadolinium enhancement beyond 3 months. This could help in distinguishing MS lesions from CNS tumors of the brain or spinal cord that can sometimes clinically mimic early MS.

Advantages of Using Gadolinium

The use of gadolinium can help to detect new MS lesion activity or to rule out confounding diagnoses that could be missed by PD/T2W imaging alone. Some diagnoses include meningiomas, small neoplasm, vascular malformations, and leptomeningeal disease such as sarcoidosis. Leptomeningeal enhancement is very rare in MS (48). In contrast, enhancement of the optic sheath is quite common at the time of optic neuritis when specialized MRI sequences are used to view the optic nerves (49,50). A potential false positive MRI finding is gadolinium within a vessel situated in a deep sulcus. Verifying the presence of a lesion on the corresponding T2W, PD, or FLAIR image or a follow-up scan can help clarify this.

T2 Lesion Natural History: Reactivation and Accumulation

Complementary information on new lesion development can be detected on the PD/T2 and FLAIR sequences. New or enlarging T2 lesions also represent new inflammation. They increase in size during the acute phase, mostly due to edema associated with inflammatory infiltrates, reaching their maximum size within four weeks (51). The process is self-limiting, and the lesions slowly decrease in size over the next six to eight weeks as edema resolves and remyelination occurs (Fig. 9-4). Unlike gadolinium enhancement, which is transient and disappears, most new lesions leave a smaller residual T2 lesion (52).

On average, MS patients will develop four to five new MRI lesions per year, with great variability amongst individuals (53). Pre-existing T2 lesions can reactivate with re-enhancement only, enlargement on T2W imaging, or both. Eventually, after many reactivations, lesions will fuse with adjacent lesions. Thus, what may have started out as several small lesions may end up forming one large, confluent lesion (54).

Annually, there is net accumulation of new and enlarging lesions that increases the total T2 volume or burden of disease (T2 BOD) of 5% to 10% per year (55). However, the variability among individuals is enormous. Monthly, the T2 BOD can fluctuate due to the changes in disease activity, especially if the baseline BOD is rather small (56).

Role of Spinal Cord Imaging

For patients who have presenting symptoms involving the spinal cord, both a brain MRI and a spinal cord MRI are recommended, especially if the symptoms have not resolved to exclude structural diseases that can mimic MS, such as spinal stenosis, vascular malformations, and neoplasm. Spinal MRI may be useful when the head MRI is normal (57) and it is recommended for patients suspected of having MS when the brain MRI results are equivocal. Early in MS, brain MRI is more likely to be positive than spinal MRI, even if the initial symptoms

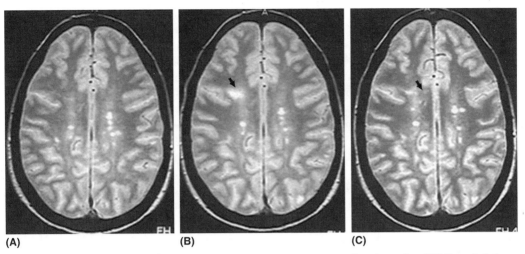

(A)   **(B)**   **(C)**

FIG. 9-4. MRI can provide evidence for dissemination in time by detecting T1W gadolinium-enhancing lesions (not shown) or by detecting new T2 lesions on follow-up studies, as shown in this time series of monthly MRIs from the same patient at the same level. **(A)** is the baseline MRI and **(B)** and **(C)** are one and two months after baseline, respectively. Gadolinium enhancement is transient, resolving within one to three months. New T2 lesions are initially large [*arrow,* **(B)**], then decrease in size as edema resolves [*arrow,* **(C)**]. They almost always leave a permanent T2 lesion that can be detected on future follow-up scans.

involve the cord. In patients presenting with spinal cord symptoms, 55% had lesions that could be detected on spinal cord imaging, while 91% of the patients had an abnormal brain MRI (58).

Spinal cord lesions can be found in 50% to 90% of clinically definite MS (CDMS) patients, and in one study of 68 patients, 38 had multiple lesions (56%) (59). Spinal cord lesions are more common in the cervical cord (Fig. 9-3) than the thoracic cord (60). These lesions tend to involve the posterior and lateral regions, are asymmetric, and occupy less than half the area of the cord on axial images (61). These lesions rarely extend beyond two vertebral segments (59).

In 115 patients with optic neuritis, 27% had lesions on spinal cord imaging, compared to 70% who had brain lesions (62). Twelve percent of CIS patients with a normal brain MRI had a spinal cord lesion, compared to 45% of those patients who had nine or more brain lesions. Using the current International Panel Diagnostic Criteria, spinal cord imaging only improved the evidence for dissemination in space (DIS) for 3/44 patients. Followed prospectively, 11/63 CIS patients developed new spinal cord lesions at one

year. Compared to using brain imaging alone, the detection of spinal cord lesions had little impact on the number of patients being diagnosed with definite MS, changing the diagnosis for one additional patient within 1 year and two additional patients within 3 years of follow-up.

In diagnostically uncertain cases, the addition of spinal cord imaging can be extremely useful. The combination of spinal cord lesions with an abnormal brain MRI can improve the diagnostic confidence when other diseases are under consideration. In contrast to brain MRI studies, T2W spinal cord lesions do not develop with normal aging or chronic hypertension and diabetes (63). Spinal cord lesions were only found in 6% of patients with other neurological diseases, including vasculitis and other inflammatory conditions (60). Spinal cord lesions are often asymptomatic in MS patients, in contrast to those caused by vasculitis or other inflammatory, infectious, and metabolic disorders. A partial list of conditions that sometimes mimic the appearance of a spinal cord presentation of MS clinically and radiologically include tumors (primary, metastatic, lymphoma); inflammatory disorders (systemic lupus, Sjögren's disease, sarcoidosis); atypical demyelinating diseases (neuromyelitis optica, Devic's disease, recurrent transverse myelitis); infection; and nutritional (vitamin B$_{12}$ deficiency). Occasionally, a solitary MS lesion in the cord can mimic the appearance of a spinal cord tumor. A brain MRI, along with CSF studies, can prevent unnecessary surgical removal or biopsy.

MRI Features of MS with Unknown Diagnostic Value

"Black Holes"

On the accompanying unenhanced T1W image, (Fig. 9-5) most T2 lesions are isointense to surrounding white matter and are therefore undetectable. Approximately one-third of T2 lesions will appear hypointense on the T1W image (T1 hypointensity or "black hole"). A proportion of these black holes are acute lesions that enhance when gadolinium is given, and almost half of these will resolve slowly over months (64). Black holes that do not enhance represent (a) subacute or resolving lesions, and (b) chronic or stable lesions. Chronic black holes are lesions that are nonenhancing, hypointense T1W lesions having a signal intensity less than or equal to grey matter; they persist for a minimum of six months after their first appearance. The chronic, T1W hypointense black holes are associated with greater tissue destruction and axonal loss (65) compared to chronic, stable T2 lesions without a corresponding black hole. T1W black holes are more prevalent in MS than seen with white matter lesions caused by vascular disease (66). While these lesions may have a better correlation with clinical disability because of their greater pathological specificity for severe

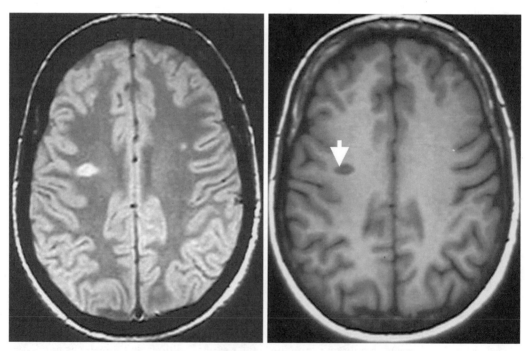

FIG. 9-5. Axial PD and corresponding pre-gadolinium T1W brain image showing multiple sclerosis lesion that appears as both a bright T2 lesion and as a hypointense T1W "black hole" *(arrow)*. Approximately 30% of T2 lesions will appear as a T1W black hole. T1W black holes that persist for at least 6 months (chronic black holes) are associated with greater tissue destruction pathologically.

axonal loss (67), they have no additional role in the diagnosis of MS.

Atrophy

Brain atrophy is an important MRI feature that underscores the neurodegenerative impact of MS (68). Brain and spinal cord atrophy has been recognized on autopsy material in MS patients prior to the current use of neuroimaging techniques. MRI studies can readily detect atrophy, ranging from 47% to 100% of MS patients (69,70). It is more severe in patients with secondary progressive MS than relapsing remitting MS (71) and can sometimes be detected after a single attack of demyelination (clinically isolated syndrome) before the diagnosis of MS is made, and in the presence of only a small T2 lesion burden (72).

It is likely that axonal loss accounts for the irreversible and progressive clinical disability that occurs in MS (73), and that atrophy is the result of axonal loss, in addition to myelin loss, and shrinkage due to gliosis. Brain volume changes, however, are complex and may also be affected by inflammation, edema, and hydration. Atrophy is progressive during the course of MS. Annually, MS patients lose 0.6% to 0.8% of brain volume compared to 0.3% for healthy controls (74–77). There is an associated increase in ventricle size of 1.6 mL/year in MS compared to 0.3 mL/year in healthy controls. In one study, this was equivalent to 17–24 mL of tissue loss per year (78). Despite efforts to develop clinically validated automated brain volume rendering software, atrophy remains a qualitative assessment by the radiologist and has very little role in the interpretation of a diagnostic clinical scan for MS.

"Dirty White Matter"

Not all lesions are discrete on MRI. There can be large, diffuse lesions visible on brain MRI with poorly defined boundaries. These areas of dirty-appearing white matter (DWM) are most common around the ventricles, especially adjacent to the occipital horn. DWM can extend over several contiguous slices and was present in 17% of relapsing-remitting MS (RRMS)

patients in one study (79). The specificity and utility in the diagnosis of MS is unknown.

Rationale for Using MRI in Early Diagnosis

The clinical diagnosis of multiple sclerosis requires two attacks or relapses consistent with demyelination of the central nervous system that are confirmed by a physician with adequate knowledge of the disease (80,81) and has an accuracy of approximately 95% (82). However, the interval between attacks is often years, and this leads to a period of uncertainty for many patients who have suffered a single attack of demyelination (CIS). Although this group of people is at risk for developing MS, a substantial number never go on to have another attack. At the time of CIS, 50% to 65% of patients will have lesions on their baseline MRI (83,84). The brain MRI findings at the time of a single clinical attack are the best predictors of developing clinical MS within the next 10 to 14 years (18,85).

The Optic Neuritis Treatment Trial (ONTT) systematically followed patients from multiple centers after a single event of optic nerve demyelination. Approximately 50% of those who had a baseline brain MRI had one or more T2 lesions. The abnormal MRI at the time of optic neuritis was the best predictor of converting to Poser criteria clinically definite MS (CDMS) at 10 years, with 56% of that group developing CDMS. Only 22% of those patients with a normal brain MRI at baseline subsequently developed CDMS (83). Similar results have been found by several groups investigating the natural history of developing MS after CIS, including O'Riordan et al. (86) after 10 years of follow-up. Subsequently, Brex et al. (18) followed the same natural history cohort for up to 14 years after the first attack. This group included other typical forms of demyelination in addition to optic neuritis, such as brainstem and spinal cord syndromes. In this population, approximately 88% of patients with an abnormal brain MRI at baseline converted to Poser CDMS or laboratory-supported definite MS. Only 19% of those with a normal brain MRI at the time of their initial attack subsequently went on to CDMS within 14 years. Although these studies differ in selection criteria and patients lost to follow-up, they support the prognostic value of early MRI abnormalities in MS. It is also important to note that several patients with an abnormal brain MRI at the time of CIS did not develop Poser CDMS. Also, a normal brain MRI does not exclude the diagnosis of MS for all CIS patients.

The Paty criteria were among the simplest MRI criteria applied to patients at risk for MS (87). An MRI that was strongly suggestive of MS required either four white matter lesions or three lesions if one was periventricular. All lesions had to be larger than 3 mm. One hundred eighty-four patients with suspected MS were prospectively followed for 2.1 years (mean), 30% of whom developed Poser CDMS. The baseline MRI was abnormal in 94% (46/55) in those who developed MS. However, the MRI was strongly suggestive of MS in 51% of those who did not develop MS during the study (58). Thus, the Paty criteria had good overall sensitivity of 94% for identifying those patients with MS at early presentation, but the specificity limited it usefulness. The specificity may be underestimated, in part, by the relatively short follow-up, as it can take up to 5 years or more before patients develop CDMS. However, as seen by the ONTT and other studies, a significant number of CIS patients do not develop MS despite having an abnormal brain MRI. The Fazekas criteria (88), though more complex, had the same sensitivity but had better specificity (100%) in a retrospective study. When evaluated prospectively in a CIS population, it performed no differently from the Paty criteria—both had identical sensitivity, specificity, and accuracy (89).

Barkhof et al. developed diagnostic MRI criteria based on a prospective study of 74 CIS patient followed for a minimum of two years (median follow-up, 39 months) (30). Thirteen (13/74) had a normal brain MRI and only one of those patients developed Poser CDMS. Sixty-one patients had an abnormal brain MRI, and half of those (32/61) developed CDMS. Fifteen MRI abnormalities were tested by logistic regression to determine which parameters or combination of parameters best predicted MS at follow-up. Most of these abnormalities were present in at least one-third of the patients (range 14% to 53%). The final model included juxtacortical lesions, gadolinium enhancement, and infratentorial and periventricular lesions. Eighty-two percent (50/61) of patients with an abnormal MRI met at least one of the four criteria. The model had a sensitivity of 82%, a specificity of 78%, and an accuracy of 80% for diagnosing MS after a single attack. In the same study, the Paty and Fazekas criteria were identical in terms sensitivity (88%), specificity (54%), and accuracy (69%). Thus, the Barkhof criteria had a greater specificity and accuracy than the other two criteria, with little to no impact on sensitivity. Interestingly, corpus callosum lesions did not make it into the final model despite a relatively high prevalence of 38%. It is also noteworthy that 10 patients were excluded from participating in the study after an alternative diagnosis was determined: three ischemia, two neoplasm, two Lyme disease, one acute disseminated encephalomyelitis (ADEM), one cervical stenosis, and one ocular disease. None of these patients fulfilled the current International Panel MRI criteria for dissemination in space (90).

Tintore et al. reproduced Barkhof's results in a prospective study of 70 CIS patients followed for a mean of 28 months (91). The Barkhof criteria were modified so that a threshold of three of the four Barkhof criteria had to be met in order to be a diagnostic scan. Again, the Paty and Fazekas criteria had identical performance (sensitivity 86%, specificity 54%, and accuracy 64%). In this study, the modified Barkhof criteria had a sensitivity of 73%, specificity of 73%, and accuracy of 75%. In the absence of gadolinium-enhancing T1 lesions, requiring that ≥ 9 T2 lesions provided a similar accuracy of 77%. The modified Barkhof criteria (92) were also validated using the MRI data from a therapeutic trial for the treatment of CIS patients with an abnormal baseline brain MRI with interferon-beta 1a SC QW (ETOMS study) (77). There was a linear relationship between the numbers of positive MRI criteria at study entry with the development of Poser CDMS at two years of follow-up. Using the modified Barkhof criteria with a cutoff of three of the four MRI criteria need to be positive, only 22% of patients below this developed Poser CDMS within two years, compared to 42% of patients above this cutoff. Thus, the more abnormal the baseline MRI is in CIS, the greater the risk of having a second clinical attack within two years.

Role of MRI in the International Panel Diagnostic Criteria for MS

MRI technology was not readily available for the investigation of MS when the Poser diagnostic criteria were proposed. An international panel of MS experts met in London, UK in 2000 to update and simplify the diagnostic criteria, and created the International Panel (IP) or McDonald diagnostic criteria for MS (81). Incorporated into the diagnostic criteria was the predictive value of MRI in high-risk CIS patients, along with the observations from natural history studies that MRI changes in MS are common and that the majority of new MS lesions seen on MRI are asymptomatic (93). In the appropriate clinical setting, MRI can support the diagnosis by providing additional evidence for disease dissemination that is separated in space and in time, especially in those patients who have only had the disease for a short period of time and sufficient clinical evidence to make the diagnosis is lacking. The MRI evidence required to support the diagnosis varies depending on the strength of the clinical findings. A patient who has had two documented clinical attacks of demyelination consistent with MS and clinical evidence of two lesions does not need to meet the MRI criteria for dissemination in space. The added value of the IP diagnostic comes, in part, from the new MRI definition of temporal dissemination not available with previous definitions including diagnostic criteria proposed by Poser, Paty, Fazekas, and Barkhof. This important feature provides temporal evidence required to make the diagnosis of MS before the second clinical attack occurs. In CIS, 20% of patients who eventually develop Poser CDMS may have a normal brain MRI at the time of their first attack (18). There needs to be careful consideration of

alternative diagnoses if the MRI is completely normal in patients with clinically definite MS (i.e., two clinical attacks), or those that do not develop new lesions in time consistent with the diagnosis of MS.

MRI Criteria for Dissemination in Space: RRMS

The modified Barkhof criteria were selected for evidence of dissemination in space (DIS) by the IP committee because of its greater specificity (73% to 78%) for diagnosing MS after a single attack while maintaining good sensitivity (73% to 82%) compared with the Paty and Fazekas criteria (sensitivity 88%, specificity 54%). In addition to the number of lesions seen, it is important to recognize that the type and strategic location of these lesions are also critical. The modified Barkhof criteria require three of four of the following: (a) one gadolinium-enhancing lesion on a T1W image or nine T2 lesions (brain and spinal cord); (b) ≥ 1 infratentorial lesion (brainstem or cerebellum T2 lesions are best seen with T2W); (c) ≥ 1 juxtacortical lesion that involves the subcortical "U fibers" (these lesions usually abut the cortex and are best seen with FLAIR); or (d) ≥ 3 periventricular lesions (also best seen with FLAIR or PD). All lesions should be larger than 3 mm. Although a spinal cord lesion can substitute for one of the nine brain lesions, if required, it cannot substitute for a juxtacortical or infratentorial criteria lesion. Refer to Table 9-3.

For centers that routinely use gadolinium for a diagnostic MRI, the minimum number of lesions necessary to fulfill the dissemination in space criteria is two: one juxtacortical lesion and one infratentorial lesion, as long as one of the two lesions is enhanced with gadolinium (Fig. 9-2). For centers that do not use gadolinium, or if no gadolinium lesions are present, the minimum number of lesions required is five: three periventricular, one juxtacortical, and one infratentorial. The alternative criteria for dissemination in space only require two MRI lesions in the brain, providing that the CSF analysis is positive for oligoclonal banding or elevated immunoglobu-

TABLE 9-3 *International panel mri criteria for dissemination of lesions in space and in time[5]*

Relapsing onset MS dissemination in space MRI criteria[4]		Primary progressive MS dissemination in space criteria	
Modified Barkhoff	Three of four criteria required	Paraclinical requirements	One of five criteria required
	1 gadolinium-enhancing lesion OR 9 T2 brain lesions[1]	Positive CSF[3]	≥ 9 T2 brain lesions
	≥ 3 Periventricular lesions	Positive CSF[3]	≥ 2 spinal cord lesions
	≥ 1 Juxtacortical lesions	Positive CSF[3]	1 spinal cord lesion and ≥ 4 brain lesions
	≥ 1 Infratentorial lesions	Positive CSF[3] and abnormal VEP[2]	≥ 4 brain lesions
		Positive CSF[3] and abnormal VEP[2]	1 spinal cord lesion and ≤ 4 brain lesions
Alternative MRI Criteria for DIS	Positive CSF[3] and > 2 brain lesions[1]	Positive CSF[3] and abnormal VEP[2]	1 spinal cord lesion and ≤ 4 brain lesions

MRI studies should be performed using a standardized protocol. An important role of MRI is to supplement clinical evidence to establish an earlier diagnosis after a single clinical attack (CIS).

[1]One spinal cord lesion can substitute for one brain lesion. A spinal cord lesion does not count as an infratentorial lesion.

[2]Positive visual-evoked potentials, delayed but well-preserved wave form.

[3]Positive CSF, oligoclonal IgG bands or elevated IgG index.

[4]The American Academy of Neurology Therapeutics and Technology Assessment Subcommittee MRI criteria for relapsing onset MS:
(a) ≥ 3 brain lesions or
(b) ≥ 2 gadolinium-enhancing lesions or
(c) new T2 or gadolinium-enhancing lesions on follow-up studies.

[5]**MRI criteria for dissemination of lesions in time require one of:**
(a) New gadolinium-enhancing lesion detected on any follow-up study that is a minimum of three months after the onset of the clinical attack. The active lesion should not be in a site implicated in the original clinical attack.
(b) New T2 lesion detected on any follow-up study that is a minimum of three months after the previous MRI. A new spinal cord lesion can substitute for a new brain lesion.

lin G (IgG) index. In this case, one spinal cord lesion can also substitute for one brain lesion.

MRI Criteria for Dissemination in Space: PPMS

The majority of MS patients have multiple attacks of neurological dysfunction (RRMS) and a minority will have a slow, progressive early course (primary progressive MS or PPMS) (94). There tend to be fewer T2 lesions in PPMS, as well as less-frequent occurrence of gadolinium enhancement. The MRI requirements are therefore less stringent than for relapsing-onset MS. One of the following five criteria is required for a diagnostic MRI in PPMS for dissemination in space: (a) ≥ 9 brain lesions; (b) ≥ 4 brain lesions and abnormal visual-evoked potentials (VEPs); (c) ≥ 2 brain and one spinal cord lesion; (d) ≥ 2 spinal cord lesions; or (e) one spinal cord lesion and abnormal VEP when there are < 4 brain lesions. Positive CSF for oligoclonal banding or elevated IgG index is also required. As seen by these five scenarios, the dissemination in space criteria can be met by brain MRI alone or spinal cord MRI alone. In most cases, both should be obtained. It would be unusual not to have some brain MRI abnormalities in established PPMS. Even in the presence of an abnormal brain MRI, spinal cord imaging is helpful to rule out alternative diagnosis such as spinal stenosis or low-grade tumors (ependymoma) in patients with a progressive spinal cord syndrome.

MRI Criteria for Dissemination in Time

The previous diagnostic MRI criteria, including those of Paty, Fazekas, and Barkhof, were all, in essence, criteria for dissemination of lesions in space. One important advantage of the IP diagnostic criteria is the substitution of a clinical attack with a new MRI lesion as evidence fulfilling the dissemination in time criteria. New MRI lesions are inevitable in MS. Serial MRI studies demonstrate that new MS lesions develop frequently in the absence of clinical symptoms (51,93,95,96). The evidence for a clinically silent MRI attack includes a gadolinium-enhancing lesion or a new T2 lesion. The advantage of using a gadolinium-enhancing lesion is that comparison with a previous MRI is not necessarily required, providing that the enhancing lesion is detected a minimum of 3 months after the presenting clinical symptoms, and the lesion is not in the same anatomical location causing those symptoms. It would be unusual for an MS lesion to persistently enhance with gadolinium for more than 3 months, and the presence of a persistently enhancing lesion on serial studies warrants investigation for alternative diagnosis such as a tumor or vascular malformation.

In a clinical trial of interferon-beta 1a sc TIW for the treatment of RRMS (PRISMS), patients who enrolled in the study had clinically active disease with at least two clinical relapses in the 2 years prior to randomization. A PD/T2W brain MRI was performed every 6 months. For the 184 patients in the placebo cohort, 75% of the MRIs had evidence of new disease activity (new or enlarging T2 lesion) and most (92%) of the placebo patients had at least one active scan during the 2 years of observation. The placebo patients had a median number of 2.25 new lesions per scan in this study (97).

The rate of MRI activity is similar in CIS. At the time of their clinical attack, 38% of CIS patients from natural history studies will have a gadolinium-enhancing lesion (30). The CHAMPS clinical trial of interferon-beta 1a IM once weekly for the treatment of patients with early-onset MS enrolled CIS patients who had a single clinical attack and an abnormal brain MRI that put them at high risk for MS (98).

MRIs were performed at baseline and every 6 months. Their percentage of placebo patients who had a gadolinium-enhancing scan ranged from 39% to 43% for each of the MRI visits. Fifty-nine percent of placebo patients had new T2 lesions by 6 months, and 82% of those followed to 18 months. In the ETOMS study of high-risk CIS patients, 94% of the placebo patients had new MRI activity during the 2 years of observation with annual MRIs (77). In a prospective cohort of CIS patients, including those with and without abnormalities on their baseline MRI, the rate of new lesion development appeared lower (99). In this study, the percentage of CIS patients with new MRI activity at 3 months was 23%, 1 year was 53%, and at 3 years was 68%.

Gadolinium enhancement is transient and easily missed. In the absence of detecting a gadolinium-enhancing lesion on a diagnostic scan, the presence of a new T2 lesion on a follow-up MRI will provide similar evidence for dissemination in time, reflecting the observation that new T2 lesions almost always are permanent (Fig. 9-4). The detection of new T2 lesions depends on a standardized MRI protocol with careful attention to repositioning. It is important to identify lesions that clearly represent new pathology to fulfill the dissemination in time criterion (100). The timing of the follow-up scan is not crucial but there must be a minimum of 3 months between MRI studies to confidently identify these new T2 lesions. New lesions developing in the spinal cord are also sufficient for the dissemination in time MRI criteria.

The timing of the first MRI after the onset of an episode consistent for demyelination dictates the minimum number of further MRIs needed to fulfill the dissemination in time criteria. Any MRI done within 3 months of the clinical onset can only serve as a baseline scan and cannot be used to fulfill dissemination in time criteria even if a gadolinium-enhancing lesion is detected. The second MRI could be done as early as 3 months after the clinical onset to demonstrate a gadolinium-enhancing lesion. A new T2 lesion at this time would not suffice since it has been less than 3 months between scans. A follow-up MRI that is at least 3 months after the previous MRI would fulfill the dissemination in time if either a gadolinium-enhancing lesion or a new T2 lesion was present. A single MRI could be used to fulfill the dissemination in time criteria if it is delayed by 3 months after the onset of the first clinical attack and it detects a gadolinium-enhancing lesion in a location different from the symptoms. MRI criteria for dissemination in time are only required if an early diagnosis is required. It is not required in the event of a second clinical attack.

The IP dissemination in time MRI criteria apply to primary progressive MS as well as relapsing-onset MS. Gadolinium-enhancing lesions are less common, seen in only 14% of 943 PPMS patients at entry into a clinical trial with glatiramer acetate (PROMISE trial) (101). Furthermore, new T2 lesion development is also much less frequent, with only 48% of PPMS patients showing a new lesion within two years of follow-up (102).

Validation of the International Panel Diagnostic Criteria

The important implication of using serial MRI to detect clinically silent disease activity is that many CIS patients with MS can be diagnosed earlier. A prospective natural history study of 119 patients with a clinically isolated syndrome included patients with optic neuritis, brainstem, or spinal cord syndromes (99). Of the 119 patients, 85 (71%) had abnormalities on their baseline brain MRI. Within 3 months 7% had a clinical attack and met Poser criteria for CDMS, compared with 21% who met IP diagnostic criteria for definite MS. The sensitivity when using the MRI criteria of dissemination in space and in time at 3 months based on those patients who developed Poser CDMS at 3 years was 59%, with a specificity of 93%. Within 1 year only 20% of patients had a second clinical attack (CDMS), whereas 43% had new, clinically silent MRI activity. When those patients who had a new MRI lesion or a new clinical attack were combined, 48% met the IP diagnostic criteria for definite MS within 1 year. When only using the MRI criteria for dissemination in time and in space, the IP criteria at 12 months had a sensitivity of 83%, specificity of 83%, and accu-

racy of 83% (103). Using the full IP criteria that include clinical signs as well as MRI increased the sensitivity to 94%, while the specificity remained high at 83%. The detection of new spinal cord lesions did not improve the sensitivity for diagnosing definite MS (IP diagnostic criteria) (62). Including new T2 lesions at three months after the clinical onset would increase sensitivity while maintaining specificity (104). However, the interval between MRI studies with this scheme is less than three months and, in clinical practice, the detection of new T2 lesions (unlike gadolinium-enhancing lesions) can be sensitive to repositioning of patients during follow-up MRI, as well as slice thickness and interslice gap, particularly in this short interval.

A similar study by Tintore et al. prospectively followed 139 CIS patients for a mean follow-up of 39 months (105). Forty-two percent had optic neuritis, 24% brainstem syndromes, 28% transverse myelitis, and 6% were polysymptomatic attacks. Thirty-eight (27%) had a normal brain MRI, two of whom developed Poser CDMS. Seventy-seven patients (56%) met criteria for dissemination in space by either MRI alone (58/77) or MRI along with abnormal CSF (19/77). At 12 months, 15 patients had a second attack and met Poser CDMS (11%) compared to 62 patients (45%) who had a new T2 lesion (gadolinium was not consistently used in this study). Fifty-one out of 139 patients developed IP criteria definite MS by month 12 using MRI criteria only for determining dissemination in space and in time, for an overall sensitivity of 74%, specificity of 86%, and accuracy of 80%.

New T2 lesions may develop in CIS patients who do not develop CDMS. One hundred and eight patients from the Optic Neuritis Treatment Trial who did not develop Poser CDMS within 10 to 14 years of follow-up were available for an MRI study. Sixty-one (56%) patients had a normal baseline MRI and 27 of those (44%) developed at least one new T2 lesion ≥ 3 mm. Twenty-six (74%) patients with at least one lesion > 3 mm on their baseline MRI also developed a new T2 lesion at follow-up (106). The follow-up scans were not assessed for dissemination in space criteria. These new lesions may not necessarily be the result of subsequent episodes of clinically silent CNS inflammation. Many of these lesions may have been present at baseline but were missed by the older MRI technology and protocol that used PD/T2 only, with thicker slices (5 mm) and an interslice gap of 2.5 mm compared to the follow-up MRI that had contiguous 3-mm slices and FLAIR. Finally, the mean age of patients at follow-up was 45 years, an age at which UBOs are commonly encountered.

Recommendations of the American Academy of Neurology

The report of the therapeutics and technology assessment subcommittee of the American Academy of Neurology (107) extensively reviewed the relevant literature concerning the utility of MRI in suspected MS, including studies published that have validated the IP diagnostic criteria. The committee was made up of international MS and MRI experts. They also emphasized the importance of ruling out alternative diagnosis since MRI lesions are pathologically nonspecific. The use of MRI for detecting dissemination in time was recommended as being highly predictive of the subsequent development of Poser CDMS. The other recommended MRI criteria that were highly predictive of MS included three or more white matter lesions ≥ 3 mm, or two gadolinium-enhancing lesions. Overall, the criteria are more lenient than the modified Barkhof MRI criteria used by IP diagnostic criteria for dissemination in space. Even the recommendation for only three lesions is more lenient than the Paty criteria, which required that at least one of these needed to be periventricular. This would increase sensitivity for diagnosing MS early, though most likely at the risk of decreased specificity, and it has not been validated prospectively, unlike the IP diagnostic criteria.

The committee's recommendations do reflect current practice in North America that patients with a well-documented CIS who also have two characteristic T2 lesions ≥ 3 mm in diameter (one of which is ovoid or periventricular) often are started on disease-modifying therapy. According to the clinical trial with interferon-beta 1a IM once weekly for the treatment of CIS

(CHAMPS) (98), these patients were at high risk for a second clinical attack, or the development and accumulation of new MRI lesions. Even in the presence of a few T2 lesions, 42% of optic neuritis patients still did not develop Poser CDMS within 10 years of follow-up (108). In another study that included patients with a variety of CIS syndromes, 12% of those with an abnormal brain MRI did not develop Poser CDMS within 14 years of follow-up (18).

The MRI criteria for dissemination in space and time that are components of the IP diagnostic criteria, and the recommendations of Therapeutics and Technology Assessment Subcommittee of the American Academy of Neurology were developed in patients with a classic demyelination syndrome (CIS). The sensitivity and specificity of the validation studies are similarly based on patients with definite CIS. Improved imaging techniques and stronger field strengths (3 Tesla and greater) will detect more MS lesions and will most likely increase the risk of false positive scans due to a higher number of nonspecific UBOs that will also be seen. MS can also be diagnosed in patients over the age of 50, where the incidence of nonspecific MRI abnormalities is high. An overreliance on MRI abnormalities in isolation of clinical findings can produce both false positive and false negative diagnosis of multiple sclerosis. In a study from 1993, 99 MRIs of suspected MS patients were reviewed. Thirty-nine percent of patients had a false positive diagnosis of MS when only MRI criteria were used without any clinical information (109). Since then, both MRI availability and sensitivity for detecting lesions have improved. MRI lesions lack pathologic specificity and, when only MRI criteria are used, there is an increased risk of false positive diagnosis (110). To avoid overdiagnosing isolated CIS as MS, or misdiagnosis of a non-MS syndrome, a conservative approach that emphasizes specificity is preferred.

Development of a Secondary Diagnosis

Patients diagnosed with MS occasionally develop unexpected symptoms or sudden deterioration. Whenever a secondary diagnosis is suspected, or the original diagnosis is under review, additional brain and spinal cord imaging can provide valuable diagnostic information in addition to CSF studies, visual evoked potentials, or other paraclinical testing.

Misdiagnosis at the time of clinical presentation is less likely with the routine use of brain and spinal cord MRI to exclude common structural diseases that can clinically mimic MS, such as spinal stenosis, vascular malformation, and most neoplasia. Other inflammatory diseases such as Sjögren's disease, systemic lupus, and sarcoidosis can be more challenging due to the nonspecific nature of MRI lesions. It is not uncommon to come across case series, such as with CNS involvement with Sjögren's disease (111) where the MRI appearance and the clinical evolution resemble MS.

Patients diagnosed with MS based on nonspecific symptoms and UBOs on a diagnostic scan warrant reinvestigation and careful follow-up. MS can also mimic other diseases, especially when it begins as a solitary lesion. Some MS lesions present as a tumor-like mass with or without crossing of the corpus callosum, resembling a glioblastoma multiforma or lymphoma (112). The open-ring sign of gadolinium enhancement is more common in large, tumor-like MS lesions (45) and demyelinating lesions tend to have less mass effect and surrounding edema compared to similar-sized tumors.

The aging MS population is at risk for ischemic stroke as a secondary diagnosis. Spinal stenosis can coexist with secondary progressive or primary progressive MS, and can go undetected without appropriate spinal cord imaging. MS patients can also develop brain abscesses and primary brain tumors (Fig. 9-6) (113). With the ongoing development of potent, new immunomodulatory therapies for MS, there remains the risk of unexpected complications as seen with the development of progressive multifocal leukoencephalopathy (PML) in patients treated with a combination of natalizumab and interferon-beta 1a IM once weekly (114). Many of these conditions can have a similar MRI appearance to MS lesions early in their development, and can be challenging to sort out clinically as well as radiologically.

SUMMARY

There is no single test that is diagnostic of MS, including MRI. The lesions detected with MRI

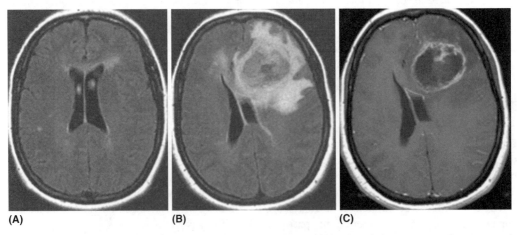

(A)   **(B)**   **(C)**

FIG. 9-6. MRI is indicated in MS patients with an unexpected deterioration or concern for a secondary diagnosis. **(A)** is a baseline, axial FLAIR image from an MS patient with relapsing-remitting disease course for 9 years, demonstrating a new periventricular lesion that looks typical of MS. **(B)** is a follow-up FLAIR image 1 year later, during which time the patient developed worsening fatigue, cognitive decline, nausea, and anorexia. **(C)** demonstrates gadolinium enhancement. MS lesions typically have minimal mass effect and transient enhancement with an open-ring sign when large. Biopsy confirmed that the new lesion is a grade IV astrocytoma.

are pathologically nonspecific. The principles of MS diagnosis are based on showing dissemination of white matter lesions in space and time. MRI is the most sensitive method for revealing asymptomatic dissemination of lesions in space and time. The pattern and evolution of MRI lesions, in the appropriate clinical setting, has made MRI abnormalities invaluable criteria for the early diagnosis of MS.

The first important role for MRI in the diagnosis of MS allows for an early diagnosis of MS for CIS patients using the IP diagnostic criteria, including MRI for dissemination in space (DIS) and time (DIT). The sensitivity of diagnosing MS within the first year after a single attack is 94%, with a specificity of 83%. The MRI evidence required to support the diagnosis varies, depending on the strength of the clinical findings. Allowing a new MRI lesion to substitute for a clinical attack doubles the number of CIS patients who can be diagnosed as having MS within 1 year of symptom onset. Increasing the sensitivity of the test with more lenient criteria, as recommended by the AAN subcommittee, can result in decreased specificity.

The second important role for MRI in the diagnostic work-up of suspected MS patients is to rule out alternative diagnoses obvious on MRI, such as spinal stenosis and most brain tumors. Characteristic lesions that favor MS include Dawson Fingers, ovoid lesions, corpus callosum lesions, and asymptomatic spinal cord lesions. However, other white matter diseases can have similar appearances on MRI. Persistent gadolinium enhancement greater than three months, lesions with mass effect, and meningeal enhancement suggest other disorders.

A standardized MRI protocol for brain and spinal cord is crucial for comparing across studies or between centers. T2W MRI cannot distinguish between acute and chronic lesions. Gadolinium provides useful information about new lesion activity and is helpful in ruling out alternative diagnoses such as neoplasm, vascular malformations, and leptomeningeal disease. A single gadolinium-enhanced MRI can potentially provide evidence for dissemination in space and time. Spinal cord imaging is equally valuable to rule out spinal stenosis or tumor, and

for detecting asymptomatic lesions when brain imaging is nondiagnostic in patients suspected of having MS.

Precise criteria may be too suggestive that MS can be diagnosed by MRI and a negative MRI at the time of CIS does not rule out MS. MRI evidence plays a supportive role in what is ultimately a clinical diagnosis of MS, in the appropriate clinical situation, and always at the exclusion of alternative diagnoses (81).

REFERENCES

1. Simon JH, Li D, Traboulsee A, et al. Standardized MRI protocol for multiple sclerosis: Consortium of MS Centers (CMSC) Consensus Guidelines. *Am J Neuroradiol* 2005. In press.
2. Filippi M, Marciano N, Capra R, et al. The effect of imprecise repositioning on lesion volume measurements in patients with multiple sclerosis. *Neurology* 1997; 49(1):274–276.
3. Rovaris M, Rocca MA, Capra R, et al. A comparison between the sensitivities of 3-mm and 5-mm thick serial brain MRI for detecting lesion volume changes in patients with multiple sclerosis. *J Neuroimag* 1998; 8(3):144–147.
4. Rydberg JN, Riederer SJ, Rydberg CH, et al. Contrast optimization of fluid-attenuated inversion recovery (FLAIR) imaging. *Magn Reson Med* 1995;34(6): 868–877.
5. Filippi M, Yousry T, Baratti C, et al. Quantitative assessment of MRI lesion load in multiple sclerosis. A comparison of conventional spin-echo with fast fluid-attenuated inversion recovery. *Brain* 1996;119(Pt 4):1349–1355.
6. Gawne-Cain ML, O'Riordan JI, Thompson AJ, et al. Multiple sclerosis lesion detection in the brain: a comparison of fast fluid-attenuated inversion recovery and conventional T2-weighted dual spin echo. *Neurology* 1997;49(2):364–370.
7. Filippi M, Yousry T, Campi A, et al. Comparison of triple dose versus standard dose gadolinium-DTPA for detection of MRI enhancing lesions in patients with MS. *Neurology* 1996;46(2):379–384.
8. Silver NC, Good CD, Barker GJ, et al. Sensitivity of contrast enhanced MRI in multiple sclerosis. Effects of gadolinium dose, magnetization transfer contrast and delayed imaging. *Brain* 1997;120(Pt 7):1149–1161.
9. Young IR, Hall AS, Pallis CA, et al. Nuclear magnetic resonance imaging of the brain in multiple sclerosis. *Lancet* 1981;2(8255): 1063–1066.
10. Lukes SA, Crooks LE, Aminoff MJ, et al. Nuclear magnetic resonance imaging in multiple sclerosis. *Ann Neurol* 1983;13:592–601.
11. Runge VM, Price AC, Kirshner HS, et al. Magnetic resonance imaging of multiple sclerosis: a study of pulse-technique efficacy. *Am J Roentgenol* 1984;143(5): 1015–1026.
12. Kirshner HS, Tsai SI, Runge VM, et al. Magnetic resonance imaging and other techniques in the diagnosis of multiple sclerosis. *Arch Neurol* 1985;42(9):859–863.

13. Robertson WD, Li DK, Mayo JR, et al. Assessment of multiple sclerosis lesions by magnetic resonance imaging. *Can Assoc Radiol J* 1987;38(3):177–182.

14. Stewart JM, Houser OW, Baker HL Jr., et al. Magnetic resonance imaging and clinical relationships in multiple sclerosis. *Mayo Clinic Proc* 1987;62(3):174–184.

15. Osborn AG, Harnsberger HR, Smoker WR, et al. Multiple sclerosis in adolescents: CT and MR findings. *Am J Roentgenol* 1990;155(2):385–390.

16. Yetkin FZ, Haughton VM, Papke RA, et al. Multiple sclerosis:specificity of MR for diagnosis. *Radiology* 1991;178(2):447–451.

17. Haughton VM, Yetkin FZ, Rao SM, et al. Quantitative MR in the diagnosis of multiple sclerosis. *Magn Res Med* 1992;26(1):71–78.

18. Brex PA, Ciccarelli O, O'Riordan JI, et al. A longitudinal study of abnormalities on MRI and disability from multiple sclerosis. *N Engl J Med* 2002;346(3):158–164.

19. Kidd D, Barkhof F, McConnell R, et al. Cortical lesions in multiple sclerosis. *Brain* 1999;122(Pt 1):17–26.

20. Boggild MD, Williams R, Haq N, et al. Cortical plaques visualised by fluid-attenuated inversion recovery imaging in relapsing multiple sclerosis. *Neuroradiology* 1996;38[Suppl 1]:S10–S13.

21. Horowitz AL, Kaplan RD, Grewe G, et al. The ovoid lesion: a new MR observation in patients with multiple sclerosis. *AJNR* 1989;10:303–305.

22. Wilms G, Marchal G, Kersschot E, et al. Axial vs sagittal T2-weighted brain MR images in the evaluation of multiple sclerosis. *J Comput Assist Tomogr* 1991; 15:359–364.

23. Simon JH, Holtas SL, Schiffer RB. Corpus callosum and subcallosal-periventricular lesions in multiple sclerosis: derection with MR. *Radiology* 1986;160: 363–367.

24. Gean-Marton AD, Vezina LG, Marton KI, et al. Abnormal corpus callosum: a sensitive and specific indicator of multiple sclerosis. *Radiology* 1991;180(1): 215–221.

25. Giroud M, Dumas R. Clinical and topographical range of callosal infarction: a clinical and radiological correlation study. *J Neurol Neurosurg Psychiatry* 1995;59(3): 238–242.

26. Abe K, Murakami T, Matsubara E, et al. Clinical Features of CADASIL. *Ann NY Acad Sci* 2002;977:266–272.

27. Buhring U, Herrlinger U, Krings T, et al. MRI features of primary central nervous system lymphomas at presentation. *Neurology* 2001;57(3):393–396.

28. Morgen K, McFarland HF, Pillemer SR. Central nervous system disease in primary Sjögren's syndrome: the role of magnetic resonance imaging. *Semin Arthritis Rheum* 2004;34(3):623–630.

29. Whiteman ML, Post MJ, Berger JR, et al. Progressive multifocal leukoencephalopathy in 47 HIV-seropositive patients: neuroimaging with clinical and pathologic correlation. *Radiology* 1993;187(1):233–240.

30. Barkhof F, Filippi M, Miller DH, et al. Comparison of MRI criteria at first presentation to predict conversion to clinically definite multiple sclerosis. *Brain* 1997;120(Pt 11):2059–2069.

31. Tien RD, Hesselink JR, Szumowski J. MR fat suppression combined with Gd-DTPA enhancement in optic neuritis and perineuritis. *J Comput Assist Tomogr* 1991;15:223–227.

32. Davies MB, Williams R, Haq N, et al. MRI of optic nerve and postchiasmal visual pathways and visual evoked potentials in secondary progressive multiple sclerosis. *Neuroradiology* 1998;40(12):765–770.

33. Stewart WA, Hall LD, Berry K, et al. Magnetic resonance imaging (MRI) in multiple sclerosis (MS): pathological correlation studies in eight cases. *Neurology* 1986;36[Suppl 1]:S320.

34. Barnes D, Munro PM, Youl BD, et al. The long-standing MS lesion. A quantitative MRI and electron microscopic study. *Brain* 114 1991;(Pt 3):1271–1280.

35. Newcombe J, Hawkins CP, Henderson CL, et al. Histopathology of multiple sclerosis lesions detected by magnetic resonance imaging in unfixed postmortem central nervous system tissue. *Brain* 1991;114 (Pt 2):1013–1023.

36. Hunt AL, Orrison WW, Yeo RA, et al. Clinical significance of MRI white matter lesions in the elderly. *Neurology* 1989;39:1470–1474.

37. de Leeuw FE, de Groot JC, Achten E, et al. Prevalence of cerebral white matter lesions in elderly people: a population based magnetic resonance imaging study. The Rotterdam Scan Study. *J Neurol Neurosurg Psychiatry* 2001;70(1):9–14.

38. van Swieten JC, Geyskes GG, Derix MMA, et al. Hypertension in the elderly is associated with white matter lesions and cognitive decline. *Ann Neurol* 1991;30:825–830.

39. Jungreis CA, Kanal E, Hirsch WL, et al. Normal perivascular spaces mimicking lacunar infarction: MR imaging. *Radiology* 1988;169(1):101–104.

40. Takao M, Koto A, Tanahashi N, et al. Pathologic findings of silent hyperintense white matter lesions on MRI. *J Neurol Sci* 1999;167(2):127–131.

41. Williams DWI, Elster AD, Kramer SI. Neurosarcoidosis: gadolinium-enhanced MR imaging. *J Comput Assist Tomogr* 1990;14:704–707.

42. Lai M., Hodgson T, Gawne-Cain M, et al. A preliminary study into the sensitivity of disease activity detection by serial weekly magnetic resonance imaging in multiple sclerosis. *J Neurol Neurosurg Psychiatry* 1996;60(3): 339–341.

43. Miller DH, Rudge P, Johnson G, et al. Serial gadolinium enhanced magnetic resonance imaging in multiple sclerosis. *Brain* 1988;111:927–939.

44. Nesbit GM, Forbes GS, Scheithauer BW, et al. Multiple sclerosis: histopathologic and MR and/or CT correlation in 37 cases at biopsy and three cases at autopsy. *Radiology* 1991;180(2):467–474.

45. Masdeu JC, Quinto C, Olivera C, et al. Open-ring imaging sign: highly specific for atypical brain demyelination. *Neurology* 2000;54(7):1427–1433.

46. Kermode AG, Tofts PS, Thompson AJ, et al. Heterogeneity of blood-brain barrier changes in multiple sclerosis: an MRI study with gadolinium-DTPA enhancement. *Neurology* 1990;40(2):229–235.

47. Cotton F, Weiner HL, Jolesz FA, Guttmann CR. MRI contrast uptake in new lesions in relapsing-remitting MS followed at weekly intervals. *Neurology* 2003; 60(4):640–646.

48. Barkhof F, Valk J, Hommes OR, et al. Meningeal Gd-DTPA enhancement in multiple sclerosis [see comments]. *Am J Neuroradiol* 1992;13:397–400.

49. Hickman SJ, Miszkiel KA, Plant GT, et al. The optic nerve sheath on MRI in acute optic neuritis. *Neuroradiology* 2005;47(1):51–55.

50. Demaerel P, Robberecht W, Casteels I, et al. Focal leptomeningeal MR enhancement along the chiasm as a

presenting sign of multiple sclerosis. *J Comput Assist Tomogr* 1995;19:297–298.

51. Willoughby EW, Grochowski E, Li DKB, et al. Serial magnetic resonance scanning in multiple sclerosis: a second prospective study in relapsing patients. *Ann Neurol* 1989;25:43–49.

52. Koopmans RA, Li DK, Oger JJ, et al. The lesion of multiple sclerosis: imaging of acute and chronic stages. *Neurology* 1989;39(7):959–963.

53. Paty DW. Magnetic resonance imaging in the assessment of disease activity in multiple sclerosis. *Can J Neurol Sci* 1988;15(3):266–272.

54. Koopmans RA, Li DKB, Grochowski E, et al. Benign versus chronic progressive multiple sclerosis: magnetic resonance imaging features. *Ann Neurol* 1989;25: 74–81.

55. Paty DW, Li DK, Oger JJ, et al. Magnetic resonance imaging in the evaluation of clinical trials in multiple sclerosis. *Ann Neurol* 1994;36[Suppl]:S95–S96.

56. Stone LA, Albert PS, Smith ME, et al. Changes in the amount of diseased white matter over time in patients with relapsing-remitting multiple sclerosis. *Neurology* 1995;45(10):1808–1814.

57. Thorpe JW, Kidd D, Moseley IF, et al. Spinal MRI in patients with suspected multiple sclerosis and negative brain MRI. *Brain* 1996;119(Pt 3):709–714.

58. Lee KH, Hashimoto SA, Hooge JP, et al. Magnetic resonance imaging of the head in the diagnosis of multiple sclerosis: a prospective 2-year follow-up with comparison of clinical evaluation, evoked potentials, oligoclonal banding, and CT. *Neurology* 1991;41(5):657–660.

59. Tartaglino LM, Friedman DP, Flanders AE, et al. Multiple sclerosis in the spinal cord: MR appearance and correlation with clinical parameters. *Radiology* 1995;195(3):725–732.

60. Bot JC, Barkhof F, Lycklama G, et al. Differentiation of multiple sclerosis from other inflammatory disorders and cerebrovascular disease: value of spinal MR imaging. *Radiology* 2002;223(1):46–56.

61. Thielen KR, Miller GM. Multiple sclerosis of the spinal cord: magnetic resonance appearance. *J Comput Assist Tomogr* 1996;20(3):434–438.

62. Dalton CM, Brex PA, Miszkiel KA, et al. Spinal cord MRI in clinically isolated optic neuritis. *J Neurol Neurosurg Psychiatry* 2003;74(11):1577–1580.

63. Lycklama G, Thompson A, Filippi M, et al. Spinal-cord MRI in multiple sclerosis. *Lancet Neurology* 2003;2(9): 555–562.

64. Bagnato F, Jeffries N, Richert ND, et al. Evolution of T1 black holes in patients with multiple sclerosis imaged monthly for 4 years. *Brain* 2003;126(Pt 8): 1782–1789.

65. van Walderveen MA, Barkhof F, Pouwels PJ, et al. A. Neuronal damage in T1-hypointense multiple sclerosis lesions demonstrated in vivo using proton magnetic resonance spectroscopy. *Ann Neurol* 1999;46(1):79–87.

66. Uhlenbrock D, Herbe E, Seidel D, et al. One-year MR imaging follow-up of patients with multiple sclerosis under cortisone therapy. *Neuroradiology* 1989;31:3–7.

67. Truyen L, van Waesberghe JH, van Walderveen MA, et al. Accumulation of hypointense lesions ("black holes") on T1 spin-echo MRI correlates with disease progression in multiple sclerosis. *Neurology* 1996; 47(6):1469–1476.

68. Miller DH, Barkhof F, Frank JA, et al. Measurement of atrophy in multiple sclerosis: pathological basis, methodological aspects and clinical relevance. *Brain* 2002;125(Pt 8):1676–1695.

69. Liu C, Edwards S, Gong Q, et al. Three dimensional MRI estimates of brain and spinal cord atrophy in multiple sclerosis. *J Neurol Neurosurg Psychiatry* 1999; 66(3):323–330.

70. Filippi M, Mastronardo G, Rocca MA, et al. Quantitative volumetric analysis of brain magnetic resonance imaging from patients with multiple sclerosis. *J Neurol Sci* 1998;158(2):148–153.

71. van Walderveen MA, Barkhof F, Tas MW, et al. Patterns of brain magnetic resonance abnormalities on T2-weighted spin echo images in clinical subgroups of multiple sclerosis: a large cross-sectional study. *Eur Neurol* 1998;40(2):91–98.

72. Brex PA, Jenkins R, Fox NC, et al. Detection of ventricular enlargement in patients at the earliest clinical stage of MS. *Neurology* 2000;54(8):1689–1691.

73. McDonald WI, Ron MA. Multiple sclerosis: the disease and its manifestations. *Philos Trans R Soc Lond B Biol Sci* 1999;354(1390):1615–1622.

74. Fox NC, Jenkins R, Leary SM, et al. J. Progressive cerebral atrophy in MS: a serial study using registered, volumetric MRI. *Neurology* 2000;54(4): 807–812.

75. Rudick RA, Fisher E, Lee JC, et al. Use of the brain parenchymal fraction to measure whole brain atrophy in relapsing-remitting MS. Multiple Sclerosis Collaborative Research Group. *Neurology* 1999;53(8): 1698–1704.

76. Rovaris M, Comi G, Rocca MA, et al. Short-term brain volume change in relapsing-remitting multiple sclerosis: effect of glatiramer acetate and implications. *Brain* 2001;124(Pt 9):1803–1812.

77. Comi G, Filippi M, Barkhof F, et al. Effect of early interferon treatment on conversion to definite multiple sclerosis: a randomised study. *Lancet* 2001;357(9268): 1576–1582.

78. Ge Y, Grossman RI, Udupa JK, et al. Brain atrophy in relapsing-remitting multiple sclerosis and secondary progressive multiple sclerosis: longitudinal quantitative analysis. *Radiology* 2000;214(3):665–670.

79. Zhao GJ, Li DK, Wang XY, et al. MRI of dirty-appearing white matter in MS. *Neurology* 2000;54:A121.

80. Poser CM, Paty DW, Scheinberg L, et al. New Diagnostic Criteria for Multiple Sclerosis. Guidelines for Research Protocols. In: Poser CM, Paty DW, Scheinberg L, Ebers GC, eds. *The Diagnosis of Multiple Sclerosis*. New York: Thieme-Stratton, 1984:225–233.

81. McDonald WI, Compston A, Edan G, et al. Recommended diagnostic criteria for multiple sclerosis: guidelines from the International Panel on the diagnosis of multiple sclerosis. *Ann Neur* 2001;50(1):121–127.

82. Engell T. A clinico-pathoanatomical study of multiple sclerosis diagnosis. *Acta Neurol Scand* 1988;78:39–44.

83. Beck RW, Trobe JD, Moke PS, et al. High- and low-risk profiles for the development of multiple sclerosis within 10 years after optic neuritis: experience of the optic neuritis treatment trial. *Arch Ophthal* 2003;121(7): 944–949.

84. Morrissey SP, Miller DH, Kendall BE, et al. The significance of brain magnetic resonance imaging abnormalities at presentation with clinically isolated syndromes suggestive of multiple sclerosis. A 5-year follow-up study. *Brain* 1993;116(Pt 1):135–146.

85. Cole SR, Beck RW, Moke PS, et al. The National Eye Institute Visual Function Questionnaire: experience of the ONTT. Optic Neuritis Treatment Trial. *Invest Ophthalmol Vis Sci* 2000;41(5):1017–1021.

86. O'Riordan JI, Thompson AJ, Kingsley DP, et al. The prognostic value of brain MRI in clinically isolated syndromes of the CNS. A 10-year follow-up. *Brain* 1998;121(Pt 3):495–503.

87. Paty DW, Oger JJ, Kastrukoff L, et al. MRI in the diagnosis of MS: a prospective study with comparison of clinical evaluation, evoked potentials, oligoclonal banding, and CT. *Neurology* 1988;38(2):180–185.

88. Fazekas F, Offenbacher H, Fuchs S, et al. Criteria for an increased specificity of MRI interpretation in elderly subjects with suspected multiple sclerosis. *Neurology* 1988;38(12):1822–1825.

89. Tas MW, Barkhof F, van Walderveen MA, et al. The effect of gadolinium on the sensitivity and specificity of MR in the initial diagnosis of multiple sclerosis. *Am J Neuroradiol* 1995;16:259–264.

90. Uitdehaag BM, Geurts JJ, Barkhof F, et al. The utility of MRI in suspected MS: report of the Therapeutics and Technology Assessment Subcommittee. *Neurology* 2004;63(6):1140.

91. Tintore M, Rovira A, Martinez MJ, et al. Isolated demyelinating syndromes: comparison of different MR imaging criteria to predict conversion to clinically definite multiple sclerosis. *Am J Neuroradiol* 2000; 21(4):702–706.

92. Barkhof F, Rocca M, Francis G, et al. Validation of diagnostic magnetic resonance imaging criteria for multiple sclerosis and response to interferon beta 1a. *Ann Neurol* 2003;53(6):718–724.

93. Isaac C, Li DKB, Genton M., et al. Multiple sclerosis: a serial study using MRI in relapsing patients. *Neurology* 1988;38(10):1511–1515.

94. Lublin FD, Reingold SC. Defining the clinical course of multiple sclerosis: results of an international survey. National Multiple Sclerosis Society (USA) Advisory Committee on Clinical Trials of New Agents in Multiple Sclerosis. *Neurology* 1996;46(4): 907–911.

95. Harris JO, Frank JA, Patronas N, et al. Serial gadolinium-enhanced magnetic resonance imaging scans in patients with early, relapsing-remitting multiple sclerosis: implications for clinical trials and natural history. *Ann Neurol* 1991;29:548–555.

96. McFarland HF, Frank JA, Albert PS, et al. Using gadolinium-enhanced magnetic resonance imaging lesions to monitor disease activity in multiple sclerosis. *Ann Neurol* 1992;32:758–766.

97. PRISMS (Prevention of Relapses and Disability by Interferon beta-1a Subcutaneously in Multiple Sclerosis) Study Group. Randomised double-blind placebo-controlled study of interferon beta-1a in relapsing/remitting multiple sclerosis. *Lancet* 1998; 352(9139): 1498–1504.

98. Jacobs LD, Beck RW, Simon JH., et al. Intramuscular interferon beta-1a therapy initiated during a first demyelinating event in multiple sclerosis. CHAMPS Study Group. *N Engl J Med* 2000;343(13):898–904.

99. Dalton CM, Brex PA, Jenkins R, et al. Progressive ventricular enlargement in patients with clinically isolated syndromes is associated with the early development of multiple sclerosis. *J Neurol Neurosurg Psychiatry* 2002;73(2):141–147.

100. Polman CH, Wolinsky JS, Reingold SC. Multiple sclerosis: should MR criteria for dissemination in time be less stringent. *Ann Neurol* 2004;55(2):297.

101. Wolinsky JS. The PROMiSe trial: baseline data review and progress report. *Mult Scler* 2004;10 [Suppl 1]:S65–S71.

102. Furrows SJ, Hartley JC, Bell J, et al. Chlamydophila pneumoniae infection of the central nervous system in patients with multiple sclerosis. *J Neurol Neurosurg Psychiatry* 2004;75(1):152–154.

103. Dalton CM, Brex PA, Miszkiel KA, et al. Application of the new McDonald criteria to patients with clinically isolated syndromes suggestive of multiple sclerosis. *Ann Neurol* 2002;52(1):47–53.

104. Dalton CM, Brex PA, Miszkiel KA, et al. New T2 lesions enable an earlier diagnosis of multiple sclerosis in clinically isolated syndromes. *Ann Neurol* 2003;53(5):673–676.

105. Tintore M, Rovira A, Rio J, et al. New diagnostic criteria for multiple sclerosis: application in first demyelinating episode. *Neurology* 2003;60(1):27–30.

106. Optic Neuritis Study Group. Long-term brain magnetic resonance imaging changes after optic neuritis in patients without clinically definite multiple sclerosis. *Arch Neurol* 2004;61(10):1538–1541.

107. Frohman EM, Goodin DS, Calabresi PA, et al. The utility of MRI in suspected MS: report of the Therapeutics and Technology Assessment Subcommittee of the American Academy of Neurology. *Neurology* 2003; 61(5):602–611.

108. Beck RW, Trobe JD, Moke PS, et al. High- and low-risk profiles for the development of multiple sclerosis within 10 years after optic neuritis: experience of the optic neuritis treatment trial. *Arch Ophthalmol* 2003;121(7):944–949.

109. Schiffer RB, Giang DW, Mushlin A, et al. Perils and pitfalls of magnetic resonance imaging in the diagnosis of multiple sclerosis. *J Neuroimag* 1993;3: 81–88.

110. Carmosino MJ, Brousseau KM, Arciniegas DB, et al. Initial evaluations for multiple sclerosis in a university multiple sclerosis center: outcomes and role of magnetic resonance imaging in referral. *Arch Neurol* 2005;62(4):585–590.

111. de Seze J, Devos D, Castelnovo G, et al. The prevalence of Sjogren syndrome in patients with primary progressive multiple sclerosis. *Neurology* 2001;57(8): 1359–1363.

112. Giang DW, Grow VM, Mooney C, et al. Clinical diagnosis of multiple sclerosis. The impact of magnetic resonance imaging and ancillary testing. Rochester-Toronto Magnetic Resonance Study Group. *Arch Neurol* 1994;51(1):61–66.

113. Traboulsee A, Laule C, Keogh C, et al. Development of a brain tumor in MS: case report. *Can J Neurol Sci* 2002;69[Suppl 1]:S29.

114. Kleinschmidt-DeMasters, BK, Tyler, Kenneth L, Progressive multifocal leukoencephalopathy complicating treatment with natalizumab and interferon beta-1a for multiple sclerosis. *N Engl J Med* 2005; 353:369-374.

10

Cerebrospinal Fluid Analysis in the Diagnosis of Multiple Sclerosis

Edward J. Thompson[1] and Mark S. Freedman[2]

[1]Department of Neuroimmunology, National Hospital for Neurology & Neurosurgery, Queen Square, London; [2]Department of Medicine (Neurology), University of Ottawa, The Ottawa Hospital, Ottawa, Ontario, Canada

INTRODUCTION

A diagnosis of multiple sclerosis (MS) still requires there to be evidence for dissemination of lesions both in space and time. Cerebrospinal fluid (CSF) analysis has been recognized as the cornerstone of paraclinical evidence supporting a diagnosis of MS long before imaging techniques advanced the field enough to surpass this test marginally in terms of sensitivity (but not specificity). More importantly, magnetic resonance imaging (MRI) is the single most important test to ensure that no diagnosis other than MS could explain the clinical presentation. Still, the results of proper CSF analysis, together with imaging, add to the overall specificity and even sensitivity of a correct diagnosis. Prior to setting a standard for MRI findings, the CSF results were used as part of diagnostic criteria for the past few decades, so much so that previous criteria used the detection of heightened intrathecal immunoglobulin G (IgG) synthesis or the presence of oligoclonal bands (OCBs) to substitute for clinical evidence for dissemination in time [refer to Poser criteria, (1)]. Now, new diagnostic criteria, often referred to as the McDonald criteria, incorporate both MRI and CSF (2). While we still await an agreed-upon international standard for MRI, we have recently published a consensus reviewing how CSF should be analyzed in order to gain the most sensitive and specific information for diagnosing MS (3,4).

Rather than the traditional exercise of listing all the options for analysis and allowing the readers to make their own decisions about what is best, we decided to state things in a fairly straightforward manner. We thus describe, in practical terms, what we feel represents the best current standard of practice in analysing CSF when a sample is sent requesting testing for a possible diagnosis of MS.

METHODOLOGY

Qualitative CSF analysis is vastly superior to quantitative analysis. This was agreed upon in an earlier European consensus that resulted in the Poser criteria (1) as well as in a more recent international consensus that resulted in the McDonald criteria (2). This refers to the testing for the presence of intrathecal-specific OCB compared with serum (i.e., qualitative analysis) compared with attempting to quantitate the amount of IgG present within the intrathecal component. It follows from this that no quantitative measure of IgG is sufficiently sensitive to make a diagnosis of MS, since the IgG index typically finds only about 75% of cases, as opposed to the wide consensus that more than 95% of patients are detected using isoelectric focusing (IEF) followed by immunofixation for IgG (5). Sensitivity of quantitative measures is marred by the number of false positives (using the IgG index, for instance, especially when there is a substantial disruption of the blood-CSF barrier) (6). The U.S. Food and Drug Administration (FDA) has recently approved a CSF diagnostic kit for combined isoelectric focusing plus immunofixation (4) and, hence, neurologists can now check that CSF is sent to a laboratory that not only utilizes this kit, but also classifies the results according to the agreed-upon international consensus of the five types of IgG patterns (1,2), as shown in Figure 10-1.

- Type 1 shows the normal pattern with diffuse polyclonal IgG present in both CSF and parallel serum.
- Type 2 is the classical pattern for local synthesis in which there are oligoclonal bands present in CSF while the parallel serum shows a normal polyclonal distribution.
- Type 3 is local and additional systemic synthesis in which oligoclonal bands are present in serum and are passively transferred down a concentration gradient into the CSF. However, in addition to these bands, there some extra bands that are found only in CSF, and thus locally synthesized, giving rise to the "greater than" pattern.
- Type 4 is the so-called "mirror" pattern in which there is mainly systemic synthesis of oligoclonal bands in serum, which are passively transferred into the CSF.
- Type 5 is the paraprotein type, which is essentially the same as Type 4, since the principal source is in the serum and the bands are again transferred into the CSF. However, in this particular case the banding pattern shows a regular, periodic spacing with the most prominent band near the cathode, and successively smaller amounts as one looks toward the anode.

In fairness, quantitative analysis may still be a useful adjunct to the presence of OCB, but must be considered of secondary significance. Should a discrepancy arise, the results of the qualitative analysis (OCB) should always be accepted as the more accurate result compared to quantitative analysis. We make these statements based on our combined practical experience of over 45 years of measuring IgG on thousands of samples (in excess of 5,000 per annum). One of us (EJT) measures IgG quantitatively only by specific request, usually reserved for patients who are studied sequentially (i.e., looking for a response to a given treatment). Although the false negatives with quantitative analysis are widely known, careful studies have also revealed the false positives; one of the most comprehensive has been from the neurologists working with the Danish Central Serum Laboratory, who stated, "Isoelectric focusing is of value when increased levels of one of the formulae are found in the absence of oligoclonal bands as it appears that such patients rarely, if ever, have MS." (7)

There is also a basic problem between immunochemistry and biochemistry in that one cannot reliably quantify IgG of pathological origin, which has been understood for many years by our haematology colleagues in the case of monoclonal bands (in myeloma) or, in our case, OCB (in MS). Indeed, we are still perplexed over the inability to find a single, common antibody in MS CSF or the antigen to which it might be directed. In the absence of knowing which antibody is the most important to measure, we opted instead to express a much wider range of IgG that encompasses a broad spectrum of values [i.e., from 20 to 1,200 ng IgG (5)]. There are only a

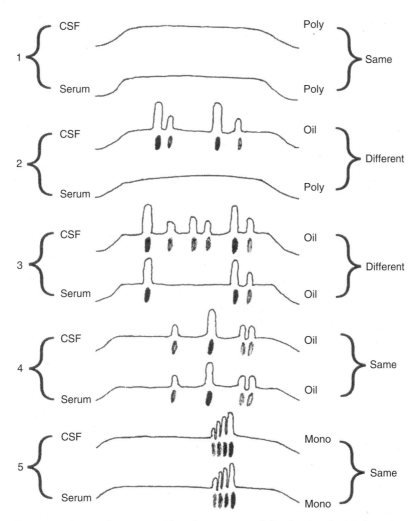

FIG. 10-1. The agreed-upon five types of banding patterns following isoelectric focusing of CSF and parallel serum. Poly, polyclonal; Oli, oligoclonal; Mono, monoclonal.

few cases where the level of IgG is too low (usually ventricular fluid from a child with hydrocephalus) or too high (typically visible with the naked eye as a brown color, looking rather like diluted serum) to be accurately measured; the latter can be diluted with distilled water as required.

Some methodological aspects of the qualitative assessment of OCB warrant further discussion in order to ensure high-quality results. The fundamental concept agreed upon by most investigators in determining the presence of OCB is that, "by eye," one should see a similar amount of staining in parallel CSF and serum from the same patient in order to interpret the patterns correctly.

Some laboratories actually measure how much IgG is applied to the gel, recommending 50 ng of IgG from parallel CSF and serum of all patients. Technically, this may play out in the older (and, some consider, the less-specific) qualitative assay such as the silver staining technique, which typically reveals significant discrepancies in up to 4 in 20 tracks on an isoelectric focusing plate, whereas the incidence of repeat staining when the technique involves visualization using the currently recommended ethylaminocarbazole is less than 1 in 20 (5). This is illustrated in Figure 10-2, with three samples having too much IgG, and one having too little. In this silver technique,

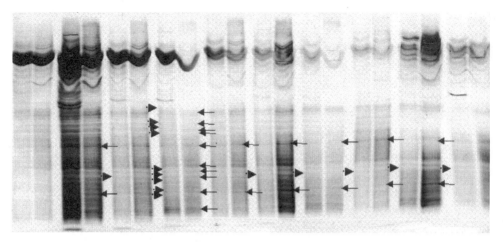

FIG. 10-2. Silver staining of all CSF and serum proteins following isoelectric focusing, where each sample ostensibly contains 50 ng of IgG.

the concentrations of IgG are measured in CSF and parallel serum before focusing, and then the appropriate dilution of serum is calculated to yield 50 ng of IgG. This is applied to the gel in parallel with the appropriate volume of CSF to achieve the same 50 ng of IgG.

Figure 10-2 shows 20 lanes, each of which is calculated to contain 50 ng of IgG.

- There are 10 consecutive pairs of samples, each consisting of CSF on the left and its corresponding serum on the right. The larger arrowheads (*pointing to the right*) illustrate the deficiencies in ampholytes which appear as horizontal white bands, or so-called white snakes. These regional weaknesses in conductivity therefore lead to an accumulation of IgG on either side of the white snakes, which appear as common artefactual bands and are easily seen in all samples. It would clearly make no physiological sense for all patients to have IgG bands with exactly the same isoelectric points.
- In Lane 7, the CSF sample from the fourth pair, nine arrowheads indicate the most prominent white snakes.
- The corresponding serum in Lane 8 from the fourth pair shows the derived artefactual bands (*arrows pointing to the left*). Two of the bands are marked in the other samples and are seen to run all the way across the gel. One of these has an isoelectric point in the middle of the range and another band is near the bottom or

cathodic end of the range. Just above the latter band, the arrowheads pointing to the right also demonstrate one of the more prominent white snakes running across all the other samples.

- Note also the gross overload of CSF IgG in Lane 3, where all bands merge and obliterate the white snakes.
- There is also an excessive amount of IgG in the serum in Lanes 12 and 18.
- At the other extreme, Lane 19 shows gross underloading of CSF IgG, such that the three white snakes nearest to the anode are not seen due to the fact that insufficient amounts of IgG were applied.

Overall, it is quite clear that, by visual inspection, equivalent amounts of IgG are not being applied; these visual inequalities are readily confirmed by densitometry on the scan of the gel (data not shown). This therefore illustrates not only the well-known difficulty in measuring the amounts of IgG from pathological specimens (notorious in myeloma or monoclonal bands), but the same problem occurring with OCB.

There is second fundamental problem that is revealed in Figure 10-2: only a relatively narrow range of IgG values can be accommodated by the silver staining technique. This is in contrast with the very broad range acceptable when staining with ethylaminocarbazole, which is precipitated by the horseradish peroxidase enzyme. This enzyme is attached to the secondary antibody that will bind to the primary antibody (which is directed against the heavy chain of the IgG molecule) (5). These two basic problems can combine to give reduced sensitivity and/or specificity, which is manifested by poor results for quality control, as we shall see below.

If we do not bother to make appropriate dilutions on the basis of elevated total protein (for which we use a 2-minute colorimetric assay for samples from our own hospital), we may then have to subsequently dilute up to 2 out of 20 CSF samples. Most of these samples containing high levels of IgG are received from other hospitals, and we are not always told their estimated total protein, so it is just as simple for us to apply a routine volume of 3 μL of CSF as an initial screen, and then dilute the occasional sample on the following day, should the IgG visually appear to be too high to interpret safely. Once we have decided that the IgG is not too high (it is rarely too low), then, in order to interpret the pattern as local synthesis, we require there to be at least two bands present in CSF, which are not apparent in a corresponding serum. If there is only a single band, or if the pattern is equivocal, we then stain with antisera directed against "whole," "intact," or "total" κ/λ light chains (i.e., not just free light chains), since the κ versus λ pattern will invariably settle the equivocal

IgG patterns. This is because the light chains allow a further level of distinction going beyond the less-discriminating, heavy chains of IgG.

Figure 10-3A shows parallel CSF (*top*) and serum (*bottom*) from four patients. These samples have been applied in accordance with the prior run in which similar amounts of IgG staining were visually observed (5). The antibodies against light chains have not been preabsorbed with intact IgG and are, therefore, directed against epitopes in both free and bound light chains. This gives a much more sensitive stain, as well as reacting with both intact IgG and with any fragments or free light chains. The different samples demonstrate that in blot A, only the fourth patient's CSF showed a common band stained with both κ and λ, which therefore probably represents an intact IgG immune complex. However, in blot B (in samples from three other patients) only the middle CSF band is stained with λ but not with κ. This is unequivocal evidence in this patient for local synthesis of antibody within the central nervous system.

This κ/λ staining is also useful in investigating abnormalities in IgA or IgM. These are routinely detected by screening all serum samples stained with Coomassie Blue after agarose electrophoresis. This is particularly helpful in detecting these in patients with neuropathy (8).

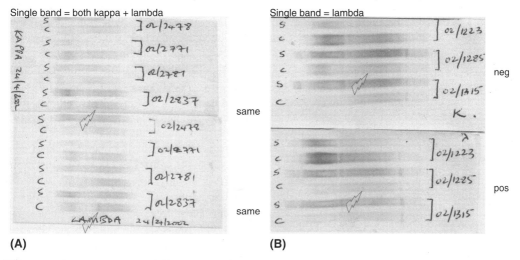

(A) **(B)**

FIG. 10-3. Immunostaining of free + bound kappa (*top*) as opposed to lambda (*bottom*) light chains following isoelectric focusing. This figure shows single bands in CSF which are either common to both light chains (**A**, *left*) or unique to one light chain (**B**, *right*). Neg, negative; Pos, positive.

The recent McDonald criteria (2), which are more explicit than the earlier Poser criteria (1), set out an additional recommendation that *immunofixation should be performed after the isoelectric focusing step (4)*. Although many laboratories have been using silver staining successfully, there is, unfortunately, a growing tendency (particularly amongst the less-experienced laboratories) toward lower standards of quality control, as noted by the Dutch survey reported in *Clinical Chemistry* by Verbeek et al. (9) The data in the supplementary web version of that paper reveal that when using the Fisher exact test, there is a clear statistical significance between those laboratories that use silver staining versus those using IgG-specific immunofixation. Table 10-1 shows the number of laboratories that correctly reported the presence of oligoclonal patterns in CSF, namely 32/35 (94%), using the gold standard technique of isoelectric focusing with immunofixation. However, using the silver technique (which requires a much greater degree of expertise and experience) the results were only 14/26 (54%). The difference between the two techniques resulted in a loss of sensitivity of about 40%.

In addition, a number of kits that employ the silver stain also have a signal-to-noise problem, (i.e., the regularity of the ampholine patterns causes most patients to show so-called common bands (the white snakes) derived from the fundamental chemistry by which the different ampholyte populations are synthesized by their particular manufacturers). All patients show an absence of the polyclonal IgG at these particular isoelectric points (pIs). There is simply an insufficient amount of the ampholytes at the respective pIs, such that the normal polyclonal IgG is effectively pushed aside to pIs just above and below the sites of the pIs of the deficient ampholytes, therefore giving a pseudobanding effect on either side of the white snakes. The overall picture is that of a very high background, such that essentially all patients have quite an excessive amount of this nonspecific banding. It is therefore very difficult to see any pathologically based oligoclonal bands since they are, in effect, lost in the plethora of artefactual bands. The net result is lower sensitivity and therefore poor quality control.

THE ONTOGENY OF THE IMMUNE RESPONSE

We have found that about half the patients with single bands will eventually develop a full-blown oligoclonal pattern. We therefore suggest to neurologists that they perform another lumbar puncture in about six months, if clinically indicated.

There is a completely separate story about the so-called free light chains (FLCs), which cannot be discussed in sufficient detail in this particular chapter. Since the antisera used to detect these free light chains are extensively preabsorbed, they will only pick up a minority of the immunoglobulins. It was shown several years ago that these same antisera, ostensibly directed against free light chains, can cross-react with bound as well as free light chains when they have been adsorbed on to nitrocellulose membranes (10). This binding to membranes is in contradistinction to the much older technique with the primary aim of in-gel agarose immunofixation, in which these antisera must form precipitates before allowing visualization of any bands (including problems with pro-zoning, namely, excessively high amounts of antigen). Thankfully, nitrocellulose adsorption (by definition) avoids these problems. Therefore we use unadsorbed (i.e. "anti-whole," which is "bound" plus "free" κ and λ rather than "anti-free" light chains.

For research purposes, levels of FLCs were quantitatively measured in CSF, serum, and urine; there proved to be a correlation between CSF and urine, but not with serum. It is again

TABLE 10-1 *Fischer exact test on silver staining of total proteins versus immunofixation for IgG*

	PAGE/IEF with silver staining	IEF with immunoblotting
True positive	14	33
False positive	12	2
Fisher exact test	$p < 0.02$	

Quality assurance data from the National Survey in Holland on laboratories using silver staining of total proteins versus immunofixation for IgG.

beyond the scope of this chapter to deal with these technical issues. These assays have therefore been used for longitudinal studies in patients receiving different types of therapy for MS and other diseases (11,12). An example is shown in Table 10-2, which also illustrates the same principle that quantitative analysis of FLCs is useful for monitoring therapy, whereas qualitative analysis is more useful for diagnosis. Table 10-2 shows the number of FLC bands found according to an earlier, semiquantitative band-counting method (13), in which nitrocellulose blots were applied following polyacrylamide gel electrophoresis (in the absence of sodium dodecyl sulphate). Any bands that moved beyond IgG, namely those with relative flow (Rf) > 0.33, were not moving as intact immunoglobulins, whose Rf was < 0.33. This antiserum was not absorbed and therefore had full sensitivity against the free and/or bound light chains. However the distinction was on the basis of physical chemistry, namely, physical size. The light chains must have been sufficiently small to travel much farther into the polyacrylamide gel with its molecular sieving effect. We therefore found statistically significant changes in both bound and free light chains.

DIAGNOSIS

Making a diagnosis of MS using paraclinical evidence involves different levels of clinical certitude (i.e., definite versus possible), as per the McDonald criteria. Typically, a higher percentage of positive findings parallels increasing clinical confidence of the diagnosis. We will now consider the different ancillary techniques used in making the diagnosis of MS, which will then lead us into the question of differential diagnosis for other specific diseases.

Looking at the results of visual-evoked potentials (VEPs), for instance, delayed visual-evoked responses can be observed in patients with cataracts, yet this group of patients is not likely to show CSF OCB. In this sense, the positive VEP would be a misleading false positive if one is interpreting that the delay is due to demyelination. In magnetic resonance imaging (MRI), we know that "a man is as old as his arteries" and, thus, there are practical concerns with patients in their forties and fifties showing white matter lesions (as part of normal aging), which might be interpreted as being due to demyelination in a patient with perhaps clinically less-convincing evidence. There is no similar problem in terms of age-related occurrences of OCB. It is well known that so-called benign paraproteins are typically found in the elderly, but these give a monoclonal, rather than an oligoclonal, pattern. MS still can rarely appear for the first time in the elderly, and investigating such patients requires a careful interpretation of the results of paraclinical tests.

The crucial difference between MRI and CSF is neither the cost nor the sensitivity (due to the false positives already alluded to as part of normal aging); it is the specificity. This is best understood from the molecular basis of the two techniques. MRI essentially measures water, which is bound to varying degrees in separate parts of the brain in different diseases. On the other hand, isoelectric focusing (IEF) measures IgG, which is the molecular product of the antigenically-stimulated B-cell (i.e., the plasma cell). There have been many retrospective studies but few prospective studies with an adequate number of patients. These prospective studies are shown in Table 10-3, and they give a specificity for CSF in the range of 87%. Specificity was based upon prospective studies in which patients had been followed-up for at least 2 years. Table 10-3 also shows the sensitivity of three retrospective studies, each of which had in excess of 500 patients, of whom more than 50 had multiple sclerosis.

TABLE 10-2 *Fisher exact test on free versus bound kappa and lambda light chains following molecular sieving on acrylamide gel in a double-blind study of cyclosporin*

	Increased κ		Increased λ	
	+ve	−ve	+ve	−ve
Cyclosporin	2	7	2	7
Placebo	7	3	8	2
Fisher exact test	$p < 0.05$		$p < 0.02$	

Following molecular sieving on acrylamide gel in a double-blind study of cyclosporin.

TABLE 10-3 *Sensitivity and specificity of CSF in diagnosing MS*

	Total	MS	Reference
Sensitivity			
100%	1,114	58	Kostulas et al. (31)
95%	1,007	82	McLean et al. (32)
96%	558	112	Ohman et al. (33)
Specificity			
87%	189	98	Beer et al. (34)
86%	44	26	Paolino et al. (35)

Data are from large and/or prospective studies.

The differential diagnoses are given in Table 10-4. This shows how oligoclonal bands can be synthesized within the central nervous system in other diseases; however, note the strikingly lower incidence among the bottom four diseases, especially neurosarcoidosis (14).

TABLE 10-4 *Incidence of oligoclonal bands as part of the differential diagnosis for MS*

Disorder	Approximate incidence of oligoclonal bands (%)	Suggested supplementary investigation
MS	97	MRI
SSPE	100	Anti-measles antibody
Neurosyphilis	95	Anti-treponemal antibody
Neuro-AIDS	80	Anti-HIV antibody
Neuro-Lyme disease	80	Anti-Borrelia antibody
Ataxia-telangiec-tasia	60	Serum IgA
Adrenoleukody-strophy	100	Long-chain fatty acids
Harada meningitis-uveitis	60	Serum CRP
Neuro-SLE	50	Antinuclear factor
Neuro-Behçet's	20	C'3 & CSF polymorphs
Neuro-sarcoidosis	< 5	Kveim test
Acute encephalitis (< 7 days)	< 5	Viral antibody
Acute meningitis (< 7 days)	< 5	CSF lactate, serum CRP
Tumor	< 5	Brain scan

Along with their associated distinguishing tests.

It is worth considering yet again the molecular basis for the serum oligoclonal pattern as part of the differential diagnosis, specifically in relation to systemic antigenic stimulation, which is passively transferred from serum into the CSF (the so-called mirror pattern). This is seen in Table 10-5 (15). The presence of serum bands can sometimes be helpful for neurologists (e.g., in Guillain–Barré syndrome, which typically has a mirror pattern). Table 10-5 shows that the local + systemic response (on the right) is a "greater than" pattern (i.e., having a greater number of bands in CSF than serum). This is principally found only in multiple sclerosis and infections, whereas the mirror pattern (on the left) is much less discriminating and only shows a slight preference for infections, neoplasia, and neuropathy.

Returning once more to the so-called white snakes shown in Figure 10-2—these give rise to a signal-to-noise problem which, when coupled with the lack of immunofixation (which are the recent McDonald criteria), has the final effect of blurring what are the true negative diseases in which oligoclonal bands are rarely synthesized locally in the CSF. These conditions are listed in Table 10-6.

Printed laboratory reports for patients in whom a diagnosis of MS is being queried, typically should state, *"Although the results are character-*

TABLE 10-5 *The differential diagnosis of serum bands*

	"Mirror"		"Greater than"	
	No.	%	No.	%
Infections	8	14	13	29
Inflammations	10	18	4	9
Paraneoplastic	3	5	2	4
Neoplastic	9	16	1	2
Guillain–Barré syndrome	9	16	0	0
Other peripheral neuropathies	10	18	0	0
Multiple sclerosis	1	2	26	57
Vascular	`3	5	0	0
Degenerative	3	5	0	0
Totals	56	99	46	100

Bands show either systemic synthesis ("mirror" pattern) or systemic + local synthesis ("greater than" pattern).

TABLE 10-6 *Diseases in which oligoclonal bands are rarely found*

Disease Category
Exclusion of infectious disorders:
Congenital disorders
Vascular disorders
Headache and pain syndromes
Metabolic disorders
Paroxysmal disorders
Traumatic and sequelae
Skeletal and sequelae including myelopathy
Systematic disorders
Psychiatric disorders
Degenerative disorders
Parkinson disease
Autonomic failure
Alzheimer disease and other dementias
Motor neurone disease
Spinal muscular dystrophy
Hereditary degenerations
Idiopathic cerebellar, spinocerebellar degenerations
Exclusion of complicating cases:
Neuropathies and myopathies
Peripheral neuropathies (hereditary and acquired)
Radicular syndromes
Isolated peripheral nerve lesions
Metabolic neuropathies
Other groups:
Isolated myelopathies
Guillain-Barré syndrome
Isolated intracranial hypertension

istic of MS, the underlying pathophysiology relates to an intrathecal immune response, and thus one should rule out other inflammatory causes." The most common and important inflammatory cause of an intrathecal OCB response other than MS is that of infection. There are a number of neurotropic agents which, for various reasons, choose to gravitate to the brain where they can then multiply. These include measles, mumps, rubella, varicella, herpes, cytomegalovirus, toxoplasma, syphilis, and the tuberculosis bacterium. Antibody reactivity to these organisms can be screened in so-called dot-blots, using equal amounts "by eye" of IgG (based upon the prior isoelectric focusing and immunofixation that are performed on all patients). Antigens are applied in what is called the first dimension, using one trough for each of the antigens, which are then incubated overnight on top of a square piece of nitrocellulose membrane. The mold is then rotated through 90 degrees and parallel samples of serum and CSF

are applied such that any positive reaction appears as a square, as shown in Figure 10-4, where there is an intersection between the individual patient's CSF or serum with each specific antigen. Figure 10-4 shows strong activity present in CSF but not in the parallel serum sample, which contained the same amount of total IgG "by eye" (this can easily be confirmed objectively by scanning densitometry). In addition, the reaction is confined to only one antigen—varicella in this example—which is quite unlike the situation in multiple sclerosis where multiple antigens show cross-reactivity, albeit at a lower level.

The dot-blot is just a screening test in which the unfractionated antibodies are revealed by the technique. Final confirmation is made by isoelectric focusing, since this is universally accepted as a much more sensitive and discriminating technique. Focusing can easily distinguish between an oligoclonal response in CSF and a polyclonal response in serum (see inset at bottom of Figure 10-4). This again illustrates the principle that if one were solely using a quantitative technique for the antigen in question (varicella), it could give the wrong answer. This is not only because one is not comparing like with like but, as haematologists have known for many years, the monoclonal immunoglobulin typically gives spurious results when compared with polyclonal standards. Figure 10-4 shows four pairs of serum (left) with corresponding CSF (right). The only positive sample, CSF in the fourth patient (No. 5454) was then run by isoelectric focusing with the serum on top and the CSF underneath. Below these was a positive control for varicella zoster.

Patients with multiple sclerosis typically have positive reactions against a number of antigens, but this may be simply representative of a more activated immune state characterized by hypergammaglobulinemia. Some people believe in the MRZ (measles, rubella, zoster) reaction but, in our experience and where appropriate, it is safer to screen for all the neurotropic agents. Our primary aim is to diagnose infectious diseases other than MS, rather than just selecting these three specific antigens as an ancillary method for the diagnosis of MS alone. In

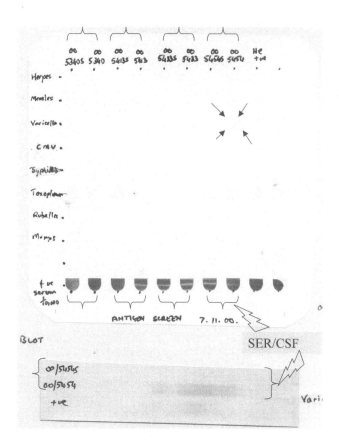

FIG. 10-4. Dot-blots of the eight neurotropic antigens (herpes, measles, varicella, CMV, syphilis, toxoplasma, rubella, mumps) in the initial incubation, followed by a 90-degree rotation and second incubation with parallel CSF and serum. Ser, serum; CSF, cerebrospinal fluid.

addition, there is international consensus that, as with other quantitative tests, the MRZ reaction is less reliable than the gold standard technique of qualitative isoelectric focusing with immunofixation (3).

In summary, for MS, the dot-blot screening test shows a mild reaction to multiple antigens, whereas in specific brain infections there is typically a very strong reaction against a single antigen (although there is sometimes a dual reaction between herpes simplex and varicella zoster, since both viruses have many proteins in common). However, by far the most important test is the qualitative comparison of CSF and serum by isoelectric focusing after binding to the antigen in question, instead of looking at the total IgG population with routine isoelectric focusing and immunofixation.

There is one further variation for identification of specific antigens that can usefully be applied to the latter technique, namely, immunofixation against IgM (rather than IgG), since the natural history of infections shows a sequential increase in IgM followed by its tailing off during the convalescent phase. One can therefore distinguish an acute or early infection from one which has occurred in the distant past, by the respective presence or absence of IgM for the antigen in question (16).

Last but not least, with any antigen one can use the presence of sodium thiocyanate (17) to remove any nonspecific antibodies [i.e., low-affinity binding (18,19)], as previously shown using quantitative enzyme-linked immunosorbent assays (ELISAs). The same principle can be applied using thiocyanate with isoelectric focusing (20,21). As we shall see below, a number of different antigens have been considered to play a role in the etiology of MS, but these have invariably been shown to demonstrate only low-affinity or nonspecific binding. The same can also be said of the so-called autoimmune etiology of MS, in which extensive studies of the animal model of experimental allergic encephalomyelitis (EAE) immunized against myelin basic protein (MBP) have shown that only a small proportion of the IgG will bind to MBP. This binding has also been shown to be low-affinity and nonspecific (22). Figure 10-5 shows that when there is a correct fit between antigen and antibody (shown on the left), there will be a large number of hydrogen bonds (approximately 35 bonds are shown) to hold the antigen tightly to its antibody. If, however, there is only a weak association between the antigen and antibody (on the right side of the picture), there will be very few hydrogen bonds (approximately 7 bonds are shown) to hold the two molecules together.

RESPONSE TO THERAPY

It has been asked, "Why are neurologists such monotherapists?" For instance, cardiologists have a whole armamentarium of drugs to use at different phases following a myocardial infarction. However, there has been much recent interest in the study of agents such as interferon-beta (IFNβ), the ostensible molecular basis of its action being to stop the replication of viruses. Disappointingly, as a result of its immunomodulatory effects, the IFNβ agents have been only shown to modestly benefit a small proportion of patients (23) in terms of disability progression. It is therefore important to be able to predict a priori which patients might be the most likely to respond to this agent, not only because it is expensive and cumbersome to administer (given that it requires parenteral injection) but, more importantly, because this could lead to some more significant clues to the underlying pathophysiology of the disease and its heterogeneity. The same can be said for other types of therapy. It would also be intriguing to be able to anticipate responses of patients to different types of immunomodulation, such as:

- Corticosteroids, which cause a generalised depression of the immune response
- Mitoxantrone, a potent immunosuppressive agent
- Intravenous immunoglobulin (IVIG), which may have many potential mechanisms of action but, of interest, an anti-idiotype effect
- Glatiramer acetate, which exerts a net negative charge by the gross excess of primary amines

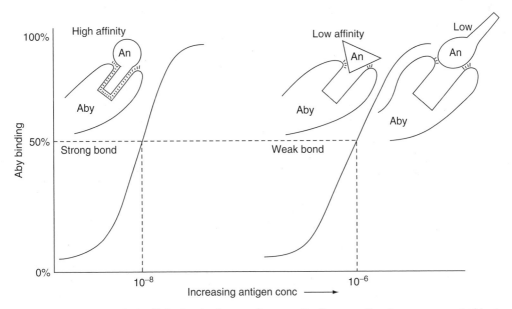

FIG. 10-5. High-versus low-affinity for the "correct" versus the "incorrect" epitopes, separated by two orders of magnitude in binding constants. An, antigen; Aby, antibody.

on the side chains of lysine, but probably functions as a so-called universal antigen that selectively activates T-cells and steers them into a more protective as opposed to a disease-causing role.

PROGNOSIS

Some investigators have tried to correlate certain features of the IgG response in the CSF with prognosis. In one study, a quantitative index of IgG synthesis (the Link Index) was linked to progression, with higher indices correlating with secondary progressive MS compared to relapsing-remitting disease (24a). Some have even suggested that prognosis correlates to the more simple measures in the CSF, such as protein elevation or lymphocytosis (24b). CSF analysis is likely to be performed on patients presenting for the first time with a demyelinating event, a clinically isolated syndrome (CIS). Some of these will turn out not to be MS, whereas others could also end up being the most benign form of disease, something that is more common if the CSF remains negative for OCB (24c). Some of these patients can also have single bands, as studied previously (25).

Quantitative measurement of IgG over many years demonstrates some correlation with disease activity. In a study by Vrethem et al., neither CSF IgA nor IgG indices correlated with disability, walking distance, or time from onset of symptoms to the need of walking aid (26a). In another study, the highest levels were associated with higher neurological disability scores [i.e., the Expanded Disability Status Scale (EDSS)] but, interestingly, not with the duration of disease (26b). In the same study, it was found that patients with the progressive subtype of MS had much greater abnormalities of the blood–CSF barrier, [i.e., either elevated total protein (26) or the presence of high molecular weight haptoglobin polymers (27)]. Another researcher has suggested that the presence of FLC of the κ variety might be a negative prognostic (12).

Much has been written about gadolinium enhancement in relapsing-remitting MS (as opposed to progressive MS, which typically does not show such discrete foci for gadolin-

ium). We will not deal here with the reasons behind the reported discrepancies in studies linking the presence of active enhancing MRI lesions and any measure of blood–brain barrier dysfunction, but a neat correlation has simply not been found. In fact, it has been generally difficult to correlate the presence of enhancing lesions and measures of blood–brain barrier dysfunction (28). Total CSF protein was statistically higher in progressive MS, even though we know that there is a tendency toward less gadolinium enhancement at that stage. This elevation of total protein may represent a more diffuse barrier damage. The corollary of this is that the presence of focal-enhancing lesions represents only a localized change in barrier permeability, which is unlikely to change global measures of barrier leakiness.

Concerning pathophysiology, there remains at least one more clue that we have yet to understand, which is revealed by the gold standard technique for assessing the presence of OCB, namely the presence of serum bands in about half of MS patients (29). It is worth stressing immediately that these bands do not come from the CSF. Of course, CSF bands are present in the serum, but they are totally swamped by the dilution effect of a 10,000-fold higher amount of IgG in the serum. This can be quickly calculated by the 400-fold higher concentration of IgG in serum relative to CSF, and by the 20-fold difference in total volume between the two fluids: 150 mL CSF versus 3,000 mL serum. Cross-multiplying these two factors gives essentially four orders of magnitude. Given this dramatic synthesis of systemic IgG in MS patients, although it is clinically a brain disease, we must nevertheless acknowledge our humility. Yet again, the positive attraction to continuing investigations is the pursuit of the molecular basis for this pathophysiological fact. These serum oligoclonal bands can be detected in almost half the MS patients (44%). They clearly do not represent the return of CSF IgG into the serum, as total CSF IgG would constitute only 3% of the total serum IgG, and thus would be totally swamped by the polyclonal background. Once again, the area under the curve for the serum oligoclonal bands is disproportionately higher than the expected 3%, which one could calculate from the CSF contribution, since dilution experiments have shown that concentrations of CSF IgG (which are < 9% of serum IgG) become lost in the background. What is clinically intriguing is that the serum bands are 10 times more common in female patients (19/27, 70%) than male patients, (1/14, 7%). The patients were also significantly older (46 years versus 38 years) and had a later age of onset (39 years versus 33 years). Immunologically, they had a two-fold increase in the IgG index (2.2 versus 1.3). Serum bands are also more commonly associated with other serum markers of autoantibody production and therefore may represent a different constitution (e.g., genetic background) for the individual concerned, or perhaps a different phase during the course of the evolution of the disease.

We must finally double back to therapy and reiterate questions about the different approaches taken and whether these alter any systemic response. Could there really be a relationship between the presence of serum IgM antibodies and myelin proteins such as myelin oligodendrocyte glycoprotein (MOG) or myelin basic protein (MBP) (30)? Are similar findings noted in the CSF and, if so, would this be due to antibody formation outside or inside the central nervous system (CNS)? It is intriguing to speculate that we may someday have tests that can be performed on CSF at the start of disease that could help confirm a diagnosis of MS, predict its course, and even anticipate a response to a particular therapy.

CONCLUSION

In summary, the gold standard technique for measuring intrathecal antibody synthesis of IgG is not only tightly coupled to the diagnosis of MS (> 95% sensitive and > 87% specific), but there are very few other diseases for which there is such a good indicator of disease. The best analogy is the specific enzyme deficiencies, which represent almost tautological evidence for the respective diseases in question. We encourage neurologists to become familiar with the techniques involved in CSF analysis much in the way they are versed in the interpretation of MRI scans, in order to better understand the true meaning of the test results. Just as not all MRI machines yield the same quality studies, laboratories analyzing CSF do not all use the same techniques and their interpretation of the results may also differ. In the hope of striving for some uniformity in analysis, we have published consensus statements (3,4) aimed at neurologists so that they may appreciate the differences in analyses and demand that the best test be used for their patients.

ACKNOWLEDGMENT

Edward J. Thompson gives special thanks to Jan Alsop, personal assistant, for her caring and intelligent work on the manuscript.

REFERENCES

1. Poser CM, Paty DW, Scheinberg L, et al. New diagnostic criteria for multiple sclerosis: guidelines for research protocols. *Ann Neurol* 1983;13(3):227–231.
2. McDonald WI, Compston A, Edan G, et al. Recommended diagnostic criteria for multiple sclerosis: guidelines from the International Panel on the Diagnosis of Multiple Sclerosis. *Ann Neurol* 2001;50:121–127.
3. Andersson M, Alvarez-Cermeno J, Cogato I, et al. The role of cerebrospinal fluid analysis in the diagnosis of multiple sclerosis: a consensus report. *J Neurol Neurosurg Psychiatry* 1994;57:897–903.
4. Freedman MS, Thompson EJ, Deisenhammer F, et al. Recommended standard of cerebrospinal fluid analysis in the diagnosis of multiple sclerosis—a consensus statement. *Arch Neurol* 2005;62:865–870.
5. Keir G, Luxton RW, Thompson EJ. Isoelectric focusing of cerebrospinal fluid immunoglobulin G: an annotated update. *Ann Clin Biochem* 1990;27(Pt 5):436–443.
6. Reiber H, Peter JB. Cerebrospinal fluid analysis: disease-related data patterns and evaluation programs. *J Neurol Sci* 2001;184:101–122.
7. Sellebjerg F, Christiansen M, Rasmussen LS, et al. The cerebrospinal fluid in multiple sclerosis: quantitative assessment of intrathecal immunoglobulin synthesis by empirical formulae. *Eur J of Neurol* 1996;3:548–559.
8. Kahn SN, Riches PG, Kohn J. Paraproteinaemia in neurological disease: incidence, associations, and classification of monoclonal immunoglobulins. *J Clin Pathol* 1980;33:617–621.
9. Verbeek MM, de Reus HP, Weykamp CW. Comparison of methods for the detection of oligoclonal IgG bands in cerebrospinal fluid and serum: results of the Dutch Quality Control survey. *Clin Chem* 2002;48:1578–1580.

10. Walker RW, Keir G, Thompson EJ. Assessment of cerebrospinal fluid immunoglobulin patterns after isoelectric focusing. Use of kappa and lambda light chain immunoperoxidase staining. *J Neurol Sci* 1983;58: 123–134.

11. McLean BN, Rudge P, Thompson EJ. Cyclosporin A curtails the progression of free light chain synthesis in the CSF of patients with multiple sclerosis. *J Neurol Neurosurg Psychiatry* 1989;52:529–531.

12. Rudick RA, Medendorp SV, Namey M, et al. Multiple sclerosis progression in a natural history study: predictive value of cerebrospinal fluid free kappa light chains. *Mult Scler* 1995;1:150–155.

13. Thompson EJ, Keir G. Improved detection of oligoclonal and Bence-Jones proteins by kappa/lambda immunoblotting. *Clin Chim Acta* 1984;143:329–335.

14. Thompson EJ. Cerebrospinal fluid. *J Neurol Neurosurg Psychiatry* 1995;59:349–357.

15. Zeman A, McLean BN, Keir G, et al. The significance of serum oligoclonal bands in neurological diseases. *J Neurol Neurosurg Psychiatry* 1993;56:32–35.

16. Coren ME, Buchdahl RM, Cowan FM, et al. Imaging and laboratory investigation in herpes simplex encephalitis. *J Neurol Neurosurg Psychiatry* 1999;67: 243–245.

17. Luxton RW, Thompson EJ. Affinity distributions of antigen-specific IgG in patients with multiple sclerosis and in patients with viral encephalitis. *J Immunol Meth* 1990;131:277–282.

18. Luxton RW, Zeman A, Holzel H, et al. Affinity of antigen-specific IgG distinguishes multiple sclerosis from encephalitis. *J Neurol Sci* 1995;132:11–19.

19. Monteyne P, Albert F, Weissbrich B, et al. The detection of intrathecal synthesis of anti-herpes simplex IgG antibodies: comparison between an antigen-mediated immunoblotting technique and antibody index calculations. *J Med Virol* 1997;53:324–331.

20. Luxton RW, McLean BN, Thompson EJ. Isoelectric focusing versus quantitative measurements in the detection of intrathecal local synthesis of IgG. *Clin Chim Acta* 1990;187:297–308.

21. Luxton RW, Thompson EJ. Differential oligoclonal band patterns on polyvinyldifluoride membranes. *J Immunol Meth* 1989;121:269–274.

22. O'Connor KC, Chitnis T, Griffin DE, et al. Myelin basic protein-reactive autoantibodies in the serum and cerebrospinal fluid of multiple sclerosis patients are characterized by low affinity interactions. *J Neuroimmunol.* 2003;136:140–148.

23. Filippini G, Munari L, Incorvaia B, et al. Interferons in relapsing remitting multiple sclerosis: a systematic review. *Lancet* 2003;361:545–552.

24a. Izquierdo G, Angulo S, Garcia-Moreno JM, et al. Intrathecal IgG synthesis: marker of progression in multiple sclerosis patients. *Acta Neurol Scand* 2002; 105(3):158–163.

24b. Rudick RA, Cookfair DL, Simonian NA, et al. Cerebrospinal fluid abnormalities in a phase III trial of Avonex (IFNbeta-1a) for relapsing multiple sclerosis. The Multiple Sclerosis Collaborative Research Group. *J Neuroimmunol* 1999;93(1–2):8–14.

24c. Zeman AZ, Kidd D, McLean BN, et al. A study of oligoclonal band negative multiple sclerosis. *J Neurol Neurosurg Psychiatry* 1996;60(1):27–30.

25. Davies G, Keir G, Thompson EJ, et al. The clinical significance of an intrathecal monoclonal immunoglobulin band: a follow-up study. *Neurology* 2003;60: 1163–1166.

26a. Vrethem M, Fernlund I, Ernerudh J, Ohman S. Prognostic value of cerebrospinal fluid IgA and IgG in multiple sclerosis. Mult Scler 2004;10:469–471.

26b. Walker RW, Thompson EJ, McDonald WI. Cerebrospinal fluid in multiple sclerosis: relationships between immunoglobulins, leucocytes and clinical features. *J Neurol* 1985;232:250–259.

27. McLean BN, Zeman AZ, Barnes D, et al. Patterns of blood-brain barrier impairment and clinical features in multiple sclerosis. *J Neurol Neurosurg Psychiatry* 1993;56:356–360.

28. Bruck W, Bitsch A, Bruck Y, et al. Inflammatory central nervous system demyelination: correlation of magnetic resonance imaging findings with lesion pathology. *Ann Neurol* 1997;42:783–793.

29. Zeman AZ, Keir G, Luxton R, et al. Serum oligoclonal IgG is a common and persistent finding in multiple sclerosis, and has a systemic source. *Q J Med* 1996;89: 187–193.

30. Berger T, Rubner P, Schautzer F, et al. Antimyelin antibodies as a predictor of clinically definite multiple sclerosis after a first demyelinating event. *N Engl J Med* 2003;349:139–145.

31. Kostulas VK, Link H, Lefvert A-K. Oligoclonal IgG bands in cerebrospinal fluid: principles for demonstration and interpretation based on findings in 1114 neurological patients. *Arch Neurol* 1987;44: 1041–1044.

32. McLean BN, Luxton RW, Thompson EJ. A study of immunoglobulin G in the cerebrospinal fluid of 1007 patients with suspected neurological disease using isoelectric focusing and the Log IgG-Index. A comparison and diagnostic applications. *Brain* 1990;113: 1269–1289.

33. Ohman S, Ernerudh J, Forsberg P, et al. Comparison of seven formulae and isoelectrofocusing for determination of intrathecally produced IgG in neurological diseases. *Ann Clin Biochem* 1992;29:417–418.

34. Beer S, Rosler KM, Hess CW. Diagnostic value of paraclinical tests in multiple sclerosis: relative sensitivities and specificities for reclassification according to the Poser committee criteria. *J Neurol Neurosurg Psychiatry* 1995;59:152–159.

35. Paolino E, Fainardi E, Ruppi P, et al. A prospective study on the predictive value of CSF oligoclonal bands and MRI in acute isolated neurological syndromes for subsequent progression to multiple sclerosis. *J Neurol Neurosurg Psychiatry* 1996;60:572–575.

11

Multiple Sclerosis Mimics

Robert M. Herndon

Department of Neurology, University of Mississippi Medical School, Jackson, Mississippi

Nothing shuts off critical neurologic thought processes faster than a diagnosis of multiple sclerosis.

Despite the addition of new and improved diagnostic testing, the false positive diagnostic error rate in multiple sclerosis (MS) appears to remain in the 5% to 10% range and is typically higher in referral centers, since they tend to receive the more difficult cases in consultation. The extreme variability of MS often makes diagnosis difficult and a number of rare and exotic conditions can mimic MS closely enough that they meet formal diagnostic criteria except for the caveat of "no better explanation" (1,2). When the disease is typical, magnetic resonance imaging (MRI) is typical and there is an elevated cerebrospinal fluid (CSF) immunoglobulin (IgG) index or synthesis rate and oligoclonal bands, few errors are made. On the other hand, when we are dealing with atypical cases, it is all too easy to make the diagnosis of possible or probable MS and forget any doubts present at the time the diagnosis was first considered. This chapter addresses some of the conditions that mimic MS and with factors that should induce repeated reconsideration of the diagnosis.

When a new patient presents to the clinic with a diagnosis of MS, it is not safe to presume the diagnosis is correct. Rather, you should assume that the diagnosis may be incorrect and do what is necessary to satisfy yourself that the diagnosis is correct. It is neither effective nor efficient to automatically put all patients through a new battery of tests to confirm the diagnosis, nor is it feasible to repeat a thorough work-up on all of your existing patients. It is usually feasible to review the basis for the diagnosis and satisfy yourself that the work-up was adequate and confirmatory or to decide if additional tests are needed. This chapter addresses the diagnosis and points out a number of features referred to as "red flags" (3). These are features, findings, or the absence of findings that should cause periodic reconsideration of the diagnosis. A red flag does not mean the patient does not have MS, and most of those misdiagnosed as MS have more than one red flag (4).

MS mimics can be divided into genetic disorders, infections, other autoimmune inflammatory disorders, vascular disease, nutritional disorders, and toxic conditions. Which alternative diagnoses need to be considered in a given case will depend on the history and presentation. Progressive spinal cord syndromes usually present the most difficult differential, whereas acute optic neuritis in a young adult generally presents the easiest.

PRESENTATIONS

Optic Neuritis

Optic neuritis is typically an acute disease beginning with visual blurring and pain on eye movement, followed by visual loss progressing over several hours up to a week or so with development of a central or paracentral scotoma and with a normal funduscopic examination. A relative afferent pupillary defect should be present. In older patients (generally over age 40) and those with vascular risk factors, it is necessary to consider the possibility of ischemic optic neuropathy (5,6). Ischemic optic neuropathy is usually painless, the scotoma is usually large, and the onset more acute. Additionally, MS presenting as optic neuritis is much less common in the older age group. In cases of suspected optic neuritis, imaging is necessary to rule out compressive lesions and to look for other evidence of demyelination. If the optic neuritis goes to complete blindness in one or both eyes and there is bilateral involvement, Devic syndrome (neuromyelitis optica) must be considered, particularly if the brain MRI is normal (7). When typical, isolated optic neuritis is good evidence of a focal demyelinating lesion. If the MRI shows the typical findings of MS and other neurologic signs and symptoms are present, one can be fairly confident in the diagnosis.

Acute Transverse Myelitis and Progressive Myelopathies

Transverse myelitis as a presenting symptom of MS is typically incomplete. Bladder and bowel involvement are usual. Early acute inflamma-

tory demyelinating polyneuropathy (Guillain-Barré syndrome) may need to be considered since it can look remarkably like transverse myelitis early in the course, but the differential here becomes clear within a few days as the disorder progresses. If the transverse myelitis is complete and the brain MRI is normal, Devic syndrome needs to be considered since transverse myelitis in MS is rarely complete. Additionally, it is unusual for the lesions in MS to involve more than three spinal segments. Other differentials include collagen vascular diseases, particularly disseminated lupus erythmatosis and Sjögren's syndrome (8,9).

Brain Stem Syndromes

These include patients presenting with one or more of the following: vertigo, nystagmus, diplopia, ataxia, and *tic doloreux*. The major differentials here are brainstem stroke, posterior fossa tumor, syringobulbia, acephalgic migraine, and Chiari malformation (10). Before the advent of MRI, posterior fossa disease was the neurologist's nemesis, but MRI will usually provide a clear answer. You should look for demyelinating lesions using the T2 sequence as the lesions do not show as well on fluid-attenuated inversion-recovery (FLAIR) sequences in the posterior fossa as they do above the tentorium. You should be aware of the possibility of ischemic lesions in young people as coagulopathies, particularly lupus anticoagulant, can cause ischemic lesions in relatively young people. A history of multiple miscarriages can be an important clue, since this problem is more common in women and multiple miscarriages can be caused by lupus anticoagulant (11).

Genetic Disorders

There are a number of genetic disorders that can masquerade as MS. These include cerebral autosomal dominant arteriopathy with strokes and leukoencephalopathy (CADASIL) (12) that causes strokes in young to middle-aged adults. The deep, cerebral white matter changes on MRI resemble the white matter lesions of MS. Here a strong family history may provide the clue necessary to indicate the need for a skin biopsy or for genetic testing for the Notch-3 mutation associated with this disease.

The dominantly inherited spinocerebellar atrophies (SCAs), of which there are now more than 22 identified genetic types, are often misdiagnosed as MS (13). Even when a family has been informed that a family member has been diagnosed with one of the SCAs, there may be considerable denial and they may report it as MS to avoid the stigma of having a genetic disease in the family. Friedreich's ataxia can also be mistaken for MS, as can familial spastic paraplegia. In these cases, the MRI may assist in finding the correct diagnosis, but in patients with vascular risk factors care must be taken to avoid misdiagnosis based on white matter ischemic changes.

Leigh's encephalopathy is another condition that may be mistaken for MS or for Devic disease, especially in its later-onset forms (14). It usually resembles a Wernicke's encephalopathy occurring in the absence of evidence of alcoholism or malnutrition. Findings may include ataxia, oculomotor palsies, and stupor. Computed tomography (CT) often shows edema in the upper brainstem, thalamus, and basal ganglia, and MRI may show T2 and FLAIR high signal in these areas. Unlike Wernicke's, the mammillary bodies are usually spared. Diagnosis is based on the occurrence of lactic acidosis and the characteristic MRI picture.

Infections

In the case of progressive myelopathy, human T-cell lymphotropic virus (HTLV)-associated myelopathy, (tropical spastic paraplegia or HAM-TSP) may be mistaken for primary progressive spinal MS (PPMS) (15). The spinal fluid is typically positive with an elevated IgG index and oligoclonal bands on the MS panel, and the diagnosis will be missed if you do not look for antibody to HTLV-1 and 2. HTLV associated myelopathy is fairly common in the Caribbean, in Native Americans of the Pacific Northwest, and in Japan. Human immunodeficiency virus (HIV) myelopathy and dementia can also be mistaken for MS (16).

Lyme disease (neuroborreliosis) is another infection with protean manifestation that is easily mistaken for MS, but also is overdiagnosed in the MS population. A history of the typical local rash before the onset of neurologic symptoms is a useful clue to this diagnosis, but is not always present (17). Diagnosis is based on the presence of antibody to *Borrelia burgdorferi* with confirmation by Western blot.

Central nervous system (CNS) involvement in tertiary syphilis, though now fairly rare, must be considered, particularly given the recent rise in the frequency of primary syphilis. Because of its rarity, routine serologic testing is no longer done. The diagnosis of CNS syphilis is often not considered, but cases still appear and are easily missed because the diagnosis is not considered. In patients with chronic spinal cord disease and in cases presenting with dementia (18), serologic testing for syphilis is warranted.

Autoimmune Disorders

Disseminated lupus erythematosus and Sjögren's syndrome can present with neurologic symptoms, particularly transverse myelitis. Similarly, central nervous system vasculitis and vasculitis associated with cocaine abuse can be mistaken for MS. A careful history, tests for antinuclear antibodies (ANAs) and antineutrophilic cytoplasmic antibodies (ANCAs), and a drug screen will usually eliminate these possibilities. Additionally, in rheumatoid arthritis, the possibility of atlanto-axial dislocation with compression of the cord at the craniocervical junction may need to be considered.

Nutritional Disorders

Nutritional disorders are rarely mistaken for MS, but in cases presenting as a slowly progressive myelopathy with or without cognitive features, vitamin B_{12} deficiency should be considered; a B_{12} level is indicated in all cases presenting with a chronic myelopathy (19). This will usually be evident on a complete blood count (CBC) but needs to be in the differential. In acute presentations with ataxia, nystagmus, and diplopia, thiamin deficiency should also be considered. This

TABLE 11-1 *Red flags*

- Absence of long tract signs
- Absence of bowel and bladder involvement
- Absence of fatigue as a significant symptom
- Positive family history
- Absence of eye findings
- Unifocal disease
- Posterior fossa
- Craniocervical junction
- Spinal cord
- Diagnosis based solely on MRI
- Normal MRI

is most commonly seen in alcoholics but, given some of the current diet fads, thiamin deficiency can be seen in individuals who do not appear to be poor or particularly malnourished. Here the severe acute onset, possibly with evidence of heart disease with congestive failure, should provide an important clue to the diagnosis. History of a diet deficient in thiamin should also be useful in picking up these cases.

RED FLAGS

There is a series of features (summarized in Table 11-1) that either should be present and are not, or are atypical for MS and serve as a reminder that the diagnosis may be in error and should be reviewed. We refer to these as red flags (3,4). They do not mean the patient does not have MS, but they indicate the need for caution in the diagnosis and the need for periodic re-evaluation. Particularly in MS clinics, it is easy for a patient initially considered as "possible MS" to be accepted as such in the absence of further evidence for the diagnosis. After several visits, these patients are accepted as part of the group of MS patients and the initial doubts vanish, even though there has been no new evidence establishing the diagnosis.

Absence of Long Tract Signs

The long spinal pathways are the largest targets for demyelination in the nervous system. By the time the disease is well-established, there should

be evidence of involvement of the long motor or sensory pathways or both. As the disease evolves, absence of clear evidence of spinal cord involvement provides an excellent reason to carefully re-evaluate the diagnosis. Again, there are cases that do not develop long tract involvement until the disease is moderately advanced, but it is an indicator that the diagnosis should not be accepted uncritically (20).

Absence of Bowel and Bladder Involvement

Both bowel and bladder function are almost always abnormal in well-established MS. A neurogenic bladder with urinary frequency and urgency or other abnormalities is so frequent, particularly if there is any spinal cord involvement, that its absence is a cause for concern. The bladder problem may be a small, spastic bladder with failure to store, a large, hypotonic bladder with overflow incontinence, or dyssynergia with both urgency and hesitancy; normal bladder function in someone with well-established MS is a rarity and deserves scrutiny.

Similarly, constipation is almost a given in MS. Autonomic dysfunction with reduced bowel motility and decreased physical activity resulting in a sluggish bowel with constipation is extremely common. There is a slightly increased incidence of inflammatory bowel disease in association with MS, so that should not be a problem as regards diagnosis. However, normal bowel function without any special measures to aid bowel function is a cause for concern regarding the diagnosis.

Absence of Fatigue as a Significant Symptom

Fatigue is the most common single symptom of MS, occurring in excess of 95% of patients. It is typically variable from day to day and is worst in the afternoon. It is a very troubling symptom in that it is invisible to others but, nevertheless, is so characteristic of the disease that the absence of significant fatigue should give one pause. Interestingly and counterintuitively, one of the most effective treatments is regular physical exercise. It usually responds to treatment with either amantadine or modafinil, but it is very troubling to the patients and its absence should cause careful reconsideration of the diagnosis.

Positive Family History

The risk of MS in first-order relatives is variously estimated at from 2% to 5%. If this is true, why should this be a red flag? The reason is that many hereditary diseases get labeled MS. If there is anything resembling a dominant inheritance pattern, great care should be taken in accepting the diagnosis. Diseases such as X-linked adrenoleukodystrophy/adrenomyeloneuropathy and the dominantly inherited spinocerebellar atrophies are frequently mistaken for MS, as is CADASIL. These conditions need to be considered in the differential when there is a family history of neurologic disease. Given the protean manifestations of adrenoleukodystrophy/adrenomyeloneuropathy, the occurrence of neurologic diseases with different manifestations within the family may require careful consideration.

Absence of Eye Findings

Eye findings are extremely common in MS. They may be subtle, as a partial internuclear ophthalmoplegia, saccadic pursuit, or a little rebound nystagmus but, with the exception of primary progressive spinal MS, it is quite rare to have a well-established MS without any visual or eye movement abnormalities.

Unifocal Disease

Unifocal disease can appear multifocal when the focus is located in the posterior fossa or at the craniocervical junction. In the past, this was the neurologist's nemesis. Now, with MRI, this problem is much less common but it is important to have a good look at the MRI to rule out a single posterior fossa lesion or a Chiari malformation. Spinal cord lesions can also present a problem, particularly in individuals with ischemic white matter changes related to small vessel disease.

Diagnosis Based on MRI Alone

One problem that has arisen since MRI became available is overinterpretation and misinterpretation of MRI. Patients with migraine and those with small vessel vascular disease who have an MRI done for other purposes may have their MRI read as indicating MS. Migraine patients often have multiple, punctate high-signal areas and, since they may have numbness, weakness, or speech and language problems as a migraine aura, may erroneously get diagnosed. Acephalgic migraine can be particularly problematic in this regard. In general, one would expect to find other indications of MS, either by history or on examination or CSF examination. In the absence of evidence beyond the MRI, considerable caution in making the diagnosis is warranted.

Normal MRI

A normal brain and spinal MRI can occur in MS but should be a cause for concern regarding the diagnosis. The brain MRI is usually normal in neuromyelitis optica but spinal cord involvement can usually be seen. When the MRI is entirely normal, considerable skepticism is warranted. Be sure there are objective signs of neurologic disease. In early cases of suspected MS with a normal MRI, evoked potentials and CSF analysis may provide important information.

SUMMARY

Even with all the newer diagnostic tools, including MRI with multiple sequences, evoked potentials, CSF studies, and so forth, multiple sclerosis remains a clinical diagnosis. In the past it was, to a large extent, a wastebasket diagnosis. Since we really could not do much about it, if our diagnosis was wrong it really didn't matter a great deal. Now, with an increasing number of effective therapies and with good therapies for some of the MS mimics, accurate diagnosis is a must. In addition to the cost of treatment, many of the current treatments such as Mitoxantrone (Novantrone®) are not benign and we should not subject our patients to unnecessary harmful therapies.

REFERENCES

1. Schumacher FA, Beeve GW, Kibler RF, et al. Problems of experimental trials of therapy in multiple sclerosis. *Ann NY Acad Sci* 1965;122:552–568

2. Poser CM, Paty DW, Scheinberg LC, et al. New diagnostic criteria for multiple sclerosis: guidelines for research protocols. *Ann Neurol* 1983;13:227–231

3. Rudick RA, Schiffer RB, Schwetz KM, et al. Multiple sclerosis: the problem of misdiagnosis. *Arch Neurol* 1986;43:578–593.

4. Herndon RM. The Changing Pattern of Misdiagnosis in Multiple Sclerosis. In: Herndon, RM, Seil FJ, eds. *Multiple Sclerosis: Current Status of Research and Treatment,* New York: Demos Publications, 1994: 149–156.

5. Beck, RW. Optic Neuritis. In: Miller NR, Newman NJ, eds. *Walsh and Hoyt's Neuro-Ophthalmology.* 4th ed. Baltimore: Williams and Wilkins, 1982: 599–648.

6. Kelman, SE. Ischemic Optic Neuropathies. In: Miller NR, Newman NJ, eds. *Walsh and Hoyt's Neuro-Ophthalmology.* 4th ed. Baltimore: Williams and Wilkins, 1982: 549–598.

7. Ghezzi A, Bergamaschi R, Martinelli V, et al. Clinical characteristics, courses and prognosis of relapsing Devic neuromyelitis optica. *J Neurol* 2004;251:47–52.

8. Harzheim M, Schlegel U, Urbach H, et al. Discriminatory features of acute transverse myelitis: a retrospective analysis of 45 patients. *J Neurolo Sci* 2004;217:217–223.

9. Scotti G, Gerevini S. Diagnosis and differential diagnosis of acute transverse myelopathy. The role of neuroradiological investigations and review of the literature. *Neurol Sci* 2001;22[Suppl 2]:S69–S73.

10. Rudick RA, Ransohoff R, Herndon RM. Demyelinating Disorder. In: Joynt RJ, Griggs RC, eds. *Clinical Neurology.* Philadelphia: J.B. Lippincott Co., 1998: Chap. 33:1–106.

11. Brey RL, Hart RG, Sherman DG, et al. Anti-phospholipid antibodies and cerebral ischemia in young people. *Neurology* 1990;40:1190–1196.

12. Bousser M-G, Biousse V. Small vessel vasculopathies affecting the central nervous system. *J Neuro-ophthalmol* 2004;24(1):56–61.

13. Schöls L, Bauer P, Schmidt T, et al. Autosomal dominant cerebellar ataxias: clinical features, genetics and pathogenesis. *Lancet Neurol* 2004;3L291–304.

14. Swaiman KF, Breningstall G. Inborn Metabolic Errors Affecting the Nervous System. In: Joynt RJ, Griggs RC, eds. *Clinical Neurology.* Philadelphia: J.B. Lippincott Co., 1998: Vol. 4, Ch. 56: 68–69.

15. Orland, JR, Engstrom J, Fridey J, et al. HTLV Outcomes Study. *Neurology* 2003;61:1588–1594.

16. Berger JR, Sabet A. Infectious myelopathies. *Semin Neurol* 2002;22(2):133–142.

17. Reik L Jr., Burgdorfer W, Donaldson JO. Neurologic abnormalities in Lyme disease without erythema chronicum migrans. *Am J Med* 1986;81(1):73–78.

18. Nitrini R. The history of tabes dorsalis and the impact of observational studies in neurology. *Arch Neurol* 2000;57(4):605–606.

19. Hemmer B, Glocker FX, Schumacher M, et al. Subacute combined degeneration: clinical, electrophysiological, and magnetic resonance imaging findings. *J Neurol Neurosurg Psychiatry* 1998;65(6):822–827.

20. Krupp LB, Coyle PK, LaRocca NG. Fatigue in multiple sclerosis. *Arch Neurol* 1995;45:435–437

12

The Use of Modern Magnetic Resonance Techniques to Monitor Disease Evolution in Multiple Sclerosis

Massimo Filippi[1] and Maria A. Rocca

Neuroimaging Research Unit, Department of Neurology, Scientific Institute and University Ospedale San Raffaele, Milan, Italy
([1]Corresponding Author)

INTRODUCTION

The application of conventional magnetic resonance imaging (cMRI) to the study of multiple sclerosis (MS) has greatly improved our ability to diagnose MS and to monitor its evolution. The sensitivity of T2-weighted MRI in the detection of MS lesions and that of post-contrast T1-weighted images to identify lesions with an increased blood–brain barrier permeability associated with inflammatory activity make it possible to demonstrate the dissemination of MS lesions in space and time earlier than with clinical assessment, and to detect disease activity with an increased sensitivity with respect to clinical evaluation of relapses (1). However, the magnitude of the relationship between cMRI measures of disease activity or burden and the clinical manifestations of the disease is weak (2,3). This clinical/MRI discrepancy is likely to be the result, at least partially, of the inability of cMRI to quantify the extent and to define the nature of MS-related tissue damage.

Modern quantitative MR techniques have the potential to overcome some of the limitations of cMRI. Metrics derived from magnetization transfer (MT) (4) and diffusion-weighted (DW) (5) MRI enable us to quantify the extent and severity of structural changes occurring within and outside cMRI-visible lesions of patients with MS. Proton MR spectroscopy (^{1}H-MRS) (6) can add information on the biochemical nature of such changes. Functional MRI (fMRI) (7) can provide new insights into the role of cortical adaptive changes in limiting the clinical consequences of MS structural damage.

This chapter provides an update of the current state of the art of the application of structural, metabolic, and functional MR-based techniques to the study of MS pathophysiology.

Basic Principles of Modern MRI Techniques

Magnetization Transfer (MT) MRI

Magnetization transfer MRI is based on the interactions between protons in a relatively free environment and those where motion is restricted. Off-resonance irradiation is applied, which saturates the magnetization of the less-mobile protons, but this is transferred to the mobile protons, thus reducing the signal intensity from the observable magnetization (Fig. 12-1). Thus, a low MT ratio (MTR) indicates a reduced capacity of the macromolecules in the central nervous system (CNS) to exchange magnetization with the surrounding water molecules, reflecting damage to myelin or to the axonal membrane. The most compelling evidence indicating that markedly decreased MTR values correspond to areas where severe and irreversible tissue loss has occurred comes from a postmortem study showing a strong correlation of MTR values from MS lesions and normal-appearing white matter (NAWM) with the percentage of residual axons and the degree of demyelination (8). More recently, a study performed on human specimens has confirmed the sensitivity of this technique toward the different pathological substrates of the disease, by showing that MTR values of remyelinated lesions are higher than those of demyelinated lesions and lower than those of the NAWM (9).

Diffusion-Weighted (DW) MRI

Diffusion is the microscopic random translational motion of molecules in a fluid system. In the CNS, diffusion is influenced by the microstructural components of tissue, including cell membranes and organelles. The diffusion coefficient of biological tissues (which can be measured in vivo by MRI) is, therefore, lower than the diffusion coefficient in free water and is thus named apparent diffusion coefficient (ADC) (10). Pathological processes that modify tissue integrity, thus resulting in a loss or increased permeability of "restricting" barriers, can determine an increase of the ADC. Since some cellular structures are aligned on the scale of an image pixel, the measurement of diffusion is also dependent on the direction in which diffusion is measured. As a consequence, diffusion measurements can give information about the size, shape, integrity, and orientation of tissues (11). A measure of diffusion that is independent of the orientation of structures is provided by the mean diffusivity (MD), the average of the ADCs measured in three orthogonal directions. A full characterization of diffusion can be obtained in terms of a tensor (12), a 3×3 matrix that accounts for the correlation existing between molecular displacement along orthogonal directions. From the tensor, it is possible to derive MD, equal to the one-third of its trace, and some other dimensionless indices of anisotropy. One of the most often-used of these indices is named fractional anisotropy (FA) (13) (Fig. 12-1). The pathological elements of MS have the potential to alter the permeability or geometry of structural barriers to water molecular diffusion in the brain. The application of DW MRI technology to MS is, therefore, appealing to provide quantitative estimates of the degree of tissue damage and, as a consequence, to improve the understanding of the mechanisms leading to irreversible disability.

Proton MR Spectroscopy (^{1}H-MRS)

Water-suppressed proton MR spectra of normal human brain at long echo times reveal four major resonances: one at 3.2 ppm from tetramethylamines [mainly from choline-containing phospholipids (Cho)], one at 3.0 ppm from creatine and phosphocreatine (Cr), one at 2.0 ppm from *N*-acetyl groups [mainly *N*-acetyl aspartate (NAA)], and one 1.3 ppm from the methyl resonance of lactate (Lac). NAA is a marker of axonal integrity, while Cho and Lac are considered chemical correlates of acute inflammatory/demyelinating changes (6). ^{1}H-MRS studies with shorter echo times can detect additional metabolites, such as lipids and myoinositol (mI), which are also regarded as markers of ongoing myelin damage. ^{1}H-MRS can complement conventional MRI in the assessment of MS patients by simultaneously defining several chemical correlates of the pathological changes occurring within and outside T2-visible lesions.

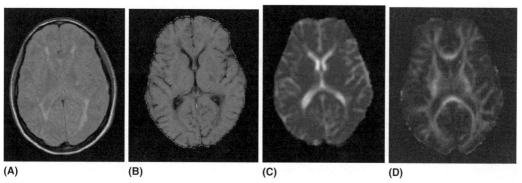

FIG. 12-1. Axial magnetic resonance (MR) images from a patient with multiple sclerosis (MS). The proton density-weighted scan **(A)** shows multiple lesions. On the magnetization transfer (MT) map **(B)**, lesions appear as hypointense areas. The degree of hypointensity is related to decrease in MT ratio and indicates damage to the myelin or to the axonal membranes. On the mean diffusivity (MD) map **(C)**, lesions appear as hyperintense areas. The degree of hyperintensity is related to increase in MD and indicates a loss of structural barriers to water molecular motion. On the fractional anisotropy (FA) map **(D)**, white matter pixels are bright because of the directionality of the white matter fiber tracts. Dark areas corresponding to macroscopic lesions indicate a loss of FA and suggest the presence of structural disorganization.

An immunopathologic study has shown that a decrease in NAA levels is correlated with axonal loss, while an increase in Cho correlates with the presence of active demyelination and gliosis (14).

Functional MRI (fMRI)

The signal changes seen during fMRI studies depend on the blood oxygenation level-dependent (BOLD) mechanism, which in turn involves changes of the transverse magnetization relaxation time—either $T2^*$ in a gradient echo sequence, or T2 in spin echo sequence. These changes are attributable to differences in deoxyhemoglobin subsequent to variations of neuronal activity (15). The application of fMRI to the study of the motor, visual, and cognitive systems in patients with MS has provided new insights into the factors with the potential to contribute to limit the progressive clinical worsening of these patients.

Quantification of Intrinsic Lesion Damage

Although cMRI has a great sensitivity in detecting the presence and extent of macroscopic

lesions in MS, it lacks specificity toward the heterogeneous pathological substrates of these lesions, which range from edema to demyelination, remyelination, gliosis, and axonal loss, as demonstrated by several pathological studies (16–19).

The following are the main findings obtained by the application of modern, MR-based techniques for the study of individual MS lesions:

1. In chronic lesions that appear as hyperintense on T2-weighted scans, MT- and DW-MRI studies have shown variable degrees of MTR, FA, and NAA reductions and MD increase (4,5,20). All these values vary dramatically across individual lesions, but are typically more pronounced in lesions that are hypointense on T1-weighted images and in patients with the most disabling courses of the disease (4,5,21,22). The variability of MTR, MD, and FA values seen in MS lesions also suggests that different proportions of lesions with different degrees of structural changes might contribute to the evolution of the disease. This concept is supported by a three-year follow-up study (23) showing that newly formed lesions from secondary progressive MS (SPMS)

patients have more severe MTR deterioration than those from mildly disabling, relapsing-remitting MS (RRMS) patients (Fig. 12-2).

2. New enhancing lesions have different range of MTR values, according to their size, modality, and duration of enhancement. In particular, MTR is higher in homogeneously enhancing lesions than in ring-enhancing lesions (24); it is also higher in lesions enhancing on a single scan than in those enhancing on two or more serial scans (25) and in lesions enhancing after the injection of a triple dose of gadolinium than in those enhancing after the injection of a standard dose (26). DW-MRI characteristics of enhancing lesions are less well-defined. While FA values are consistently lower in enhancing than in nonenhancing lesions (27,28), conflicting results have been achieved when comparing ADC or MD between these two lesion populations. While some studies reported higher ADC or MD values in nonenhancing than in enhancing lesions (27,29), others, based on larger samples of patients and lesions, did not report any significant difference between these two lesion populations (28,30). The heterogeneity of enhancing lesions has been also underlined by the demonstration that water diffusivity is markedly increased in ring-enhancing lesions when compared to homogeneously enhancing lesions (31), or in the nonenhancing portions of enhancing lesions when compared with enhancing portions (31). ^{1}H-MRS of acute MS lesions at both short and long echo times reveals increases in Cho and Lac resonance intensities (20,32), which reflect the releasing of membrane phospholipids and the metabolism of inflammatory cells, respectively. In large, acute demyelinating lesions, decreases of Cr can also be seen (20). Short echo time spectra can detect transient increases in visible lipids, released during myelin breakdown and mI (33). All these changes are usually associated with a decrease in NAA. After the acute phase and over a period of days to weeks, there is a progressive reduction of raised Lac resonance intensities to normal levels. Resonance intensities of Cr also return to normal within a few days. Cho, lipid, and mI resonance intensities return to normal over months. The signal intensity of NAA may remain decreased or show partial recovery, starting soon after the acute phase and lasting for several months (20,32,34).

3. A progressive decrease of MTR values, and an increase of MD (Fig. 12-3) values can be detected in regions that will develop new lesions (35–40). Using MRS, Cho increase, probably reflecting an altered myelin chemistry or the presence of inflammation, and a decrease in NAA have been also shown in prelesional NAWM (33,41,42).

4. Average lesion MTR has been found to be lower in patients with RRMS than in those with clinically isolated syndromes (CIS) suggestive of MS (43,44), whereas no differences have been found in cross-sectional studies between patients with RRMS and those with SPMS (43) or between patients with SPMS and those with primary progressive MS (PPMS) (45).

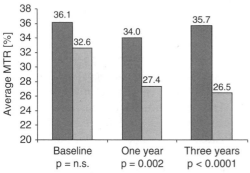

FIG. 12-2. The bars show average magnetization transfer ratio (MTR) values of newly enhancing lesions from patients with relapsing-remitting MS (RRMS) (*dark gray*) and secondary progressive MS (SPMS) (*light gray*) MS at baseline and over a 3-year follow-up period. At each time point, the MTR values of new enhancing lesions were lower in SPMS than in RRMS patients. During the 3-year follow-up, while the MTR values of new enhancing lesions of RRMS patients remained stable, those of SPMS patients showed a progressive reduction (p = 0.0005).

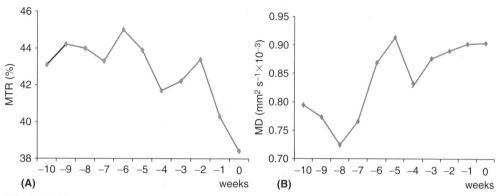

FIG. 12-3. Progressive decrease of magnetization transfer ratio (MTR) values **(A)** and increase of mean diffusivity (MD) values **(B)** as seen on weekly MT and diffusion-weighted MRI scans in regions of normal-appearing white matter that will be subsequent sites of new lesion development (time 0). These changes tend to become significant six weeks before the appearance of a new lesion.

Assessment of Normal-Appearing Brain Tissue (NABT) and Normal-Appearing White Matter (NAWM) Damage

Postmortem studies have shown subtle and widespread abnormalities in the NAWM from MS patients, which include diffuse astrocytic hyperplasia, patchy edema, and perivascular cellular infiltration, as well as axonal damage (16,17,46). The application of modern, MR-based techniques to the assessment of MS patients has allowed the in vivo quantification of the extent of NAWM involvement in this disease, which can be obtained using either a region-of-interest (ROI) analysis or a histogram-based approach. The main advantage of ROI analysis is that it enables one to obtain detailed information on the characteristics of clinically eloquent NAWM sites; however, in histogram analysis the amount of operator intervention is reduced, thus limiting both the measurement variability in serial studies and the time needed for the analysis. In addition, the recent development of fully automated techniques to segment the various components of brain parenchyma has enabled us to obtain histograms from the NAWM in isolation, by preliminarily excluding from the analysis those pixels belonging to T2-visible lesions and gray matter (GM).

The following are the main results obtained by the application of modern, MR-based techniques to the study of the NABT and NAWM of MS patients:

1. Using ROI analysis, reduced MTR, FA, and NAA and increased ADC and MD values have been shown in the NABT and NAWM of MS patients with all the major MS phenotypes (27–30,39–41,47–54). Diffusely elevated Cho, Cr, and Ins concentrations have been described in the NAWM of RRMS (55,56) and PPMS (57) patients. Elevated levels of Ins have also been detected in the NAWM of patients with early RRMS (58) and in patients at presentation with CIS suggestive of MS (59). Recently, MTR changes of a lower magnitude than those observed in T2-visible lesions have been detected in the dirty-appearing white matter of MS patients (60).

2. The application of histogram analysis (43–45,50,51,61–64) to the study of the NABT and of the NAWM, confirmed and extended the previous findings obtained with ROI analysis, by showing that these abnormalities can be detected even in patients with CIS suggestive of MS (44,63) and in those with early-onset MS (65), are more

pronounced in SPMS and PPMS patients than in patients with the other disease phenotypes (62) (Fig. 12-4), and are similar between patients with SPMS and those with PPMS (45). Consistent with this is the demonstration that NAA reduction is more pronounced in the NAWM of SPMS and PPMS patients than in those with RRMS (53,57). Nevertheless, reduced NAWM NAA can also be detected in patients with no overt clinical disability (54) and in those in the early phase of the disease (66). The recent development of an unlocalized ^{1}H-MRS sequence for measuring NAA levels in the whole brain (WBNAA) (67) has made it possible to extend the previous findings by showing the presence of marked axonal pathology in clinically definite MS (68–70) and in patients at the earliest clinical phases of MS (71) (Fig. 12-5).

3. Longitudinal studies have demonstrated that modern MR techniques are useful for monitoring disease evolution. On average, these studies have shown that NABT changes tend to worsen over time in all MS phenotypes (44,53,72–74), including patients with PPMS (75), and that these changes seem to be more pronounced in SPMS patients (72). In patients with CIS, the extent of NABT changes has been found to be an independent predictor of subsequent evolution to clinically definite MS (44), whereas in patients with established MS, NAWM-MTR reduction has been shown to predict the accumulation of clinical disability over the subsequent five years (73,74). In patients with RRMS, longitudinal decrease over time of NAA:Cr ratios in the NAWM correlates strongly with Expanded Disability Status Scale (EDSS) worsening (53,76), suggesting that progressive axonal damage or loss may be responsible for functional impairment in MS. More recently, it has been demonstrated that brain axonal damage begins in the early stages of MS, develops rapidly in this phase of the disease, and correlates more strongly with disability in patients with mild disability than in those with more severe disability (66).

4. NABT MTR, MD, and NAA values are only partially correlated with the extent of macroscopic lesions and the severity of intrinsic lesion damage (28,30,50,51,62,69,71,77–80), thus suggesting that NABT pathology does not only reflect Wallerian degeneration of axons traversing large focal abnormalities, but they may also represent small focal abnormalities beyond the resolution of conventional scanning and independent of larger lesions.

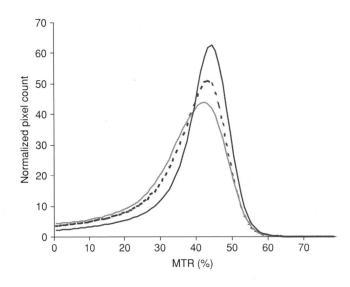

FIG. 12-4. Average magnetization transfer ratio (MTR) histograms of normal-appearing brain tissue (NABT) from patients with clinically isolated syndromes (CISs) suggestive of MS *(black line),* relapsing-remitting MS (RRMS) *(dotted line)* and secondary progressive MS (SPMS) *(gray line).* The decrease of average NABT MTR values is more pronounced in SPMS than in the two other groups of patients (CIS versus RRMS: p = 0.0009; RRMS versus SPMS: p = 0.05).

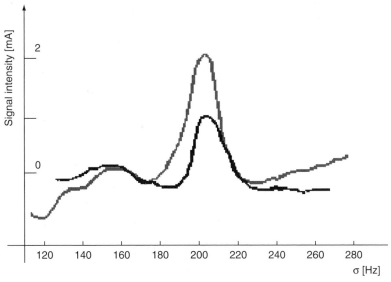

FIG. 12-5. Whole-brain *N*-acetylaspartate (WBNAA) spectra from a healthy subject *(gray line)* and from a patient with a clinically isolated syndrome suggestive of MS *(black line)*. In the latter, a decrease of the WBNAA peak is clearly visible.

5. The quantification of the extent of NABT and NAWM involvement has allowed us to increase the strength of the relationship between MRI metrics and the clinical manifestations of the disease. Moderate to strong correlations between various brain MTR and MD histogram-derived metrics and the severity of physical disability have been shown by several studies (28,61,64,79,81–85). These correlations have been found to be stronger in patients with RRMS and SPMS than in other disease phenotypes (61,82). Subtle MTR changes in the NABT (86,87) and in the cortical/subcortical (88) brain tissue are well-correlated with the presence of neuropsychological impairment in MS patients. In addition, a multivariate analysis of several MRI and MT MRI variables has demonstrated that average NABT–MTR is more strongly associated to cognitive impairment in MS patients than the extent of T2-visible lesions and their intrinsic tissue damage (89). More recently, the reduction of the NAA:Cr ratio in MS patients NAWM has been related to the presence of fatigue (90).

6. MT-MRI, DW-MRI, and MRS metrics of specific brain structures, such as the cerebellum (52,81,91), the brainstem (81), or the pyramidal tracts (92,93) of MS patients are significantly associated with impairment of these functional systems (52,81,91–93). More recently, Gadea et al. (94) found a relationship between attentional dysfunction in early RRMS patients and NAA:Cr values in the locus coeruleus nuclei of the pontine ascending reticular activation system.

Assessment of Gray Matter Damage

Several postmortem studies (95–98) have shown the presence of MS-related damage, including axonal and neuronal loss, in the cortical and deep gray matter (GM) of MS patients. Such abnormalities usually go undetected when using conventional imaging because of their relatively small size, their relaxation characteristics which result in poor contrast with the surrounding normal GM, and because of partial volume effects with the surrounding cerebrospinal fluid (CSF). The application of modern, MR-based techniques for the assessment of normal-appearing gray matter (NAGM) pathology has undoubtedly allowed overcoming some of the limitations of conventional imaging. Consistent with pathological findings, these techniques have shown that:

1. Using ROI (51) and histogram analysis (51,85,99–102), MT- and DT-MRI abnormalities have been shown in the NAGM of MS patients, including those with PPMS (85,101), whereas no MD abnormalities have been detected in the NAGM and NAWM of patients with early RRMS (103). As shown for the NABT and the NAWM, NAGM changes are also more pronounced in patients with SPMS than in those with RRMS (100,102), while no differences in the extent and severity of NAGM involvement have been identified between patients with SPMS and those with PPMS (85). However, recently an 18-month follow-up study performed on patients with RRMS showed that NAGM changes worsen over time (104). This suggests a progressive accumulation of GM damage already in the relapsing-remitting phase of the disease, which was previously unrecognized and which might be one of the factors responsible for the development of brain atrophy (105).
2. Metabolite abnormalities, including decrease of NAA, Cho, and glutamate, have also been shown in the cortical GM of MS patients (56,58,106,107), since the early phases of the disease (58), but not in CIS patients (108). These changes are more pronounced in patients with SPMS than in those with RRMS (106,109). More recently, reduction of NAA values and increase of ADC values have also been demonstrated in the thalamus of SPMS (98,110) and RRMS patients (110,111). As shown for cortical changes, even deep GM abnormalities are more pronounced in SPMS than in RRMS patients (110).
3. Significant correlations have been reported between MT- and DT-MRI changes and T2-lesion volume (51,85,99,102). This fits with

the notion that at least part of the GM pathology in MS is secondary to retrograde degeneration of fibers traversing WM lesions.
4. A precise and accurate quantification of NAGM damage might help to explain some of the clinical manifestations of MS, such as cognitive impairment, and might contribute to increase the strength of the correlation between clinical and MRI findings. Recent studies have indeed found a correlation between the severity of cognitive impairment and the degree of MTR (88) and MD (112) changes in the GM of MS patients. In addition, NAGM MTR metrics have been shown to correlate with the severity of clinical disability in patients with RRMS (99) and PPMS (101). Disappointingly, no correlation has been demonstrated between the extent of GM pathology, measured using MT- and DW-MRI, and fatigue (113). On the contrary, a marked reduction of NAA was found in highly fatigued in comparison with low-fatigued patients (114).

Assessment of Optic Nerve and Spinal Cord Damage

Reliable MTR measurements can be obtained from the optic nerve (ON) (115–118) and spinal cord, which shows the feasibility of the application of this technique for the assessment of the involvement of these critical structures. Two ROI-based studies (115,116) reported abnormal MTR values in the ON after an acute optic neuritis, independently from the presence of T2-visible abnormalities (116). In the study by Thorpe et al. (115), MTR of the ON has been found to be correlated with the visual-evoked potential latency, whereas, more recently, Inglese et al. (117) showed a correlation between MTR changes and the degree of visual function recovery after an acute episode of optic neuritis in 30 MS patients. In a one-year follow-up study of patients with acute optic neuritis, Hickman et al. (118) showed a progressive decline of average MTR of the affected ON, which reached a nadir after about eight months despite the rapid initial visual recovery, thus demonstrating the feasibility of using this technique in longitudinal studies of the ON in MS patients. Although more technically demanding, successful DW-MRI of the ON (119,120) has also been obtained in healthy individuals (119,120) and MS patients (119). Iwasawa et al. (119) assessed water diffusion in the ON of patients with optic neuritis, demonstrating significantly different ON ADC values between controls and patients. In addition, this study demonstrated that ADC values are decreased in the acute (inflammatory) stage of optic neuritis and increased in the chronic phase. Several studies used MT-MRI for the quantification of cervical cord damage in MS, whereas the implementation of DW-MRI technology for cord imaging is still in a preliminary phase.

Using ROIs analysis, Silver et al. (121) found reduced MTR values in the cervical cord of 12 MS patients in comparison with healthy volunteers. However, no correlation was found between cord MTR and disability, probably due to the small number of subjects enrolled and the limited portion of cord studied. These results have been partially confirmed by a subsequent study performed on 65 MS patients (122), where a weak correlation ($r = -0.25$) between the reduction of MTR values and the increase of clinical disability has been found.

More recently, the use of histogram analysis has allowed one to obtain, as already demonstrated for the brain, a more global picture of cord pathology in patients with MS and different disease phenotypes. Histograms analysis has demonstrated that cord MTR histogram metrics in RRMS patients are similar to those of healthy individuals (123), even in patients with early-onset MS (65). On the contrary, cord MTR metrics are similarly and markedly reduced in patients with SPMS and PPMS (45,124) (Fig. 12-6). A recent study has compared cervical cord MTR histogram metrics of patients with PPMS and SPMS and found no significant difference between these two groups (45) (Fig. 12-6). In PPMS, a model including cord area and cord MTR histogram peak height was significantly, albeit modestly, associated with the level of disability (45). Average cervical cord MTR is lower in MS patients with locomotor disability than in those without (123). Interestingly, in

patients with MS, cord MTR is only partially correlated with brain MTR (124) (Fig. 12-7), suggesting that MS pathology in the cord is not a mere reflection of brain pathology and, as a consequence, measuring cord pathology might be a rewarding exercise in terms of understanding MS pathophysiology.

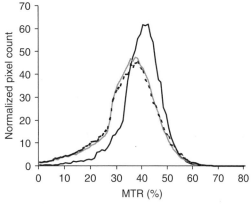

FIG. 12-6. Average magnetization transfer ratio (MTR) histograms of the cervical cord from healthy subjects *(black line),* secondary progressive MS (SPMS) *(dotted line)* and primary progressive (PPMS) *(gray line).* Compared to healthy subjects, SPMS and PPMS patients have similar reductions of cord average MTR (PPMS versus healthy subjects: p = 0.001; SPMS versus healthy subjects: p = 0.003).

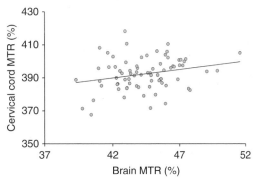

FIG. 12-7. Scatterplot showing the correlation between average brain and cervical cord MTR values in patients with MS. The lack of a significant correlation suggests that MS cord pathology is at least partially independent from brain pathology.

With increasing technical advances, it has also become possible to study cord MS pathology using DW-MRI (125–130). A preliminary study, which assessed water diffusion in seven cord lesions of three MS patients with locomotor disability (127), found increased MD values in MS cord lesions in comparison to the cord tissue from healthy volunteers. More recently, Valsasina et al. (129) used DW histogram analysis to assess cervical cord damage in a cohort of 44 patients with either RRMS or SPMS and found reduced average cord FA in MS patients compared to controls. Interestingly, in MS patients the reduction of cord FA was moderately correlated ($r = -0.48$) with the degree of disability. Altered MD and FA cord histogram-derived metrics have also been found in patients with PPMS (130).

Mechanisms of Recovery

The resolution of acute inflammation, remyelination, redistribution of voltage-gated sodium channels in persistently demyelinated axons, and recovery from sublethal axonal injury are all factors likely to limit the clinical impact of damaging MS pathology (131,132). However, other mechanisms have been recently recognized as potential contributors to the recovery or maintenance of function in the presence of irreversible, MS-related axonal damage. Brain plasticity is a well-known feature of the human brain that is likely to have several pathologic substrates, including an increased axonal expression of sodium channels (133), synaptic changes, increased recruitment of parallel existing pathways or latent connections, and reorganization of distant sites. All these changes might have a major adaptive role in limiting the functional consequences of axonal loss.

The following are the main findings derived from the application of fMRI to the assessment of MS patients:

1. Functional cortical changes have been demonstrated in all MS phenotypes, using different fMRI paradigms. A study of the visual system (134) in patients who had recovered from a single episode of acute

optic neuritis demonstrated that such patients had an extensive activation of the visual network compared to healthy volunteers. An altered brain pattern of movement-associated cortical activations, characterized by an increased recruitment of the contralateral primary sensorimotor cortex (SMC) during the performance of simple tasks (135,136) and by the recruitment of additional so-called classical and higher-order sensorimotor areas during the performance of more complex tasks (136), has been demonstrated in patients with CIS. An increased recruitment of several sensorimotor areas, mainly located in the cerebral hemisphere ipsilateral to the limb that performed the task, has also been demonstrated in patients with early MS and a previous episode of hemiparesis (137). Interestingly, in patients with similar characteristics but who presented with optic neuritis, this increased recruitment involved sensorimotor areas that were mainly located in the contralateral cerebral hemisphere (138). In patients with established MS and a relapsing-remitting course, functional cortical changes have been shown during the performance of visual (139), motor (140–144), and cognitive (145–148) tasks. Movement-associated cortical changes, characterized by the activation of highly specialized cortical areas, have also been described in patients with SPMS (149) during the performance of a simple motor task. Finally, two fMRI studies of the motor system (150,151) of patients with PPMS suggested a lack of classical adaptive mechanisms as a potential additional factor contributing to the accumulation of disability.

The results of all these studies suggest that there might be a natural history of the functional reorganization of the cerebral cortex in MS patients, which might be characterized, at the beginning of the disease, by an increased recruitment of those areas normally devoted to the performance of a given task, such as the primary SMC and the supplementary motor area (SMA) in the case of a motor task. At a later stage, bilateral activation of these regions is first seen, followed by a widespread recruitment of additional areas, which are usually recruited in normal people to perform novel or complex tasks. This notion has been supported by the results of a recent study (152) that has provided a direct demonstration that MS patients, during the performance of a simple motor task, activate cortical regions that are part of a fronto-parietal circuit, whose activation typically occurs in healthy subjects during object manipulation (152) (Fig. 12-8).

2. Functional and structural changes of MS brain are strictly correlated. Several moderate to strong correlations have been demonstrated between the activity of given cortical and subcortical areas and the extent of brain T2-visible lesions (137,140,144,149,151), the severity of intrinsic lesion damage (138,144), the severity of NABT damage measured using ^{1}H-MRS (135,142), MT-MRI or DW-MRI (144,149,150), the extent of NAGM damage (149,153) (Fig. 12-9) and, finally, the severity of cervical cord damage (150,154).

3. Although the actual role of cortical reorganization in the clinical manifestations of MS remains unclear, there are several pieces of evidence (in addition to the strong correlation found between functional and structural changes) that suggest that cortical adaptive changes are likely to contribute in limiting the clinical consequences of MS-related structural damage. Specifically, in a patient with an acute hemiparesis following a new, large, demyelinating lesion located in the corticospinal tract, dynamic changes of the brain pattern of activation of the classical motor areas, ending in a full recovery of function, have been observed (141). The correlation found between the extent of functional cortical changes and NAA levels suggests that dynamic reorganization of the motor cortex can occur in response to axonal injury associated with MS activity. In patients complaining of fatigue, when compared to matched, nonfatigued MS patients (143), a reduced activation of a complex movement-associated cortical/subcortical network, including the cerebellum, the rolandic operculum, the thalamus, and the middle frontal gyrus has been found. In fatigued patients, a strong correlation between the reduction of thalamic activity and the clinical severity of fatigue was also found, indicating that a less-marked cortical recruitment might be associated to the appearance of clinical symptomatology in MS. Finally, preliminary work has shown that the pattern of movement-associated cortical activations in MS is determined by both the extent of brain injury and disability and that these changes are distinct (155).

CONCLUSIONS

The extensive application of modern, MR-based techniques to the assessment of brain and cord pathology in patients with MS has considerably improved our understanding of MS pathophysiology and has provided new, objective metrics that might be useful to monitor disease evolution, either in natural history studies or in treatment trials. The large body of available literature clearly shows, however, that none of these quantitative techniques, taken in isolation, is able to provide a complete picture of the complexity of the MS process. There are several pieces of evidence indicating that a multiparametric

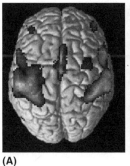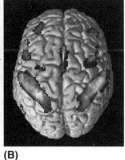

(A)   **(B)**

FIG. 12-8. Brain patterns of cortical activations on a rendered brain in right-handed patients with relapsing-remitting MS during the performance of a simple motor task **(A)** and in healthy subjects during the performance of a more complex task, consisting in object manipulation **(B)**. During the simple task, MS patients tend to activate some frontal regions that are activated by healthy subjects during object manipulation.

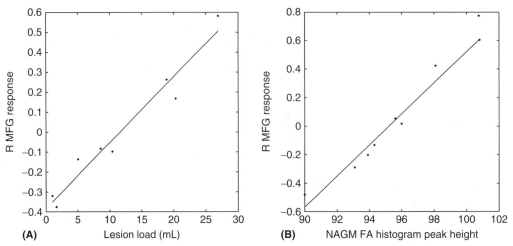

FIG. 12-9. Scatterplots of the correlations between the relative activation of the ipsilateral middle frontal gyrus during the performance of a simple motor task with the dominant right-upper limb and brain dual-echo lesion load **(A)** (r = 0.87, p < 0.001) and peak height of the fractional anisotropy histogram of the normal-appearing gray matter **(B)** (r = 0.88, p < 0.001) in patients with secondary progressive MS. These correlations suggest a possible adaptive role of functional cortical changes in MS.

approach, combining aggregates of different MR quantities, might improve our ability to monitor the disease (45,81,128,156). Such an approach should include not only the assessment of brain damage, but also that of cord pathology. This was suggested by a recent study in which, putting together brain and cord measures reflecting the severity of MS-related abnormalities, it was possible to explain about 50% of the variance of patients' disability (128). Finally, in the evaluation of the relationship between clinical and MRI markers of disease severity and evolution, the presence and efficacy of functional cortical changes should also be considered.

REFERENCES

1. McDonald WI, Compston A, Edan G, et al. Recommended diagnostic criteria for multiple sclerosis: guidelines from the International Panel on the diagnosis of multiple sclerosis. *Ann Neurol* 2001;50:121–127.
2. Rovaris M, Filippi M. Magnetic resonance techniques to monitor disease evolution and treatment trial outcomes in multiple sclerosis. *Curr Opin Neurol* 1999;12:337–344.
3. Molyneux PD, Barker GJ, Barkhof F, et al. Clinical-MRI correlations in a European trial of interferon beta-1b in secondary progressive MS. *Neurology* 2001;57:2191–2197.
4. Filippi M, Grossman RI, Comi G, eds. Magnetization transfer in multiple sclerosis. *Neurology* 1999;53[Suppl 3].
5. Filippi M, Inglese M. Overview of diffusion-weighted magnetic resonance studies in multiple sclerosis. *J Neurol Sci* 2001;186[Suppl 1];S37–S43.
6. Filippi M, Arnold DL, Comi G, eds. *Magnetic Resonance Spectroscopy in Multiple Sclerosis.* Milan: Springer-Verlag, 2001.
7. Filippi M, Rocca MA. Disturbed function and plasticity in multiple sclerosis as gleaned from functional magnetic resonance imaging. *Curr Opin Neurol* 2003;16:275–282. Review.
8. van Waesberghe JH, Kamphorst W, De Groot CJ, et al. Axonal loss in multiple sclerosis lesions: magnetic resonance imaging insights into substrates of disability. *Ann Neurol* 1999;46:747–754.
9. Barkhof F, Bruck W, De Groot CJ, et al. Remyelinated lesions in multiple sclerosis: magnetic resonance image appearance. *Arch Neurol* 2003;60:1073–1081.
10. Le Bihan D, Breton E, Lallemand D, et al. MR imaging of intravoxel incoherent motions: application to diffusion and perfusion in neurologic disorders. *Radiology* 1986;161:401–407.
11. Le Bihan D, Turner R, Pekar J, et al. Diffusion and perfusion imaging by gradient sensitization: design, strategy and significance. *J Magn Reson Imaging* 1991;1:7–8.
12. Basser PJ, Mattiello J, Le Bihan D. Estimation of the effective self-diffusion tensor from the NMR spin-echo. *J Magn Reson* 1994;103:247–254.

13. Pierpaoli C, Jezzard P, Basser PJ, et al. Diffusion tensor MR imaging of the human brain. *Radiology* 1996;201:637–648.

14. Bitsch A, Bruhn H, Vougioukas V, et al. Inflammatory CNS demyelination: histopathologic correlation with in vivo quantitative proton MR spectroscopy. *Am J Neuroradiol* 1999;20:1619–1627.

15. Ogawa S, Menon RS, Tank DW, et al. Functional brain mapping by blood oxygenation level-dependent contrast magnetic resonance imaging. A comparison of signal characteristics with a biophysical model. *Biophys J* 1993;64:803–812

16. Allen IV, McKeown SR. A histological, histochemical and biochemical study of the macroscopically normal white matter in multiple sclerosis. *J Neurol Sci* 1979;41:81–91.

17. Evangelou N, Esiri MM, Smith S, et al. Quantitative pathological evidence for axonal loss in normal appearing white matter in multiple sclerosis. *Ann Neurol* 2000;47:391–395.

18. Ferguson B, Matyszak MK, Esiri MM, et al. Axonal damage in acute multiple sclerosis lesions. *Brain* 1997;120:393–399.

19. Trapp BD, Peterson J, Ransohoff RM, et al. Axonal transection in the lesions of multiple sclerosis. *N Engl J Med* 1998;338:278–285.

20. De Stefano N, Matthews PM, Antel JP, et al. Chemical pathology of acute demyelinating lesions and its correlation with disability. *Ann Neurol* 1995;38:901–909.

21. van Walderveen MA, Barkhof F, Pouwels PJ, et al. Neuronal damage in T1-hypointense multiple sclerosis lesions demonstrated in vivo using proton magnetic resonance spectroscopy. *Ann Neurol* 1999;46:79–87.

22. Falini A, Calabrese G, Filippi M, et al. Benign versus secondary progressive multiple sclerosis: the potential role of ¹H MR spectroscopy in defining the nature of disability. *Am J Neuroradiol* 1998;19:223–229.

23. Rocca MA, Mastronardo G, Rodegher M, et al. Long-term changes of magnetization transfer-derived measures from patients with relapsing-remitting and secondary progressive multiple sclerosis. *Am J Neuroradiol* 1999;20:821–827.

24. Silver NC, Lai M, Symms MR, et al. Serial magnetization transfer imaging to characterize the early evolution of new MS lesions. *Neurology* 1998;51:758–764.

25. Filippi M, Rocca MA, Comi G. Magnetization transfer ratios of multiple sclerosis lesions with variable durations of enhancement. *J Neurol Sci* 1998;159:162–165.

26. Filippi M, Rocca MA, Rizzo G, et al. Magnetization transfer ratios in multiple sclerosis lesions enhancing after different doses of gadolinium. *Neurology* 1998;50:1289–1293.

27. Werring DJ, Clark CA, Barker GJ, et al. Diffusion tensor imaging of lesions and normal-appearing white matter in multiple sclerosis. *Neurology* 1999;52:1626–1632.

28. Filippi M, Cercignani M, Inglese M, et al. Diffusion tensor magnetic resonance imaging in multiple sclerosis. *Neurology* 2001;56:304–311.

29. Droogan AG, Clark CA, Werring DJ, et al. Comparison of multiple sclerosis clinical subgroups using navigated spin echo diffusion-weighted imaging. *J Magn Reson Imaging* 1999;17:653–661.

30. Filippi M, Iannucci G, Cercignani M, et al. A quantitative study of water diffusion in multiple sclerosis lesions and normal-appearing white matter using echo-planar imaging. *Arch Neurol* 2000;57:1017–1021.

31. Roychowdhury S, Maldijan JA, Grossman RI. Multiple sclerosis: comparison of trace apparent diffusion coefficients with MR enhancement pattern of lesions. *Am J Neuroradiol* 2000;21:869–874.

32. Davie CA, Hawkins CP, Barker GJ, et al. Serial proton magnetic resonance spectroscopy in acute multiple sclerosis lesions. *Brain* 1994;117:49–58.

33. Narayana PA, Doyle TJ, Lai D, et al. Serial proton magnetic resonance spectroscopic imaging, contrast-enhanced magnetic resonance imaging, and quantitative lesion volumetry in multiple sclerosis. *Ann Neurol* 1998;43:56–71.

34. Arnold DL, Matthews PM, Francis GS, et al. Proton magnetic resonance spectroscopic imaging for metabolic characterization of demyelinating plaques. *Ann Neurol* 1992;31:235–241.

35. Filippi M, Rocca MA, Martino G, et al. Magnetization transfer changes in the normal appearing white matter precede the appearance of enhancing lesions in patients with multiple sclerosis. *Ann Neurol* 1998;43:809–814.

36. Goodkin DE, Rooney WD, Sloan R, et al. A serial study of new MS lesions and the white matter from which they arise. *Neurology* 1998;51:1689–1697.

37. Pike GB, De Stefano N, Narayanan S, et al. Multiple sclerosis: magnetization transfer MR imaging of white matter before lesion appearance on T2-weighted images. *Radiology* 2000;215:824–830.

38. Fazekas F, Ropele S, Enzinger C, et al. Quantitative magnetization transfer imaging of pre-lesional white-matter changes in multiple sclerosis. *Mult Scler* 2002;8:479–484.

39. Rocca MA, Cercignani M, Iannucci G, et al. Weekly diffusion-weighted imaging of normal-appearing white matter in MS. *Neurology* 2000;55:882–884.

40. Werring DJ, Brassat D, Droogan AG, et al. The pathogenesis of lesions and normal-appearing white matter changes in multiple sclerosis. A serial diffusion MRI study. *Brain* 2000;123:1667–1676.

41. Sarchielli P, Presciutti O, Pelliccioli GP, et al. Absolute quantification of brain metabolites by proton magnetic resonance spectroscopy in normal-appearing white matter of multiple sclerosis patients. *Brain* 1999;122:513–521.

42. Tartaglia MC, Narayanan S, De Stefano N, et al. Choline is increased in pre-lesional normal appearing white matter in multiple sclerosis. *J Neurol* 2002;249:1382–1390.

43. Filippi M, Iannucci G, Tortorella C, et al. Comparison of MS clinical phenotypes using conventional and magnetization transfer MRI. *Neurology* 1999;52:588–594.

44. Iannucci G, Tortorella C, Rovaris M, et al. Prognostic value of MR and magnetization transfer imaging findings in patients with clinically isolated syndromes suggestive of multiple sclerosis at presentation. *Am J Neuroradiol* 2000;21:1034–1038.

45. Rovaris M, Bozzali M, Santuccio G, et al. In vivo assessment of the brain and cervical cord pathology of patients with primary progressive multiple sclerosis. *Brain* 2001;124:2540–2549.

46. Bjartmar C, Kinkel RP, Kidd G, et al. Axonal loss in normal-appearing white matter in a patient with acute MS. *Neurology* 2001;57:1248–1252.

47. Filippi M, Campi A, Dousset V, et al. A magnetization transfer imaging study of normal-appearing white matter in multiple sclerosis. *Neurology* 1995;45:478–482.

48. Loevner LA, Grossman RI, Cohen JA, et al. Microscopic disease in normal-appearing white matter on conventional MR images in patients with multiple sclerosis: assessment with magnetization-transfer measurements. *Radiology* 1995;196:511–515.

49. Horsfield MA, Lai M, Webb SL, et al. Apparent diffusion coefficients in benign and secondary progressive multiple sclerosis by nuclear magnetic resonance. *Magn Reson Med* 1996;36:393–400.

50. Cercignani M, Iannucci G, Rocca MA, et al. Pathologic damage in MS assessed by diffusion-weighted and magnetization transfer MRI. *Neurology* 2000;54:1139–1144.

51. Cercignani M, Bozzali M, Iannucci G, et al. Magnetisation transfer ratio and mean diffusivity of normal-appearing white and gray matter from patients with multiple sclerosis. *J Neurol Neurosurg Psychiatry* 2001;70:311–317.

52. Ciccarelli O, Werring DJ, Wheeler-Kingshott CA, et al. Investigation of MS normal-appearing brain using diffusion tensor MRI with clinical correlations. *Neurology* 2001;56:926–933.

53. Fu L, Matthews PM, De Stefano N, et al. Imaging axonal damage of normal-appearing white matter in multiple sclerosis. *Brain* 1998;121:103–113.

54. De Stefano N, Narayanan S, Francis SJ, et al. Diffuse axonal and tissue injury in patients with multiple sclerosis with low cerebral lesion load and no disability. *Arch Neurol* 2002;59:1565–1571.

55. Inglese M, Li BS, Rusinek H, et al. Diffusely elevated cerebral choline and creatine in relapsing-remitting multiple sclerosis. *Magn Reson Med* 2003;50:190–195.

56. Kapeller P, McLean MA, Griffin CM, et al. Preliminary evidence for neuronal damage in cortical grey matter and normal appearing white matter in short duration relapsing-remitting multiple sclerosis: a quantitative MR spectroscopic imaging study. *J Neurol* 2001;248:131–138.

57. Suhy J, Rooney WD, Goodkin DE, et al. 1H MRSI comparison of white matter and lesions in primary progressive and relapsing-remitting MS. *Mult Scler* 2000;6:148–155.

58. Chard DT, Griffin CM, McLean MA, et al. Brain metabolite changes in cortical grey and normal-appearing white matter in clinically early relapsing-remitting multiple sclerosis. *Brain* 2002;125:2342–2352.

59. Fernando KT, McLean MA, Chard DT, et al. Elevated white matter myo-inositol in clinically isolated syndromes suggestive of multiple sclerosis. *Brain* 2004;127:1361–1369.

60. Ge Y, Grossman RI, Babb JS, et al. Dirty-appearing white matter in multiple sclerosis: volumetric MR imaging and magnetization transfer ratio histogram analysis. *Am J Neuroradiol* 2003;24:1935–1940.

61. Kalkers NF, Hintzen RQ, van Waesberghe JH, et al. Magnetization transfer histogram parameters reflect all dimensions of MS pathology, including atrophy. *J Neurol Sci* 2001;184:155–162.

62. Tortorella C, Viti B, Bozzali M, et al. A magnetization transfer histogram study of normal-appearing brain tissue in MS. *Neurology* 2000;54:186–193.

63. Traboulsee A, Dehmeshki J, Brex PA, et al. Normal-appearing brain tissue MTR histograms in clinically isolated syndromes suggestive of MS. *Neurology* 2002;59:126–128.

64. Nusbaum AO, Tang CY, Wei TC, et al. Whole-brain diffusion MR histograms differ between MS subtypes. *Neurology* 2000;54:1421–1426.

65. Mezzapesa DM, Rocca MA, Falini A, et al. A preliminary diffusion tensor and magnetization transfer magnetic resonance imaging study of early-onset multiple sclerosis. *Arch Neurol* 2004;61:366–368.

66. De Stefano N, Narayanan S, Francis GS, et al. Evidence of axonal damage in the early stages of multiple sclerosis and its relevance to disability. *Arch Neurol* 2001;58:65–70.

67. Gonen O, Viswanathan AK, Catalaa I, et al. Total brain N-acetylaspartate concentration in normal, age-grouped females: quantitation with non-echo proton NMR spectroscopy. *Magn Reson Med.* 1998;40:684–689.

68. Gonen O, Catalaa I, Babb JS, et al. Total brain N-acetylaspartate. A new measure of disease load in MS. *Neurology* 2000;54:15–19.

69. Bonneville F, Moriarty DM, Li BS, et al. Whole-brain N-acetylaspartate concentration: correlation with T2-weighted lesion volume and expanded disability status scale score in cases of relapsing-remitting multiple sclerosis. *Am J Neuroradiol* 2002;23:371–375.

70. Inglese M, Ge Y, Filippi M, et al. Indirect evidence for early widespread gray matter involvement in relapsing-remitting multiple sclerosis. *NeuroImage* 2004;21:1825–1829.

71. Filippi M, Bozzali M, Rovaris M, et al. Evidence for widespread axonal damage at the earliest clinical stage of multiple sclerosis. *Brain* 2003;126:433–437.

72. Filippi M, Inglese M, Rovaris M, et al. Magnetization transfer imaging to monitor the evolution of MS: a 1-year follow-up study. *Neurology* 2000;55:940–946.

73. Santos AC, Narayanan S, De Stefano N, et al. Magnetization transfer can predict clinical evolution in patients with multiple sclerosis. *J Neurol* 2002;249:662–668.

74. Rovaris M, Agosta F, Sormani MP, et al. Conventional and magnetization transfer MRI predictors of clinical multiple sclerosis evolution: a medium-term follow-up study. *Brain* 2003;126:2323–2332.

75. Schmierer K, Altmann DR, Kassim N, et al. Progressive change in primary progressive multiple sclerosis normal-appearing white matter: a serial diffusion magnetic resonance imaging study. *Mult Scler* 2004;10:182–187.

76. De Stefano N, Matthews PM, Fu L, et al. Axonal damage correlates with disability in patients with relapsing-remitting multiple sclerosis. Results of a longitudinal magnetic resonance spectroscopy study. *Brain* 1998;121:1469–1477.

77. Ciccarelli O, Werring DJ, Barker GJ, et al. A study of the mechanisms of normal-appearing white matter damage in multiple sclerosis using diffusion tensor imaging—evidence of Wallerian degeneration. *J Neurol* 2003;250:287–292.

78. Caramia F, Pantano P, Di Legge S, et al. A longitudinal study of MR diffusion changes in normal appearing white matter of patients with early multiple sclerosis. *Magn Reson Imaging* 2002;20:383–388.

79. Cercignani M, Inglese M, Pagani E, et al. Mean diffusivity and fractional anisotropy histograms of patients with multiple sclerosis. *Am J Neuroradiol* 2001;22:952–958.

80. Iannucci G, Rovaris M, Giacomotti L, et al. Correlation of multiple sclerosis measures derived from T2-weighted, T1-weighted, magnetization transfer, and diffusion tensor MR imaging. *Am J Neuroradiol* 2001;22:1462–1467.

81. Iannucci G, Minicucci L, Rodegher M, et al. Correlations between clinical and MRI involvement in multiple sclerosis: assessment using T1, T2 and MT histograms. *J Neurol Sci* 1999;171:121–129.

82. Dehmeshki J, Ruto AC, Arridge S, et al. Analysis of MTR histograms in multiple sclerosis using principal components and multiple discriminant analysis. *Magn Reson Med* 2001;46:600–609.

83. Traboulsee A, Dehmeshki J, Peters KR, et al. Disability in multiple sclerosis is related to normal appearing brain tissue MTR histogram abnormalities. *Mult Scler* 2003;9:566–573.

84. Castriota Scanderbeg A, Tomaiuolo F, Sabatini U, et al. Demyelinating plaques in relapsing-remitting and secondary-progressive multiple sclerosis: assessment with diffusion MR imaging. *Am J Neuroradiol* 2000;21:862–868.

85. Rovaris M, Bozzali M, Iannucci G, et al. Assessment of normal-appearing white and gray matter in patients with primary progressive multiple sclerosis. *Arch Neurol* 2002;59:1406–1412.

86. Rovaris M, Filippi M, Falautano M, et al. Relation between MR abnormalities and patterns of cognitive impairment in multiple sclerosis. *Neurology* 1998;50:1601–1608.

87. van Buchem MA, Grossman RI, Armstrong C, et al. Correlation of volumetric magnetization transfer imaging with clinical data in MS. *Neurology* 1998;50:1609–1617.

88. Rovaris M, Filippi M, Minicucci L, et al. Cortical/subcortical disease burden and cognitive impairment in multiple sclerosis. *Am J Neuroradiol* 2000;21:402–408.

89. Filippi M, Tortorella C, Rovaris M, et al. Changes in the normal appearing brain tissue and cognitive impairment in multiple sclerosis. *J Neurol Neurosurg Psychiatry* 2000;68:157–161.

90. Tartaglia MC, Narayanan S, Francis SJ, et al. The relationship between diffuse axonal damage and fatigue in multiple sclerosis. *Arch Neurol* 2004;61:201–207.

91. Davie CA, Barker GJ, Webb S, et al. Persistent functional deficit in multiple sclerosis and autosomal dominant cerebellar ataxia is associated with axon loss. *Brain* 1995;118:1583–1592.

92. Lee MA, Blamire AM, Pendlebury S, et al. Axonal injury or loss in the internal capsule and motor impairment in multiple sclerosis. *Arch Neurol* 2000;57:65–70.

93. Wilson M, Tench CR, Morgan PS, et al. Pyramidal tract mapping by diffusion tensor magnetic resonance imaging in multiple sclerosis: improving correlations with disability. *J Neurol Neurosurg Psychiatry* 2003;74:203–207.

94. Gadea M, Martinez-Bisbal MC, Marti-Bonmati L, et al. Spectroscopic axonal damage of the right locus coeruleus relates to selective attention impairment in early stage relapsing-remitting multiple sclerosis. *Brain* 2004;127:89–98.

95. Lumsden CE. The Neuropathology of Multiple Sclerosis. In: Vinken PJ, Bruyn GW, eds. *Handbook of Clinical Neurology*. Amsterdam: North-Holland, 1970, Vol 9: 217–309.

96. Kidd D, Barkhof F, McConnell R, et al. Cortical lesions in multiple sclerosis. *Brain* 1999;122:17–26.

97. Peterson JW, Bo L, Mork S, et al. Transected neurites, apoptotic neurons, and reduced inflammation in cortical multiple sclerosis lesions. *Ann Neurol* 2001;50:389–400.

98. Cifelli A, Arridge M, Jezzard P, et al. Thalamic neurodegeneration in multiple sclerosis. *Ann Neurol* 2002;52:650–653.

99. Ge Y, Grossman RI, Udupa JK, et al. Magnetization transfer ratio histogram analysis of gray matter in relapsing-remitting multiple sclerosis. *Am J Neuroradiol* 2001;22:470–475.

100. Ge Y, Grossman RI, Udupa JK, et al. Magnetization transfer ratio histogram analysis of normal-appearing gray matter and normal-appearing white matter in multiple sclerosis. *J Comput Assist Tomogr* 2002;26:62–68.

101. Dehmeshki J, Chard DT, Leary SM, et al. The normal appearing grey matter in primary progressive multiple sclerosis: a magnetisation transfer imaging study. *J Neurol* 2003;250:67–74.

102. Bozzali M, Cercignani M, Sormani MP, et al. Quantification of brain gray matter damage in different MS phenotypes by use of diffusion tensor MR imaging. *Am J Neuroradiol* 2002;23:985–988.

103. Griffin CM, Chard DT, Ciccarelli O, et al. Diffusion tensor imaging in early relapsing-remitting multiple sclerosis. *Mult Scler* 2001;7:290–297.

104. Oreja-Guevara C, Rovaris M, Iannucci G, et al. Progressive grey matter damage in patients with relapsing remitting MS: a longitudinal diffusion tensor MRI study. *Arch Neurol* 2004. In press.

105. Miller DH, Barkhof F, Frank JA, et al. Measurement of atrophy in multiple sclerosis: pathological basis, methodological aspects and clinical relevance. *Brain* 2002;125:1676–1695. Review.

106. Sarchielli P, Presciutti O, Tarducci R, et al. Localized (1) H magnetic resonance spectroscopy in mainly cortical gray matter of patients with multiple sclerosis. *J Neurol* 2002;249:902–910.

107. Sharma R, Narayana PA, Wolinsky JS. Grey matter abnormalities in multiple sclerosis: proton magnetic resonance spectroscopic imaging. *Mult Scler* 2001;7:221–226.

108. Kapeller P, Brex PA, Chard D, et al. Quantitative 1H MRS imaging 14 years after presenting with a clinically isolated syndrome suggestive of multiple sclerosis. *Mult Scler* 2002;8:207–210.

109. Adalsteinsson E, Langer-Gould A, Homer RJ, et al. Gray matter N-acetyl aspartate deficits in secondary progressive but not relapsing-remitting multiple sclerosis. *Am J Neuroradiol* 2003;24:1941–1945.

110. Fabiano AJ, Sharma J, Weinstock-Guttman B, et al. Thalamic involvement in multiple sclerosis: a diffusion-weighted magnetic resonance imaging study. *J Neuroimaging* 2003;13:307–314.

111. Wylezinska M, Cifelli A, Jezzard P, et al. Thalamic neurodegeneration in relapsing-remitting multiple sclerosis. *Neurology* 2003;60:1949–1954.

112. Rovaris M, Iannucci G, Falautano M, et al. Cognitive dysfunction in patients with mildly disabling relapsing-remitting multiple sclerosis: an exploratory study with diffusion tensor MR imaging. *J Neurol Sci* 2002;195:103–109.

113. Codella M, Rocca MA, Colombo B, et al. Cerebral grey matter pathology and fatigue in patients with multiple sclerosis: a preliminary study. *J Neurol Sci* 2002;194:71–74.

114. Tartaglia MC, Narayanan S, Francis SJ, et al. The relationship between diffuse axonal damage and fatigue in multiple sclerosis. *Arch Neurol* 2004;61:201–207.

115. Thorpe JW, Barker GJ, Jones SJ, et al. Magnetisation transfer ratios and transverse magnetisation decay curves in optic neuritis: correlation with clinical findings and electrophysiology. *J Neurol Neurosurg Psychiatry* 1995;59:487–492.

116. Boorstein JM, Moonis G, Boorstein SM, et al. Optic neuritis: imaging with magnetization transfer. *Am J Roentgenol* 1997;169:1709–1712.

117. Inglese M, Ghezzi A, Bianchi S, et al. Irreversible disability and tissue loss in multiple sclerosis: a conventional and magnetization transfer magnetic resonance imaging study of the optic nerves. *Arch Neurol* 2002;59:250–255.

118. Hickman SJ, Toosy AT, Jones SJ, et al. Serial magnetization transfer imaging in acute optic neuritis. *Brain* 2004;127:692–700.

119. Iwasawa T, Matoba H, Ogi A, et al. Diffusion-weighted imaging of the human optic nerve: a new approach to evaluate optic neuritis in multiple sclerosis. *Magn Reson Med* 1997;38:484–491.

120. Wheeler-Kingshott CA, Parker GJ, Symms MR, et al. ADC mapping of the human optic nerve: increased resolution, coverage, and reliability with CSF-suppressed ZOOM-EPI. *Magn Reson Med* 2002;47:24–31.

121. Silver NC, Barker GJ, Losseff NA, et al. Magnetisation transfer ratio measurement in the cervical spinal cord: a preliminary study in multiple sclerosis. *Neuroradiology* 1997;39:441–445.

122. Lycklama a Nijeholt GJ, Castelijns JA, Lazeron RH, et al. Magnetization transfer ratio of the spinal cord in multiple sclerosis: relationship to atrophy and neurologic disability. *J Neuroimaging* 2000;10:67–72.

123. Filippi M, Bozzali M, Horsfield MA, et al. A conventional and magnetization transfer MRI study of the cervical cord in patients with MS. *Neurology* 2000;54:207–213.

124. Rovaris M, Bozzali M, Santuccio G, et al. Relative contributions of brain and cervical cord pathology to multiple sclerosis disability: a study with magnetisation transfer ratio histogram analysis. *J Neurol Neurosurg Psychiatry* 2000;69:723–727.

125. Wheeler-Kingshott CA, Hickman SJ, Parker GJ, et al. Investigating cervical spinal cord structure using axial diffusion tensor imaging. *NeuroImage* 2002;16: 93–102.

126. Bammer R, Augustin M, Prokesch RW, et al. Diffusion-weighted imaging of the spinal cord: interleaved echo-planar imaging is superior to fast spin-echo. *J Magn Reson Imaging* 2002;15:364–373.

127. Clark CA, Werring DJ, Miller DH. Diffusion imaging of the spinal cord in vivo: estimation of the principal diffusivities and application to multiple sclerosis. *Magn Reson Med* 2000;43:133–138.

128. Cercignani M, Horsfield MA, Agosta F, et al. Sensitivity-encoded diffusion tensor MR imaging of the cervical cord. *Am J Neuroradiol* 2003;24:1254–1256.

129. Valsasina P, Rocca MA, Agosta F, et al. Mean diffusivity and fractional anisotropy histogram analysis of the cervical cord in MS patients. *NeuroImage* 2005. In press.

130. Agosta F, Benedetti B, Rocca MA, et al. Quantification of cervical cord pathology in primary progressive MS using diffusion tensor MRI. *Neurology* 2005;64:631–635.

131. Waxman SG, Ritchie JM. Molecular dissection of the myelinated axon. *Ann Neurol* 1993;33:121–136.

132. De Stefano N, Matthews PM, Arnold DL. Reversible decreases in *N*-acetylaspartate after acute brain injury. *Magn Reson Med* 1995;34:721–727.

133. Waxman SG. Demyelinating diseases: new pathological insights, new therapeutic targets. *N Engl J Med* 1998;338:323–326

134. Werring DJ, Bullmore ET, Toosy AT, et al. Recovery from optic neuritis is associated with a change in the distribution of cerebral response to visual stimulation: a functional magnetic resonance imaging study. *J Neurol Neurosurg Psychiatry* 2000;68:441–449.

135. Rocca MA, Mezzapesa DM, Falini A, et al. Evidence for axonal pathology and adaptive cortical reorganisation in patients at presentation with clinically isolated syndromes suggestive of MS. *NeuroImage* 2003;18:847–855.

136. Filippi M, Rocca MA, Mezzapesa DM, et al. Simple and complex movement-associated functional MRI changes in patients at presentation with clinically isolated syndromes suggestive of MS. *Human Brain Mapping* 2004;21:108–117.

137. Pantano P, Iannetti GD, Caramia F, et al. Cortical motor reorganization after a single clinical attack of multiple sclerosis. *Brain* 2002;125:1607–1615.

138. Pantano P, Mainero C, Iannetti GD, et al. Contribution of corticospinal tract damage to cortical motor reorganization after a single clinical attack of multiple sclerosis. *NeuroImage* 2002;17:1837–1843.

139. Rombouts SA, Lazeron RH, Scheltens P, et al. Visual activation patterns in patients with optic neuritis: an fMRI pilot study. *Neurology* 1998;50:1896–1899.

140. Lee M, Reddy H, Johansen-Berg H, et al. The motor cortex shows adaptive functional changes to brain injury from multiple sclerosis. *Ann Neurol* 2000;47:606–613.

141. Reddy H, Narayanan S, Matthews PM, et al. Relating axonal injury to functional recovery in MS. *Neurology* 2000;54:236–239.

142. Reddy H, Narayanan S, Arnoutelis R, et al. Evidence for adaptive functional changes in the cerebral cortex with axonal injury from multiple sclerosis. *Brain* 2000;123:2314–2320.

143. Filippi M, Rocca MA, Colombo B, et al. Functional magnetic resonance imaging correlates of fatigue in multiple sclerosis. *NeuroImage* 2002;15:559–567.

144. Rocca MA, Falini A, Colombo B, et al. Adaptive functional changes in the cerebral cortex of patients with non-disabling MS correlate with the extent of brain structural damage. *Ann Neurol* 2002;51:330–339.

145. Staffen W, Mair A, Zauner H, et al. Cognitive function and fMRI in patients with multiple sclerosis: evidence for compensatory cortical activation during an attention task. *Brain* 2002;156:1275–1282.

146. Hillary FG, Chiaravalloti ND, Ricker JH, et al. An investigation of working memory rehearsal in multiple sclerosis using fMRI. *J Clin Exp Neuropsychol* 2003;25:965–978.

147. Parry AM, Scott RB, Palace J, et al. Potentially adaptive functional changes in cognitive processing for patients with multiple sclerosis and their acute modulation by rivastigmine. *Brain* 2003;126:2750–2760.

148. Mainero C, Caramia F, Pozzilli C, et al. fMRI evidence of brain reorganization during attention and memory tasks in multiple sclerosis. *NeuroImage* 2004;21:858–867.

149. Rocca MA, Gavazzi C, Mezzapesa DM, et al. A functional magnetic resonance imaging study of patients with secondary progressive multiple sclerosis. *NeuroImage* 2003;19:1770–1777.

150. Filippi M, Rocca MA, Falini A, et al. Correlations between structural CNS damage and functional MRI changes in primary progressive MS. *NeuroImage* 2002;15:537–546.

151. Rocca MA, Matthews PM, Caputo D, et al. Evidence for widespread movement-associated functional MRI changes in patients with PPMS. *Neurology* 2002;58:866–872.

152. Filippi M, Rocca MA, Mezzapesa DM, et al. A functional MRI study of cortical activations associated with object manipulation in patients with MS. *NeuroImage* 2004;21:1147–1154.

153. Rocca MA, Pagani E, Ghezzi A, et al. Functional cortical changes in patients with MS and non-specific conventional MRI scans of the brain *NeuroImage* 2003;19:826–836.

154. Rocca MA, Mezzapesa DM, Ghezzi A, et al. Cord damage elicits brain functional reorganization after a single episode of myelitis. *Neurology* 2003;61:1078–1085.

155. Reddy H, Narayanan S, Woolrich M, et al. Functional brain reorganization for hand movement in patients with multiple sclerosis: defining distinct effects of injury and disability. *Brain* 2002;125:2646–2657.

156. Mainero C, De Stefano N, Iannucci G, et al. Correlates of MS disability assessed in vivo using aggregates of MR quantities. *Neurology* 2001;56:1331–1334.

13

The Role of MRS and fMRI in Multiple Sclerosis

Maria Carmela Tartaglia[1] and Douglas L. Arnold[2]

[1]Department of Neurology, University of Western Ontario, London, Ontario, Canada; [2]Department
of Neurology and Neurosurgery, McGill University, Montreal, Quebec, Canada

Medical imaging of the brain has altered our perception of neurological illness. Some physicians have embraced imaging as a tool to facilitate care of the patient, in which case its primary function resides in diagnosis, lesion location, and following disease evolution. For others, however, imaging provides a window onto pathogenesis, answering some questions and giving rise to new ones. Imaging is one of the few means at our disposal for investigating the pathophysiology of multiple sclerosis (MS), as there is no completely analogous animal model. Multiple sclerosis is usually considered an inflammatory, demyelinating disease characterized by the recurrent formation of multifocal plaques located primarily in the white matter. These white matter lesions are readily visible on MRI and, as of 2001, imaging of these lesions has been incorporated into the diagnostic criteria for MS (1).

Conventional MRI enables the visualization of MS lesions as hyperintensities on T2-weighted (T2W) and proton density-weighted (PD) MRI. These plaques represent a variable combination of demyelination, inflammation, axonal loss, and remyelination (2,3). The visibility of plaques has made them a convenient marker of disease progression, and it is now well-known that patients can accumulate lesion burden (i.e., increased plaque volume) in the absence of clinically evident activity (4,5). This notion has forced a new way of thinking about MS in which relapses and remissions correspond to clinical phenomenon that do not necessarily correlate with what is happening in the brain, and thus MS may be more appropriately considered a progressive illness, even in the setting of clinical quiescence. With this in mind, it is now becoming apparent that MS may be more similar to neurodegenerative diseases than was once appreciated.

The visualization of MS lesions has provided important insight into the disease process; however, the frequency and volume of plaque formation fail to explain much of the variance in clinical disability. A number of nonconventional MRI techniques have emerged that have helped to fill this gap—proton magnetic resonance spectroscopy (^{1}H-MRS) and functional magnetic resonance imaging (fMRI) are two of these techniques. The focus of this chapter will be on the aspects of MS that have come to light or are better understood as a result of imaging MS patients with these techniques. Other MRI techniques, including magnetization transfer (MT) and diffusion-weighted imaging (DWI), have been reviewed elsewhere (6). Refer also to Chapter 12 by Filippi and Rocca.

INTRODUCTION TO MAGNETIC RESONANCE SPECTROSCOPY

Magnetic resonance spectroscopy (MRS) allows the in vivo assessment of brain metabolites. Proton magnetic resonance spectroscopy (^{1}H-MRS) has, in conjunction with neuropathology, radically changed the way we view MS and has shed light on several important concepts about MS that will be discussed below:

1. MS pathology extends beyond the confines of the lesions that can be appreciated both clinically and by conventional MRI.
2. Axonal pathology is a prominent feature of MS that begins early in the disease course.
3. There is more to MS than inflammation; there is neurodegeneration.
4. Some of the pathology is reversible.
5. Gray matter pathology in MS.
6. Cognitive changes and fatigue in MS.

We will begin with a brief overview of the nature of the information that ^{1}H-MRS has provided and then focus on the novel insights it has allowed us to acquire. ^{1}H-MRS enables the in vivo assessment of the biochemical pathology that characterizes MS and has been used to noninvasively measure metabolic changes in the brains of MS patients (6–11). Four major resonances are revealed with water-suppressed ^{1}H-MRS of the healthy human brain at long echo times (TE = 136 to 288 ms, most commonly). At 3.2 parts per million (ppm) from the resonance frequency of tetramethylsilane (the standard), there is a resonance from choline-containing phospholipids (Cho). This peak is believed to represent a combination of free choline,

phosphorylcholine, glycerylphosphorylcholine, and possibly taurine and betaine (12). Choline-containing compounds are normal constituents of myelin and membranes.

^{1}H-MRS of acute MS lesions reveals increased resonance intensities from choline and lactate in the early phases of the new T2W lesion appearance on MRI, which may be associated with gadolinium enhancement (13). If acquisition parameters are suitable (i.e., relatively short echo times), resonances from neutral lipids released from membranes can also be observed (14,15). An increase of choline within acute plaques has been interpreted as resulting from demyelination, as well as increased membrane turnover associated with inflammatory or glial cell reactions (7,8,12,16,17). The Cho/creatine (Cr) ratio has been shown to be elevated in areas of normal-appearing white matter (NAWM) that go on to develop plaque even a year later (Fig. 13-1) (18,19). In addition, this ratio was increased in plaques that increased in size 6 and 12 months later (19). The return of Cho/Cr ratios toward normal is concurrent with a reduction in inflammation and the beginning of remyelination (17).

At 3.0 ppm, there is a resonance usually referred to as Cr, which originates from both Cr and phosphocreatine. Cr is relatively homogeneously distributed throughout the brain, and thus can be used as an internal reference standard to normalize the intensity of other resonances such as N-acetyl aspartate (NAA) and Cho in situations where the concentration of Cr is not significantly altered by the pathology. There is inconsistency in the literature on this point (20–25). In a meta-analysis of published results (26), Cr values in MS NAWM were compared to those in the WM of normal control (NC) in 26 comparisons that appeared in 13 publications (18,20,25,27–36). NAWM Cr was not clearly different from normal in most reports, but was slightly increased relative to normal control white matter (NCWM) in a small number of comparisons. The summary statistic for all these reports suggested a statistically significant alteration of Cr in MS NAWM of approximately 3%. This small change is not likely to be practically significant in most circumstances.

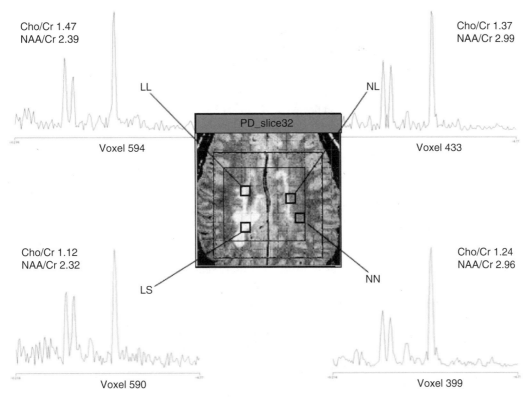

Cho/Cr 1.47
NAA/Cr 2.39

LL

Voxel 594

Cho/Cr 1.37
NAA/Cr 2.99

NL

Voxel 433

PD_slice32

Cho/Cr 1.12
NAA/Cr 2.32

LS

Voxel 590

Cho/Cr 1.24
NAA/Cr 2.96

NN

Voxel 399

FIG. 13-1. Proton density image from an RR Patient seen at Time point 1 with examples of spectroscopic data from a voxel of NAWM that remains as NAWM on subsequent scan at 6 months (NN), from a voxel of NAWM that develops a lesion on subsequent scan at 6 months (NL), from a voxel of lesion that remains stable on subsequent scan at 6 months (LS), and from a voxel of lesion that increases in size on subsequent scan at 6 months (LL). There was a significantly lower Cho/Cr level in voxels of normal control subjects compared with Lesion voxels but not NAWM voxels in MS patients. The NAA/Cr of control subjects was significantly higher than the NAA/Cr ratio in both NAWM and Lesion voxels of MS patients. Cho/Cr was significantly higher in voxels that either developed a lesion or increased in lesion size as compared with their stable counterpart.

At 2.0 ppm, the resonance arising from N-acetyl groups (mainly NAA in the cerebral hemispheres) dominates the spectrum. NAA is synthesized by neuronal mitochondria from L-aspartate and acetyl-CoA and requires intact mitochondrial metabolism (37–39). It is the second-most abundant amino acid in the adult central nervous system (CNS) after glutamate (40–42). The function of NAA remains elusive. It has been speculated that it participates in lipid synthesis, osmotic regulation, myelination, and metabolism of neurotransmitters such as aspartate and *N*-acetyl-glutamate (37,40,43,44). Immunohistochemical studies have clearly shown that NAA is neuron-specific (41,45). Although there are reports that NAA is also found in O2A progenitor cells in vivo, there is no evidence that this is relevant in the adult brain in vivo. Bjartmar et al. (45), using a model of rat optic nerve transection, have demonstrated that loss of NAA reflects axonal degeneration and that the oligodendroglial cell precursors that become prevalent in the optic nerve after injury do not affect the NAA resonance intensity.

NAA is decreased 30% to 80% in T2W lesions, whether they be acute or chronic WM lesions (7–9,14,21,46). Decreases are greater in acute lesions and may show partial recovery (47), at least outside the very core of the lesions (8). Reversible decreases in NAA can be produced in cultures of neuronal cell lines by transient serum deprivation and after reversal of mitochondrial poisoning with the mitochondrial toxin 3-nitropropionate (48). Although the function of NAA is unclear, its specificity for neurons and neuronal processes in the normal mature brain render it an ideal surrogate marker of neuronal integrity (42). Decreased NAA reflects neuronal/axonal injury and can be due to impaired neuronal mitochondrial metabolism or a decreased neuronal/axonal relative partial volume (density) in the MRS voxels. The latter could be secondary to neuronal/axonal loss or atrophy (45). Decreases due to dilution by edema or cellular infiltration also can affect NAA density and must be taken into account. Normalizing to intravoxel Cr is largely immune to this.

At 1.3 ppm, there is a resonance from lactate that is usually not seen above the level of the noise in the spectrum from a normal brain performing aerobic metabolism. Lactate can be seen if its concentration is increased due to increased anaerobic metabolism associated with local ischemia, neuronal mitochondrial dysfunction, or infiltration by macrophages, which rely on anaerobic glycolysis (49,50). Lactate has been reported with higher frequency in enhancing than in nonenhancing lesions, and this is thought to reflect primarily the invasion of macrophages (14,15). After the acute phase, over a period of days to weeks the lactate resonance intensity returns to normal.

Short echo times (TE = 20 to 30 ms) can be used to visualize additional metabolites, including mobile lipids at 0.9 to 1.3 ppm, myo-inositol at 3.65 and 3.77 ppm, and glutamate and glutamine between 2.1 and 2.45 ppm. Transient increases in lipids are attributed to the breakdown of myelin since the myelin sheaths consist of a lipid-bilayer membrane (18). The time course of ^{1}H-MRS lipid detection seems to be compatible with the time course of disappearance of lipid-laden macrophages from areas of acute myelin destruction. Recently, Fernando et al. (51) have reported increased myo-inositol as well as elevated Cr in the NAWM of clinically isolated syndrome (CIS) patients without concomitant increase of other metabolites. The early increase in myo-inositol may reflect a process of pathogenic importance in multiple sclerosis NAWM.

EXTENT OF MS PATHOLOGY

MS pathology extends beyond the confines of the lesions that can be appreciated both clinically and by conventional MRI. Although the primary pathology of MS is usually viewed as demyelination, it alone cannot account for the functional impairments experienced by MS patients. Demyelinated axons reorganize their sodium channels and reestablish conduction (52,53). A clinical example is recovery from optic neuritis, which cannot be explained by remyelination alone since recovery of conduction has been demonstrated in chronically demyelinated regions of the optic nerve (54).

As previously stated, NAA is decreased in lesions seen on T2W MRI. These lesions are associated with axonal transection, the occurrence of which is related to the degree of inflammation within the lesion (11,55). The interesting and more troublesome discovery is that decreases in NAA concentration are not restricted to MS lesions, but also occur in the NAWM adjacent to and distant from these lesions (24,56). Note in Figure 13-1 that voxels in the lesion have a lower NAA/Cr than voxels in NAWM, and that both groups have a lower NAA/Cr ratio than normal controls (19). The NAA in the NAWM is not as low as in the lesions, but it is significantly lower than in healthy control subjects (56). Chard et al. (57) also noted increased myo-inositol in the NAWM. The elevated myo-inositol was interpreted as reflecting glial proliferation (57). NAA/Cr is lower in lesions than in the NAWM in both relapsing-remitting MS (RRMS) and secondary progressive MS (SPMS) patients. Although lesions displayed a similar NAA/Cr reduction in both patient groups, the NAA/Cr in the NAWM was significantly lower in SPMS patients, who were more disabled, suggesting that the diffuse, nonlesional axonal pathology was more strongly related to disability than the lesional pathology (56).

Another troubling discovery was that diffuse WM pathology is apparent early on in the course of RRMS, and may even be present at disease onset (58,59). A diffuse decrease in NAA can be detected in MS patients with very short disease duration, in the absence of extensive brain demyelination and before clinical disability becomes evident.

Axons generally project through lesions, so any axonal interruption that occurs within lesions will be associated with Wallerian degeneration, axonal dysfunction, and volume loss that extend beyond the borders of MS lesions. Evangelou et al. (60) assessed axonal loss in the NAWM of the corpus callosum in postmortem brains of patients with MS and showed that the corpus callosum was atrophied and also had a decreased density of axons in the remaining tissue. Pathology studies have demonstrated alterations in neurofilament phosphorylation and substantial loss of axon density well outside the demyelinating lesions (61). The pathological abnormalities noted in postmortem and biopsy studies reveal abnormalities in the NAWM that include diffuse astrocytic hyperplasia, patchy edema, perivascular cellular infiltration, abnormally thin myelin sheaths, axonal loss, and gliosis.

Genetic studies have demonstrated the importance of genetic predisposition to the evolution of MS. For example, patients with the epsilon4 allele of apolipoprotein E (APOE epsilon4) have a relatively more rapid clinical worsening and more severe tissue damage on MRI (62–64). Patients with MS and an epsilon4 allele also had a significantly lower NAA/Cr ratio than those without an epsilon4 allele. Furthermore, the drop in the NAA/Cr ratio of epsilon4 carriers was significantly larger and was paralleled by a higher number of relapses and a faster (although nonsignificant) progression of disability.

The above-mentioned results establish MS as a more diffuse disease than has been generally appreciated, even at an early stage. The evidence implies also that the disease is present before the first clinical manifestation and in patients with very low lesion burden, suggesting that there may be a component of MS that is neurodegenerative.

AXONAL PATHOLOGY

Axonal pathology is a prominent feature of MS that begins early on in the disease course. Over a century ago, Charcot noted that MS pathology

included axons (65). However, this observation was overshadowed by the overwhelming myelin and oligodendrocyte pathology, and the fact that axons were *relatively* spared. Decreases in the concentration of the biomarker NAA have proven invaluable in reemphasizing the importance and prevalence of axonal pathology in MS. A number of histopathology studies have demonstrated the axonal pathology in MS (11,60,66–68). A strong correlation of decreased NAA with axonal degeneration in transected nerves has been demonstrated in a model of rat optic nerve transection (45). In a postmortem study of MS patients, spinal cord NAA density, measured by high-performance liquid chromatography (HPLC), correlated with axonal density, as determined by immunohistochemistry (66). The decrease in axonal density of 49% to 78% in the inactive spinal cord lesions supports axonal loss as a major cause of decreased white matter NAA in SPMS. The fact that average NAA/axonal volume was decreased by 30% in myelinated axons and by 42% in demyelinated axons in MS lesions indicates that axonal mitochondrial dysfunction is also an important factor in determining NAA concentration in MS.

Loss of axons in MS has become a focus of interest, as it has become increasingly clear that axonal loss is the substrate of chronic, irreversible disability (11,69–71). Axonal transection is a common feature of MS lesions and begins at disease onset. Cumulative axonal loss appears to be responsible for the progressive disability observed in patients with MS (11,72). Axonal injury has been quantified in early and chronic MS lesions, and reductions in axonal density of up to 60% have been demonstrated (73,74). Axonal loss has also been demonstrated in NAWM (74). Losses of approximately 45% of nerve fibers in the corpus callosum and optic nerve have been demonstrated on postmortem examination of MS patients (60,75).

Using NAA as a marker of axonal integrity, a number of researchers have demonstrated a strong link between the degree of axonal dysfunction and permanent disability in MS patients (69). Recent ^{1}H-MRS studies have shown that NAA decreases can occur very early in the course of MS (58), and can be detected in subcortical (76,77) and neocortical (78) brain regions and throughout the NAWM (79,80). De Stefano et al. (58) found that decreases in NAA compatible with diffuse cerebral axonal injury are present in the early stages of MS when there is little or no disability. NAA density actually decreases more rapidly in the earlier, relapsing-remitting stage of MS, and correlates more strongly with disability in patients with mild disease than in patients with more severe, secondary progressive disease. NAA concentrations in the brain are significantly correlated with patients' clinical disability (81), selective motor impairment (82), and cognitive dysfunction (83). There is an inverse correlation between the NAA of the NAWM and disability (7). Davie et al. (84) showed that MS patients with greater cerebellar dysfunction had lower cerebellar NAA.

The evidence for early neuronal loss or dysfunction in MS increases steadily. Ge et al. (85) showed a disparity between atrophy and whole-brain NAA, with the conclusion that neuronal/axonal dysfunction precedes parenchymal loss. In another study, decreases in NAA signal intensity were noted in acute, enhancing lesions in patients with benign and SPMS, but the chronic lesions in patients with benign MS had much higher NAA concentrations than the chronic lesions in patients with SPMS (86). Those authors concluded that acute lesions in patients with less disability displayed improved recovery.

In summary, multiple lines of evidence suggest that neuro-axonal pathology is an early event of MS that does not proceed in parallel with white matter demyelination, and that axonal injury underlies the accumulation of irreversible disability in MS.

NEURODEGENERATION IN MS

MS has traditionally been considered an inflammatory disease that eventually develops a neurodegenerative phase. More recently, the idea that neurodegeneration may be an early and separate process in MS is becoming more accepted. Recent data from MRI and pathologic studies have shown that axonal loss and atrophy are common, begin at disease onset, and provide the pathological substrate for irreversible functional neurological and neurobehavioral impairments (11,61,69,70,72).

The relationship between inflammation and neurodegeneration is unclear at this time. Gadolinium enhancement, an indicator of inflammation, appears to be one factor that predicts the development of brain atrophy, suggesting a link between inflammation and subsequent tissue destruction (87). Longitudinal studies have suggested that enhancement is 5 to 10 times more common than overt clinical attacks or progression of disability, indicating the continuous nature of the MS disease process and the sensitivity of MRI to ongoing disease activity (88,89). A correlation exists between the persistence of T1W black holes and the duration of the lesion's inflammatory phase (90).

A link between inflammation and neurodegeneration has also been supported pathologically (91). Amyloid precursor protein (APP), an index of injury, is seen in axons of active MS lesions and at the border of chronic, active MS lesions. The number of APP-positive axons correlates with the degree of inflammation (91). Trapp et al. (11) showed that axonal transection occurred in active MS lesions, even in patients with very short disease duration (72). Autopsy data reveal that MS lesions show a loss of 45% to 84% of their axons, with an average decrease in axonal density of more than 50% (66,74).

Axonal loss has been noted in the NAWM so that axons distal to the site of transection undergo Wallerian degeneration. A 19% to 42% decrease in axonal density in the lateral corticospinal tract of MS patients with lower extremity weakness has been observed (92). Simon et al. (93) noted Wallerian degeneration in the corticospinal tract remote from a classic-appearing focal demyelinating events in the brain in patients presenting with their first symptoms suggestive of MS. Using APP again, Kuhlmann et al. (55) demonstrated that acute axonal damage occurred early during the disease and lesion formation, and that APP-positive axons could be detected at all stages of the demyelinating activity as well as in the periplaque white matter. They reported that acute axonal damage was most prominent within the first year after disease onset. In both RRMS and SPMS patients they found acute axonal damage to be significantly higher in the early stages of disease than after a duration of 10 years or more. They also found a correlation between acute axonal damage and the number of CD8-positive T-cells and macrophages/microglia.

The notion that neurodegeneration is not necessarily a consequence of inflammation is supported by autopsy data that identified pathological changes that preceded leukocyte infiltration and demyelination (94). Those authors proposed that apoptotic oligodendrocyte death in a circumscribed area could be the initial event in lesion formation. This oligodendrocyte death is what they propose may initiate the cascade that results in inflammation and development of a focal lesion. The failure of immunomodulatory and immunosuppressive drugs to prevent disease progression provides indirect evidence for neuronal and/or axonal degeneration in MS (95).

Imaging techniques provide further evidence of neurodegeneration in MS. NAA is markedly decreased in lesions but is still lower than controls in the NAWM. The decrease of NAA per lesion volume was significantly higher in SPMS patients with irreversible neurological disability than in RRMS patients with mild disability (96). Whole-brain NAA measurements revealed widespread axonal pathology that was independent of MRI enhancement and was present from the earliest clinical stage of the disease (97). Neurodegeneration of subcortical structures (as measured by MRI) has been noted, with a substantial neocortical volume loss reported and confirmed in the thalamus of RRMS and SPMS (76,77,98). Neuronal death in cortical MS lesions has also been observed (99). Figure 13-2 illustrates the possible interaction of inflammatory and degenerative changes in the pathological evolution of MS.

REVERSIBILITY OF SOME OF THE PATHOLOGY

The decrease in NAA in patients with MS is partly reversible in acute demyelinating lesions (18). This implies that some of the axonal pathology observed is reversible. The mechanisms proposed for the recovery of NAA include resolution of inflammation, remyelination, recovery of neuronal mitochondrial dysfunction, and/or redistribution of axolemmal ion channels. The increasing NAA after an attack is loosely associated with the clinical recovery observed after a relapse (which also depends on cerebral plasticity, as discussed below).

The NAA decrease observed in the NAWM also is not necessarily permanent. Reversible changes in NAA concentration can be detected in the NAWM of the hemisphere contralateral to solitary acute lesions (100), as well as in lesions, suggesting that sublethal axonal injury is a contributing factor to acute, potentially reversible MS disability (8,47,101).

One study of an MS patient with a large, demyelinating lesion and acute, relapse-related disability used combined MRS and fMRI to demonstrate a subacutely increased area of activation and a decreased NAA that subsequently showed partial recovery in parallel with the recovery of functional impairment (102). Upon full recovery, the patient's volume of activation was similar to controls; the NAA, however, was still abnormally low at the final scan. Decreases in activation area were associated with normalization of the impairment, in parallel with the progressive recovery of NAA.

GRAY MATTER PATHOLOGY IN MS

The GM pathology of MS patients has often been overlooked. An autopsy study in the 1960s noted macroscopic GM pathology and a recent study has described the microscopic features of GM pathology seen in MS-neuronal apoptosis and characteristic inflammatory infiltrates in cortical lesions (99,103–105). Although it is more difficult to appreciate GM pathology compared with WM

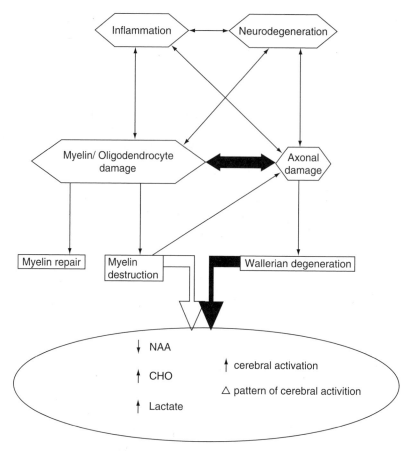

FIG. 13-2. Flow diagram illustrating the dynamic nature of the pathological process in MS as well as the effect on MRS and fMRI.

pathology using conventional MRI, new MRI techniques are providing evidence of GM involvement in MS. Kapeller et al. (31) showed in 16 MS patients with short-duration, mild MS [1.8 years, Expanded Disability Status Scale (EDSS) median 1] that their cortical gray matter displayed lower NAA and myo-inositol compared with controls, implying widespread neuronal dysfunction or loss early on in RRMS patients. Chard et al. (57) confirmed and expanded on these results to conclude that the cortical gray matter of MS patients also showed decreased choline, NAA, glutamate, and glutamine. These changes were unrelated to white matter lesion load (31,78,106). The reduced Cho was interpreted as possibly representing both reduced cellular density and metabolic activity. The reduced NAA was felt to represent cell loss and/or metabolic dysfunction. The reduced glutamate and glutamine were also felt to represent neuronal metabolic dysfunction. Those researchers found a correlation between clinical impairment and cortical gray matter glutamate and glutamine, but not with NAA, and suggested that it is more closely associated with neuronal dysfunction than loss in clinically early RRMS. The pathology in deep gray structures may be different, as thalamic neurodegeneration has been demonstrated in MS patients with a decreased NAA that could be accounted for by neuronal loss alone (76,77).

COGNITIVE CHANGES AND FATIGUE IN MS

It is accepted that cognitive changes occur in MS, even early on in the disease. Although Cristodoulou et al. (107) found that central atrophy displayed the highest correlation with cognition, NAA ratios in the right hemisphere also correlated quite significantly. Recently, Gadea et al. (108) showed (using MRS) that axonal damage in the NAWM of the right locus coeruleus relates to selective attention impairment in the early stage of RRMS.

A strong relationship also has been demonstrated between left and right hemispheric cognitive function and lateralized concentrations of periventricular NAA (83). The Selective Reminding Test, a measure of verbal function and memory, correlated significantly with left hemispheric periventricular NAA. The Tower of Hanoi, a test of conceptual planning, correlated significantly with right hemispheric periventricular NAA.

Tartaglia et al. (109) found that diffuse, periventricular axonal injury is associated with increased fatigue in MS patients. Independent of EDSS, T2 lesion volume, age, and disease duration, the NAA/Cr ratio was significantly lower in the high-fatigue group as compared to the low-fatigue group. Moreover, a significant correlation was present between fatigue and the NAA/Cr ratio.

Foong et al. (110) found that patients who had more severe abnormalities in their NAA/Cr ratios performed significantly worse than the other patients on the more difficult levels of the spatial working memory test, despite similar frontal lesion load among the groups. The deficit in working memory performance in these patients would suggest that decreases in NAA density may reflect the presence of subtle pathological processes that also contribute to cognitive deficits.

FUNCTIONAL MRI

Functional MRI (fMRI) can be used to localize brain activation associated with cognitive, visual, auditory, motor, and sensory tasks. The most widely used method is based on contrast that is blood oxygenation level-dependent (BOLD). Localized brain activation leads to an increase in local synaptic activity that is associated with an increase in blood flow and oxygen consumption. Since blood flow increases in excess of oxygen consumption, the blood oxyhemoglobin:deoxyhemoglobin ratio increases. This causes a change in the T2 relaxation of water that results in an increase in signal intensity (111). fMRI has provided a window onto the functioning brain and allowed the discovery of a process once thought to be confined to the developing or young brain—plasticity or reorganization. Cortical plasticity or reorganization is an adaptive mechanism that refers to changes in the distribution of cortical function. This phenomenon may be important for understanding the poor correlation reported between EDSS and conventional MRI markers of disease burden, such as T1 and T2 lesion volumes (112). Expanding the area of neural tissues dedicated to a given functional area and recruiting additional support is a basic compensatory mechanism that allows normal performance to continue despite injury to parts of the functional system. Cortical reorganization of motor areas has been reported in many neurological diseases including stroke (113–115), brain tumors (116), and amyotrophic lateral sclerosis (117).

With the help of well-designed fMRI experiments, it is now appreciated that patients with MS display altered activation patterns as compared to normal subjects. Most interesting is the notion that altered, and not only increased, activation is implicated in this continued functionality. Changes in activation have been observed both within the normal circuitry associated with a given function and outside it (i.e., involving the recruitment of brain regions not normally associated with the function) (118). Moreover, fMRI experiments are confirming that patients with MS undergo significant cognitive changes.

CORTICAL REORGANIZATION

Functional MRI has been used to establish that functional reorganization occurs in patients with RRMS (119), SPMS (120), and PPMS

(121,122). Even patients with clinically isolated syndromes have been shown to display altered brain activation patterns (59).

Simple motor tasks are often used to assess functional reorganization. fMRI studies typically reveal a larger volume of activation both in the contralateral and ipsilateral motor areas. An early case report serves to illustrate the current perspective of compensation observed in MS patients (102). An RRMS patient with a very large demyelinating lesion in the left hemisphere and an associated right hemiplegia displayed a larger volume of activation both in the contralateral and ipsilateral motor areas at three and six weeks (Fig. 13-3). ^{1}H-MRS done on this patient revealed a decreased NAA initially, with subsequent partial recovery in the area of the left corticospinal tract in parallel with recovery of its associated functional impairment. Upon functional recovery, the patient's volume of activation had apparently normalized, but the NAA density remained low.

These dynamic changes suggest that unmasking of latent motor pathways provides an important adaptive mechanism in MS.

Lee et al. (123) used fMRI to show that changes in cortical activation patterns are directly related to relevant disease burden. In patients with MS, the increase in ipsilateral motor cortex activation was related to increased T2-lesion load in the contralateral hemisphere. In addition, the authors described a posterior shift in the center of activation of the sensorimotor cortex in the patients relative to controls. Reddy et al. (124) found a high correlation between the extent of reorganization of sensorimotor cortex activation during finger movement and decreases of NAA in voxels localized to the descending corticospinal tracts. Therefore, cortical reorganization appears to be an adaptive response to tissue injury.

In trying to differentiate between the effects related to disability as opposed to those related to disease burden, Reddy et al. (125), in an

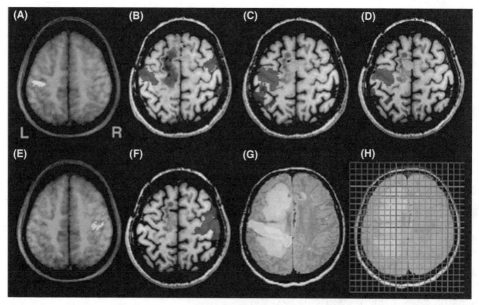

FIG. 13-3. Axial images for functional MRI motor activations for normal controls and the patient, and chosen areas of interest for MR spectroscopic imaging. "Hot metal" representation of the proportion of normal controls exhibiting activation in the motor cortex with right **(A)** or left **(E)** hand movements. Pixel brightness increases with frequency of activation at that location. **B-D,** Areas activated by the patient during movements of the impaired right hand at the first, second, and third fMRI examinations, respectively. **F,** Areas activated by the patient with movement of the unimpaired (left) hand. These did not change significantly during the study. Segmented activations: sensorimotor (red), supplementary motor (yellow), or other cortex (blue). **G,** The corticospinal tract mask used to select voxels of interest **(H)** for analysis of spectroscopy data.

elegant study, demonstrated that the effect of brain injury was distinct from that of disability. Their study involved three patient groups: one with no evidence of either substantial injury (normal NAA) or functional impairment (no disability); one with significant WM injury (low NAA) but no upper limb impairment (no disability); and one with a similar degree of tissue injury (low NAA) and substantial upper limb impairment (high disability). Comparing the two groups that differed in brain injury (NAA) but had similar functional abilities revealed significant activation increases in ipsilateral premotor cortex and the supplementary motor area bilaterally in the group with the greater brain injury. To assess whether disability itself can alter patterns of cortical activation associated with hand weakness, a comparison was made between patients with decreased NAA and either impaired or unimpaired hand function. This contrast demonstrated greater bilateral primary and secondary somatosensory cortex activation with greater limb disability. The authors concluded that the pattern of cerebral activity changes independently, both with increasing injury and with increasing disability. Furthermore, by having patients also do a passive task and noting that there was a significant correlation between the activation of the active and passive tasks, they were able to show that true brain reorganization occurs. A recent study by Rocca et al. (121) also demonstrated a strong relationship between patterns of brain activation change in MS patients and disability. These authors also noted that in some of the activated cortical areas there was a correlation between extent of fMRI activation changes and MRI lesion burden.

The mechanisms contributing to reorganization were explored by Mainero et al. (126), who found overexcitation of the ipsilateral hemisphere when paired-pulse transcranial magnetic stimulation (TMS) and single-dose 3,4 3,4-diaminopyridine (a potassium channel-blocking agent) were given. This provides support for the hypothesis that reorganization is associated with reduced inhibition from the contralateral motor cortex that results in disinhibition of the ipsilateral corticospinal tract.

Cortical motor reorganization has even been shown in patients who were very early in their disease course (127). During both right- and left-hand movement, these patients with previous right or left hemiparesis activated significantly greater cortical areas in both contralateral and ipsilateral cerebral hemispheres compared with controls. During right-hand movement, the MS patients displayed an altered pattern of activation in the ipsilateral sensorimotor cortex, lateral premotor cortex, inferior parietal lobule, insula, and contralateral inferior parietal lobule. The left hand also displayed an altered pattern of activation that was different from that seen in the right hand. Time since clinical onset was positively associated with extent of activation in ipsilateral motor areas during right-hand movement and with extent of activation in both ipsilateral and contralateral motor area during left-hand movements. The T1 lesion volume along the motor pathway was significantly associated with extent of activation in the contralateral motor areas during right-hand movement. Filippi et al. (128) also found increased and altered activation in CIS patients in areas of the brain not displaying damage clinically. The fact that the brain has a reserve capacity that can be recruited to compensate for focal injury may mask the accumulation of axonal loss and damage, at least early in the course of MS (129).

Most of the studies report altered activity of areas that have been recognized as playing a role in motor reorganization or compensation: increased contralateral primary sensorimotor cortex, secondary somatosensory cortex, and inferior frontal gyrus (112). The supplementary motor area is often implicated in functional reorganization, it is involved in movement programming and execution, and is responsible for modulating the activity of the primary sensorimotor cortex throughout its extensive connections with this area. The supplementary motor area is known to activate in healthy control when asked to do complex motor tasks (112).

COGNITIVE CHANGES IN MS

Most of the studies to evaluate functional reorganization in MS have focused on the motor system for convenience, but it has become apparent that all aspects of brain function may be capable of utilizing this mechanism of adaptation. Cognitive function has also been shown to display compensatory reorganization and, once again, this begins early in the disease course. Wishart et al. (118) showed that patients with mild RRMS asked to perform an n-back task (assesses working memory) showed shifts in brain activation patterns within and beyond typical components of working memory circuits. Their patients showed less activation than controls in prefrontal and parietal regions of working memory circuitry and greater activation in bilateral medial frontal, cingulate, parietal, bilateral middle temporal, and occipital regions. The patients' performance on the tasks was not statistically worse than that of controls. Staffen et al. (130) found an altered pattern of activation in MS patients with short duration of disease (less than three years) and a normal Paced Visual Serial Addition Task (test for concentration and attention) with patients displaying significant activation in left Brodmann's area (BA) 39, right prefrontal regions (BA 6, 8, 9) in contrast to controls who displayed significant activation in BA 32. A striking study of patients with CIS suggestive of MS revealed an altered pattern of activation for the Paced Auditory Serial Addition Task (PASAT). Compared with controls, these patients showed greater activation in right frontopolar cortex, bilateral lateral prefrontal cortices, and right cerebellum. They argue for compensatory cortical activation in regions involved in executive processing in patients (131).

Parry et al. (132) not only assessed activation differences between MS patients and controls performing a cognitive task, but also attempted to elucidate some of the physiology underlying these changes. They acquired fMRI data while subjects performed the Stroop Task, which tests selective attention or interference/inhibition. MS patients and age-matched controls activated distinct brain regions during the Stroop Task, despite similar performance. MS patients displayed greater activation primarily in the left middle frontal gyrus/left superior frontal sulcus and bilateral superior frontal gyrus (BA 8, 9, 10), whereas controls showed greater activation

in the right inferior frontal cortex (BA 95) and the right basal ganglia. The extent of differences in the pattern of brain activation in MS patients was correlated with total brain disease burden. The maximum signal change in the left medial frontal region correlated with the magnitude of the Stroop Effect and was thus felt to be relevant to the interference task. The authors propose that the increased activation observed in the patients in this region relates to the need for increased internal performance monitoring as the relative impairment of primary processing relevant to task performance worsens with increased disease burden. Similar responses are seen in controls doing cognitive tasks requiring the generation of an internal response, inhibition with selection of a response from among alternatives, or self-monitoring while maintaining multiple contingencies on-line (133–135). Rivastigmine (a cholinesterase inhibitor) led to the normalization of the brain activation pattern, thus implying that cholinergic modulation may be involved in compensatory/adaptive mechanisms. Unmasking of latent pathways and not structural reorganization may be the substrate for concentration (132).

Mainero et al. (136) also noted altered patterns of activation during a cognitive task. All their patients exhibited a greater extent of fMRI brain activation than healthy controls and recruited brain areas not normally activated for the performance of the PASAT and recall task. Patients with MS activated larger areas in the bilateral prefrontal and inferior parietal cortex, right temporal cortex, and additional foci in the supplementary motor area (SMA) and anterior cingulate of the right hemisphere. Prefrontal cortex activation tended to be more extensive and less lateralized in patients than in controls. Significantly greater brain activation also involved the bilateral middle and superior temporal cortex. Finally, additional foci were activated in the right lateral premotor area, left thalamus, and in both basal ganglia. Once again the interpretation suggested was that this represented a compensatory mechanism for reduction in the response efficiency of canonical task-related brain areas, allowing a normal performance despite the presence of neuronal injury. In support of this hypothesis, they found that brain overactivation was more significant among patients with MS whose performance matched that of healthy controls both in the PASAT and in the recall task. Conversely, patients who performed worse showed less-extensive brain activation. It is possible that the fMRI changes observed may, at least partially, reflect underlying neural disorganization or disinhibition associated with MS that is directly related to task performance. Support for this hypothesis comes from finding that the extent of activation in some cerebral areas increased with increasing lesion burden on conventional MRI.

Compensatory changes in brain activation also have been noted in the visual system. Rombouts et al. (137) showed that patients with unilateral optic neuritis activated a smaller volume of the visual cortex after stimulation of either the affected or the unaffected eye compared with healthy individuals. However, patients with good recovery from optic neuritis showed higher visual cortex activation than patients who had poor recovery or no recovery at all. A subsequent study of nine patients with previous optic neuritis confirmed these findings (138) and showed that patients with optic neuritis not only have a low activation of the primary visual cortex but also have a reduced fMRI signal change in this region, suggestive of an abnormality in synaptic input. Altered activation patterns also have been noted in visual tasks performed by patients recovering from optic neuritis (139). Compared with healthy volunteers, patients with a single episode of acute unilateral optic neuritis had extensive activations of the claustrum, lateral temporal and posterior parietal cortices, and the thalamus, in addition to activation of the primary visual cortex when the clinically affected eye was studied. Stimulation of the unaffected eye activated only the visual cortex and the right insula claustrum. The volume of extraoccipital activation in these patients was strongly related to the latency of the visual evoked potentials. The results from these cognitive fMRI studies are consistent with the notion that changes in brain activation help mitigate the effects of the diffuse neuronal injury present even at the first signs of MS.

FATIGUE

Fatigue is a common and distressing symptom of MS patients. There is growing evidence that fatigue in MS has a central nervous system component and is at least partially related to diffuse axonal injury. It has been demonstrated that fatigued and nonfatigued MS patients display different activation patterns (140). The nonfatigued MS patients displayed increased activation of ipsilateral cerebellar hemisphere, ipsilateral rolandic operculum, ipsilateral precuneus, contralateral thalamus, and contralateral middle frontal gyrus. Fatigued MS patients displayed greater activation of the contralateral cingulate motor area. In addition, Fatigue Severity Scale scores correlated with activity in the contralateral intraparietal sulcus, thalamus, and ipsilateral rolandic operculum. Fatigue in MS may be related to impaired interaction between functionally related cortical and subcortical areas. In an attempt to understand whether these altered activations were static or could be modulated by other cognitive or psychological phenomena, we investigated the effects of fatigue on this compensatory activity (141). We asked patients to perform a motor task, the PASAT, and then redo the motor task. We noted that patients changed and increased their pattern of activation after performing the fatiguing PASAT, but the controls did not. Although compensatory/adaptive cortical reorganization is advantageous for mitigating the effects of diffuse axonal injury, the price of increased activation may be fatigue.

SUMMARY

Multiple sclerosis is now recognized as more than simply a disease of inflammation and demyelination in the brain and spinal cord. Conventional MRI has been established as the most important paraclinical tool in the diagnostic assessment of patients with suspected MS, and in the monitoring of treatment efficacy in clinical trials, at least in relapsing disease. Magnetization-transfer, diffusion-weighted MRI, ^{1}H-MRS, and fMRI improve our ability to quantify the pathological changes in MS in vivo.

Although we have gained some insight into the disease and are starting to uncover some of the structural and physiological substrates for the disability that develops in MS patients, we are far from understanding what causes MS and how to prevent its progression. Imaging can be used as a tool to better understand the pathophysiology of MS and ultimately improve on the treatment of MS.

REFERENCES

1. McDonald WI, Compston A, Edan G, et al. Recommended diagnostic criteria for multiple sclerosis: guidelines from the International Panel on the diagnosis of multiple sclerosis. *Ann Neurol* 2001;50(1):121–127.
2. Miller DH, Albert PS, Barkhof F, et al. Guidelines for the use of magnetic resonance techniques in monitoring the treatment of multiple sclerosis. U.S. National MS Society Task Force. *Ann Neurol* 1996;39(1):6–16.
3. Stewart WA, Hall LD, Berry K, et al. Correlation between NMR scan and brain slice data in multiple sclerosis [letter]. *Lancet* 1984;2(8399):412.
4. O'Riordan JI, Thompson AJ, Kingsley DP, et al. The prognostic value of brain MRI in clinically isolated syndromes of the CNS. A 10-year follow-up. *Brain* 1998;121(Pt 3):495–503.
5. Jacobs LD, Cookfair DL, Rudick RA, et al. Intramuscular interferon beta-1a for disease progression in relapsing multiple sclerosis. The Multiple Sclerosis Collaborative Research Group (MSCRG) [See comments.] [Published erratum appears in *Ann Neurol* 1996;40(3):480.] *Ann Neurol* 1996;39(3):285–294.
6. Miller DH, Grossman RI, Reingold SC, et al. The role of magnetic resonance techniques in understanding and managing multiple sclerosis. *Brain* 1998;121(Pt 1):3–24.
7. Arnold DL, Matthews PM, Francis G, et al. Proton magnetic resonance spectroscopy of human brain in vivo in the evaluation of multiple sclerosis: assessment of the load of disease. *Magn Reson Med* 1990;14(1):154–159.
8. Arnold DL, Matthews PM, Francis GS, et al. Proton magnetic resonance spectroscopic imaging for metabolic characterization of demyelinating plaques. *Ann Neurol* 1992;31(3):235–241.
9. Matthews PM, Francis G, Antel J, et al. Proton magnetic resonance spectroscopy for metabolic characterization of plaques in multiple sclerosis. [Published erratum appears in *Neurology* 1991;41(11):1828.] *Neurology* 1991;41(8):1251–1256.
10. Richards TL. Proton MR spectroscopy in multiple sclerosis: value in establishing diagnosis, monitoring progression, and evaluating therapy. *Am J Roentgenol* 1991;157(5):1073–1078.
11. Trapp BD, Peterson J, Ransohoff RM, et al. Axonal transection in the lesions of multiple sclerosis [see comments]. *N Engl J Med* 1998;338(5):278–285.
12. Brenner RE, Munro PM, Williams SC, et al. The proton NMR spectrum in acute EAE: the significance of the change in the Cho:Cr ratio. *Magn Reson Med* 1993;29(6):737–745.
13. Simone IL, Tortorella C, Federico F, et al. Axonal damage in multiple sclerosis plaques: a combined magnetic resonance imaging and 1H-magnetic resonance spectroscopy study. *J Neurol Sci* 2001;182(2):143–150.
14. Davie CA, Hawkins CP, Barker GJ, et al. Serial proton magnetic resonance spectroscopy in acute multiple sclerosis lesions. *Brain* 1994;117(Pt 1):49–58.
15. De Stefano N, Matthews PM, Antel JP, et al. Chemical pathology of acute demyelinating lesions and its correlation with disability. *Ann Neurol* 1995;38(6):901–909.
16. Bitsch A, Bruhn H, Vougioukas V, et al. Inflammatory CNS demyelination: histopathologic correlation with in vivo quantitative proton MR spectroscopy. *Am J Neuroradiol* 1999;20(9):1619–1627.
17. Degaonkar MN, Khubchandhani M, Dhawan JK, et al. Sequential proton MRS study of brain metabolite changes monitored during a complete pathological cycle of demyelination and remyelination in a lysophosphatidyl choline (LPC)-induced experimental demyelinating lesion model. *NMR Biomed* 2002;15(4):293–300.
18. Narayana PA, Doyle TJ, Lai D, et al. Serial proton magnetic resonance spectroscopic imaging, contrast-enhanced magnetic resonance imaging, and quantitative lesion volumetry in multiple sclerosis. *Ann Neurol* 1998;43(1):56–71.
19. Tartaglia MC, Narayanan S, De Stefano N, et al. Choline is increased in pre-lesional normal appearing white matter in multiple sclerosis. *J Neurol* 2002;249(10):1382–1390.
20. Davies SE, Newcombe J, Williams SR, et al. High resolution proton NMR spectroscopy of multiple sclerosis lesions. *J Neurochem* 1995;64(2):742–748.
21. Husted CA, Goodin DS, Hugg JW, et al. Biochemical alterations in multiple sclerosis lesions and normal-appearing white matter detected by in vivo 31P and 1H spectroscopic imaging. *Ann Neurol* 1994;36(2):157–165.
22. Pan JW, Hetherington HP, Vaughan JT, et al. Evaluation of multiple sclerosis by 1H spectroscopic imaging at 4.1 T. *Magn Reson Med* 1996;36(1):72–77.
23. Rooney WD, Goodkin DE, Schuff N, et al. 1H MRSI of normal appearing white matter in multiple sclerosis. *Mult Scler* 1997;3(4):231–237.
24. Sarchielli P, Presciutti O, Pelliccioli GP, et al. Absolute quantification of brain metabolites by proton magnetic resonance spectroscopy in normal-appearing white matter of multiple sclerosis patients. *Brain* 1999;122(Pt 3):513–521.
25. van Walderveen MA, Barkhof F, Pouwels PJ, et al. Neuronal damage in T1-hypointense multiple sclerosis lesions demonstrated in vivo using proton magnetic resonance spectroscopy. *Ann Neurol* 1999;46(1):79–87.
26. Caramanos Z, Le Nezet P, Matos A, et al. MRI evidence for primary degeneration of myelin and axons in patients with multiple sclerosis. *Proceedings of the International Society for Magnetic Resonance in Medicine.* Twelfth Scientific Meeting, May, 2004, Kyoto, Japan.
27. Cucurella MG, Rovira A, Rio J, et al. Proton magnetic resonance spectroscopy in primary and secondary progressive multiple sclerosis. *NMR Biomed* 2000;13(2):57–63.

28. Helms G. Volume correction for edema in single-volume proton MR spectroscopy of contrast-enhancing multiple sclerosis lesions. *Magn Reson Med* 2001;46(2):256–263.

29. Helms G, Stawiarz L, Kivisakk P, et al. Regression analysis of metabolite concentrations estimated from localized proton MR spectra of active and chronic multiple sclerosis lesions. *Magn Reson Med* 2000; 43(1):102–110.

30. Kapeller P, Brex PA, Chard D, et al. Quantitative 1H MRS imaging 14 years after presenting with a clinically isolated syndrome suggestive of multiple sclerosis. *Mult Scler* 2002;8(3):207–210.

31. Kapeller P, McLean MA, Griffin CM, et al. Preliminary evidence for neuronal damage in cortical grey matter and normal appearing white matter in short duration relapsing-remitting multiple sclerosis: a quantitative MR spectroscopic imaging study. *J Neurol* 2001;248(2):131–138.

32. Mader I, Roser W, Kappos L, et al. Serial proton MR spectroscopy of contrast-enhancing multiple sclerosis plaques: absolute metabolic values over 2 years during a clinical pharmacological study. *Am J Neuroradiol* 2000;21(7):1220–1227.

33. Mader I, Seeger U, Weissert R, et al. Proton MR spectroscopy with metabolite-nulling reveals elevated macromolecules in acute multiple sclerosis. *Brain* 2001;124(Pt 5):953–961.

34. Sarchielli P, Presciutti O, Tarducci R, et al. 1H-MRS in patients with multiple sclerosis undergoing treatment with interferon beta-1a: results of a preliminary study. *J Neurol Neurosurg Psychiatry* 1998;64(2):204–212.

35. Schubert F, Seifert F, Elster C, et al. Serial 1H-MRS in relapsing-remitting multiple sclerosis: effects of interferon-beta therapy on absolute metabolite concentrations. *Magma* 2002;14(3):213–222.

36. Suhy J, Rooney WD, Goodkin DE, et al. 1H MRSI comparison of white matter and lesions in primary progressive and relapsing-remitting MS. *Mult Scler* 2000;6(3):148–155.

37. Clarke DD, Greenfield S, Dicker E, et al. A relationship of N-acetyl-L-aspartate biosynthesis to neuronal protein synthesis. *J Neurochem* 1975;24(3):479–485.

38. Patel TB, Clark JB. Synthesis of N-acetyl-L-aspartate by rat brain mitochondria and its involvement in mitochondrial/cytosolic carbon transport. *Biochem J* 1979;184(3):539–546.

39. Truckenmiller ME, Namboodiri MA, Brownstein MJ, et al. N-Acetylation of L-aspartate in the nervous system: differential distribution of a specific enzyme. *J Neurochem* 1985;45(5):1658–1662.

40. Birken DL, Oldendorf WH. N-acetyl-L-aspartic acid: a literature review of a compound prominent in 1H-NMR spectroscopic studies of brain. *Neurosci Biobehav Rev* 1989;13(1):23–31.

41. Moffett JR, Namboodiri MA, Cangro CB, et al. Immunohistochemical localization of N-acetylaspartate in rat brain. *Neuroreport* 1991;2(3):131–134.

42. Simmons ML, Frondoza CG, Coyle JT. Immunocytochemical localization of N-acetyl-aspartate with monoclonal antibodies. *Neuroscience* 1991;45(1):37–45.

43. Cangro CB, Namboodiri MA, Sklar LA, et al. Immunohistochemistry and biosynthesis of N-acetylaspartylglutamate in spinal sensory ganglia. *J Neurochem* 1987;49(5):1579–1588.

44. Lee JH, Arcinue E, Ross BD. Brief report: organic osmolytes in brain of an infant with hypernatremia. *N Engl J Med* 1994;331:439–442.

45. Bjartmar C, Battistuta J, Terada N, et al. N-acetylaspartate is an axon-specific marker of mature white matter in vivo: a biochemical and immunohistochemical study on the rat optic nerve. *Ann Neurol* 2002;51(1):51–58.

46. Arnold DL, Riess GT, Matthews PM, et al. Use of proton magnetic resonance spectroscopy for monitoring disease progression in multiple sclerosis. *Ann Neurol* 1994;36(1):76–82.

47. De Stefano N, Matthews PM, Arnold DL. Reversible decreases in N-acetylaspartate after acute brain injury. *Magn Reson Med* 1995;34(5):721–727.

48. Dautry C, Vaufrey F, Brouillet E, et al. Early N-acetylaspartate depletion is a marker of neuronal dysfunction in rats and primates chronically treated with the mitochondrial toxin 3-nitropropionic acid. *J Cereb Blood Flow Metab* 2000;20(5):789–799.

49. Matthews PM, Pioro E, Narayanan S, et al. Assessment of lesion pathology in multiple sclerosis using quantitative MRI morphometry and magnetic resonance spectroscopy. *Brain* 1996;119(Pt 3):715–722.

50. Posse S, Schuknecht B, Smith ME, et al. Short echo time proton MR spectroscopic imaging. *J Comput Assist Tomogr* 1993;17(1):1–14.

51. Fernando KT, McLean MA, Chard DT, et al. Elevated white matter myo-inositol in clinically isolated syndromes suggestive of multiple sclerosis. *Brain* 2004;127(Pt 6):1361–1369.

52. Waxman SG, Craner MJ, Black JA. Na(+) channel expression along axons in multiple sclerosis and its models. *Trends Pharmacol Sci* 2004;25(11): 584–591.

53. Moll C, Mourre C, Lazdunski M, et al. Increase of sodium channels in demyelinated lesions of multiple sclerosis. *Brain Res* 1991;556(2):311–316.

54. Youl BD, Turano G, Miller DH, et al. The pathophysiology of acute optic neuritis. An association of gadolinium leakage with clinical and electrophysiological deficits. *Brain* 1991;114 (Pt 6):2437–2450.

55. Kuhlmann T, Lingfeld G, Bitsch A, et al. Acute axonal damage in multiple sclerosis is most extensive in early disease stages and decreases over time. *Brain* 2002;125(Pt 10):2202–2212.

56. Fu L, Matthews PM, De Stefano N, et al. Imaging axonal damage of normal-appearing white matter in multiple sclerosis. *Brain* 1998;121(Pt 1):103–113.

57. Chard DT, Griffin CM, McLean MA, et al. Brain metabolite changes in cortical grey and normal-appearing white matter in clinically early relapsing-remitting multiple sclerosis. *Brain* 2002;125(Pt 10): 2342–2352.

58. De Stefano N, Narayanan S, Francis GS, et al. Evidence of axonal damage in the early stages of multiple sclerosis and its relevance to disability. *Arch Neurol* 2001;58(1):65–70.

59. Rocca MA, Mezzapesa DM, Falini A, et al. Evidence for axonal pathology and adaptive cortical reorganization in patients at presentation with clinically isolated syndromes suggestive of multiple sclerosis. *Neuroimage* 2003;18(4):847–855.

60. Evangelou N, Konz D, Esiri MM, et al. Regional axonal loss in the corpus callosum correlates with cerebral white matter lesion volume and distribution in multiple sclerosis. *Brain* 2000;123(Pt 9):1845–1849.

61. Bjartmar C, Trapp BD. Axonal and neuronal degeneration in multiple sclerosis: mechanisms and functional consequences. *Curr Opin Neurol* 2001;14(3):271–278.

62. Enzinger C, Ropele S, Strasser-Fuchs S, et al. Lower levels of *N*-acetylaspartate in multiple sclerosis patients with the apolipoprotein E epsilon4 allele. *Arch Neurol* 2003;60(1):65–70.

63. Fazekas F, Strasser-Fuchs S, Kollegger H, et al. Apolipoprotein E epsilon 4 is associated with rapid progression of multiple sclerosis. *Neurology* 2001;57(5):853–857.

64. Enzinger C, Ropele S, Smith S, et al. Accelerated evolution of brain atrophy and "black holes" in MS patients with APOE-epsilon 4. *Ann Neurol* 2004;55(4):563–569.

65. Charcot JM. Histologie de la sclerose en plaques. *Gaz Hosp* 1868;141:554–558.

66. Bjartmar C, Kidd G, Mork S, et al. Neurological disability correlates with spinal cord axonal loss and reduced *N*-acetyl aspartate in chronic multiple sclerosis patients. *Ann Neurol* 2000;48(6):893–901.

67. Evangelou N, Esiri MM, Smith S, et al. Quantitative pathological evidence for axonal loss in normal appearing white matter in multiple sclerosis. *Ann Neurol* 2000;47(3):391–395.

68. Trapp BD, Bo L, Mork S, et al. Pathogenesis of tissue injury in MS lesions. *J Neuroimmunol* 1999; 98(1):49–56.

69. Matthews PM, De Stefano N, Narayanan S, et al. Putting magnetic resonance spectroscopy studies in context: axonal damage and disability in multiple sclerosis. *Semin Neurol* 1998;18(3):327–336.

70. Arnold DL, Matthews PM. MRI in the diagnosis and management of multiple sclerosis. *Neurology* 2002;58(8)[Suppl 4]:S23–S31.

71. Lassmann H, Bruck W, Lucchinetti C. Heterogeneity of multiple sclerosis pathogenesis: implications for diagnosis and therapy. *Trends Mol Med* 2001;7(3):115–121.

72. Ferguson B, Matyszak MK, Esiri MM, et al. Axonal damage in acute multiple sclerosis lesions. *Brain* 1997;120(Pt 3):393–399.

73. Mews I, Bergmann M, Bunkowski S, et al. Oligodendrocyte and axon pathology in clinically silent multiple sclerosis lesions. *Mult Scler* 1998;4(2):55–62.

74. Lovas G, Szilagyi N, Majtenyi K, et al. Axonal changes in chronic demyelinated cervical spinal cord plaques. *Brain* 2000;123(Pt 2):308–317.

75. Evangelou N, Konz D, Esiri MM, et al. Size-selective neuronal changes in the anterior optic pathways suggest a differential susceptibility to injury in multiple sclerosis. *Brain* 2001;124(Pt 9):1813–1820.

76. Wylezinska M, Cifelli A, Jezzard P, et al. Thalamic neurodegeneration in relapsing-remitting multiple sclerosis. *Neurology* 2003;60(12):1949–1954.

77. Cifelli A, Arridge M, Jezzard P, et al. Thalamic neurodegeneration in multiple sclerosis. *Ann Neurol* 2002;52(5):650–653.

78. Sarchielli P, Presciutti O, Tarducci R, et al. Localized (1)H magnetic resonance spectroscopy in mainly cortical gray matter of patients with multiple sclerosis. *J Neurol* 2002;249(7):902–910.

79. De Stefano N, Narayanan S, Francis SJ, et al. Diffuse axonal and tissue injury in patients with multiple sclerosis with low cerebral lesion load and no disability. *Arch Neurol* 2002;59(10):1565–1571.

80. Bjartmar C, Kinkel RP, Kidd G, et al. Axonal loss in normal-appearing white matter in a patient with acute MS. *Neurology* 2001;57(7):1248–1252.

81. De Stefano N, Matthews PM, Fu L, et al. Axonal damage correlates with disability in patients with relapsing-remitting multiple sclerosis. Results of a longitudinal magnetic resonance spectroscopy study. *Brain* 1998;121(Pt 8):1469–477.

82. Lee MA, Blamire AM, Pendlebury S, et al. Axonal injury or loss in the internal capsule and motor impairment in multiple sclerosis. *Arch Neurol* 2000;57(1):65–70.

83. Pan JW, Krupp LB, Elkins LE, et al. Cognitive dysfunction lateralizes with NAA in multiple sclerosis. *Appl Neuropsychol* 2001;8(3):155–160.

84. Davie CA, Barker GJ, Webb S, et al. Persistent functional deficit in multiple sclerosis and autosomal dominant cerebellar ataxia is associated with axon loss. *Brain* 1995;118(Pt 6):1583–1592.

85. Ge Y, Gonen O, Inglese M, et al. Neuronal cell injury precedes brain atrophy in multiple sclerosis. *Neurology* 2004;62(4):624–627.

86. Falini A, Calabrese G, Filippi M, et al. Benign versus secondary-progressive multiple sclerosis: the potential role of proton MR spectroscopy in defining the nature of disability. *Am J Neuroradiol* 1998;19(2):223–229.

87. Molyneux PD, Filippi M, Barkhof F, et al. Correlations between monthly enhanced MRI lesion rate and changes in T2 lesion volume in multiple sclerosis. *Ann Neurol* 1998;43(3):332–339.

88. Kappos L, Moeri D, Radue EW, et al. Predictive value of gadolinium-enhanced magnetic resonance imaging for relapse rate and changes in disability or impairment in multiple sclerosis: a meta-analysis. Gadolinium MRI Meta-analysis Group. *Lancet* 1999;353(9157):964–969.

89. McFarland HF, Frank JA, Albert PS, et al. Using gadolinium-enhanced magnetic resonance imaging lesions to monitor disease activity in multiple sclerosis. *Ann Neurol* 1992;32(6):758–766.

90. Bagnato F, Jeffries N, Richert ND, et al. Evolution of T1 black holes in patients with multiple sclerosis imaged monthly for 4 years. *Brain* 2003;126(Pt 8): 1782–1789.

91. Bitsch A, Schuchardt J, Bunkowski S, et al. Acute axonal injury in multiple sclerosis. Correlation with demyelination and inflammation. *Brain* 2000;123(Pt 6):1174–1183.

92. Ganter P, Prince C, Esiri MM. Spinal cord axonal loss in multiple sclerosis: a post-mortem study. *Neuropathol Appl Neurobiol* 1999;25(6):459–467.

93. Simon JH, Kinkel RP, Jacobs L, et al. A Wallerian degeneration pattern in patients at risk for MS. *Neurology* 2000;54(5):1155–1160.

94. Barnett MH, Prineas JW. Relapsing and remitting multiple sclerosis: pathology of the newly forming lesion. *Ann Neurol* 2004;55(4):458–468.

95. Secondary Progressing Efficacy Clinical Trial of Recombinant Interferon-beta-1a in MS (SPECTRIMS) Study Group. Randomized controlled trial of interferon-beta-1a in secondary progressive MS: clinical results. *Neurology* 2001;56(11): 1496–1504.

96. Tourbah A, Stievenart JL, Gout O, et al. Localized proton magnetic resonance spectroscopy in relapsing remitting versus secondary progressive multiple sclerosis. *Neurology* 1999;53(5):1091–1097.

97. Filippi M, Bozzali M, Rovaris M, et al. Evidence for widespread axonal damage at the earliest clinical stage of multiple sclerosis. *Brain* 2003;126(Pt 2):433–437.

98. De Stefano N, Matthews PM, Filippi M, et al. Evidence of early cortical atrophy in MS: relevance to white matter changes and disability. *Neurology* 2003;60(7):1157–1162.

99. Peterson JW, Bo L, Mork S, et al. Transected neurites, apoptotic neurons, and reduced inflammation in cortical multiple sclerosis lesions. *Ann Neurol* 2001;50(3): 389–400.

100. De Stefano N, Narayanan S, Matthews PM, et al. In vivo evidence for axonal dysfunction remote from focal cerebral demyelination of the type seen in multiple sclerosis. *Brain* 1999;122(Pt 10):1933–1939.

101. Vion-Dury J, Nicoli F, Salvan AM, et al. Reversal of brain metabolic alterations with zidovudine detected by proton localised magnetic resonance spectroscopy. *Lancet* 1995;345(8941):60–61.

102. Reddy H, Narayanan S, Matthews PM, et al. Relating axonal injury to functional recovery in MS. *Neurology* 2000;54(1):236–239.

103. Brownell B, Hughes JT. The distribution of plaques in the cerebrum in multiple sclerosis. *J Neurol Neurosurg Psychiatry* 1962;25:315–320.

104. Kidd D, Barkhof F, McConnell R, et al. Cortical lesions in multiple sclerosis. *Brain* 1999;122(Pt 1):17–26.

105. Revesz T, Kidd D, Thompson AJ, et al. A comparison of the pathology of primary and secondary progressive multiple sclerosis. *Brain* 1994;117(Pt 4):759–765.

106. Sharma R, Narayana PA, Wolinsky JS. Grey matter abnormalities in multiple sclerosis: proton magnetic resonance spectroscopic imaging. *Mult Scler* 2001;7(4):221–226.

107. Christodoulou C, Krupp LB, Liang Z, et al. Cognitive performance and MR markers of cerebral injury in cognitively impaired MS patients. *Neurology* 2003; 60(11):1793–1798.

108. Gadea M, Martinez-Bisbal MC, Marti-Bonmati L, et al. Spectroscopic axonal damage of the right locus coeruleus relates to selective attention impairment in early stage relapsing-remitting multiple sclerosis. *Brain* 2004;127(Pt 1):89–98.

109. Tartaglia M, Narayanan S, Francis SJ, et al. The relationship between diffuse axonal damage and fatigue in MS. *Arch Neurol* 2004;61(2):201-207.

110. Foong J, Rozewicz L, Davie CA, et al. Correlates of executive function in multiple sclerosis: the use of magnetic resonance spectroscopy as an index of focal pathology. *J Neuropsychiatry Clin Neurosci* 1999;11(1):45–50.

111. Ogawa S, Menon RS, Tank DW, et al. Functional brain mapping by blood oxygenation level-dependent contrast magnetic resonance imaging. A comparison of signal characteristics with a biophysical model. *Biophys J* 1993;64(3):803–812.

112. Filippi M, Rocca MA, Mezzapesa DM, et al. Simple and complex movement-associated functional MRI changes in patients at presentation with clinically isolated syndromes suggestive of multiple sclerosis. *Human Brain Mapping* 2004;21(2):108–117.

113. Chollet F, DiPiero V, Wise RJ, et al. The functional anatomy of motor recovery after stroke in humans: a study with positron emission tomography. *Ann Neurol* 1991;29(1):63–71.

114. Weiller C, Chollet F, Friston KJ, et al. Functional reorganization of the brain in recovery from striatocapsular infarction in man. *Ann Neurol* 1992;31(5):463–472.

115. Cao Y, D'Olhaberriague L, Vikingstad EM, et al. Pilot study of functional MRI to assess cerebral activation of motor function after poststroke hemiparesis. *Stroke* 1998;29(1):112–122.

116. Yoshiura T, Hasuo K, Mihara F, et al. Increased activity of the ipsilateral motor cortex during a hand motor task in patients with brain tumor and paresis. *Am J Neuroradiol* 1997;18(5):865–869.

117. Kew JJ, Goldstein LH, Leigh PN, et al. The relationship between abnormalities of cognitive function and cerebral activation in amyotrophic lateral sclerosis. A neuropsychological and positron emission tomography study. *Brain* 1993;116(Pt 6):1399–1423.

118. Wishart HA, Saykin AJ, McDonald BC, et al. Brain activation patterns associated with working memory in relapsing-remitting MS. *Neurology* 2004;62(2):234–238.

119. Rocca MA, Falini A, Colombo B, et al. Adaptive functional changes in the cerebral cortex of patients with nondisabling multiple sclerosis correlate with the extent of brain structural damage. *Ann Neurol* 2002;51(3):330–339.

120. Rocca MA, Gavazzi C, Mezzapesa DM, et al. A functional magnetic resonance imaging study of patients with secondary progressive multiple sclerosis. *NeuroImage* 2003;19(4):1770–1777.

121. Rocca MA, Matthews PM, Caputo D, et al. Evidence for widespread movement-associated functional MRI changes in patients with PPMS. *Neurology* 2002;58(6):866–872.

122. Filippi M, Rocca MA, Falini A, et al. Correlations between structural CNS damage and functional MRI changes in primary progressive MS. *NeuroImage* 2002;15(3):537–546.

123. Lee M, Reddy H, Johansen-Berg H, et al. The motor cortex shows adaptive functional changes to brain injury from multiple sclerosis. *Ann Neurol* 2000;47(5): 606–613.

124. Reddy H, Narayanan S, Arnoutelis R, et al. Evidence for adaptive functional changes in the cerebral cortex with axonal injury from multiple sclerosis. *Brain* 2000;123(Pt 11):2314–2320.

125. Reddy H, Narayanan S, Woolrich M, et al. Functional brain reorganization for hand movement in patients with multiple sclerosis: defining distinct effects of injury and disability. *Brain* 2002;125 (Pt 12):2646–2657.

126. Mainero C, Inghilleri M, Pantano P, et al. Enhanced brain motor activity in patients with MS after a single dose of 3,4-diaminopyridine. *Neurology* 2004;62(11): 2044–2050.

127. Pantano P, Iannetti GD, Caramia F, et al. Cortical motor reorganization after a single clinical attack of multiple sclerosis. *Brain* 2002;125(Pt 7):1607–1615.

128. Filippi M, Rocca MA, Mezzapesa DM, et al. A functional MRI study of cortical activations associated with object manipulation in patients with MS. *NeuroImage* 2004;21(3):1147–1154.

129. Cifelli A, Matthews PM. Cerebral plasticity in multiple sclerosis: insights from fMRI. *Mult Scler* 2002;8(3):193–199.

130. Staffen W, Mair A, Zauner H, et al. Cognitive function and fMRI in patients with multiple sclerosis: evidence

for compensatory cortical activation during an attention task. *Brain* 2002;125(Pt 6):1275–1282.

131. Audoin B, Ibarrola D, Ranjeva JP, et al. Compensatory cortical activation observed by fMRI during a cognitive task at the earliest stage of MS. *Human Brain Mapping* 2003;20(2):51–58.

132. Parry AM, Scott RB, Palace J, et al. Potentially adaptive functional changes in cognitive processing for patients with multiple sclerosis and their acute modulation by rivastigmine. *Brain* 2003;126(Pt 12):2750–2760.

133. Schlosser R, Hutchinson M, Joseffer S, et al. Functional magnetic resonance imaging of human brain activity in a verbal fluency task. *J Neurol Neurosurg Psychiatry* 1998;64(4):492–498.

134. Ruff CC, Woodward TS, Laurens KR, et al. The role of the anterior cingulate cortex in conflict processing: evidence from reverse Stroop interference. *NeuroImage* 2001;14(5):1150–1158.

135. Leung HC, Skudlarski P, Gatenby JC, et al. An event-related functional MRI study of the Stroop color word interference task. *Cereb Cortex* 2000;10(6):552–560.

136. Mainero C, Caramia F, Pozzilli C, et al. fMRI evidence of brain reorganization during attention and memory tasks in multiple sclerosis. *NeuroImage* 2004;21(3):858–867.

137. Rombouts SA, Lazeron RH, Scheltens P, et al. Visual activation patterns in patients with optic neuritis: an fMRI pilot study. *Neurology* 1998;50(6):1896–1899.

138. Langkilde AR, Frederiksen JL, Rostrup E, et al. Functional MRI of the visual cortex and visual testing in patients with previous optic neuritis. *Eur J Neurol* 2002;9(3):277–286.

139. Werring DJ, Bullmore ET, Toosy AT, et al. Recovery from optic neuritis is associated with a change in the distribution of cerebral response to visual stimulation: a functional magnetic resonance imaging study. *J Neurol Neurosurg Psychiatry* 2000;68(4): 441–449.

140. Filippi M, Rocca MA, Colombo B, et al. Functional magnetic resonance imaging correlates of fatigue in multiple sclerosis. *NeuroImage* 2002;15(3): 559–567.

141. Tartaglia M, Narayanan S, Arnold DL. Fatigue in MS is Associated with an Altered Pattern and Increased Volume of Cerebral Activation. Supplement to *Neurology* 2004;7(62):A294.

14

The Use of MRI as an Outcome Measure in Clinical Trials

David K.B. Li,[1] Mary Jane Li,[1] Anthony Traboulsee,[2] Guojun Zhao,[3] Andrew Riddehough,[4] and Donald Paty[3]

[1]Department of Radiology, University of British Columbia Hospital, Vancouver, British Columbia, Canada; [2]Division of Neurology, Department of Medicine, University of British Columbia Hospital, Vancouver, British Columbia, Canada; [3]Division of Neurology, Department of Medicine, University of British Columbia, Vancouver, British Columbia, Canada; [4]MS/MRI Research Group, Department of Medicine, University of British Columbia, Vancouver, British Columbia, Canada.

INTRODUCTION

Magnetic resonance imaging (MRI) has had a major impact on our understanding of multiple sclerosis (MS). The sensitivity of MRI in detecting clinically asymptomatic lesions is an important aid in the earlier diagnosis of the disease (1). Despite a limited correlation with clinical findings, MRI has been used in most recent clinical trials to support the primary clinical outcome measures by providing an index of the underlying pathological process.

Rationale for Using MRI as an Outcome Measure

Biomarkers

The generic term *biomarker* has been applied to any detectable biologic parameter, whether biochemical, genetic, histological, anatomic, physi-ologic, functional, or metabolic (2) that can be objectively measured and evaluated as an indicator of normal biological processes, pathogenic processes, or pharmacologic responses to a therapeutic intervention (3). In recent years, there has been great interest within regulatory agencies such as the U.S. Food and Drug Administration (FDA), as well as amongst clinical scientists and industry researchers, regarding the evaluation and the use of biomarkers, including imaging biomarkers such as MRI, as surrogate endpoints to help speed the development of safe and effective medical therapies (4). To be an effective and reliable surrogate measure (2,5), the biomarker should be biologically plausible, closely linked, and able to reflect the severity of disease. The detection and/or measurement of the biomarker must be accurate, reproducible, and feasible over time, and measured changes should be closely related to success or failure of the therapeutic effect of the product being evaluated. It must improve rapidly with treatment and correlate with true clinical outcomes (6).

Difficulties with Clinical Measures

Performing clinical trials in MS is difficult. The clinical course of the disease is highly unpredictable, characterized by relapses and remissions with a variable time course for the development of irreversible disability, which often extends over decades (longer than the duration of most clinical trials). Clinical assessments are intrinsically subjective and are prone to bias despite the use of so-called blinded evaluators and attempts to standardize clinical methods. The reproducibility of the assessment of the clinical scales commonly used for quantifying disability [e.g., the Expanded Disability Status Scale (EDSS)] have been improved by training but still suffer from limited sensitivity in capturing all of the patient's functional disability and the true progression of disability. Nevertheless, the definitive evaluation of new treatments must be based on clinically meaningful outcomes such as relapse rate or progression in disability (as measured by sustained increase in EDSS). The reference standard for clinical trials in MS is the prospective, randomized, controlled, double-blind study, which is expensive. Such studies require large patient numbers (usually several hundreds) and follow-up of at least two to three years—a long time frame for a clinical trial, but relatively short compared to the usual course of MS, which evolves over several decades. While placebo-controlled trials were previously standard for MS trials, the presence of several clinically accepted treatments for MS in recent years has necessitated the design of trials employing an active treatment control arm. When there are differences in the route of administration and side effects of the treatment and active control, the ability to achieve blinding for the patient and the evaluator may be compromised. Clearly, having surrogate outcome measures would be useful in allowing for faster, smaller, and less-costly trials with the added value of using endpoints that have the potential for increased objectivity, ease of blinding, and sensitivity to detect earlier and smaller changes.

Surrogacy

The issue of surrogacy is extremely complex and the criteria for a validated surrogate are stringent (7). First, the surrogate must predict future clinical disease. Second, the effect of treatment on clinical disease must be explained by the treatment on the surrogate, with the effect of the treatment on the clinical outcomes being through mechanisms working through the surrogate. Third, for a surrogate not restricted to use with a single, specific treatment, there must be evidence that different treatments also affect the surrogate in the same and predictable manner. As will be discussed below, studies to date that have examined the relationship between MRI measures of disease and clinical status have shown, at best, only a modest relationship. Therefore, currently there is insufficient evidence to support any single or combination of MRI measures as a fully validated surrogate (8,9). Yet, because the changes on MRI likely reflect various aspects of the underlying pathology of MS, there may be a rationale for the use of MRI measures as an unvalidated surrogate. An unvalidated surrogate is defined as a surrogate that is reasonably likely to predict the clinical benefit of interest, but for which there is insufficient evidence to establish that such an effect does, in fact, result in the desired clinical outcome. In fact, Section 506(b) of the FDA Modernization Act permits the regulatory agency to approve a drug product "...upon determination that the product has an effect on a clinical endpoint or on a surrogate endpoint that is reasonably likely to predict clinical benefit." (10) This was the case in 1993 when interferon β-1b (IFN β-1b, Betaseron; Berlex Laboratories, Montville, NJ) became the first biotechnology product to be licensed under the FDA's accelerated approval regulations. The news release stated: "The accelerated approval policy allows for expediting the approval of therapies that provide a meaningful therapeutic benefit for patients with serious illnesses. It enables FDA to approve therapies as soon as their safety and effectiveness can be reasonably established. Accelerated approval relies solely or in part on 'surrogate endpoints'—laboratory measurements or physical signs—for evidence of effectiveness. The surrogate endpoints are believed to be likely to predict benefit for the patient. The surrogate endpoints used in licensing Interferon β-1b were data from magnetic resonance imaging (MRI) scans of the brain, which supported the clinical findings. MRI scans indicated that after 2 years of treatment, there was a greater increase in the multiple sclerosis lesion areas in the brains of patients treated with a placebo than in patients treated with Interferon β-1b. The trials did not demonstrate, however, that the findings on MRI scans correlate with slower disease progression. The accelerated approval regulations require the product's manufacturer, Chiron Corp. of Emeryville, Calif., to conduct postmarketing studies to investigate the effectiveness of Interferon β-1b in slowing or preventing progression of multiple sclerosis." (11) Ever since that landmark decision, MRI outcome measures have been used in many MS clinical trials to provide objective, supportive evidence for the clinical endpoints by providing measurements of some aspects of the pathological status of the disease, and not necessarily to substitute for the clinical measures.

MRI Outcome Measures

For therapeutic trials of MS, reduction in relapse rate and slowing the progression of irreversible disability (as measured by sustained change in EDSS) are the most commonly used, meaningful, and relevant clinical endpoints. In a sense, these clinical endpoints can be thought of as markers for the underlying pathological process. The pathological basis for relapses is believed to be acute inflammatory lesions occurring in clinically eloquent locations resulting in blood–brain barrier disruption, edema, myelin breakdown, and a degree of axonal destruction (12,13). The main pathological substrate for progression of disability is undoubtedly chronic axonal loss. However, the underlying pathogenic mechanisms and the relationship to the focal inflammatory demyelinating lesions are

still not fully understood. MRI biomarkers or outcome measures that reflect and predict these important clinical outcomes and the underlying pathological changes thus fall into the following two categories:

1. MRI biomarkers of relapses and acute inflammation
2. MRI biomarkers of progressive disability and chronic axonal loss

Table 14-1 is a summary of the current literature regarding the use of MRI outcomes in clinical trials.

MRI Biomarkers of Relapses and Acute Inflammation

Lesion Activity Measures

Acute inflammatory lesions on MRI include *enhancing* lesions on gadolinium (Gd)-enhanced, T1-weighted (T1) scans and/or *new*, *enlarging*, and *recurrent* lesions on PD/T2-weighted (T2) scans. To avoid double-counting lesions that both enhance and are morphologically active, some studies perform an additional analysis to link these simultaneously active lesions in order to determine a *combined, unique, active* lesion count (14–18). MRI disease activity can be expressed in terms of (a) numbers or rates of active lesions; (b) the percentage of scans that are active per patient (percent active scans); and (c) percentage of patients with active scans (percent active patients). The activity may be assessed on frequent, serial MRI performed most commonly every 4 to 6 weeks or with less-frequent annual or semiannual intervals. The frequent serial scans may be obtained throughout the duration of the study (e.g., 6 months to 3 years) or only at the beginning (e.g., initial 6 to 9 months) or at the beginning and end (e.g., initial and last 6 months) of the study. The number of active lesions identified (particularly enhancing lesions) can be increased [e.g., through magnetization transfer (19,20), more frequent (such as weekly) scanning (21), higher doses (double or triple) of gadolinium (19,20,22), delayed scanning (20), or thinner slices (23)]. However, these

Text continues on p. 214.

TABLE 14-1 *Summary of clinical trials using MRI as an outcome measure*

Reference	Treatment and study design	No. of Patients/ type MS	Study duration	Number of MRI scans	MRI Outcomes					Clinical result
					Activity	Volume	Black holes	Other	MRI result	
Ristori G, et al. 1999 (156)	**BCG** Vaccine 0.1 ml intracut.; single CO	12 RR	12 mos	Baseline, monthly: 6 run-in, 6 post	T1: pre/post Gd, T2				+	±
Paolillo A, et al. 2003 (121)	Sub-study	12 RR	Further 18 mos	3 further scans q 6 mos			% evolving		+	na
	Cladribine									
Beutler E, et al.1996 (45)	Cladribine 2.8 mg IV total/yr; then to crossover group: 1.4 mg IV total/yr; PC; DB; CO	51 CP	24 mos	Baseline, q 6 mos		T1Gd, T2			+	+
Rice GP, et al. 2000 (68)	Cladribine 0.7 mg/kg or 2.1 mg/kg or placebo, in 8 monthly courses; DB; PC; PG	159 PP, SP	12 mos (with 6 yr extension)	Baseline, mos 6, 12, 18, 24	T1Gd, T2	T1, T2			+	–
Filippi M, et al. 2000 (104)	Sub-study	159 PP, SP	12 mos (with 6 yr extension)	Baseline, mos 6, 12		Brain			–	na
Gobbini MI, et al. 1999 (157)	**Cyclophosphamide** 1g/m2 IV monthly; OL	5; refractory RR	28 mos (mean)	Monthly (mean 28)	T1Gd	T2			+	na
Kappos, et al. 1988 (70,158)	Cyclosporine 5 mg/kg/day vs. AZA 2.5 mg/kg/day; DB; CS	75 RR, RP, CP	24–32 mos	Baseline, end of 24–32 mos		T2		Qualitative rating	–	–
MS Study Group 1990; Zhao GJ, et al. 1997 (69)	**Cyclosporine** at blood level 300–500 ηg/ml; DB; PC	163 CP	24 mos	Baseline, 24 mos	T2	T2			–	–
	Glatiramer Acetate									
Mancardi GL, et al. 1998 (159)	Glatiramer Acetate 20 mg SC daily; BT	10 RR	21–40	Monthly	T1Gd	T1, T2			+	na
Ge Y, et al. 2000 (160)	Glatiramer Acetate 20 mg SC daily; PC	27 RR	24 mos	Baseline, annual	T1Gd, T2	T1, T2, brain			T1+ brain – vol+ T2	na
Comi G, et al. 2001 (36)	Glatiramer Acetate 20 mg SC daily; DB; PC	239 RR	9 mos	Monthly	T1Gd, T2	T1, T2	Volume		+	relapse

Reference	Design / Treatment	N	Duration	Frequency	MRI sequence	Measure	Result	Clinical
Filippi M, et al. 2001 (122)	Sub-study	239 RR	9 mos	Monthly	T1Gd, T2	Number, % evolving	+	na
Rovaris M, et al. 2001 (105)	Subgroup, OL; CO	227 RR	18 mos	q 3 mos	T1Gd, Brain T2	Volume	−	na
Wolinsky JS, et al. 2002 (161)	Subgroup, OL; CO	224 RR	18 mos	q 3 mos			+	relapse +
Sormani MP, et al. 2004 (107)	Sub-study; OL; CO	207 RR	18 mos	Baseline, 9, 18 mos	Brain		+	na
Wolinsky JS, et al. 2001 (162)	Glatiramer Acetate 20 mg SC daily; OL	135 RR	2447 ± 61 d after randomiz.	1	T1Gd, T2; T1, T2	Number, volume	±	na
Rovaris M, et al. 2002 (163)	Glatiramer Acetate 20 mg SC daily; BT; SX	20 RR	12+ mos	Monthly: 5× pre and 5× aft 3 mos trment	T1Gd diff doses, T2; T1	% CSF volume, Z4 composite	+	na
IFN a								
Kastrukoff LF, et al. 1990 (164)	Human lymphoblastoid IFN 5miu SC daily × 6 mos; DB; PC	100 CP	24	Baseline, 6, 24 mos	T2		−	−
Durelli L, et al. 1994 (165)	rIFN α-2a 9 miu IM alt days; DB; PC	20 RR	6 mos	Baseline, 6 mos	T2		+	+
Myhr KM, et al. 1999 (166)	IFN a-2a 4.5 miu or 9 miu SC 3×/week for 6 mos; DB; PC	97 RR	12 mos	Baseline, monthly × 6, 12 mos	T1Gd, T2		+	−
IFN β-1a								
Pozzilli C, et al. 1996 (167)	IFN β-1a 3 miu or 9 miu SC 3×/week for 6 mos; BT	68 RR	12 mos	Monthly: baseline × 6, treatmt × 6	T1Gd, T2; T1, T2		+	relapse
Paolillo A, et al. 1999 (168)	Sub-study	68 RR	24 mos	Baseline: 2 scans treatmt: 2 scans 1 yr follow up: 1	T1Gd, T2	Evolving	+	na
Gasperini C, et al. 1999 (117)	Sub-study	67 RR	Further 6 mos	Baseline, monthly		Volume	+	na
Gasperini C, et al. 2002 (98)	Subgroup	52 RR	24 mos	Baseline, monthly × 9, 12, 24 mos	T2, brain	Volume	T2+ bl holes ± brain vol −	na
Jacobs LD, et al. 1996; Simon JH, et al. 1998 (169,170)	IFN β-1a 6 miu IM weekly; DB; PC	301 RR	24 mos	Baseline, 12, 24 mos	T1Gd, T2; T1, T2		+	+

(continued)

TABLE 14-1 *Summary of clinical trials using MRI as an outcome measure* **Continued**

Reference	Treatment and Study Design	No. of Patients/ Type MS	Study Duration	Number of MRI Scans	MRI Outcomes Activity	Volume	Black Holes	Other	MRI Result	Clinical Result
Rudick RA, et al. 1999 (96)	Sub-study	140 RR	24 mos	Baseline, 12, 24 mos		Brain			2nd yr only +	na
Simon JH, et al. 2000 (119)	Sub-study	160 RR	24 mos	Baseline, 12, 24 mos			Volume		–	na
PRISMS Study Gr 1998 (171)	IFN β-1a 6 miu or 12 miu SC 3×/wk; DB; PC	560 RR	24 mos	Baseline, q 6 mos	T2	T2			+	+
Li DKB, et al. 1999 (14)	Subgroup	205 RR	24 mos	Baseline ×2, monthly ×9	T1Gd, T2, CUA				+	na
Sarchielli P, et al. 1998 (172)	IFN β-1a 6 miu (30 mcg) IM weekly	5 treated, 5 untreated, 6 healthy controls; RR	6 mos	Baseline, 1, 3, 6 mos	T1Gd	T2 qualitative		MRS	T1 Gd/T2: – Cho: +	–
OWIMS Study Gr 1999 (17)	IFN β-1a 22 mcg or 44 mcg SC once weekly; DB; PC	293 RR	12 mos	Baseline, q 4 wks × 6, wk 48	T1Gd, T2, CUA	T2			+	–
Kita M, et al. 2000 (152)	IFN β-1a 6 miu IM weekly; BT	8	20 mos	Monthly	T1Gd			Lesion MTR	+	na
Li DKB, et al. 2001 (16)	IFN β-1a 22 mcg or 44 mcg SC 3×/week; DB; PC	618 SP	36 mos	Baseline, q 6 mos; plus subgroup: monthly ×11	all: T2, subgroup: T1Gd, T2, CUA	All: T2			+	±
Comi G, et al. 2001 (173)	IFN β-1a 22 mcg SC weekly; DB; PC	308 1st episode neurol. Dysfn.	24 mos	Baseline, 12, 24 mos	T1Gd, T2	T2			+	+
CHAMPS Study Group 2001 (174)	IFN β-1a 30 mcg IM weekly, PC	192 optic neuritis	36 mos	Baseline, 6, 12, 18 mos	T1Gd, T2	T2			+	+
Clanet M, et al. 2002 (175)	IFN β-1a 30 mcg vs. 60 mcg IM weekly; DB; PG; DC	802 RR	36 mos	Baseline,12, 24, 36 mos	T1Gd, T2	T2	Volume		no diff. except T2 at 36 mos	no diff.

Reference	Treatment	N / type	Duration	Schedule	MRI	MRI region	Measure	Results
Cohen JA, et al. 2002 (176)	IFN β-1a 60 mcg 60 mcg IM weekly; DB; PC	436 SP	24 mos	Baseline, 12, 24 mos	T1Gd, T2			+; +; (MSFC)
Panitch H, et al. 2002 (EVIDENCE) (18)	IFN β-1a: Rebif 44 mcg SC 3×/wk vs. Avonex 30 mcg IM weekly; C; CS	677 RR	48 wks	Baseline, q 4 wks up to 24th; 48th.	T1Gd, T2, CUA			favors Rebif; favors Rebif
Leary SM, et al. 2003 (101)	IFN β-1a 30 mcg or 60 mcg IM weekly; PC	50 PP	24 mos	Baseline, 6, 12, 24 mos	T1, T2,	T1, T2 spinal cord, brain, ventricle		±; —
Lin X, et al. 2003 (90)	IFN β-1a 22 mcg or 44 mcg SC 3×/wk, as per PRISMS and SPECTRIMS protocol	20 RR, 18 SP, 31 healthy	48 mos	Baseline, 6, 12, 18, 48 mos		Spinal cord		—; na
Parry A, et al. 2003 (138)	IFN β-1a –9 pts: 22 mcg SC 3×/wk; 1 pt: 6 miu IM weekly; 1 pt: 8 miu SC alt days	11 active RR	12 mos	Baseline, 3, 6, 12 mos	T2	T2	MRS, T2 water relaxation	NAA/Cr – relapse; lesion vol +; T2 relaxn + EDSS; relapse +
Polman C, et al. 2003 (177)	Oral IFN β-1a 0.06 or 0.6 or 6 miu alt days up to 6 mos; DB; PC	194 RR	6 mos	Baseline, monthly	T1Gd	T1, T2		—; —
IFN β-1b								
IFNB Multiple Sclerosis Study Group 1993, 1995 (178)	IFN β-1b 1.6 miu or 8 miu SC alt days; DB; PC	372 RR	24–36 mos (up to 60)	Baseline, and annual (4)	T2	T2		+; relapse +
Paty DW, et al. 1993 (179)	Subgroup	52 RR	24 mos	17 (q 6 wks)	T2	T2		+; na
Zhao GJ, et al. 2000 (180)	Sub-study	342 RR	60 mos	Annual	T2	T2		+; na
Stone LA, et al. 1997 (46)	IFN β-1b 8 miu SC alt. days; BT	29 RR	6 mos	Baseline, monthly × 6	T1Gd			+; na
Richert ND, et al. 1998 (181)	Subgroup	8 pts, 4 healthy controls; RR	12 mos	Monthly, (total 11)	T1Gd		Whole-brain MTR	MTR –; MRI +; na
European Study Gr on IFN β-1b in SPMS 1998 (182)	IFN β-1b 8 miu SC alt. days; DB; PC	718 SP	24 mos	Annual × 3	T1Gd, T2	T2		+; +
Miller DH, et al. 1999 (67)	Subgroup	125 SP	24 mos	Monthly 0–6, 18–24 mos	T1Gd, T2	T2		+; na
Barkhof F, et al. 2001 (118)	Subgroup	95 SP	36 mos	Baseline, q 6 mos		T2	Volume, Number, % evolving	+; number +; na
Brex PA, et al. 2001 (125)	Sub-study	125 SP	24 mos	Baseline, mos 1–6, 19–24		T2		+ evolving –; na

(continued)

TABLE 14-1 *Summary of clinical trials using MRI as an outcome measure* **Continued**

Reference	Treatment and Study Design	No. of Patients/ Type MS	Study Duration	Number of MRI Scans	MRI Outcomes Activity	Volume	Black Holes	Other	MRI Result	Clinical Result
Inglese M, et al. 2003 (154)	Subgroup	75 SP	75 at 12 mos 54 at 24 mos 47 at 36 mos	Baseline, 12, 24, 36 mos				Whole-brain MTR	−	na
Narayanan S, et al. 2001 (139)	IFN β-1b 8 miu SC alt. days	10 (+ 6 untreated controls); RR	12 mos	All: baseline, 12 mos (8 pts: 1 more at 6 mos)		T2		Multivoxel MRS	100 + lesion vol −	+
Richert ND, et al. 2001 (153)	IFN β-1b 8 miu SC alt. Days; BT	4 RR	Baseline 15 mos, treatmt 16 mos (mean)	Monthly	T1Gd	T1		Lesion MTR	MTR + MRI +	na
Durelli L, et al. 2002 (INCOMIN) (183)	IFN β-1b 250 mcg SC alt days vs. IFN β-1a 30 mcg IM weekly; CS	188 RR	24 mos	Baseline, q 12 mos	T2	T2			favors INFβ-1b	Favors INFβ-1b
Teksam M, et al. 2000 (184)	**Immunoglobulin** IgG 0.4 mg/kg/day IV ×5 days, then monthly ×9; DB; PC	13 RR	9+ mos	Baseline, 3, 6 mos	T2	T2			+	na
Milligan NM, et al. 1994 (185)	Methylprednisolone 0.5 g IV day 6–10, then day 20: **Isoprinosine** 3 g oral daily; DB; PC	52 RR, SP, PP	24 mos	Day 2, day 16, 24 mos	T2				−	−
Lenercept MS Study Gr 1999 (186)	**Lenercept** (sTNFR-IgG p55) 10,50, or 100 mg IV q 4 wks ×6; DB; PC	168 RR	48 wks	Baseline, then q 4 wks up to 24 wks	T1Gd, T2	T2			−	−
Karussis DM, et al. 1996 (187)	**Linomide** Linomide 2.5 mg oral daily; DB; PC	30 SP	6 mos	Baseline, monthly ×6	% pts with activity				+	+

Reference	Treatment	Patients	Duration	MRI schedule	MRI sequence	MRI measure		MRI outcome	Clinical outcome
Tan IL, et al. 2000 (188)	Linomide 2.5 or 5 mg oral daily; PC	413 RR, SP	3 mos (d/c due to CV events)	Baseline, 3 mos	T1Gd	T1		+	na
Wolinsky JS, et al. 2000 (189)	Linomide 1.0,2.5 or 7.5 mg oral daily; PC	718 RR, SP	d/c due to cardiac toxicity	Baseline, q 3 mos	T1Gd	T1, T2, brain	#, volume / MRI composite	+	na
Lugaresi A, et al. 2001 (190)	Methotrexate 7.5 mg/wk (oral)	20 CP	23 mos	Baseline, ann	T1Gd		not specified	–	–
Oliveri RL, et al. 1998 (191)	Methylprednisolone 0.5g/day or 2.0 g/day IV for 5 days; DB; DC	31 RR in relapse	2 mos	Baseline, day 7, 15, 30, 60	T1Gd brain + spinal cord			higher dose +	higher dose +
Zivadinov R, et al. 2001 (103)	Methylprednisolone 1g/day IV ×5 days q 4 mos for 3 yrs, then q 6 mos for 2 yrs; SB; C; Ph.II	88 RR	5 yrs	Baseline, 5 yrs	T2, brain	T2, brain	volume	brain vol + bl. hole +	EDSS +
Metz LM, et al. 2004 (41)	Minocycline 100 mg oral twice daily ×6 mos; BT	10 RR	9 mos	Baseline, q 4 wks	T1Gd			+	–
Millefiorini E, et al. 1997 (192)	Mitoxantrone 8 mg/m2/month IV for 1 yr; PC	51 RR	24 mos	Baseline, 12, 24 mos	T2			–	±
van de Wyngaert FA, et al. 2001 (193)	Mitoxantrone 12 mg/m2 IV or Methylprednisolone 1 g IV: 13 infusions /32 mos; DB; CS	49 relapsing SP	32 mos	Q 6 mos	T1Gd			mitoxantrone +	mitoxantrone +
Miller DH, et al. 2003 (39)	Natalizumab 3 mg/kg or 6 mg/kg IV q 28 days ×6 mos; DB; PC	213; RR, relapsing SP	12 mos	Baseline, monthly 0–6; 9, 12 mos	T1Gd, T2	T1		+	+
Dalton CM, et al. 2004 (123)	Subgroup	78; RR, relapsing SP	12 mos	Baseline, 0, 6, 12 mos	T1Gd		Number, % evolving	+	na
Vollmer T, et al. 2004 (40)	Simvastatin 80 mg oral daily ×6 mos; OL; SA	30 RR	9 mos	Baseline ×3, trment ×3	T1Gd	T1, T2, brain		+	–
Combination Therapy Sorensen PS, et al. 1996 (194)	Plasma exchange q1 wk ×4, q2wk ×10; AZA 2 mg/kg; SB; CO	11 SP	9+ mos	Baseline, q 3 wks	T1Gd	T2		–	na

(continued)

TABLE 14-1 Summary of clinical trials using MRI as an outcome measure **Continued**

Reference	Treatment and Study Design	No. of Patients/Type MS	Study Duration	Number of MRI Scans	MRI Outcomes			MRI Result	Clinical Result
					Activity	Black VolumeHoles	Other		
Edan G, et al. 1997 (195)	**Mitoxantrone** 20 mg IV and **Methylprednisolone** 1g IV monthly × 6, vs. Methylprednisolone alone	42 RR, SP	6 mos	Monthly: baseline × 3, treatment × 6	T1Gd, T2			combin +	combin +
Patti F, et al. 2001 (71)	**IFN β-1a** 6 pts-6 miu IM weekly, 4 pts-8 miu SC alt days; **Cyclophosphamide** 500 mg-1500 mg/m2 IV/month for 12 mos, then @14, 16, 18mos	10 rapidly transitional MS	18 mos	Baseline, early phase, end of study	T2	T2		+	+
Puri BK, et al. 2001 (196)	**Lofepramine** 70 mg bid and **L-phenylalanine** 500 mg bid oral; **Vit. B12** 1 mg IM/wk; PC	15 MS patients +7 healthy	6 mos	Baseline, 6 mos	T1, T2	Ventricle		+	−
Fernandez O, et al. 2002 (197)	**IFN β-1b** 8 miu SC alt days and **AZA** oral 50 mg tid; NC	8; SP (> 2 relapses on IFN alone)	24 mos	Baseline, 12, 24 mos	T1, T2	T2		−	−
Markovic-Plese S, et al. 2003 (198)	**IFN β-1b** 8 miu SC alt days, and **AZA** titrated to 2 mg/kg/day oral; OL; SA	6 refractory RR	Varied (median 15 mos)	Monthly	T1Gd	T2		±	±
Lus G, et al. 2004 (199)	**IFN β-1a** 6 miu SC alt days and **AZA** oral 50–250 mg daily	23 RR not resp to mono ther.	24 mos	Baseline, and after 2 yrs	T1Gd, T2		Number new	+	+
Wiles CM, et al. 1994 (200)	**Miscellaneous** **Total lymphoid irradiation**; DB; PC	27 SP, PP	24+ mos	Baseline, q 6 mos	T2			±	−
van Oosten BW, et al. 1997 (42)	**Monoclonal anti-CD4 antibody cM-T412** 50 mg IV, monthly × 6 mos; DB; PC	71 RR, SP	18 mos	Baseline, monthly to 9 mos, 12, 18 mos	T1 Gd, T2			−	−

Reference	Treatment	Patients	Follow-up	MRI timing	MRI measures	Analysis	MRI outcome	Clinical outcome
Bowen JD, et al. 1998 (201)	Hu23F2G one dose (anti-CD11/CD18 monoclonal antibody) 0.01 to 4.0 mg/kg IV; Phase I; dose escal.; NC.	24 PP, SP	30 days	Baseline, day 10		Qualitative only	–	na
Paolillo A, et al. 1999 (75)	Monoclonal antibody Campath 1H 20 mg IV daily for 5 days; BT	25 treated, 4 untreated SP	18 mos	Monthly: 3 run-in; mos 1–6, mos 12–18	T1Gd; T1, T2, brain, spinal cord	Volume	T1Gd + brain vol – spinal cord – T1/T2 lesion volume –	EDSS –
Goodkin DE, et al. 2000 (202)	DR2:MBP84–102 (AG248)-Human leukocyte antigen with myelin basic protein. Dose escal.: 0.6, 2.0, 6.0, 20, 60, 105, 150 mcg/kg IV × 3 alt days; PC; DB; Phase 1	33 SP	12 wks observation after 1st IV	4 (2 pre-, 2 posttreatment)	T1Gd, T2		–	–
Skurkovich S, et al. 2001 (203)	Antibodies to IFN γ or TNF a; DB; PC; PG	45 SP	12 mos	Baseline, 6 mos	T1Gd, T2		(IFN γ)+	(IFN γ) +
Mancardi GL, et al. 2001 (204)	Autologous hematopoietic stem cell transplantation	10; rapidly evolving SP	Median follow-up 15 mos	Monthly: 3× pre, 6× post, then q 3 mos	T1Gd (triple dose), T2		+	na
Saiz A, et al. 2001 2004 (205 206)	Autologous hematopoietic stem cell transplantation	14; severe SP/RR	36 mos	Baseline, 1, 3, 6, 12; then q 6 mos	T1Gd; T2, ventricle width, callosum area	Number	+	+
Frank JA, et al. 2002 (43)	rhIGF-1 (recombinant Insulin-like growth factor) 50 mg SC bid for 24 wks; OL; CO	7 SP	48 wks	Monthly (6× before, 6× after treatmt)	T1Gd; T1, spinal cord	Volume; MTR, MRS	–	–

AZA, Azathioprine; BT, baseline vs. treatment; C, controlled; Cho, Choline; CO, cross-over; CP, chronic progressive; CS, comparative study; CUA, combined unique active; DB, double-blind; EDSS, Expanded Disability Status Scale; Gd, Gadolinium; DC, dose comparison; IFN, Interferon; Ins, Inositol; MRS, magnetic resonance spectroscopy; MSFC, MS functional composite; MTR, magnetization transfer ratio; na, not applicable; NAA:Cr, N-acetyl aspartate:creatinine ratio; NAWM, normal-appearing white matter; NC, noncontrolled; OL, open label; PC, placebo-controlled; PG, parallel group; PP, primary progressive; RP, relapsing-progressive; RR, relapsing-remitting; SA, single arm; SB, single-blind; SP, secondary progressive; SX, single crossover; +, positive treatment effect; –, negative treatment effect.

additional strategies are seldom used because of the limited impact on sample size requirements, as the increased sensitivity for activity is accompanied by a cost of increased variability of lesion numbers between patients. Although fewer numbers of active lesions are generally identified on the PD/T2 scans than on the Gd-T1-enhanced scans, and although their identification may be more difficult and tedious (requiring careful and laborious comparison of sequential studies), in some cases T2 activity appears better able to detect a treatment effect. For example, in the PRISMS (Prevention of Relapses and Disability by Interferon β-1a Subcutaneously in Multiple Sclerosis Study Group) IFN β-1a trial, a dose difference was observed, with a lower number of new T2 lesions favoring the high-dose group, but not for the number of new Gd-T1-enhancing lesions (14). This increased sensitivity is probably due to the lower standard deviation of the number of T2 active lesions compared with Gd-T1-enhanced lesions. One other advantage of T2 activity analysis is the ability to provide a running count of activity, especially when the scanning interval is prolonged (e.g., every 6 to 12 months). Because Gd enhancement is transient [with 80% of lesions enhancing 4 weeks or less (21,24,25)], it only offers a snapshot of current inflammatory activity. Once formed, however, T2 lesions will persist. Although the occasional small, new T2 lesion may disappear (more common when older scanners and thicker slices were used), most new T2 lesions will, after their initial appearance, gradually decrease in size over the next 4 to 8 weeks, leaving a smaller, residual T2 abnormality (26) that can be identified with careful review of sequential images as evidence of lesion activity.

As Table 14-1 indicates, Gd-enhancing lesions and active T2 lesions have been the most frequently used MRI outcome measures in clinical trials. These measures are highly sensitive in detecting asymptomatic disease activity, occurring 5 to 10 times more frequently than clinical relapses (27–34) in relapsing-remitting MS (RRMS) and secondary progressive MS (SPMS). However, because their long-term relationship with progression and disability is still uncertain, the current recommendation (35) is that they be used only as secondary outcome measures in definitive, Phase III trials. The results from trials of different therapies (including campath-1H, cladribine, glatiramer acetate (GA), various interferon (IFN) β, mitoxantrone, and natalizumab) have consistently demonstrated an effect of treatment in reducing the frequency of relapses as well as the number of MRI active lesions, although the magnitude of the effects may vary. Refer to Table 14-1 for a summary of these results. For instance, patients treated with GA had 29% fewer total enhancing lesions over nine months compared to placebo patients, paralleling the 33% reduction in relapse rate (36). On the other hand, high doses of IFN β-1a and β-1b, while reducing the relapse rate to a similar degree, decreased the number of MRI active lesions by 70% or more (14,37). Generally speaking, there have been no trials with a positive clinical outcome in the absence of an MRI effect. The reverse is not true; an effect on MRI measures can be seen in the absence of a clinical effect. Most commonly, this has been attributed to increased sensitivity of the MRI activity and a lack of power with the clinical ones. However, MRI results contradicting clinical outcomes may be difficult or impossible to interpret.

It is now generally accepted that if the aim of a new therapy is to prevent relapses, new Gd-enhancing and T2 lesions can be considered an appropriate surrogate outcome measure of relapses (9). This is, in fact, what the Task Force on Use of MRI in MS Clinical Trials of the U.S. National MS Society recommended in 1996 (35). For exploratory (Phase I and II) and dose-finding studies of new agents, whose mechanism of action might be through suppression of gadolinium enhancement and new T2 lesion activity, MRI activity outcomes can be recommended as the primary measure of treatment efficacy. Failure to demonstrate a reduction in lesion activity halts further development, avoiding the time, cost, and risks of a large Phase III trial. However, if the trial was positive, there would still be the need for a definitive Phase III study in a larger cohort to evaluate for clinical efficacy, persistence of effect, and drug safety.

Recent examples of positive trials where the primary endpoint was the number of new brain lesions on monthly, Gd-enhanced MRI is the humanized monoclonal antibody against alpha4 integrin, natalizumab (38,39), oral simvastatin treatment (40), and minocycline (41). Examples of negative trials include the monoclonal anti-CD4 antibody cM-T412 (42), recombinant insulin-like growth factor-1 (43), and the altered peptide ligand myelin basic protein peptide (amino acids 83–99) (44).

For hypothesis-testing Phase I and II studies, a number of different trial designs have been used. These include (a) randomized parallel groups without crossover (42); (b) randomized parallel groups with washout and crossover (45); and (c) open-label crossover (baseline versus treatment) (43,46). The latter design, proposed by McFarland et al. (47), commonly involves serial MRI performed at two- to six-week intervals for periods of three to six months (baseline phase) to obtain information on each patient's natural history (based on the number of Gd-enhancing lesions) followed by serial MRI and clinical examinations at the same scanning interval and over the same duration while they undergo treatment (treatment phase). The patient can be carefully observed for safety and his or her response to the treatment and valuable pharmacokinetic information can be obtained. The main advantage is that, because the patient serves as his or her own control, only a small sample size is required. For a 50% reduction in lesion frequency, with a six-month baseline and six-month treatment phase, only 10 to 15 patients are required, compared to 2×40 patients to show a 60% reduction in new, enhancing lesions over six months for a parallel placebo-controlled design (47–49); this can be performed in a single institution (50). The disadvantages are that there is no placebo group to serve as a control; there is insufficient power to provide any clinical outcome data; and there is uncertainty because subjects are typically enrolled on the basis of their disease activity on baseline MRI scans, and the reduction in activity between the baseline and treatment phase may simply be due to a regression to the mean rather than treatment efficacy.

In addition to its use as a measure of treatment efficacy, MRI lesion activity measures have also been used in exploratory Phase I and II trials as a measure of safety. Because MRI measures of disease activity can be up to 10 times more sensitive than the frequency of clinical relapses (27–29,34,51), they may serve as an early warning of potential toxicity of a new agent. For example, in a Phase I study with the monoclonal antitumor necrosis factor (TNF) antibody cA2,2, treated patients showed transient increase in the number of Gd-enhanced lesions and increased cerebrospinal fluid (CSF) leukocyte counts and immunoglobulin indices, in the absence of any clinical neurologic changes (52). This suggested that the treatment caused immune activation and an increase in disease activity. Yet, in the double-blind, placebo-controlled Phase II trial of lenercept (a recombinant TNF receptor p55 immunoglobulin fusion protein), no significant group differences were detected on the MRI activity measures, whereas significantly increased exacerbations were experienced by the lenercept-treated patients compared with placebo patients, with the exacerbations also occurring earlier. Currently, no formal stopping rules based on MRI activity measures have been formulated. The National Institutes of Health (NIH) group, using data from their longitudinal natural history studies, have developed a set of guidelines for following individual patients enrolled in open-label, baseline-versus-treatment trials (48): If the number of Gd-enhanced lesions during any given month of therapy exceeds the mean enhancing lesion frequency found during the baseline period by six standard deviations plus 15 new enhancing lesions, then they recommend stopping the treatment in an individual patient.

Gadolinium-Enhanced T1 Lesion Volume

In addition to the number of enhancing lesions, the volume of Gd-enhancing lesions has also been used as an outcome measure. The intensity and size of the enhancing lesion, and hence the area/volume to be quantitatively measured, depend on the local concentration of gadolinium, which is determined by its intravascular concentration (itself dependent on the injected dose and renal excretion), the degree of blood–brain barrier permeability, the size of the leakage space (53), and the delay following injection. The enhancing pattern can also change; peripheral, ring-like enhancement often becomes more homogeneous and nodular 10 to 15 minutes later (54), and deciding what should be included in the quantification can sometimes be difficult. Generally, however, the added time and cost for quantifying the enhancing lesion volume is unnecessary because of the very high positive correlation between the number of enhancing lesions and the enhancing lesion volume (55,56).

T2 Lesion Volume

Total brain T2 lesion volume or lesion load, which is a snapshot in time of the T2 burden of disease (BOD), is determined by measuring (using various manual, semiautomatic, and fully automatic segmentation methods) the area of the MRI lesions on each slice of the PD/T2 scans and then summing the area slice by slice to obtain a total lesion area. Total lesion volume or BOD is then calculated by multiplying the area by the thickness of the slices. To detect changes on sequential follow-up scans with reliability, care in repositioning of the subjects is important (35,57,58). Operator training (59) and postprocessing measurement strategies that employ volumetric display, registration, reconstruction, reformation, and reorientation of slices all help to reduce interscan differences and improve precision and reproducibility (60–65). However, the gains of such improvements need to be balanced against the time and effort required, since the main source of variability in measuring BOD is the biologic (i.e., interpatient) variability that far exceeds the variability between different quantifying methods (66).

Although an important limitation of the hyperintense T2 MS lesions is their pathologic heterogeneity, with different aspects of the histopathological features of MS (including inflammation, edema, demyelination, axonal loss, gliosis, and remyelination) all appearing similarly hyperintense, patients in the placebo arm of clinical trials have consistently demonstrated a progressive increase in BOD compared to baseline over time (14,36,37,67,68). It is the net accumulation of new and enlarging lesions over time and the chronic enlargement of more diffuse lesions (which may not be as visually obvious) that results in an increase in total BOD. This consistent behavior of the placebo group provides an internal validation of the accuracy of the quantifying methodology. Whereas month-to-month fluctuations in BOD can occur because of changes in disease activity (as well as from inaccuracies and variations of the quantitative methods), the progressive increase in BOD occurs not only with the placebo groups but also with those treated groups in trials with negative clinical and MRI results (15,69,70). In contrast, in trials with positive effect on clinical relapses and MRI lesion activity, there have been significant reductions in BOD for the treated groups (14,36,37,67,68,71), which probably reflects the reduction in inflammatory changes from new activity by the treatment. For example, in an RRMS trial of IFN β-1a, the BOD of the high-dose treated group remained at about the same level over the subsequent 2 years of the trial following a dramatic, initial 6-month reduction. This suggested that there was not only a reduction in acute activity, but also no further net increase in the more chronic changes of demyelination and gliosis from 6 to 24 months (14). In fact, annual BOD quantification is an efficient measure of ongoing disease activity because of the significant correlation between change in lesion load over annual and more frequent (monthly) gadolinium-enhancing activity and relapse rate (72).

While the relationship between T2 BOD, Gd-enhancing, and new T2 lesions and relapses seems clear, MRI lesion activity and burden correlate poorly, if at all, with the progression of disability (8,73). In separate clinical trials of SPMS, treatment with Campath-1H (74,75), cladribine (68), and IFN β (16,76) all reduced MRI lesion activity and relapses but did not affect the progression of disability as measured by EDSS. One exception was in patients at initial presentation with isolated syndromes suggestive of multiple sclerosis: the increases in total T2 BOD in the first five years did moderately correlate with the degree of long-term disability, more so than for increases in later years (77). Therefore, apart from the early years of relapsing-remitting MS, new lesions and changes in T2 BOD are not reliable in predicting future disability and cannot be considered as a surrogate for that clinical outcome. The findings from clinical trials showing continued clinical progression despite suppression of clinical and MRI inflammatory activity have led to the suggestion that different pathogenic mechanisms may be involved in the development of relapses and persistent disability, particularly later in the disease course.

MRI Biomarkers of Progressive Disability and Chronic Axonal Loss

Brain and Spinal Cord Volume (Atrophy)

Findings on cross-sectional and longitudinal studies have consistently shown reduced brain and spinal cord volume or area in patients with multiple sclerosis, even in the earliest phases of the disease. Such changes are generally greater with increasing disease duration and with PPMS and SPMS than RRMS patients, although the rate of change can be quite variable between subjects (78–90). For the brain, a variety of regional (e.g., corpus callosum, brainstem, central 4 slice brain) and whole-brain measurements have been used. These have ranged from indirect measures (such as linear measurements of third ventricular width) to more direct and sensitive three-dimensional volumetric data acquisition with registration employing semiautomated and automated segmentation analysis algorithms and normalization (91–93). For the spinal cord, measurement of the cross-sectional upper cervical cord area (at C2–C3) has been the most robust (94,95).

While axonal loss is undoubtedly a major factor in volume loss and the reason for the intense interest in the measure as a biomarker of progressive disability, it is not the sole cause. Loss of myelin from demyelination and failure to remyelinate, as well as glial proliferation or loss, gliosis, inflammation, edema, and tissue water content can also affect brain and spinal cord volume measurements. Therefore, it is important not to equate volume loss with tissue loss and atrophy in all cases. The correlations with clinical disability and changes in disability are, at best, only moderate for brain volumes (Spearman rank correlation coefficient $r = 0.3$ to 0.4) (87,96), and somewhat better for spinal cord measures ($r = 0.3$ to 0.7) (94,95). While a greater degree of volume loss has been seen in patients with clinical worsening (97,98), this has not been invariable (99), even with the spinal cord (94). Another confounding factor is the volumetric fluctuations attributable to inflammation. It is probable that anti-inflammatory therapies such as high-dose corticosteroids (100) and interferon (101) may reduce brain volume as a result of changes in tissue water content, without there having been axonal loss.

A significant treatment effect on brain volume reduction has been reported for patients with early RRMS only in a two-year trial of IFN β-1a (102) (in the second year) and in a five-year study of long-term corticosteroid therapy (103). In most other clinical trials of RRMS and SPMS [including cladribine (104), Campath 1H (75), glatiramer acetate (105), IFN β-1a (98) and IFN β-1b (106)], none of these treatments had an effect on reducing brain volume loss, despite significant effects on clinical and MRI outcomes of disease activity. Failure to find a significant treatment benefit might be the result of the relatively short durations of the trials, which may not be adequate to reveal beneficial effects in such a chronic disease. In one case, the use of a different quantitative method with lower measurement errors permitted a treatment effect of glatiramer acetate to be detected (107). More likely, these results suggest that treatments effective in reducing MS-related inflammation are unable to do so with the same efficacy on brain atrophy, concordant with their limited effects on progressive disability (108).

"Black Holes" (T1 Hypointense Lesions)

T1 hypointense lesions or so-called black holes (BHs) are defined as areas on a conventional spin echo, T1-weighted image that are hypointense compared with surrounding normal-appearing white matter, accompanied by a hyperintense area on the PD/T2 image. BHs usually begin as regions of enhancement on Gd-enhanced T1 images appearing hypointense on the precontrast images (acute BHs). Some of these acute BHs are reversible, gradually resolving over subsequent months with resolution of edema and remyelination; others, however, evolve into persistent and stable T1 hypointensities (109,110). It is these chronic BHs that have been histopathologically linked with matrix destruction, axonal loss, and increase in extracellular fluid (111,112), and a better correlation with disability as measured by EDSS, than T2 BOD (113–115).

Changes in T1 hypointense lesion load have been monitored in several recent trials. Because of the very strong correlation ($r = 0.8$) between T2 BOD and T1 hypointense lesion load (116), the monitoring of T1 hypointense lesion load provides little additional information compared to T2 BOD (117,118). In fact, in two trials [the MSCRG trial of IFN β-1a (119) and the European/Canadian trial of glatiramer acetate (36)], the effect on T1 hypointense lesion load was not significant, despite definite treatment effects on T2 BOD. One explanation could have been that a smaller patient cohort was studied, which was the case for the former but not the latter. Another possible reason might have been the greater interobserver variability in delineating and quantifying the T1 hypointense lesion load (120). One exception was the randomized, controlled, 5-year, single-blind, Phase II clinical trial of intravenous methylprednisolone (IVMP). RRMS patients on long-term, pulsed IVMP had a reduced mean change in T1 black hole volume, reduced mean change in brain parenchymal volume, and less EDSS score worsening compared to patients receiving IVMP only for relapses, while there was no significant difference between treatment arms in the change in T2 volume or annual relapse rate (103).

A measure that is proving useful as a possible biomarker of recovery and repair is the proportion of Gd-enhancing lesions that evolve (after at least 6 months of follow-up) into chronic BHs. A treatment effect has been demonstrated

for Bacille-Calmette-Guerin vaccination (121), glatiramer acetate (122), natalizumab (123), and IFN β-1a (124), but not for IFN β-1b (125).

Magnetic Resonance Spectroscopy (MRS)

N-acetyl aspartate (NAA) is the main metabolite with the largest peak (occurring at 2.0 ppm) on the water-suppressed proton MR spectrum of the human brain. Because it is found largely in the mitochondria of neurons and their processes, measurement of NAA is a potential biomarker of axonal pathology (126). Decreases in NAA can be the result of axonal loss (127), as well as potentially reversible axonal metabolic dysfunction (128,129). In MS, decreases in NAA occur both in lesions and in normal-appearing white matter (NAWM); the loss in NAWM has the strongest correlation with disability (130–137). Despite the obvious promise of NAA as an outcome measure, it has had limited applications in clinical trials. The reasons are mainly technical, including low signal-to-noise, modest reproducibility, different approaches to quantification (ratio versus absolute concentrations), and restricted coverage (6). A single, large voxel (approximately 70 to 160 cc) centered on the corpus callosum and adjacent white matter, has been the most commonly used technique (138,139). More recently, a method to measure whole-brain NAA has been developed (140,141). However, a study by Pelletier et al.(142) showed that metabolite ratios from a central brain region-of-interest (ROI) were statistically equivalent and highly correlated with those obtained from much larger volume of supratentorial brain.

There have been two small, single-center studies of RRMS patients treated with IFN β. Results have been conflicting. In one study of 10 treated patients, the NAA:Cr ratio showed an increase of 5.5% 12 months after the start of treatment, significantly higher than in a group of six untreated patients selected to have a similar range of EDSS scores and baseline NAA:Cr (139). In another study of 16 patients, treatment was associated with a reduction in relapse rate and stabilization of T2 BOD, but the NAA:Cr ratio (which was reduced over 16% compared to healthy controls) continued to decrease over the period of observation (mean = 6.2%, p = 0.02) (138). In a pilot study of recombinant insulin-like growth factor-1 in seven patients, no significant difference was seen between 24-week baseline and 24-week treatment periods for any clinical or MRI measures of activity (43). Proton MRS using a multislice, multivoxel sequences also failed to demonstrate any difference in any metabolite ratio for 10 regions-of-interest in gray matter, NAWM, and MS lesions.

Magnetization Transfer

Magnetization transfer (MT) makes use of the equilibrium that occurs between protons associated with free water (which is MRI-visible) and protons associated with macromolecules or bound protons (normally MRI-invisible) (143,144). The MT ratio is a measure of the reduction in the signal intensity of the free protons as a result of the effect of an off-resonance saturation pulse on the bound proton pool. There is a reduction in MTR when the numbers of bound protons are decreased. Animal models (145–147) have indicated that this predominantly reflects demyelination and axonal loss, but pathological correlations in human tissues are limited. It is likely that a significant reduction in MTR occurs with any damage to the macromolecular structure, whether inflammatory, demyelinating, or axonal. MTR can also be affected to a lesser degree by edema.

There have been two general approaches to the use of MT in the study of MS: global assessment of MTR expressed as a whole-brain histogram (148–151), and assessment of MTR changes within individual lesions (110). However, the number of studies that have used MT measures as an outcome measure have been extremely limited. There have been two small, single-center studies (eight patients and four patients, respectively) that have shown that treatment with IFN β-1a (152) and treatment with IFN β-1b and intravenous methylprednisolone (153) favorably improves the recovery of MTR values in Gd-enhancing lesions. In the negative cross-over pilot study (seven patients) of recombinant insulin-like growth factor-1, there was no difference in any of the whole-brain MTR histogram measures between baseline and treatment periods (43). The first parallel-group, placebo-controlled study on the effect of IFN β-1b in SPMS using whole-brain MT histogram analysis over a three-year period in 82 patients from five centers also failed to show a treatment effect on MT measures, despite a beneficial effect on clinical progression, relapse rate, and MRI activity measures (154). Nevertheless, the results were concordant with a similar lack of efficacy with respect to brain volume measures, as discussed above (106). The study did serve to highlight challenges of standardizing MT acquisition across multiple centers and over time. Recently, specific guidelines for implementing MT imaging as part of a large, multicenter clinical trial have been published in anticipation that MT would be incorporated into future new trials (155).

Other Quantitative Measures

Other quantitative measures that have been studied in MS, such as T1 and T2 relaxation measurements and diffusion tensor imaging, have not yet been applied within the rigors of a clinical trial.

SUMMARY

Because the changes on MRI likely reflect various aspects of the underlying pathology of multiple sclerosis, MRI outcome measures have become an important component of most MS clinical trials, providing objective, supportive evidence for the clinical endpoints. Although there is currently insufficient evidence to support any single or combination of MRI measures as a fully validated surrogate, it is now generally accepted that if the aim of a new therapy is to prevent relapses, new Gd-enhancing and T2 lesions can be considered an appropriate surrogate outcome measure of relapses, and MRI activity outcomes can be recommended as the primary measure of treatment efficacy.

REFERENCES

1. McDonald WI, Compston A, Edan G, et al. Recommended diagnostic criteria for multiple sclerosis: guidelines from the International Panel on the diagnosis of multiple sclerosis. *Ann Neurol* 2001;50:121–127.
2. Smith JJ, Sorensen AG, Thrall JH. Biomarkers in imaging: realizing radiology's future. *Radiology* 2003;227:633–638.
3. Biomarkers Definitions Working Group. Biomarkers and surrogate endpoints: preferred definitions and conceptual framework. *Clin Pharmacol Ther* 2001;69:89–95.
4. Bloom JC, Dean RA. *Biomarkers in Clinical Drug Development.* New York: Marcel Dekker, 2003.
5. Brody AS. Scoring systems for ct in cystic fibrosis: who cares? *Radiology* 2004;231:296–298.
6. McFarland HF, Barkhof F, Antel J, et al. The role of MRI as a surrogate outcome measure in multiple sclerosis. *Mult Scler* 2002;8:40–51.
7. Prentice RL. Surrogate endpoints in clinical trials: definition and operational criteria. *Stat Med* 1989;8:431–440.
8. Sormani MP, Bruzzi P, Beckmann K, et al. MRI metrics as surrogate endpoints for EDSS progression in SPMS patients treated with IFN beta-1b. *Neurology* 2003;60:1462–1466.
9. Sormani MP, Bruzzi P, Comi G, et al. MRI metrics as surrogate markers for clinical relapse rate in relapsing-remitting MS patients. *Neurology* 2002; 58:417–421.
10. Katz R. Biomarkers and surrogate markers: an FDA perspective. *NeuroRx* 2004;1:189–195.
11. U.S. Food and Drug Administration. Licensing approval notice for Betaseron (July 23,1993). Available at: http://www.fda.gov/bbs/topics/NEWS/NEW00424.html. Accessed: June 23, 2004.
12. Ferguson BM, MK, Esiri MM, et al. Axonal damage in acute multiple scerosis lesions. *Brain* 1997;120(Pt 3):393–399.
13. Trapp BD, Peterson J, Ransohoff RM, et al. Axonal transection in the lesions of multiple sclerosis. *N Engl J Med* 1998;338:278–285.
14. Li DK, Paty DW. Magnetic resonance imaging results of the PRISMS trial: a randomized, double-blind, placebo-controlled study of interferon-beta1a in relapsing-remitting multiple sclerosis. Prevention of relapses and disability by interferon-beta1a subcutaneously in multiple sclerosis. *Ann Neurol* 1999;46:197–206.
15. The Lenercept Multiple Sclerosis Study Group and The University of British Columbia MS/MRI Analysis Group. TNF neutralization in MS: results of a randomized, placebo-controlled multicenter study. *Neurology* 1999;53:457–465.
16. Li DK, Zhao GJ, Paty DW. Randomized controlled trial of interferon-beta-1a in secondary progressive MS: MRI results. *Neurology* 2001;56:1505–1513.
17. The Once Weekly Interferon for MS Study Group. Evidence of interferon beta-1a dose response in relapsing-remitting MS: the OWIMS Study. *Neurology* 1999;53:679–686.
18. Panitch H, Goodin DS, Francis G, et al. Randomized, comparative study of interferon beta-1a treatment regimens in MS: the EVIDENCE trial. *Neurology* 2002;59:1496–1506.
19. van Waesberghe JH, Castelijns JA, Roser W, et al. Single-dose gadolinium with magnetization transfer versus triple-dose gadolinium in the MR detection of multiple sclerosis lesions. *Am J Neuroradiol* 1997;18:1279–1285.
20. Silver NC, Good CD, Barker GJ, et al. Sensitivity of contrast enhanced MRI in multiple sclerosis. Effects of gadolinium dose, magnetization transfer contrast and delayed imaging. *Brain* 1997;120:1149–1161.
21. Lai M, Hodgson T, Gawne-Cain M, et al. A preliminary study into the sensitivity of disease activity detection by serial weekly magnetic resonance imaging in multiple sclerosis. *J Neurol Neurosurg Psychiatry* 1996;60:339–341.
22. Filippi M, Yousry T, Campi A, et al. Comparison of triple dose versus standard dose gadolinium-DTPA for detection of MRI enhancing lesions in patients with MS. *Neurology* 1996;46:379–384.
23. Tubridy N, Barker GJ, MacManus DG, et al. Optimisation of unenhanced MRI for detection of lesions in multiple sclerosis: a comparison of five pulse sequences with variable slice thickness. *Neuroradiology* 1998;40:293–297.
24. Tortorella C, Codella M, Rocca MA, et al. Disease activity in multiple sclerosis studied by weekly triple-dose magnetic resonance imaging. *J Neurol* 1999;246:689–692.
25. Miller DH, Rudge P, Johnson G, et al. Serial gadolinium enhanced magnetic resonance imaging in multiple sclerosis. *Brain* 1988;111:927–939.
26. Koopmans RA, Li DK, Oger JJ, et al. The lesion of multiple sclerosis: imaging of acute and chronic stages. *Neurology* 1989;39:959–963.
27. Willoughby EW, Grochowski E, Li DK, et al. Serial magnetic resonance scanning in multiple sclerosis: a second prospective study in relapsing patients. *Ann Neurol* 1989;25:43–49.
28. Koopmans RA, Li DK, Oger JJ, et al. Chronic progressive multiple sclerosis: serial magnetic resonance brain imaging over six months. *Ann Neurol* 1989;26:248–256.
29. Isaac C, Li DK, Genton M, et al. Multiple sclerosis: a serial study using MRI in relapsing patients. *Neurology* 1988;38:1511–1515.
30. Thompson AJ, Kermode AG, Wicks D, et al. Major differences in the dynamics of primary and secondary progressive multiple sclerosis. *Ann Neurol* 1991;29:53–62.
31. Thompson AJ, Miller D, Youl B, et al. Serial gadolinium-enhanced MRI in relapsing/remitting multiple sclerosis of varying disease duration. *Neurology* 1992;42:60–63.
32. Barkhof F, Scheltens P, Frequin ST, et al. Relapsing-remitting multiple sclerosis: sequential enhanced MR imaging vs clinical findings in determining disease activity. *Am J Roentgenol* 1992;159:1041–1047.
33. Miller DH, Barkhof F, Nauta JJ. Gadolinium enhancement increases the sensitivity of MRI in detecting disease activity in multiple sclerosis. *Brain* 1993;116:1077–1094.
34. Harris JO, Frank JA, Patronas N, et al. Serial gadolinium-enhanced magnetic resonance imaging scans in patients with early, relapsing-remitting multiple sclerosis: implications for clinical trials and natural history [see comments]. *Ann Neurol* 1991;29:548–555.

35. Miller DH, Albert PS, Barkhof F, et al. Guidelines for the use of magnetic resonance techniques in monitoring the treatment of multiple sclerosis. U.S. National MS Society Task Force. *Ann Neurol* 1996;39:6–16.

36. Comi G, Filippi M, Wolinsky JS. European/Canadian multicenter, double-blind, randomized, placebo-controlled study of the effects of glatiramer acetate on magnetic resonance imaging—measured disease activity and burden in patients with relapsing multiple sclerosis. European/Canadian Glatiramer Acetate Study Group. *Ann Neurol* 2001;49:290–297.

37. Paty DW, Li DK, UBC MS/MRI Study Group, IFNB Multiple Sclerosis Study Group. Interferon beta-1b is effective in relapsing-remitting multiple sclerosis. II. MRI analysis results of a multicenter, randomized, double-blind, placebo-controlled trial. *Neurology* 1993;43:662–667.

38. Tubridy N, Behan PO, Capildeo R, et al. The effect of anti-alpha4 integrin antibody on brain lesion activity in MS. The UK Antegren Study Group [see comments]. *Neurology* 1999;53:466–472.

39. Miller DH, Khan OA, Sheremata WA, et al. A controlled trial of natalizumab for relapsing multiple sclerosis. *N Engl J Med* 2003;348:15–23.

40. Vollmer T, Key L, Durkalski V, et al. Oral simvastatin treatment in relapsing-remitting multiple sclerosis. *Lancet* 2004;363:1607–1608.

41. Metz LM, Zhang Y, Yeung M, et al. Minocycline reduces gadolinium-enhancing magnetic resonance imaging lesions in multiple sclerosis. *Ann Neurol* 2004;55:756.

42. van Oosten BW, Lai M, Hodgkinson S, et al. Treatment of multiple sclerosis with the monoclonal anti-CD4 antibody cM-T412: results of a randomized, double-blind, placebo-controlled, MR-monitored phase II trial. *Neurology* 1997;49:351–357.

43. Frank JA, Richert N, Lewis B, et al. A pilot study of recombinant insulin-like growth factor-1 in seven multiple sclerosis patients. *Mult Scler* 2002;8:24–29.

44. Bielekova B, Goodwin B, Richert N, et al. Encephalitogenic potential of the myelin basic protein peptide (amino acids 83–99) in multiple sclerosis: results of a phase II clinical trial with an altered peptide ligand. *Nat Med* 2000;6:1167–1175.

45. Beutler E, Sipe JC, Romine JS, et al. The treatment of chronic progressive multiple sclerosis with cladribine. *Proc Natl Acad Sci USA* 1996;93:1716–1720.

46. Stone LA, Frank JA, Albert PS, et al. Characterization of MRI response to treatment with interferon beta-1b: contrast-enhancing MRI lesion frequency as a primary outcome measure. *Neurology* 1997;49:862–869.

47. McFarland HF, Frank JA, Albert PS, et al. Using gadolinium-enhanced magnetic resonance imaging lesions to monitor disease activity in multiple sclerosis. *Ann Neurol* 1992;32:758–766.

48. Frank JA, McFarland HF. How to participate in a multiple sclerosis clinical trial. *Neuroimaging Clin North Am* 2000;10:817–830,x.

49. Tubridy N, Ader HJ, Barkhof F, et al. Exploratory treatment trials in multiple sclerosis using MRI: sample size calculations for relapsing-remitting and secondary progressive subgroups using placebo controlled parallel groups. *J Neurol Neurosurg Psychiatry* 1998;64:50–55.

50. Stone LA, Frank JA, Albert PS, et al. The effect of interferon-beta on blood-brain barrier disruptions demonstrated by contrast-enhanced magnetic resonance imaging in relapsing-remitting multiple sclerosis. *Ann Neurol* 1995;37:611–619.

51. Thorpe JW, Kidd D, Moseley IF, et al. Serial gadolinium-enhanced MRI of the brain and spinal cord in early relapsing-remitting multiple sclerosis. *Neurology* 1996;46:373–378.

52. van Oosten BW, Barkhof F, Truyen L, et al. Increased MRI activity and immune activation in two multiple sclerosis patients treated with the monoclonal anti-tumor necrosis factor antibody cA2. *Neurology* 1996;47:1531–1534.

53. Tofts PS, Kermode AG. Measurement of the blood-brain barrier permeability and leakage space using dynamic MR imaging. 1. Fundamental concepts. *Magn Reson Med* 1991;17:357–367.

54. Kermode AG, Tofts PS, Thompson AJ, et al. Heterogeneity of blood-brain barrier changes in multiple sclerosis: an MRI study with gadolinium-DTPA enhancement. *Neurology* 1990;40:229–235.

55. Miki Y, Grossman RI, Udupa JK, et al. Computer-assisted quantitation of enhancing lesions in multiple sclerosis: correlation with clinical classification. *Am J Neuroradiol* 1997;18:705–710.

56. Rovaris M, Bastianello S, Capra R, et al. Correlation between enhancing lesion number and volume on standard and triple dose gadolinium-enhanced brain MRI scans from patients with multiple sclerosis [In Process Citation]. *Magn Reson Imaging* 1999;17:985–988.

57. Gawne-Cain ML, Webb S, Tofts P, et al. Lesion volume measurement in multiple sclerosis: how important is accurate repositioning? *J Magn Reson Imaging* 1996;6:705–713.

58. Filippi M, Marciano N, Capra R, et al. The effect of imprecise repositioning on lesion volume measurements in patients with multiple sclerosis. *Neurology* 1997;49:274–276.

59. Filippi M, Gawne-Cain ML, Gasperini C, et al. Effect of training and different measurement strategies on the reproducibility of brain MRI lesion load measurements in multiple sclerosis. *Neurology* 1998;50:238–244.

60. Filippi M, Horsfield MA, Bressi S, et al. Intra- and inter-observer agreement of brain MRI lesion volume measurements in multiple sclerosis. A comparison of techniques. *Brain* 1995;118:1593–1600.

61. Grimaud J, Lai M, Thorpe J, et al. Quantification of MRI lesion load in multiple sclerosis: a comparison of three computer-assisted techniques. *Magn Reson Imaging* 1996;14:495–505.

62. Barkhof F, Filippi M, Miller DH, et al. Strategies for optimizing MRI techniques aimed at monitoring disease activity in multiple sclerosis treatment trials. *J Neurol* 1997;244:76–84.

63. Filippi M, Rovaris M, Sormani MP, et al. Intraobserver and interobserver variability in measuring changes in lesion volume on serial brain MR images in multiple sclerosis. *Am J Neuroradiol* 1998;19:685–687.

64. Filippi M, Horsfield MA, Ader HJ, et al. Guidelines for using quantitative measures of brain magnetic resonance imaging abnormalities in monitoring the treatment of multiple sclerosis. *Ann Neurol* 1998;43:499–506.

65. Molyneux PD, Tofts PS, Fletcher A, et al. Precision and reliability for measurement of change in MRI lesion volume in multiple sclerosis: a comparison of two computer assisted techniques *J Neurol Neurosurg Psychiatry* 1998;65:42–47.

66. Cover KS, Petkau J, Li DK, et al. Lesion load reproducibility and statistical sensitivity of clinical trials in multiple sclerosis. *Neurology* 1999;52:433–435.

67. Miller DH, Molyneux PD, Barker GJ, et al. Effect of interferon-beta1b on magnetic resonance imaging outcomes in secondary progressive multiple sclerosis: results of a European multicenter, randomized, double-blind, placebo-controlled trial. European Study Group on Interferon-beta1b in secondary progressive multiple sclerosis. *Ann Neurol* 1999;46:850–859.

68. Rice GP, Filippi M, Comi G. Cladribine and progressive MS: clinical and MRI outcomes of a multicenter controlled trial. Cladribine MRI Study Group. *Neurology* 2000;54:1145–1155.

69. Zhao GJ, Li DK, Wolinsky JS, et al. Clinical and magnetic resonance imaging changes correlate in a clinical trial monitoring cyclosporine therapy for multiple sclerosis. The MS Study Group. *J Neuroimaging* 1997;7:1–7.

70. Kappos L, Stadt D, Ratzka M, et al. Magnetic resonance imaging in the evaluation of treatment in multiple sclerosis. *Neuroradiology* 1988;30:299–302.

71. Patti F, Cataldi ML, Nicoletti F, et al. Combination of cyclophosphamide and interferon-beta halts progression in patients with rapidly transitional multiple sclerosis. *J Neurol Neurosurg Psychiatry* 2001;71:404–407.

72. Molyneux PD, Filippi M, Barkhof F, et al. Correlations between monthly enhanced MRI lesion rate and changes in T2 lesion volume in multiple sclerosis. *Ann Neurol* 1998;43:332–339.

73. Kappos L, Moeri D, Radue EW, et al. Predictive value of gadolinium-enhanced magnetic resonance imaging for relapse rate and changes in disability or impairment in multiple sclerosis: a meta-analysis. Gadolinium MRI Meta-analysis Group. *Lancet* 1999;353:964–969.

74. Coles AJ, Wing MG, Molyneux P, et al. Monoclonal antibody treatment exposes three mechanisms underlying the clinical course of multiple sclerosis [In Process Citation]. *Ann Neurol* 1999;46:296–304.

75. Paolillo A, Coles AJ, Molyneux PD, et al. Quantitative MRI in patients with secondary progressive MS treated with monoclonal antibody Campath 1H. *Neurology* 1999;53:751–757.

76. Secondary Progressing Efficacy Clinical Trial of Recombinant Interferon-beta-1a in MS (SPECTRIMS) Study Group. Randomized controlled trial of interferon-beta-1a in secondary progressive MS: clinical results. *Neurology* 2001;56:1496–1504.

77. Brex PA, Ciccarelli O, O'Riordan JI, et al. A longitudinal study of abnormalities on MRI and disability from multiple sclerosis. *N Engl J Med* 2002;346:158–164.

78. Bakshi R, Benedict RH, Bermel RA, et al. Regional brain atrophy is associated with physical disability in multiple sclerosis: semiquantitative magnetic resonance imaging and relationship to clinical findings. *J Neuroimaging* 2001;11:129–136.

79. Bermel RA, Bakshi R, Tjoa C, et al. Bicaudate ratio as a magnetic resonance imaging marker of brain atrophy in multiple sclerosis. *Arch Neurol* 2002;59:275–280.

80. Brex PA, Jenkins R, Fox NC, et al. Detection of ventricular enlargement in patients at the earliest clinical stage of MS. *Neurology* 2000;54:1689–1691.

81. Brex PA, Leary SM, O'Riordan JI, et al. Measurement of spinal cord area in clinically isolated syndromes suggestive of multiple sclerosis. *J Neurol Neurosurg Psychiatry* 2001;70:544–547.

82. Chard DT, Griffin CM, Parker GJ, et al. Brain atrophy in clinically early relapsing-remitting multiple sclerosis. *Brain* 2002;125:327–337.

83. Chard DT, Brex PA, Ciccarelli O, et al. The longitudinal relation between brain lesion load and atrophy in multiple sclerosis: a 14 year follow up study. *J Neurol Neurosurg Psychiatry* 2003;74:1551–1554.

84. Dastidar P, Heinonen T, Lehtimaki T, et al. Volumes of brain atrophy and plaques correlated with neurological disability in secondary progressive multiple sclerosis [In Process Citation]. *J Neurol. Sci* 1999;165:36–42.

85. De Stefano N, Matthews M, Filippi M, et al. Evidence of early cortical atrophy in MS: relevance to white matter changes and disability. *Neurology* 2003; 60:1157–1162.

86. Filippi M, Campi A, Colombo B, et al. A spinal cord MRI study of benign and secondary progressive multiple sclerosis. *J Neurol* 1996;243:502–505.

87. Fisher E, Rudick RA, Cutter G, et al. Relationship between brain atrophy and disability: an 8-year follow-up study of multiple sclerosis patients. *Mult Scler* 2000;6:373–377.

88. Ge Y, Grossman RI, Udupa JK, et al. Brain atrophy in relapsing-remitting multiple sclerosis and secondary progressive multiple sclerosis: longitudinal quantitative analysis. *Radiology* 2000;214:665–670.

89. Kalkers NF, Ameziane N, Bot JC, et al. Longitudinal brain volume measurement in multiple sclerosis: rate of brain atrophy is independent of the disease subtype. *Arch Neurol* 2002;59:1572–1576.

90. Lin X, Tench CR, Turner B, et al. Spinal cord atrophy and disability in multiple sclerosis over four years: application of a reproducible automated technique in monitoring disease progression in a cohort of the interferon beta-1a (Rebif) treatment trial. *J Neurol Neurosurg Psychiatry* 2003;74:1090–1094.

91. Miller DH, Barkhof F, Frank JA, et al. Measurement of atrophy in multiple sclerosis: pathological basis, methodological aspects and clinical relevance. *Brain* 2002;125:1676–1695.

92. Simon JH. Brain and spinal cord atrophy in multiple sclerosis. *Neuroimaging Clin North Am* 2000; 10:753–770,ix.

93. Simon JH. Brain and spinal cord atrophy in multiple sclerosis: role as a surrogate measure of disease progression. *CNS Drugs* 2001;15:427–436.

94. Stevenson VL, Leary SM, Losseff NA, et al. Spinal cord atrophy and disability in MS: a longitudinal study. *Neurology* 1998;51:234–238.

95. Losseff NA, Webb SL, O'Riordan JI, et al. Spinal cord atrophy and disability in multiple sclerosis. A new reproducible and sensitive MRI method with potential to monitor disease progression. *Brain* 1996;119:701–708.

96. Rudick RA, Fisher E, Lee JC, et al. Use of the brain parenchymal fraction to measure whole brain atrophy in relapsing-remitting MS. Multiple Sclerosis Collaborative Research Group. *Neurology* 1999;53:1698–1704.

97. Losseff NA, Wang L, Lai HM, et al. Progressive cerebral atrophy in multiple sclerosis. A serial MRI study. *Brain* 1996;119:2009–2019.

98. Gasperini C, Paolillo A, Giugni E, et al. MRI brain volume changes in relapsing-remitting multiple sclerosis patients treated with interferon beta-1a. *Mult Scler* 2002;8:119–123.

99. Fox NC, Jenkins R, Leary SM, et al. Progressive cerebral atrophy in MS: a serial study using registered, volumetric MRI. *Neurology* 2000;54:807–812.

100. Hoogervorst EL, Polman CH, Barkhof F. Cerebral volume changes in multiple sclerosis patients treated with high-dose intravenous methylprednisolone. *Mult Scler* 2002;8:415–419.

101. Leary SM, Miller DH, Stevenson VL, et al. Interferon beta-1a in primary progressive MS: an exploratory, randomized, controlled trial. *Neurology* 2003;60:44–51.

102. Rudick RA, Fisher E, Lee JC, et al. Brain atrophy in relapsing multiple sclerosis: relationship to relapses, EDSS, and treatment with interferon beta-1a. *Mult Scler* 2000;6:365–372.

103. Zivadinov R, Rudick RA, De Masi R, et al. Effects of IV methylprednisolone on brain atrophy in relapsing-remitting MS. *Neurology* 2001;57:1239–1247.

104. Filippi M, Rovaris M, Iannucci G, et al. Whole brain volume changes in patients with progressive MS treated with cladribine. *Neurology* 2000;55:1714–1718.

105. Rovaris M, Comi G, Rocca MA, et al. Short-term brain volume change in relapsing-remitting multiple sclerosis: effect of glatiramer acetate and implications. *Brain* 2001;124:1803–1812.

106. Molyneux PD, Kappos L, Polman C, et al. The effect of interferon beta-1b treatment on MRI measures of cerebral atrophy in secondary progressive multiple sclerosis. European Study Group on Interferon beta-1b in secondary progressive multiple sclerosis. *Brain* 2000;123:2256–2263.

107. Sormani MP, Rovaris M, Valsasina P, et al. Measurement error of two different techniques for brain atrophy assessment in multiple sclerosis. *Neurology* 2004;62:1432–1434.

108. Rovaris M, Filippi M. Interventions for the prevention of brain atrophy in multiple sclerosis: current status. *CNS Drugs* 2003;17:563–575.

109. van Walderveen MA, Truyen L, van Oosten BW, et al. Development of hypointense lesions on T1-weighted spin-echo magnetic resonance images in multiple sclerosis: relation to inflammatory activity. *Arch Neurol* 1999;56:345–351.

110. van Waesberghe JH, van Walderveen MA, Castelijns JA, et al. Patterns of lesion development in multiple sclerosis: longitudinal observations with T1-weighted spin-echo and magnetization transfer MR. *Am J Neuroradiol* 1998;19:675–683.

111. van Waesberghe JH, Kamphorst W, De Groot CJ, et al. Axonal loss in multiple sclerosis lesions: magnetic resonance imaging insights into substrates of disability [In Process Citation]. *Ann Neurol* 1999;46:747–754.

112. van Walderveen MA, Kamphorst W, Scheltens P, et al. Histopathologic correlate of hypointense lesions on T1-weighted spin-echo MRI in multiple sclerosis. *Neurology* 1998;50:1282–1288.

113. Truyen L, van Waesberghe JH, van Walderveen MA, et al. Accumulation of hypointense lesions ("black holes") on T1 spin-echo MRI correlates with disease progression in multiple sclerosis. *Neurology* 1996;47:1469–1476.

114. van Walderveen MA, Lycklama A Nijeholt GJ, Ader HJ, et al. Hypointense lesions on T1-weighted spin-echo magnetic resonance imaging: relation to clinical characteristics in subgroups of patients with multiple sclerosis. *Arch Neurol* 2001;58:76–81.

115. Sailer M, Losseff NA, Wang L, et al. T1 lesion load and cerebral atrophy as a marker for clinical progression in patients with multiple sclerosis. A prospective 18 months follow-up study. *Eur J Neurol* 2001;8:37–42.

116. O'Riordan JI, Gawne Cain M, Coles A, et al. T1 hypointense lesion load in secondary progressive multiple sclerosis: a comparison of pre versus post contrast loads and of manual versus semi automated threshold techniques for lesion segmentation [In Process Citation]. *Mult Scler* 1998;4:408–412.

117. Gasperini C, Pozzilli C, Bastianello S, et al. Interferon-beta-1a in relapsing-remitting multiple sclerosis: effect on hypointense lesion volume on T1 weighted images. *J Neurol Neurosurg Psychiatry* 1999;67:579–584.

118. Barkhof F, van Waesberghe JH, Filippi M, et al. T(1) hypointense lesions in secondary progressive multiple sclerosis: effect of interferon beta-1b treatment. *Brain* 2001;124:1396–1402.

119. Simon JH, Lull J, Jacobs LD, et al. A longitudinal study of T1 hypointense lesions in relapsing MS: MSCRG trial of interferon beta-1a. Multiple Sclerosis Collaborative Research Group. *Neurology* 2000;55:185–192.

120. Molyneux PD, Brex PA, Fogg C, et al. The precision of T1 hypointense lesion volume quantification in multiple sclerosis treatment trials: a multicenter study. *Mult Scler* 2000;6:237–240.

121. Paolillo A, Buzzi MG, Giugni E, et al. The effect of Bacille Calmette-Guerin on the evolution of new enhancing lesions to hypointense T1 lesions in relapsing remitting MS. *J Neurol* 2003;250:247–248.

122. Filippi M, Rovaris M, Rocca MA, et al. Glatiramer acetate reduces the proportion of new MS lesions evolving into "black holes." *Neurology* 2001;57:731–733.

123. Dalton CM, Miszkiel KA, Barker GJ, et al. Effect of natalizumab on conversion of gadolinium enhancing lesions to T1 hypointense lesions in relapsing multiple sclerosis. *J Neurol* 2004;251:407–413.

124. Paolillo A, Bastianello S, Frontoni M, et al. Magnetic resonance imaging outcome of new enhancing lesions in relapsing-remitting multiple sclerosis patients treated with interferon beta-1a [In Process Citation]. *J Neurol* 1999;246:443–448.

125. Brex PA, Molyneux PD, Smiddy P, et al. The effect of IFNbeta-1b on the evolution of enhancing lesions in secondary progressive MS. *Neurology* 2001;57:2185–2190.

126. Arnold DL, De Stefano N, Narayanan S, et al. Proton MR spectroscopy in multiple sclerosis. *Neuroimaging Clin North Am* 2000;10:789–798,ix-x.

127. Bitsch A, Bruhn H, Vougioukas V, et al. Inflammatory CNS demyelination: histopathologic correlation with in vivo quantitative proton MR spectroscopy. *Am J Neuroradiol* 1999;20:1619–1627.

128. Lassmann H. Brain damage when multiple sclerosis is diagnosed clinically. *Lancet* 2003;361:1317–1318.

129. Dautry C, Vaufrey F, Brouillet E, et al. Early N-acetyl-laspartate depletion is a marker of neuronal dysfunction in rats and primates chronically treated with the mitochondrial toxin 3-nitropropionic acid. *J Cereb Blood Flow Metab* 2000;20:789–799.

130. Brex PA, Gomez-Anson B, Parker GJ, et al. Proton MR spectroscopy in clinically isolated syndromes suggestive of multiple sclerosis. *J Neurol Sci* 1999;166:16–22.

131. De Stefano N, Narayanan S, Mortilla M, et al. Imaging axonal damage in multiple sclerosis by means of MR spectroscopy. *J Neurol Sci* 2000;21:S883–S887.

132. De Stefano N, Narayanan S, Francis SJ, et al. Diffuse axonal and tissue injury in patients with multiple sclerosis with low cerebral lesion load and no disability. *Arch Neurol* 2002;59:1565–1571.

133. De Stefano N, Guidi L, Stromillo ML, et al. Imaging neuronal and axonal degeneration in multiple sclerosis. *Neurol Sci* 2003;24[Suppl 5]:S283–S286.

134. Filippi M. In-vivo tissue characterization of multiple sclerosis and other white matter diseases using magnetic resonance based techniques. *J Neurol* 2001;248:1019–1029.

135. Pan JW, Coyle PK, Bashir K, et al. Metabolic differences between multiple sclerosis subtypes measured by quantitative MR spectroscopy. *Mult Scler* 2002;8:200–206.

136. Tourbah A, Stievenart JL, Abanou A, et al. Correlating multiple MRI parameters with clinical features: an attempt to define a new strategy in multiple sclerosis. *Neuroradiology* 2001;43:712–720.

137. Narayanan S, Fu L, Pioro E, et al. Imaging of axonal damage in multiple sclerosis: spatial distribution of magnetic resonance imaging lesions. *Ann Neurol* 1997;41:385–391.

138. Parry A, Corkill R, Blamire AM, et al. Beta-interferon treatment does not always slow the progression of axonal injury in multiple sclerosis. *J Neurol* 2003;250:171–178.

139. Narayanan S, De Stefano N, Francis GS, et al. Axonal metabolic recovery in multiple sclerosis patients treated with interferon beta-1b. *J Neurol* 2001;248:979–986.

140. Ge Y, Gonen O, Inglese M, et al. Neuronal cell injury precedes brain atrophy in multiple sclerosis. *Neurology* 2004;62:624–627.

141. Gonen O, Catalaa I, Babb JS, et al. Total brain N-acetylaspartate: a new measure of disease load in MS. *Neurology* 2000;54:15–19.

142. Pelletier D, Nelson SJ, Grenier D, et al. 3-D echo planar (1)HMRS imaging in MS: metabolite comparison from supratentorial vs. central brain. *Magn Reson Imaging* 2002;20:599–606.

143. McGowan JC. The physical basis of magnetization transfer imaging. *Neurology* 1999;53:S3–7.

144. Grossman RI. Magnetization transfer in multiple sclerosis. *Ann Neurol* 1994;36:S97–S99.

145. Rausch M, Hiestand P, Baumann D, et al. MRI-based monitoring of inflammation and tissue damage in acute and chronic relapsing EAE. *Magn Reson Med* 2003;50:309–314.

146. Gareau PJ, Rutt BK, Karlik SJ, et al. Magnetization transfer and multicomponent T2 relaxation measurements with histopathologic correlation in an experimental model of MS. *J Magn Reson Imaging* 2000;11:586–595.

147. Dousset V, Grossman RI, Ramer KN, et al. Experimental allergic encephalomyelitis and multiple sclerosis: lesion characterization with magnetization transfer imaging [Published erratum appears in *Radiology* 1992;183(3):878.] *Radiology* 1992;182:483–491.

148. van Buchem MA, Grossman RI, Armstrong C, et al. Correlation of volumetric magnetization transfer imaging with clinical data in MS. *Neurology* 1998;50:1609–1617.

149. van Buchem MA, McGowan JC, Grossman RI. Magnetization transfer histogram methodology: its clinical and neuropsychological correlates. *Neurology* 1999;53:S23–28.

150. van Buchem MA, McGowan JC, Kolson DL, et al. Quantitative volumetric magnetization transfer analysis in multiple sclerosis: estimation of macroscopic and microscopic disease burden. *Magn Reson Med* 1996;36:632–636.

151. van Buchem MA, Udupa JK, McGowan JC, et al. Global volumetric estimation of disease burden in multiple sclerosis based on magnetization transfer imaging. *Am J Neuroradiol* 1997;18:1287–1290.

152. Kita M, Goodkin DE, Bacchetti P, et al. Magnetization transfer ratio in new MS lesions before and during therapy with IFNbeta-1a. *Neurology* 2000;54:1741–1745.

153. Richert ND, Ostuni JL, Bash CN, et al. Interferon beta-1b and intravenous methylprednisolone promote lesion recovery in multiple sclerosis. *Mult Scler* 2001;7:49–58.

154. Inglese M, Van Waesberghe JH, Rovaris M, et al. The effect of interferon beta-1b on quantities derived from MT MRI in secondary progressive MS. *Neurology* 2003;60:853–860.

155. Horsfield MA, Barker GJ, Barkhof F, et al. Guidelines for using quantitative magnetization transfer magnetic resonance imaging for monitoring treatment of multiple sclerosis. *J Magn Reson Imaging* 2003;17:389–397.

156. Ristori G, Buzzi MG, Sabatini U, et al. Use of Bacille Calmette-Guerin (BCG) in multiple sclerosis. *Neurology* 1999;53:1588–1589.

157. Gobbini MI, Smith ME, Richert ND, et al. Effect of open label pulse cyclophosphamide therapy on MRI measures of disease activity in five patients with refractory relapsing-remitting multiple sclerosis. *J Neuroimmunol* 1999;99:142–149.

158. Kappos L. Clinical trials of immunosuppression and immunomodulation in multiple sclerosis. *J Neuroimmunol* 1988;20:261–268.

159. Mancardi GL, Sardanelli F, Parodi RC, et al. Effect of copolymer-1 on serial gadolinium-enhanced MRI in relapsing remitting multiple sclerosis. *Neurology* 1998;50:1127–1133.

160. Ge Y, Grossman RI, Udupa JK, et al. Glatiramer acetate (Copaxone) treatment in relapsing-remitting MS: quantitative MR assessment. *Neurology* 2000;54:813–817.

161. Wolinsky JS, Comi G, Filippi M, et al. Copaxone's effect on MRI-monitored disease in relapsing MS is reproducible and sustained. *Neurology* 2002;59:1284–1286.

162. Wolinsky JS, Narayana PA, Johnson KP. United States open-label glatiramer acetate extension trial for relapsing multiple sclerosis: MRI and clinical correlates. Multiple Sclerosis Study Group and the MRI Analysis Center. *Mult Scler* 2001;7:33–41.

163. Rovaris M, Codella M, Moiola L, et al. Effect of glatiramer acetate on MS lesions enhancing at different gadolinium doses. *Neurology* 2002;59:1429–1432.

164. Kastrukoff LF, Oger JJ, Hashimoto SA, et al. Systemic lymphoblastoid interferon therapy in chronic progressive multiple sclerosis. I. Clinical and MRI evaluation. *Neurology* 1990;40:479–486.

165. Durelli L, Bongioanni MR, Cavallo R, et al. Chronic systemic high-dose recombinant interferon alfa-2a reduces exacerbation rate, MRI signs of disease activity, and lymphocyte interferon gamma production in relapsing-remitting multiple sclerosis. *Neurology* 1994;44:406–413.

166. Myhr KM, Riise T, Green Lilleas FE, et al. Interferon-alpha2a reduces MRI disease activity in relapsing-remitting multiple sclerosis. Norwegian Study Group on Interferon-alpha in Multiple Sclerosis. *Neurology* 1999;52:1049–1056.

167. Pozzilli C, Bastianello S, Koudriavtseva T, et al. Magnetic resonance imaging changes with recombinant human interferon-beta-1a: a short term study in relapsing-remitting multiple sclerosis [see comments]. *J Neurol Neurosurg Psychiatry* 1996;61:251–258.

168. Paolillo A, Bastianello S, Frontoni M, et al. Magnetic resonance imaging outcome of new enhancing lesions in relapsing-remitting multiple sclerosis patients treated with interferon beta1a. *J Neurol* 1999;246:443–448.

169. Jacobs LD, Cookfair DL, Rudick RA, et al. Intramuscular interferon beta-1a for disease progression in relapsing multiple sclerosis. The Multiple Sclerosis Collaborative Research Group (MSCRG). *Ann Neurol* 1996;39:285–294.

170. Simon JH, Jacobs LD, Campion M, et al. Magnetic resonance studies of intramuscular interferon beta-1a for relapsing multiple sclerosis. The Multiple Sclerosis Collaborative Research Group [see comments]. *Ann Neurol* 1998;43:79–87.

171. PRISMS (Prevention of Relapses and Disability by Interferon beta-1a Subcutaneously in Multiple Sclerosis) Study Group. Randomised double-blind placebo-controlled study of interferon beta-1a in relapsing/remitting multiple sclerosis. *Lancet* 1998;352:1498–1504.

172. Sarchielli P, Presciutti O, Tarducci R, et al. 1H-MRS in patients with multiple sclerosis undergoing treatment with interferon beta-1a: results of a preliminary study. *J Neurol Neurosurg Psychiatry* 1998;64:204–212.

173. Comi G, Filippi M, Barkhof F, et al. Effect of early interferon treatment on conversion to definite multiple sclerosis: a randomised study. *Lancet* 2001;357:1576–1582.

174. Champs AC. Interferon beta-1a for optic neuritis patients at high risk for multiple sclerosis. *Am J Ophthalmol* 2001;132:463–471.

175. Clanet M, Radue EW, Kappos L, et al. A randomized, double-blind, dose-comparison study of weekly interferon beta-1a in relapsing MS. *Neurology* 2002;59:1507–1517.

176. Cohen JA, Cutter GR, Fischer JS, et al. Benefit of interferon beta-1a on MSFC progression in secondary progressive MS. *Neurology* 2002;59:679–687.

177. Polman C, Barkhof F, Kappos L, et al. Oral interferon beta-1a in relapsing-remitting multiple sclerosis: a double-blind randomized study. *Mult Scler* 2003;9:342–348.

178. TIMSS. Interferon beta-1b is effective in relapsing-remitting multiple sclerosis. I. Clinical results of a multicenter, randomized, double-blind, placebo-controlled trial. *Neurology* 1993;43:655–661.

179. Paty DW, Li DK. Interferon beta-1b is effective in relapsing-remitting multiple sclerosis. II. MRI analysis results of a multicenter, randomized, double-blind, placebo-controlled trial. UBC MS/MRI Study Group and the IFNB Multiple Sclerosis Study Group. *Neurology* 1993;43:662–667.

180. Zhao GJ, Koopmans RA, Li DK, et al. Effect of interferon beta-1b in MS: assessment of annual accumulation of PD/T2 activity on MRI. UBC MS/MRI Analysis Group and the MS Study Group. *Neurology* 2000;54:200–206.

181. Richert ND, Ostuni JL, Bash CN, et al. Serial whole-brain magnetization transfer imaging in patients with relapsing-remitting multiple sclerosis at baseline and during treatment with interferon beta-1b. *Am J Neuroradiol* 1998;19:1705–1713.

182. European Study Group on interferon beta-1b in secondary progressive MS. Placebo-controlled multicentre randomised trial of interferon beta-1b in treatment of secondary progressive multiple sclerosis. *Lancet* 1998;352:1491–1497.

183. Durelli L, Verdun E, Barbero P, et al. Every-other-day interferon beta-1b versus once-weekly interferon beta-1a for multiple sclerosis: results of a 2-year prospective randomised multicentre study (INCOMIN). *Lancet* 2002;359:1453–1460.

184. Teksam M, Tali T, Kocer B, Isik S. Qualitative and quantitative volumetric evaluation of the efficacy of intravenous immunoglobulin in multiple sclerosis: preliminary report. *Neuroradiology* 2000;42:885–889.

185. Milligan NM, Miller DH, Compston DA. A placebo-controlled trial of isoprinosine in patients with multiple sclerosis. *J Neurol Neurosurg Psychiatry* 1994;57:164–168.

186. TNF neutralization in MS: results of a randomized, placebo-controlled multicenter study. The Lenercept Multiple Sclerosis Study Group and The University of British Columbia MS/MRI Analysis Group [In Process Citation]. *Neurology* 1999;53:457–465.

187. Karussis DM, Meiner Z, Lehmann D, et al. Treatment of secondary progressive multiple sclerosis with the immunomodulator linomide: a double-blind, placebo-controlled pilot study with monthly magnetic resonance imaging evaluation. *Neurology* 1996;47:341–346.

188. Tan IL, Lycklama A Nijeholt GJ, Polman CH, et al. Linomide in the treatment of multiple sclerosis: MRI results from prematurely terminated phase-III trials. *Mult Scler* 2000;6:99–104.

189. Wolinsky JS, Narayana PA, Noseworthy JH, et al. Linomide in relapsing and secondary progressive MS: part II: MRI results. MRI Analysis Center of the University of Texas-Houston, Health Science Center,

and the North American Linomide Investigators. *Neurology* 2000;54:1734–1741.

190. Lugaresi A, Caporale C, Farina D, et al. Low-dose oral methotrexate treatment in chronic progressive multiple sclerosis. *Neurol Sci* 2001;22:209–210.

191. Oliveri RL, Valentino P, Russo C, et al. Randomized trial comparing two different high doses of methyl-prednisolone in MS: a clinical and MRI study. *Neurology* 1998;50:1833–1836.

192. Millefiorini E, Gasperini C, Pozzilli C, et al. Randomized placebo-controlled trial of mitox-antrone in relapsing-remitting multiple sclerosis: 24-month clinical and MRI outcome. *J Neurol* 1997;244:153–159.

193. van de Wyngaert FA, Beguin C, D'Hooghe MB, et al. A double-blind clinical trial of mitoxantrone versus methylprednisolone in relapsing, secondary progressive multiple sclerosis. *Acta Neurol Belg* 2001;101:210–216.

194. Sorensen PS, Wanscher B, Szpirt W, et al. Plasma exchange combined with azathioprine in multiple sclerosis using serial gadolinium-enhanced MRI to monitor disease activity: a randomized single-masked cross-over pilot study. *Neurology* 1996;46:1620–1625.

195. Edan G, Miller D, Clanet M, et al. Therapeutic effect of mitoxantrone combined with methylprednisolone in multiple sclerosis: a randomised multicentre study of active disease using MRI and clinical criteria [see comments]. *J Neurol Neurosurg Psychiatry* 1997;62:112–118.

196. Puri BK, Bydder GM, Chaudhuri KR, et al. MRI changes in multiple sclerosis following treatment with lofepramine and L-phenylalanine. *Neuroreport* 2001;12:1821–1824.

197. Fernandez O, Guerrero M, Mayorga C, et al. Combination therapy with interferon beta-1b and aza-thioprine in secondary progressive multiple sclerosis. A two-year pilot study. *J Neurol* 2002;249:1058–1062.

198. Markovic-Plese S, Bielekova B, Kadom N, et al. Longitudinal MRI study: the effects of azathioprine in MS patients refractory to interferon beta-1b. *Neurology* 2003;60:1849–1851.

199. Lus G, Romano F, Scuotto A, et al. Azathioprine and interferon beta(1a) in relapsing-remitting multiple sclerosis patients: increasing efficacy of combined treatment. *Eur Neurol* 2004;51:15–20.

200. Wiles CM, Omar L, Swan AV, et al. Total lymphoid irradiation in multiple sclerosis. *J Neurol Neurosurg Psychiatry* 1994;57:154–163.

201. Bowen JD, Petersdorf SH, Richards TL, et al. Phase I study of a humanized anti-CD11/CD18 monoclonal antibody in multiple sclerosis. *Clin Pharmacol Ther* 1998;64:339–346.

202. Goodkin DE, Shulman M, Winkelhake J, et al. A phase I trial of solubilized DR2:MBP84–102 (AG284) in multiple sclerosis. *Neurology* 2000;54:1414–1420.

203. Skurkovich S, Boiko A, Beliaeva I, et al. Randomized study of antibodies to IFN-gamma and TNF-alpha in secondary progressive multiple sclerosis. *Mult Scler* 2001;7:277–284.

204. Mancardi GL, Saccardi R, Filippi M, et al. Autologous hematopoietic stem cell transplantation suppresses Gd-enhanced MRI activity in MS. *Neurology* 2001;57:62–68.

205. Saiz A, Carreras E, Berenguer J, et al. MRI and CSF oligoclonal bands after autologous hematopoietic stem cell transplantation in MS. *Neurology* 2001;56:1084–1089.

206. Saiz A, Blanco Y, Carreras E, et al. Clinical and MRI outcome after autologous hematopoietic stem cell transplantation in MS. *Neurology* 2004;62:282–284.

15

Symptom Management

Paul O'Connor

Department of Medicine (Neurology), University of Toronto, Toronto, Ontario, Canada

INTRODUCTION

The neurologic deficits of multiple sclerosis can lead to an array of physical and cognitive symptoms, varying in kind and intensity, and depending on where the central nervous system (CNS) damage has occurred. Symptom management refers to a variety of palliative strategies that serve both to prevent complications and to improve patient quality of life generally. These approaches can be applied independently of treatments designed to arrest or reverse the course of the underlying demyelination. Patient involvement is an important component of any treatment strategy, not only in terms of level of the perceived discomfort and consequent need to treat, but also in assessing the commitment to the chosen intervention, as well as tolerance of potential side effects. While one focus of this review is the range of pharmacological interventions available, it should be noted that many symptoms can be managed using a combination of rehabilitation and counseling (1).

SPASTICITY

Spasticity refers to a velocity-dependent increase in muscle tone, derived from hyperexcitability of the stretch reflex, and is most often described by patients as a constant feeling of limb stiffness. This, in turn, reflects lesions in upper motor neurons of the CNS, and is associated with sprouting of descending motor pathways, the formation of new synaptic connections with spinal motoneurons, and denervation hypersensitivity (2). As a result, the normal physiological balance between opposing muscle groups is disrupted. Spasticity is a common symptom in MS, with one recent survey reporting that 70% of patients experienced it in mild to severe degree (3). See Table 15-1.

Spasticity occurs most commonly in lower limbs and can lead to pain, stiffness, tremor, clonus, impaired balance and spasms (1,4). Spasms, as distinct from spasticity, are spontaneous, intermittent contractions of groups of muscles, usually in the limbs, which cause unwanted and usually painful flexion or extension movements. Although spasticity can actually be helpful in early stages of MS, by assisting the patient in standing, disease progression can result in severe spasms. Extensor spasms most often occur at night or upon waking, and can even lead to ejection of the patient from a wheelchair, while flexor spasms lead to sudden falls and, as disease progresses, to a permanently flexed posture (4). In a recent report, MS-induced clonus resulted in bilateral spontaneous periacetabular fractures (5).

The most widely used measure of degree of spasticity is the Ashworth scale (6). See Table 15-2. Although it is not considered to be sufficiently sensitive to discriminate differing degrees of spasticity in many clinical situations, and in fact has been modified for some purposes (7), it continues to be employed in randomized controlled trials as the best available objective measure of treatment efficacy (8,9).

Rather than aiming for complete elimination of spasticity, management should focus on reduction of symptoms to improve patient comfort and function, as well as minimizing complications that can result from spasms or clonus. Overtreatment can interfere with wakefulness and ambulation, as well as increasing the risk of venous thromboses (1). Spasticity may be induced by a variety of noxious stimuli that increase afferent stimulation of stretch reflexes, and whose elimination should therefore be ensured through combined assessment and patient education. These include urinary tract infections, constipation, ingrown toenails, pressure ulcers, and poorly fitting braces or wheelchairs (1,10), as well as cold temperature and supine posture (1). Treatment with interferon-β may also be an exacerbating factor (11), perhaps because it may enhance nerve conduction in the spinal cord.

Physiotherapy should be instituted, including regular stretching exercises and massage, heat or cold applications to loosen muscles, and patient instruction as to adopting appropriate postural positions that minimize the likelihood of clonus or spasms. Orthoses may aid in preventing contractures of spastic limbs, and transcutaneous nerve stimulation may also be helpful in alleviating spasticity (10,12).

TABLE 15-1. *Common symptoms in MS*

Spasticity
Fatigue
Pain
Cognitive impairment
Depression and anxiety
Bladder, bowel, and sexual dysfunction
Tremor
Vertigo
Weakness
Dysphagia
Numbness
Paroxysmal attacks
Acute relapses

TABLE 15-2. *Ashworth scale for measurement of spasticity*

Grade	Description
0	Normal: no increase in tone
1	Slight increase in tone, giving a "catch" when the limb is moved in flexion or extension
2	More marked increase in tone, but limb easily flexed
3	Considerable increase in tone; passive movement difficult
4	Limb rigid in flexion or extension

Drug Therapies

The principal oral pharmacological therapies for treating spasticity are baclofen, tizanidine, diazepam, dantrolene, and gabapentin (13). In addition to these oral agents, botulinum toxin injections, as well as intrathecal administration of baclofen and phenol have been employed to good effect. The use of nerve stimulators [e.g., transcutaneous nerve stimulation (TENS)] has been suggested to decrease spasticity, but these have not been well-studied. The use of cannabinoids is discussed in a separate section devoted to this class of drugs. See Table 15-3.

Baclofen

Baclofen is a GABA analog, and acts as a $GABA_B$ receptor agonist both pre- and postsynaptically to inhibit transmission of monosynaptic and polysynaptic reflexes (14). It is the most commonly used drug in the treatment of MS-associated spasticity, showing efficacy in improving the range of joint movement, while decreasing the frequency and intensity of spasms. As patient sensitivity is highly variable, dosage titration is customarily practiced. As liver enzyme levels may be elevated in response to baclofen, hepatic screening is advised every six months. Principal side effects include weakness, fatigue, nausea, drowsiness, and dizziness. Particular caution must be exercised in cessation of baclofen treatment, as this may induce hallucinations and seizures (13) and, as with all sedating medications, discontinuation after chronic treatment should be achieved in a tapering fashion.

Tizanidine

Tizanidine is an imidazole derivative that acts centrally as an α_2-adrenergic agonist to reduce synaptic transmission both presynaptically and

TABLE 15-3. *Principal oral drugs used to treat spasticity (adapted from Kita & Goodkin, 2000)*

Drug	Starting Dosage	Maximum Recommended Dosage	Adverse Effects	Monitoring	Precautions
Baclofen	5 mg/day increasing to in 15 mg/day; 3 divided doses	80 mg/day in divided doses	Muscle weakness, sedation, fatigue, dizziness, nausea	Periodic liver function tests	Abrupt cessation associated with seizures
Tizanidine	2-4 mg/day	36 mg/day in divided doses	Drowsiness, dry mouth, dizziness, reversible dose-related elevated liver transaminases	Periodic liver function tests	Not to be used with anti-hypertensives or clonidine
Diazepam	2 mg/day bid or 5 mg qhs	40-60 mg/day in divided doses	Sedation, cognitive impairment, depression	Potential for dependence	Withdrawal syndrome
Dantrolene	25 mg/day	400 mg/day in divided doses	Hepatoxicity (potentially irreversible) weakness, sedation stomach upset	Periodic liver function tests	Hepatoxicity
Gabapentin	100 mg tid	3600 mg/day in divided doses	Stomach upset		
Clonidine	0.1 mg/day	Usual dose in hypertension 0.2-0.6 mg/day	Bradycardia, hypotension dry mouth, drowsiness, constipation, dizziness depression		Add on agent; hypotension may result; not for use with tizanidine

bid = twice daily; qhs = at bedtime; tid = three times daily.

postsynaptically, leading to inhibition of release of excitatory amino acids from spinal interneurons. Like baclofen, it is titrated for efficacy, over a period of several weeks, and has shown efficacy in reducing muscle tone and spasms associated with MS. Principal side effects are dry mouth, dizziness and drowsiness, and in 5% to 7% of patients, hepatotoxicity, manifested in increases in liver transaminases (13,15). It has been reported that muscle weakness is a less common side effect than with baclofen, though the evidence for this has been questioned (4). As tizanidine may cause hypotension, it should not be used in combination with other antihypertensives such as clonidine (13).

Diazepam

Diazepam is the benzodiazepine that is most commonly used to treat spasticity. It acts by binding to the $GABA_A$ receptor to increase chloride conductance, leading to increased presynaptic inhibition. Comparisons with baclofen suggested similar efficacy in treatment of spasticity and, depending on the study, varying patient preference in selecting between the two drugs (13). Adverse effects include cognitive impairment, sedation, and depression, with potential for developing dependence. As with baclofen, care must be taken in stopping diazepam treatment, lest seizures be induced.

Dantrolene

Dantrolene is a hydantoin derivative that acts directly on the ryanodine receptor of muscle to decrease excitation–contraction coupling (16). An early comparative trial with diazepam indicated similar efficacy in reducing spasticity (17), but varying degrees of efficacy have been seen in comparison to placebo (4). As it acts directly on muscle, rather than on synaptic transmission, muscle weakness is a common side effect of dantrolene treatment. In addition, potentially irreversible hepatotoxicity mandates careful monitoring of liver function during prolonged administration (13).

Gabapentin

Gabapentin is another GABA analog which, however, does not bind to conventional GABA receptors (13). It has shown some efficacy in treating spasticity in small-scale trials and anecdotal reports (18,19) and has proved useful in controlling MS-induced nocturnal spasms (20).

Clonidine

Clonidine acts centrally as an α_2-receptor agonist and is used primarily to treat hypertension and opiate withdrawal, but it has other actions, including reduction in muscle tone in patients with brain injuries. It is not considered to be a first-line option for spasticity, but may be used in conjunction with other drugs, such as baclofen. Side effects include bradycardia, hypotension, dry mouth, drowsiness, constipation, dizziness, and depression (13); owing to its hypotensive action, it should not be employed in conjunction with other agents, such as tizanidine, which also have the potential to lower blood pressure.

Intrathecal Baclofen

Intrathecal administration of baclofen may be useful if oral medication fails. This surgical procedure involves implantation of a pump and associated reservoir into the abdominal wall, and catheterization to permit administration of baclofen into the subarachnoid space. This permits administration of locally elevated doses to be delivered at only 1% of the oral dosage, without impact on serum concentrations and consequent systemic effects (21). The reservoir can be refilled every 6 to 12 weeks percutaneously. A series of trials has shown consistent benefit in reducing MS-associated spasticity, including lowered muscle tone, reduction in frequency of spasms, and reduced pain (4), although the attractiveness of this therapy is reduced by the possibility of accidental overdosage-associated coma and the need for special equipment to adjust the pump on an ongoing basis.

Intrathecal Phenol

Intrathecal phenol treatment is not an established option for MS-associated spasticity, though it has been employed in other contexts of CNS injury. The primary effect of phenol injection is nerve damage, resulting from protein coagulation. In a recent trial with 25 patients with severe MS-associated spasticity, Jarrett et al. (8) reported that lumbar intrathecal phenol injection on one side led to significant bilateral reduction in spasms and pain, together with reductions in limb tone, after both the initial and subsequent injections; the most notable impact was on the targeted side after the initial injection. The authors suggest that this approach may offer advantages over intrathecal baclofen in cases where patients develop tolerance, or do not wish the responsibilities inherent in continued pump installation.

Botulinum Toxin

Botulinum toxin (BTX) is a poison produced by the bacterium *Clostridium botulinum*, whose best-known attribute is its blockage of acetylcholine release from cholinergic nerve endings. Owing to retrograde axonal transport, however, a variety of other effects may ensue, including reduced motoneuronal excitability, action on central synapses such as decreased Renshaw inhibition and increased presynaptic inhibition, action on gamma motoneuronal endings, and action on most active terminals. Locally injected BTX can also spread to neighboring muscles, and BTX effects may also spread to remote muscles (22). There are seven immunologically distinct variants of BTX, with type A being most often employed for local injection to reduce spasticity in selected muscles. In two small-scale trials, it has shown efficacy in reducing MS-induced spasticity, with lowered muscle tone and frequency of spasms, reduction in pain, and improved range of motion of the hips (23,24). The principal side effect was muscle weakness. The benefits of BTX were expressed even though patients were receiving concomitant oral antispasticity and analgesic medications (24).

Overview of Current Treatments for Spasticity

In a recent overview, Beard et al. (4) evaluated the evidence for current treatments of spasticity, and concluded overall that there was weak evidence for the efficacy of the four principal oral treatments, namely, baclofen, tizanidine, diazepam, and dantrolene. While all show roughly equivalent clinical benefit, there is no evidence for functional improvement with any of these drugs. The evidence in support of intrathecal baclofen was considered to be the most compelling, though the expense associated with installation of the pump, reservoir, and catheters may well restrict its use. In some measure these conclusions are not surprising, in that there is unlikely to be a magic bullet for treating MS-associated spasticity, given the potentially widespread nature of the immune attack on the CNS. There is thus considerable room for monitoring, together with empiricism, in selecting a treatment or combination of treatments for a given patient.

FATIGUE

Fatigue in multiple sclerosis is defined as an abnormal sense of weariness and lack of energy, out of proportion to the degree of effort or level of disability, and sufficient to interfere significantly with routine intellectual and physical functioning. Depending on the survey in question, 65% to 97% of MS patients report significant fatigue, with 15% to 40% considering it to be the most disabling MS symptom (25). It is qualitatively different from the normal sense of fatigue that attends intense mental or physical exertion, and can be experienced by patients even while at rest (26). See Table 15-4. Patients sense that performance of a given task will entail an excessive expenditure of energy, leading them to reduce their overall physical activity, even while deriving little subjective sense of beneficial rest (26). Overall, fatigue makes a significant and independent contribution to diminished quality of life (27). While some reports have suggested that fatigue is correlated with the extent of the underlying neurologic disability

TABLE 15-4. *Characteristics distinguishing fatigue in MS patients and healthy controls (Krupp et al, 1988)*

Characteristic	MS (%)	Control (%)	P
Heat worsens it	92	17	<0.001
Prevents sustained physical functioning	89	0	<0.001
Comes on easily	82	22	<0.001
Interferes with physical functioning	79	28	<0.01
Interferes with responsibilities	67	0	<0.001
Causes frequent problems	63	17	<0.01

TABLE 15-5. *Fatigue Severity Scale (from Krupp et al, 1989)*

1. My motivation is lower when I am fatigued.
2. Exercise brings on my fatigue
3. I am easily fatigued.
4. Fatigue interferes with my physical functioning.
5. Fatigue causes frequent problems for me.
6. My fatigue prevents sustained physical functioning.
7. Fatigue interferes with carrying out certain duties and responsibilities.
8. Fatigue is among my three most disabling symptoms.
9. Fatigue interferes with my work, family, or social life.

Patients are instructed to choose a number from 1 to 7, to indicate their degree of agreement with each statement; 1 indicates strong disagreement, 7 indicates strong agreement.

and consequent physical impairment (28–30), with a particular link to pyramidal tract dysfunction (29), this has not been confirmed in other studies (31–34). A significant correlation with MS fatigue has been found with lowered mental health and depressed mood (32,33,35) and, in particular, with depression (30,34).

Assessment

Krupp et al. (31) identified several characteristics of MS-related fatigue that differed in kind from fatigue as experienced by healthy controls. Based on this work, they developed a questionnaire that forms the basis of the Fatigue Severity Scale (FSS) as a measure of fatigue-associated debility (Table 15-5; Figs. 15-1, 15-2) (36). Despite the subsequent elaboration of several other scales, such as the more extensive Modified Fatigue Impact Scale (MFIS), the FSS continues to be a useful tool (30). Other parameters of relevance in planning treatment include whether the symptoms are chronic (defined operationally as being present on at least 50% of days for more than 6 weeks) or acute, and whether they reflect primary fatigue, arising from the disease pathology, or secondary aspects such as disease-related lack of exercise, loss of sleep, or side effects of medications (25). Drugs that are used in treatment of MS and that can induce fatigue include type I interferons, antispasticity agents, tricyclic antidepressants, benzodiazepines, and anticonvulsants

(37,38). In addition, many drug classes employed in treating an array of common afflictions have been implicated as potential contributors to fatigue and lethargy (38). A sudden increase in fatigue, or its appearance as a new

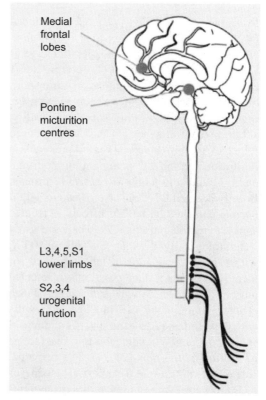

FIG. 15-1. Neuroanatomy of the bladder and its central connections.

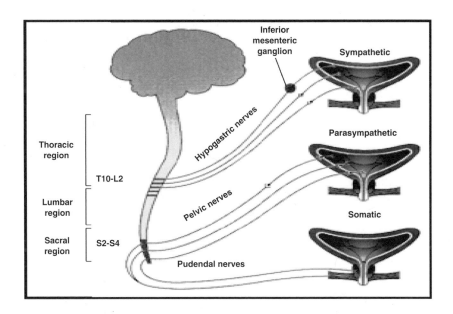

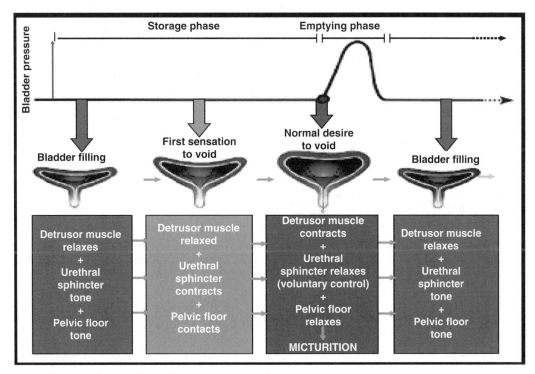

FIG. 15-2. How the bladder works.

symptom, mandates careful analysis as to possible inducing factors, including a range of laboratory analyses of thyroid, liver, and renal function, blood cell count, and glucose levels, to exclude these as possible inducing factors.

Owing to the subjectivity inherent in the patient's sense of fatigue, establishing a diagnosis may be difficult. Schwid et al. (39,40) included three aspects of fatigue as possible presenting symptoms: (a) motor fatigue; (b) lassitude; and

(c) cognitive fatigue. Motor fatigue is the most straightforward and can be assessed as decline in strength occurring during sustained contractions (41,42); in these tests, fatigue did not correlate with muscle weakness, suggesting that the two phenomena are distinct (41). Lassitude, defined as a subjective sense of reduced energy, is far less amenable to study and depends completely on patient reports; Schwid et al. (43) have devised the so-called Rochester Fatigue Diary to help systematize these reports, and achieved some success in assessing reductions in fatigue as a result of cooling vests. Attempts to assess cognitive fatigue have met with varying success, depending on experimental design. Parmenter et al. (44) found no difference between performance of MS patients during periods of high and low fatigue, whereas Schwid et al. (40) found that one measure, the Paced Serial Audition Test (PASAT), employed in a test requiring sustained attention, did yield a significant decline in performance in MS patients but not in healthy controls as the test wore on (an effect attributed to cognitive fatigability).

Pathophysiology of Fatigue

The pathophysiology of MS fatigue is not understood. The two principal mechanisms that have been proposed are (a) action of activated leukocytes or their secreted inflammatory mediators on nerve function, and (b) loss of function in central and peripheral neuronal pathways by demyelination, which could result in diminished recruitment of peripheral motor units, as well as increased central fatigue in performance on nonmotor tasks (26,40). Evidence is not strong in either instance, and certainly cannot yet form the basis for treatment strategies. While there are elevated levels of inflammatory cytokines in MS, and the administration of these molecules can induce somnolence, there is no direct evidence linking these changes to fatigue in MS patients (39). Regarding demyelination and axonal loss, magnetic resonance imaging (MRI) measurements have not shown any association between brain atrophy or lesion load and fatigue (45,46). There is evidence, however, from fluorodeoxyglucose positron emission tomography

(FDG-PET), of widespread brain hypometabolism in MS patients compared to healthy controls (47). In another report, Roelcke et al. (48) found that MS patients with fatigue had lowered glucose metabolism in the bilateral prefrontal cortex and basal ganglia, while MS patients without fatigue did not show this decrement. It is thus conceivable that dysfunction in the neural circuits of these areas is involved in MS fatigue. More recent work by Arnold et al. suggests that fatigue results from diffuse axonal damage, as measured by reduction in whole-brain N-acetyl aspartate (NAA):creatine ratios (252). Refer also to Chapter 13 by Arnold and Tartaglia.

One instance in which proposed physiological mechanisms for fatigue may explain a favorable therapeutic intervention is the case of cooling. Thermosensitivity is a common complaint in MS, and may reflect exacerbation of conduction deficits by body heat induced by exercise; any additional exertion, as would be required to overcome MS-induced conduction block, would further worsen the situation (25). In this connection, White et al. (49) found that precooling by immersion of the legs in 16 to 17°C water significantly reduced fatigue after exercise, as compared to the noncooled trial. Similarly, Schwid et al. (43) reported that wearing a cooling garment led to significant benefit with respect to several MS symptoms, including fatigue.

Management

Management of fatigue symptoms typically involves both pharmacological and nonpharmacological components. Individualized treatment strategies should be devised, taking into account the specific manifestations of MS in a given patient that may contribute to fatigue, such as spasticity, pain, depression, and urogenital complications. Other potential precipitating factors include infections, thyroid complications, medications, or sensitivity to heat (25). As part of a general management strategy, patients should eliminate smoking and adopt commonsense routines for conserving energy, such as properly spacing activities to allow for rest periods or naps, and arranging living quarters with a view to minimizing the effort required in daily tasks. If necessary, aid in developing these strategies can be provided through formal, outpatient energy conservation courses (50). Appropriate exercise programs should be undertaken both for maintenance of general health and to minimize fatigue induced by disuse (51,52). In addition, structured outpatient rehabilitation programs have also shown benefit in reducing MS fatigue (53), and specific measures, such as cooling regimes, can be implemented for those patients who show particular heat sensitivity.

In the event that pharmacological treatment is required, two oral drugs, modafinil and amantadine, have shown efficacy in reducing MS fatigue in clinical trials. Modafinil is an agent that activates brain regions that promote wakefulness (54) and is employed as an agent to treat narcolepsy (25). Two recent trials have supported its use in treating MS fatigue. In the first report, of a placebo-controlled trial involving 72 patients, modafinil was found to provide significant improvement in MS fatigue at a dosage of 200 mg/day, as measured by several scales, including the FSS and MFIS (55). Doses of 400 mg/day did not lead to improvement on these measures, though they did show efficacy on the Epworth Sleepiness Scale (ESS). Very similar results were reported by Zifko et al. (56) in an open-label trial with 50 patients, using dose titration from a starting level of 100 mg; the highest dose employed was 300 mg. Whether measured by the FSS or the ESS, patients reported significant improvement ($p < 0.0001$), with 43 of 50 reporting clear clinical improvement. Modafinil is reasonably well-tolerated; the most common side effects are nausea, headache, nervousness, and insomnia. Suggested procedures are to start at 100 mg/day and to titrate upward for maximal benefit; from the data available, the effects on fatigue in MS are realized at doses below the 400 mg/day that are recommended for narcolepsy (56). Modafinil is currently the drug of choice for treatment of fatigue in MS.

Amantadine, a dopaminergic agent, was examined in a placebo-controlled crossover trial involving 93 patients, together with pemoline, another drug that has been employed in treatment of MS fatigue (57). No improvement was seen with pemoline; in contrast, amantadine showed significant relief of patient-reported fatigue as compared to placebo, when measured by the MS-Specific Fatigue Scale, although no impact was seen on the FSS. Adverse effects include insomnia, irritability, constipation, dizziness, hallucinations, blurred vision, nausea, and headache (25).

In addition to modanifil and amantadine, there are three single reports of medications that gave evidence of reducing MS fatigue, but which require further confirmation. The agents concerned are: (a) oral 4-aminopyridine (58); (b) a transdermal patch containing histamine phosphate and caffeine citrate (59); and (c) acetyl L-carnitine (60). Finally, while they are not specifically indicated for treating fatigue in MS, two other drugs, methylphenidate and fluoxetine, may also be of use. Methylphenidate, an amphetamine, acts as a CNS stimulant and is used in treating excess sleepiness in several neurological conditions (61). Fluoxetine, a selective serotonin reuptake inhibitor, is classically indicated for depression (62), but may also be of assistance in treating refractory MS fatigue (1); its utility may reflect a linkage between fatigue and depression in MS. (34)

PAIN

Pain is a common symptom in MS. In a recent review of studies, Beard et al. (4) found that prevalence varied from 26% to 86% among MS patients, depending on the particular survey, with the majority of studies reporting a prevalence of approximately two-thirds. In survey carried out by the MS Society of the UK, 18% of patients considered pain to be among the three worst symptoms accompanying the disease (63). While one report suggested that the severity of pain correlated with the degree of disability (64), this has not been confirmed by other researchers (65,66). Despite the relevance of MS-associated pain to patients' quality of life, Beard et al. (4) were not able to identify a single randomized, controlled trial to assess the efficacy of standard treatments, with the literature consisting exclusively of small-scale studies and case reports. Ironically, the single exception appears to be the use of cannabinoids, for which one report includes benefit in patient-reported pain (9), and for which other trial data are expected in coming months (67).

Pain symptoms in MS are manifold and varied (4). They may reflect the underlying disease process (as, for example, the neuralgias, dysesthesias, optic neuritis, and the pain associated with MS-induced spasticity), or they may be secondary manifestations of MS-related debility, such as low back pain. Symptoms may be acute or chronic, and a given patient may experience several of them during the course of the disease. Unfortunately, the specific mechanisms leading to the assorted painful syndromes are, as a rule, not understood. Demyelination, the underlying physiological defect of MS, not only affects transmission through established neuronal pathways, but may also lead to secondary effects, such as dysregulation of sodium channel expression, that further perturb normal impulse trafficking (68). As it cannot be predicted how these phenomena will affect a given patient, treatment strategies are of necessity empirical.

Acute Neuropathic Pain

Trigeminal Neuralgia

Trigeminal neuralgia is associated with the second and third roots of the trigeminal nerve, and consists of brief lancinating pains, lasting for a few seconds, that can be triggered by facial movements or light touch to the face. It is not specific to MS, but occurs 400 times more frequently among MS sufferers than among the general population (69) and may be the first presenting symptom of MS (70), especially in younger patients (71). While idiopathic trigeminal neuralgia is thought to involve vascular compression of the trigeminal root, MRI examinations indicate the MS-induced syndrome involves demyelinating lesions of pontine pathways (72). It is generally treated with carbamazepine, a sodium channel blocker, although use of this drug may be limited by side effects and, occasionally, by exacerbation of MS symptoms (70,73); it has also provided relief in MS-related glossopharyngeal neuralgia (74). Alternate antileptic therapies include phenytoin (another sodium channel blocker) (75), gabapentin (76), and lamotrigine (77), with low-dose combinations involving gabapentin and either carbamazepine or lamotrigine also showing efficacy without prompting side effects (75). With all these agents, it is advisable to begin with low doses and to titrate upward, as required. If all pharmacological interventions fail, rhizotomy procedures, including percutaneous radiofrequency rhizotomy (78) and gamma knife radiosurgery (79), have proved effective.

L'hermitte Sign

L'hermitte sign is a shooting, electrical sensation from the spine into the limbs, induced upon flexing the neck; in one survey, two-thirds of patients reported experiencing such episodes (80). While distracting, it is not always considered painful, and symptoms have been successfully alleviated by intravenous administration of lidocaine, a sodium channel blocker (81).

Tonic Spasms

Painful tonic spasms are brief episodes of muscle twitching, lasting from 30 seconds to 2 minutes, that occur in localized body parts, with any region potentially affected; they are often accompanied by intense tingling or burning sensations. Between 10% and 20% of MS patients report their occurrence (82). They can be induced by stimuli such as sudden noises, hyperventilation, or pinpricks, or may occur spontaneously. In the arm, they often begin with tetanic flexion of the fingers and wrists, and may spread up to the face (83,84). Successful treatment has been reported with carbamazepine (84), gabapentin (85), and tiagabine, an inhibitor of the GABA transporter GAT-1 (86).

Paroxysmal Limb Pain

In addition to tonic spasms, MS patients often experience bursts of burning, aching, or itching, lasting for seconds to minutes in the affected limbs, with potential to spread to the pelvic area (87,88). Symptoms have been treated successfully with carbamazepine (87,88), lamotrigine (89), and gabapentin (85).

Acute Radicular Pain

There is a single report of acute radicular pain (90), occurring as the presenting symptom of MS in 11 patients (4% of the total new of MS patients over a 15-year period). No information regarding treatment was provided.

Headache

There have been several single-case reports of headaches that have been correlated with MS-related lesions (91–93). Freedman and Gray (94) also identified 44 cases in which the initial presentation or subsequent exacerbation were marked by migraine-type vascular headache. Rolak and Brown (95) also reported that a diagnosis of MS included a probability that 52% of patients would suffer from headaches, compared to only 18% of matched neurology patients; headaches included both the tension and vascular types. They did not find any correlation, however, between occurrence of headaches and particular clinical features of MS.

Acute Inflammatory Pain: Optic Neuritis

Optic neuritis is an aching pain, sometimes including stabbing-like episodes, in the orbit; it is often worsened by eye movement. It is believed to result from inflammation of the meninges surrounding the optic nerve, and it has been reported to respond to steroid treatment (96). In a formal clinical trial, oral prednisone did not differ significantly from placebo in short-term visual recovery from optic neuritis, whereas significant improvement was seen with administration of intravenous methylprednisolone (1 g/day) given over three days, followed by oral prednisone (1 mg/kg/day) for 11 days (97). At six months, visual function was not significantly different among the three treatment groups.

Chronic Neuropathic Pain

Pain Associated with Spasticity

The complications resulting from increased muscle tone in MS are often accompanied by pain, which is accordingly resolved as a consequence of successful treatment of the spasticity; these issues have been discussed above.

Dysesthetic Limb Pain

This is the most common pain syndrome in MS, consisting of a persistent burning and itching sensation. It is usually felt in the legs and feet but is capable of affecting the arms and torso, as well. Symptoms may be exacerbated by changes in weather. The pain is generally of moderate intensity and is thought to reflect demyelinating lesions in the dorsal column of the spinal cord, since it is accompanied by deficits in sensory deficits in the affected region (87,98). Small-scale studies have reported success in treatment with gabapentin (99,100) and lamotrigine (89,101); tricyclic antidepressants such as amitriptyline may also be of use for some patients (102).

Pain as a Secondary Manifestation of MS

The primary symptoms of MS can lead to assorted other painful debilities, of which the most common is low back pain. Abnormal stress on muscles, bones, and joints can result from spastic weakness, immobility, poor posture, abnormal gait, or improper compensatory adaptations to spasticity and weakness, with resultant acceleration of disc degeneration (4,102). Pressure sores may also result from immobilization. A survey of trials assessing the use of cyclobenzaprine has reported an overall superiority to placebo in alleviating low back pain, although patients on the drug were more likely to suffer from side effects, particularly drowsiness (103). Other approaches may be assayed empirically, including heat treatments, massage, standard over-the-counter analgesics, and ultrasound. Physical therapy, including strengthening exercises, should be maintained.

Steroid-induced osteoporosis may increase the potential for vertebral compression fractures (4). The potential for osteoporotic complications can be reduced by minimizing steroid use, if possible; avoidance of tobacco and excess alcohol; and care to ensure adequate daily intake of calcium and vitamin D. Where necessary, antiresorptive therapies such as alendronate and risedronate may be employed (104).

NEUROPSYCHIATRIC SYMPTOMS

Derangements in mental functioning constitute a significant aspect of the morbidity associated with multiple sclerosis. Their impacts go beyond the immediate expression of a defect, and can lead to major interference with the patients' sense of self and capacity for normal social functioning. They fall into two main classes: defects in cognition, and disorders of mood, affect, and behavior (105).

Cognitive Dysfunction

Cognitive impairment is common in MS, affecting from 40% to over 80% of patients, depending on the tests employed (105,106). In a longitudinal study of 45 patients with early-onset MS, 37 were considered cognitively unimpaired at the baseline assessment, a figure which declined to 20 (representing 56% with impairment) after 10 years (107). As a rule, the defects tend to be less striking than those found in classical cortical dementias such as Alzheimer's disease, with such syndromes as aphasia, apraxia, and agnosia being largely absent. Despite the more subtle nature of MS-related cognitive defects, their impact can nonetheless be severe for patients as well as caregivers. Compared with patients who do not experience cognitive decline, those suffering impairment exhibit more psychopathology and are less likely to be employed or to engage in social activities, while needing greater support in activities of daily living. These social limitations are correlated with the extent of cognitive decline, independent of the degree of physical disability. At the same time, affected patients and caregivers can often be unaware of the extent of their difficulties, since typical measures of disability do not detect many of the cognitive decrements (107,108). Interactions with family members can become especially difficult, leading to potential rupture, if patients' personality defects are not recognized as reflecting the underlying disease rather than being a willful lack of responsibility or acting out (109).

Instead of being part of a global debility, cognitive defects in MS are usually restricted to specific processes. The most common deficits include: (a) memory, especially recent memory, observed in 22% to 31% of patients, leading to difficulties in reading, following medication procedures, remembering recent events, and keeping appointments (110); (b) attention and information processing, leading to patients' perception of being generally slow of thought, easily distracted, and requiring excessive mental effort on routine tasks (105,110,111); (c) executive functions, leading to difficulties in decision-making, problem-solving, and orderly execution of tasks (112); (d) visual spatial abilities, usually unnoticed by patients but reflected in family comments about patients' poor driving (109); and (e) verbal fluency (105,110).

Brain Abnormalities Underlying Cognitive Defects in MS

The relative subtlety of MS-related cognitive deficits, compared to those of Alzheimer's disease, is believed to reflect the predominantly subcortical etiology of MS, with demyelination, by definition, occurring in the white matter (105). The dichotomy is far from complete, however, with up to 26% of lesions detected in MRI studies being within or adjacent to the cortex (113), including significant impact on the thalamus (114). Some mitigation of their impact may result from compensatory cortical reorganization (115). MRI scans have revealed several parameters that have been correlated with cognitive dysfunction (109,116). These include total lesion area (110,117,118), frontal lobe lesion burden (119), corpus callosum atrophy (120,121), posterior fossa lesion volume (122), and measures of brain atrophy, including increased third ventricle size (123), frontal cortex atrophy (124) and overall brain volume (118,121,125). Edwards et al. (121) reported that the correlations between decreased brain volume and cognitive defects were restricted to white matter, with no correlation observed between gray matter volumes and any cognitive test.

Detection of Cognitive Dysfunction

Defects in cognition can often be misdiagnosed as stress, depression, or psychosis (109). While depression is common in MS, the correlation between extent of depression and cognitive defects is usually weak (126), although there is evidence that depressed patients may have defects in working memory capacity (127). Similarly, there are only weak correlations between cognitive dysfunction and physical disability, disease course, gender, age, or disease duration (109,110). Cognitive defects may be accompanied by personality defects such as neuroticism and lack of empathy (128), and may be exacerbated by a variety of medications, including anticholinergics, antileptics, benzodiazepines, muscle relaxants, narcotics, tricyclic depressants, selective serotonin reuptake inhibitors (SSRIs), steroids, and drugs to counter fatigue (109).

Cognitive deficits can be present at all stages of MS, and cognitive decline is progressive (106,129). As disease-modifying therapy may slow the cognitive decline (see below), accurate assessment of cognitive defects is essential. The most accurate determination requires a formal neuropsychological examination, but this is time-consuming, fatiguing for patients, expensive, and not always available in clinical settings (105,109). While self-report scales can reliably predict neurological impairment in MS (130), patients' self-appraisals are not reliable indicators of cognitive defects of which they may be unaware (109,131). A common, rapid screening assessment, the Brief Neuropsychological Battery (110), employs four rapid tests of cognitive function, including the Controlled Oral Word Association Test (COWAT), the Paced Auditory Serial Addition Task (PASAT), and measures of verbal and nonverbal memory. It shows a sensitivity (detection of true positives) of 71% and specificity (rejection of false negatives) of 94%. Recently, an alternative test has been developed, the MS Neuropsychological Screening Questionnaire, which has reported sensitivity and specificity of 83% and 97%, respectively, in reference to caregiver-informant reports on patient cognition. Even with this superior performance, one in six impaired patients would be still missed, and further sensitivity and specificity improvement is required (131).

Therapy

There are no established drugs available for treating MS-related cognition at the symptomatic level. A small, open-label trial with donepezil hydrochloride, an inhibitor of acetylcholinesterase, given for 12 weeks to 17 MS patients resulted in significant improvement in attention, memory, and executive function (132). These data require confirmation in a proper placebo-controlled trial. Counseling programs involving direct training, compensatory strategies, and neuropsychotherapy have shown positive results in one study (133), but not in another (134).

Of the disease-modifying agents used in treating MS (interferon β-1a, interferon β-1b, and glatiramer acetate), both interferon β-1b and interferon β-1a have shown some benefits in alleviating MS-related cognitive deficits (135,136). In addition, interferon β-1a reduced the rate of brain atrophy by 55% (137). A trial with glatiramer acetate proved ineffective in treating cognitive dysfunction (138). At best, the efficacy of these agents is modest in this regard, and is not ordinarily the sole basis on which to initiate (or stop) treatment.

Disorders of Mood, Affect, and Behavior

Depression

Clinical depression is the most serious mood disorder associated with MS, affecting approximately half of all patients at some point in their lives (139,140), and is a major contributor to lowered quality of life associated with the disease (141–143). The most common depressive symptoms experienced by MS patients are irritability, discouragement, and frustration (105), and reactions can be severe. Approximately 30% of MS patients contemplate suicide, and the actual suicide rate is several-fold greater than occurs in the general population, with socially isolated patients and abusers of alcohol especially at risk (105,144).

That patients with MS should be depressed is hardly surprising, given the severity of the disease, the uncertainly as to the physical and mental effects that may lie in wait, and the lack of a cure. Several studies have found that a significant component of depression can be accounted for by stress, degree of disability, modes of coping, and uncertainty (145–147), with feelings of uncertainty being particularly acute during periods of disease exacerbation (148). The correlation with degree of disability has not always been found, however (149). Such a lack seems counterintuitive; it may reflect methodological differences in the studies or the fact that the more disabled patients, in many instances, tend to be older, with a longer history of disease, and accordingly more reconciled to their condition. Depression does appear to be closely correlated with fatigue (150,151), prompting the suggestion that common mechanisms (whether involving psychological factors or brain lesions) may be operating to generate both fatigue and depression (150). In some cases depression may present early in the course of MS, before the onset of any physical or cognitive disability (152).

There is now a substantial body of evidence that depressive symptoms are not entirely psychogenic, with degenerative brain abnormalities playing an important role. In MRI studies, Feinstein et al. (153) found that depressive MS patients had greater lesion volume in the left inferior prefrontal cortex, together with greater atrophy in the left anterior temporal region, than nondepressed MS patients; these differential lesion loads accounted for 42% of the variance in incidence of depression. Other groups have reported similar correlations involving the right temporal lobe (154–157) and left arcuate fasciculus (158). Depression has also been correlated with frontal atrophy and higher lesion scores in superior frontal, superior parietal, and temporal regions (159). In addition to these degenerative brain changes, depression has also been correlated with physiological parameters that are potentially related to central inflammatory reactions, including dysregulation of the hypothalamic–pituitary–adrenal axis (160) and production of the inflammatory cytokines tumor necrosis factor-α and interferon-γ (161,162).

Finally, the development of interferon-β treatments for disease progression was initially accompanied by concerns that they might induce depression. Subsequent studies have not confirmed this general association for either interferon-β-1a or interferon-β-1b (163,164), although depressive episodes may be triggered in patients who already have a past history of psychiatric illness (164).

Treatment of Depression

Current treatment approaches for MS-related depression include both psychotherapy and pharmacological interventions. Mohr et al. (165) reported substantial benefit of psychotherapy, matching sertraline in efficacy, and success was also achieved in telephone counseling sessions, obviating the need for transport to the clinic (166). Similar long-term benefits of psychological therapy involving counseling, relaxation, and physical exercise were observed by Tesar et al. (167). Given the strong correlation between suicidal intent and social isolation (144), maintenance of some form of social contact for patients should form part of treatment strategies.

Pharmacological interventions for MS-related depression follow those already established for depression outside the context of MS. As yet, there are no established approaches that respond to the particular etiology of the MS case other than treatments to halt the progress of the disease. Selective serotonin reuptake inhibitors (SSRIs), including fluoxetine (1) and sertraline (165,168) are effective, with their principal side effect being sexual dysfunction, potentially exacerbating a symptom already common in MS (105). One open-label trial with moclobemide, a monoamine oxidase inhibitor, led to complete remission in 9 of 10 patients, with only minor side effects (169). Tricyclic antidepressants such as amitriptyline and imipramine have historically been used as well (170), but for the most part have been supplanted because of the improved side effect profile of the SSRIs.

Pathological Laughing and Crying (PLC)

PLC is an expressive disorder in which laugher or weeping is triggered in the absence of any corresponding felt emotion. It occurs in approximately 10% of MS patients (171) and is associated with frontal lobe dysfunction (172), although in other neurological conditions disparate regions of the brain may also involved (105). PLC responds to pharmacological treatment with amitriptyline, SSRIs, and dopaminergic-enhancing drugs (105).

Anxiety

While major depression is the most disabling condition found in MS, anxiety is even more common. Feinstein et al. (173) found that clinically significant anxiety was reported by 25% of outpatients (three times the rate for depression) and that anxiety and depression together, rather than either condition on its own, significantly increased the morbidity and social dysfunction associated with MS. An MRI study by Zorzon et al. (155) reported that while depression was associated with brain abnormalities, anxiety was not, and they accordingly described it as being a reactive psychological response to MS. The diagnosis of MS is itself often accompanied by significant increases in anxiety and stress, on the part of both patients and caregivers (174). Treatment of anxiety includes psychological counseling (167) and, if necessary, pharmacological intervention. As with depression, treatment follows standard approaches, with benzodiazepines, SSRIs, and serotonin receptor-1A agonists such as buspirone all showing efficacy in the clinic (175).

Stress

While stress is not a symptom that is readily separable from other psychological consequences of MS, it is important to note that patients have long associated exacerbations of MS with stressful life events. A recent meta-analysis of 14 studies has confirmed the significance of this association, although the effect is modest and not consistent across patients or within individual patients across time. The data also do not allow correlations between exacerbations and specific triggering events (176). The authors recommend that a clinical trial be undertaken to assess whether behavioral counseling in stress reduction leads to any significant impact on exacerbations. In the absence of such definitive data, inclusion of assistance in minimizing stress as part of general patient education in responding to MS is a reasonable precaution.

BLADDER, BOWEL, AND SEXUAL DYSFUNCTION

Bladder Dysfunction

Bladder dysfunction occurs in 50% to 80% of all MS patients over the course of the disease. Severity of bladder problems is not related to disease duration, but does correlate with severity of other neurologic symptoms. Despite rarely leading to life-threatening complications, bladder dysfunction does contribute significantly to the morbidity associated with MS, resulting in considerable disability and lowered quality of life (178,179). Therapy should aim to relieve symptoms as much as possible and to prevent possible complications such as infections and renal damage (1).

Pathophysiology

Micturition involves the coordinated action of several sets of innervation of the bladder musculature. These include: (a) parasympathetic postganglionic efferents that activate the bladder detrusor muscle, while relaxing the internal sphincter, leading to emptying; (b) lumbar sympathetic innervation that relaxes the detrusor muscle while contracting the internal sphincter, promoting urine retention; and (c) voluntary cholinergic innervation to contract the external sphincter, also promoting retention. This innervation is integrated through a spinal reflex arc, and ultimately controlled by pontine structures whose proper functioning is dependent on intact efferent and afferent pathways. The pons also responds to cortical input, allowing for voluntary control of micturition.

Demyelination in MS can affect neuronal function at several of these sites, leading to loss of urinary control as well as bladder and urethral spasms. The most common syndrome, seen in 50% to 90% of MS patients, is detrusor hyperreflexia, involving spontaneous and uncontrolled detrusor contractions and leading to frequent voiding of small amounts of urine. Approximately half of these patients will also suffer from detrusor sphincter dyssynergia, caused by concomitant spontaneous contractures of the external urinary sphincter, leading to high intravesical pressure and poor emptying, and potential complications such as hydroureteronephrosis and infections (179), which can in turn trigger relapses (180). Detrusor sphincter dyssynergia may also be caused by the reverse condition, simultaneous relaxation of the bladder wall and the external sphincter, resulting in incontinence and overfilling.

Damage to sacral parasympathetic pathways can lead to a third syndrome, detrusor hyporeflexia, or flaccid bladder, in which the bladder fails to empty (postvoid volume > 150 cc). Over time, most of these patients will ultimately develop detrusor hyperreflexia and possibly dyssynergia (177). All three syndromes may be accompanied by symptoms of urgency, frequency, and incontinence; detrusor hyporeflexia and detrusor sphincter dyssynergia may also include symptoms of concomitant urgency and hesitancy. As symptoms are shared among the different conditions, determination of postmicturitional residual volumes, using a catheter or ultrasound, will usually be required to select among treatment options.

Treatment

Treatment is directed toward achieving complete bladder emptying while increasing the interval between micturition, reducing incontinence, and avoiding urinary tract infections and complications arising from high detrusor filling pressures. These complications include bladder and kidney stones, hydronephrosis, pyelonephritis, and renal insufficiency (181).

Detrusor hyperreflexia

Detrusor hyperreflexia, the most common problem, responds to several oral agents.

Anticholinergics (antimuscarinics) Blockers of muscarinic receptors are the first-line treatment for urgency and incontinence. The most widely prescribed is oxybutynin; the most common side effect is dry mouth, blurred vision, and constipation (182). Alternative muscarinic blockers include propantheline bromide and flavoxate hydrochloride (1), as well as tolterodine. Tolterodine has shown equal efficacy, with fewer side effects, than oxybutynin (183). Oxybutynin and tolterodine are available in regular (twice a day) or long-acting (once per day) formulations. A transdermal form of oxybutynin, requiring application only twice per week, is also now available.

Imipramine Imipramine is a tricyclic antidepressant with anticholinergic, alpha-adrenergic, and central nervous system effects. It can prove helpful on its own or in conjunction with oxybutynin, with both drugs being given at lower than normal doses to reduce the possibility of side effects (177).

Desmopressin Desmopressin is a vasopressin analogue; taken in tablet form or as a nasal spray, it can aid in reducing daytime frequency or nocturia in patients who do not respond to other oral therapies. As it acts to increase water reabsorption at the collecting tubule of the kidney, serum sodium levels should be monitored in the first weeks of treatment if patients show any of the adverse events (headache, nausea, or vomiting) that accompany dilutional hyponatremia (182).

Detrusor hyporeflexia

There are no truly effective pharmacological treatments for detrusor hyporeflexia. Moderate cases may be relieved through the Credé maneuver of bladder massage (177), possibly including taking an alpha-sympathetic blocking agent such as terazosin to reduce urethral outlet resistance pressure (1,177). If these measures do not reduce retention volumes below 100 cc, intermittent self-catheterization or a permanent indwelling catheter are possible options, though the latter carries the risk of urinary tract infections, urethral stricture, callus formation, or urethrocutaneous fistula (177).

Detrusor sphincter dyssynergia

Treatment of detrusor sphincter dyssynergia depends on the particular form of the faulty coordination and consequent residual urine volume. If the retention volumes are excessive, catheterization will be required; alternatively, if volumes are small, owing to hyperrflexia, anticholinergic medications can assist by relaxing the bladder wall.

Finally, if all other approaches fail, various adjunctive measures such as pads, undergarments, or condom catheters may alleviate discomfort. These measures are far from ideal, however, and carry the risk of introducing further complications, including increasing the potential for infections, skin and penile ulcerations, as well as the attendant awkwardness of changing or wearing a leg bag (177). In addition, the potential role of botulinum toxin (184), urethral stents (185), and other more radical surgical approaches to bladder dysfunction in MS remain promising areas of ongoing research.

Spasms

As with other symptoms of bladder dysfunction, bladder and urethral spasms require empirical treatment. Factors that can contribute to their alleviation include frequent emptying and treatment of lower limb spasticity and constipation. Drugs that may be of assistance include baclofen, benzodiazepines, smooth muscle relaxants such as hyoscine butylbromide, and oxybutynin. If spasms impede urethral catheterization, use of an anesthetic such as lidocaine jelly may assist in the process (1).

Bowel Dysfunction

The prevalence of bowel dysfunction in MS is significantly higher than in the general population, with surveys indicating that from 39% to 73% of patients suffer from constipation, fecal incontinence, or both (186,187). In one survey, frequency of both constipation and fecal incontinence correlated with duration of disease and genitourinary symptoms, and was common even among mildly disabled patients (186). Bowel dysfunction is a significant contributor to disability and has been ranked third among the most troublesome symptoms in limiting ability to work (187).

Pathophysiology of bowel dysfunction is not well understood, beyond the assumption that demyelinating lesions are ultimately involved. Spinal and cerebral involvement has been implicated in some electrophysiological studies, but as these did not include a MS control group, the results may have been a feature of MS rather than a specific issue related to bowel dysfunction (187). One study (188) reported that paradoxical puborectalis contraction is common among MS patients suffering from constipation, suggesting the presence of inadequate voluntary sphincter control, analogous to detrusor sphincter dyssynergia. Contributing factors may include other MS syndromes such as muscle weakness, spasticity, fatigue, and poor mobility, as well as some classes of drugs, including antidepressants, antispasticity agents, and cholinergic blockers prescribed for comorbid bladder problems (187).

Treatment is basically empirical, with patient education an important component of management. Constipation is best approached through commonsense measures including physical exercise, maintaining a high-fiber diet, drinking sufficient water, and establishing a bowel program routine. If necessary, bulk formers or softeners can help to regulate stool hardness, while mild laxatives, suppositories, and enemas can be employed (but, ideally, not on a regular basis) (1). Diarrhea and incontinence should be managed through use of bulk-forming agents and attention to routine. Biofeedback training, involving a focus on improving strength of pelvic floor muscles and rectal sensory perception, has also proved useful in decreasing urge incontinence among MS patients (189). If symptoms are not due to impaction with overflow, drugs such as loperamide or codeine phosphate are effective in treating incontinence (187). Bowel spasms that result in incontinence may be minimized with oxybutynin.

Sexual Dysfunction

Sexual dysfunction is common among MS patients, affecting up to 80% of men and over 50% of women. In addition to direct effects of demyelination on the nerve tracts controlling sexual response, sexual problems may also reflect other impacts of MS, including bladder and bowel dysfunction, pain, spasticity, and effects on personality as manifested in depression, anxiety, and cognitive changes (1). Complications may also ensue as a result of medications, many of which impair erectile function. These include tricyclic antidepressants, SSRIs, benzodiazepines, antihypertensives, antineoplastics, neuroleptics, antihistamines, anticonvulsants, anticholinergics, and hormonal therapies such as estrogens and glucocorticoids. (181). Sexual disorders may occur early in the course of the disease and tend to accompany bladder and bowel difficulties (179).

Innervation of the penis and clitoris includes somatic afferents and efferents, carried in the pudendal nerve, as well as sympathetic and parasympathetic contributions that mediate erection, ejaculation, and detumescence. In addition, several centers in the brain have been implicated in sexual feeling and erectile response, including cortex, thalamus, hippocampus, hypothalamus, limbic system, and pons (179,181,190). MS-related lesions in any of these areas, or in ascending or descending spinal cord pathways, could accordingly contribute to sexual dysfunction. In addition, disruption of the hypothalamic–pituitary axis, which is known to occur in MS (160), can contribute to sexual difficulties in women through impacts on hormonal balances (182).

Decreased libido and perineural sensation are common in both sexes. Women may also suffer from vaginal dryness and itching, failure to reach orgasm, and pain during intercourse, while problems in men include erectile dysfunction (estimated to be as high as 70% in MS) and ejaculatory disorders (in 35% to 50% of patients) (182).

Treatment

Given the importance of psychological factors in sexual response, patient education is an important component of treatment, and properly structured counseling programs can yield significant improvement (191). Measures such as appropriate scheduling of antispasticity medications to obviate spasms, proper bowel and bladder care, control of fatigue, and use of vibrators and other sexual aids all can contribute to more successful love-making (1).

Impaired vaginal lubrication can be treated with vaginal creams, with some varieties including estrogens that can improve clitoral sensitivity and reduce pain associated with intercourse (182). To date, there are no drugs that are of use for treating female sexual response. One placebo-controlled crossover trial, involving 19 women with spinal cord injuries, suggested that the phosphodiesterase inhibitor sildenafil may lead to some improvement in arousal (192), but a recent trial with MS patients resulted in only limited benefit (in the lubrication domain of sexual function) without any improvement in overall quality of life (193).

In men, sildenafil has proved useful in treating sexual dysfunction. It acts to prevent the breakdown of cyclic guanine monophospate, whose local increase is induced by release of NO, resulting in smooth muscle relaxation, penile engorgement of blood, and erection. In a trial with 217 MS patients, 90% reported better erections as compared to 24% on placebo (194); side effects were tolerable, with the principal adverse events being headache, flushing, nasocongestion, and dyspepsia. Two new agents, vardenafil and tadalafil, which have the same basic mode of action but differing in speed of onset and duration of effect, have also shown efficacy in clinical trials (195). Although they have yet to be tested in MS patients, they appear to be promising candidates, given that they also act locally on the penis and should accordingly not be affected by demyelinating lesions.

Several alternative approaches have also employed to treat erectile dysfunction (181). These include: (a) intracavernosal injection of prostaglandin E1 (196), as well as papaverine, phentolamine, and moxisylite (the potential side effects are priapism, pain, and scarring); (b) external vacuum devices that produce penile rigidity, which is subsequently maintained by constriction bands to prevent venous drainage; and (c) surgically implanted prostheses, which may be rigid, semirigid, or inflatable.

TREMOR

Tremor, defined as an involuntary, rhythmic, oscillatory movement of a body part, is one of the most disabling symptoms in MS, and is estimated to occur in 75% of patients. Precise estimates are difficult, as tremor may form only part of a complex movement disorder; it is often accompanied by gait ataxia, as well as titubation and dysarthria (37). MS-related tremor has been described in relation to the head, neck, vocal cords, trunk, and limbs. It may be postural or kinetic, occurring during directed movements. Two types of kinetic tremor have been defined: intention tremor, involving increases in amplitude during visually guided movement toward a target, often rendering the attempt impossible, and action tremor, characterized by rhythmic oscillation around the path of movement. Both types of kinetic tremor frequently coexist in the same patient. Lesions in the cerebellum are particularly associated with kinetic tremors, but tremor may also result from pyramidal and thalamic lesions (1,198).

Physiotherapy and speech therapy may aid patients in control of movements and vocalization, respectively, but results are not guaranteed. There are no standard pharmacological treatments. Various drugs have shown some utility, but rarely in more than a minority of patients. Agents that are potentially useful include benzodiazepines, propanolol, hydroxyzine, trihexyphenidyl, carbamazepam, and isoniazid (1,198). An early trial of intravenous ondansetron, a 5-HT3 antagonist, showed promise in relieving cerebellar tremor (198), but this has not been confirmed in a subsequent trial (199). Recently, gabapentin has shown

promise in a small trial (200), but these findings require confirmation. If tremor symptoms reflect the occurrence of a relapse, standard corticosteroid management may provide relief.

Surgical approaches include stereotactic thalamotomy and deep brain thalamic stimulation, using an implantable electrode. A comparison of the two approaches indicated that they were of equivalent efficacy, with tremor being substantially reduced in the great majority of patients, but that the stimulation protocol involved fewer side effects (201). A recent review of results with chronic deep brain stimulation has confirmed its overall efficacy, with approximately 87% of patients showing some sustained relief of tremor, and 76% experiencing improvement in daily functioning (202). In some cases, efficacy declines over time, and frequent reprogramming may be required to maintain control. This approach thus appears promising, but it does carry all the risks inherent in major surgery.

VERTIGO

Vertigo occurs in approximately 20% of MS patients during the course of their illness. If the condition reflects demyelinating lesions, the medial vestibular nucleus and root entry of the auditory nerve are the most common sites (203). Ondansetron, perchlorizine, and cinnarizine are pharmacological options that may provide relief (204,205). It should be noted, however, that not all MS patients suffering from vertigo have brainstem lesions, so proper diagnosis is imperative. In a recent retrospective review, one clinic reported that a majority of MS patients with vertigo suffered from benign paroxysmal positioning vertigo and responded to particle-positioning maneuvers; only 32% suffered from acute MS exacerbations resulting from lesions in the brainstem (206).

WEAKNESS

Muscle weakness is a common MS symptom, leading to reduced respiratory function, stressful alterations of posture, and difficulties in walking (1,207). Weakness is accompanied by lower motoneuron firing rates (208), which, in turn, are believed to reflect defects in central motor control pathways (209). It appears to be a separate phenomenon from MS-induced motor fatigue, since the ability of given muscles to sustain effort is not correlated with inherent muscle strength (41). Weakness is also exacerbated by the relative immobility and disuse that is common in MS.

There are no effective pharmacological therapies for treating MS weakness. An early trial of 3-4 diaminopyridine suggested that it might be effective in enhancing leg strength, though toxicity was a concern (210). This agent is currently in clinical trial to reassess this question. However, a recent review of concluded that there is still no solid evidence that diaminopyridines can be recommended as therapeutic agents in MS treatment (211). A properly structured program of physiotherapy remains the best approach to minimizing the effects of weakness and for maintaining ambulation.

DYSPHAGIA

Dysphagia is a common symptom in MS. Two recent inpatient surveys patients revealed overall prevalences of 24% and 34%, respectively; 59% of patients with permanent dysphagia experienced incidents of coughing or choking during eating (212,213). Prevalence was correlated directly with degree of disability, with 65% of the most severely disabled subjects being affected. All affected patients showed oral involvement, with pharyngeal involvement occurring in patients with Expanded Disability Status Scale (EDSS) scores higher than 7.5. Mild dysphagia was usually accompanied by difficulties in handling liquids, while more severe pharyngeal involvement led to more problems with solids.

Management of dysphagia usually consists of patient education as to proper food selection and therapeutic maneuvers to facilitate swallowing; in more severe cases, videofluoroscopy is indicated to assess the behavior of the oral cavity. In severe cases, where swallowing is likely to lead to aspiration or if intake is insufficient, percutaneous gastrostomy is indicated (205).

NUMBNESS

Numbness is one of the most commonly observed symptoms in MS. It is usually regional, affecting the trunk, an entire limb, or a set of limbs. Numbness may occur in the absence of other symptoms in the same area, or it may also be accompanied by tingling or painful stimuli, described as burning or squeezing. Regional numbness of the trunk, occurring in a suspended distribution, is common in MS and is often associated with a perception of tightness, the "MS hug." Symptoms may be of short duration or they may last for months, or even be permanent. While numbness may cause some loss of function, rendering controlled movements of a limb difficult, for instance, it is rarely seriously debilitating. As there is no treatment, patients can only be provided with counseling to aid in their adaptation to the condition.

PAROXYSMAL SYMPTOMS

The immune attack on the CNS in MS leads to a variety of symptoms that are experienced as brief bursts, lasting for a few seconds to a few minutes. It is thought that these result from short-circuiting caused by demyelinating lesions. Symptoms include pain, dysesthesia, itching, seizures, tonic spasms, loss of vision, ataxia, weakness, akinesia, chorea, dysarthria, and paresthesia. Fortunately, symptoms generally end as abruptly as they began; if necessary, drugs such as anticonvulsants, benzodiazepines, or tricyclic antidepressants can be employed with good success (37).

MANAGEMENT OF ACUTE RELAPSES

Treatment with glucocorticosteroids is the mainstay of relapse management. They exert a wide range of inhibitory actions on inflammatory processes, with the repressive action ultimately based on downregulation of transcription of several key mediators of the immune response. These include immunoglobulins, inflammatory cytokines such as interleukin-2, interferon-γ, and transforming growth factor-α, and adhesion molecules that mediate lymphocyte and macrophage migration to sites of inflammation (214). There is a wide range of potential side effects but, since relapses generally do not occur more than once every 6 months, the short courses of treatment are tolerable.

A standard protocol involves outpatient treatment with intravenous methylprednisolone (typically 1 g/day for 5 days), with or without a tapering course of oral prednisone (215). Although one trial suggested that oral prednisone is as effective as IV methylprednisolone (216), this report has been criticized on methodological grounds (217) and the optimal mode of administration remains unresolved.

Another question at issue is whether glucocorticoid treatment can slow the progress of MS. A meta-analysis of randomized clinical trials of steroid treatment of MS and optical neuritis concluded that while improvement resulted after 30 days, it was not detectable at longer-term follow-up, compared to placebo (218). In another recent report, optic nerve atrophy following optic neuritis was not prevented by a course of intravenous methylprednisone (219).

In a single countervailing study, however, Zivadinov et al. (220) examined the effect of pulsed intravenous methylprednisolone, given every 4 months for 3 years, then every 6 months for 2 more years. Compared to controls who were treated only for relapses, patients receiving regular treatments showed less disability, lower T1 lesion volume, and less brain atrophy, although annual relapse rate was the same in both groups. These results require confirmation in a larger-scale, Phase III trial; if positive outcomes are confirmed, this approach could yield another option, either alone or in combination with existing disease-modifying therapies, for slowing the course of MS.

CANNABIS USE IN MS SYMPTOM MANAGEMENT

Several lines of evidence underlie the current interest in the use of cannabis (marijuana) in the management of MS. Prior to the prohibition of its use in the twentieth century, smoking marijuana had long served as a traditional treatment for a variety of ills, and a series of anec-

dotal reports have suggested that it could alleviate symptoms associated with MS, especially pain and spasticity (221,222). In parallel with a major research effort focused on the physiological basis of cannabis action, larger-scale, randomized clinical trials are currently being conducted with the aim of more rigorously assessing its efficacy in treating MS symptoms.

Physiological Basis for Cannabis Action: The Endocannabinoid System

The hemp plant (*Cannabis sativa*) is a source of several dozen cannabinoids, a family of aromatic hydrocarbons. Work in the 1960s identified two compounds, Δ^9-tetrahydrocannabinol (Δ^9-THC) and cannabidiol (CBD) as the two principal cannabinoids, with only Δ^9-THC showing psycho-active properties (67,222). Subsequent molecular cloning research has identified two principal cannabinoid receptors, CB1 and CB2, both coupled to G-proteins, which not only respond to Δ^9-THC and CBD, but which are also the principal molecular targets for an endogenous family of fatty acid ligands, the endocannabinoids.

Research focused on the function of this system has suggested several mechanisms through which the endocannabinoids could affect symptoms of MS (67,221,222). These include: (a) regulation of excitatory and inhibitory synaptic transmission, both centrally and peripherally (222, 223,224); (b) regulation of muscle tone and prevention of spasticity (225,226); (c) alleviation of relapses, symptoms, and disease progression in animal models of MS, as well as provision of a neuroprotective action (227,228,229); (d) relief of pain, both through inhibiting nociceptive pathways (230,231,232), as well as depressing release of inflammatory cytokines by immune cells (232,233).

Clinical Findings

The clinical literature involving cannabis and MS is not extensive; for the most part it involves anecdotal studies or trials with small numbers of patients, and the results are not consistent. Several caveats are in order when attempting to assess these findings. First, there is a strong placebo effect with MS patients, as much as 65% to 70% (234). Analysis is further complicated by the fact that the strong psychoactive properties of cannabis make it is virtually impossible to conduct a properly blinded trial (9). Finally, as the various cannabinoid compounds are highly lipid-soluble, it is difficult to achieve reproducible concentrations through oral administration. While smoking cannabis is the most efficient means of drug delivery (224), leading to more reproducible blood concentrations and also avoidance of liver metabolism, the attendant risks of inhaling carcinogenic substances are sufficient as to preclude this mode of administration in formal trials (9). Studies are ongoing (2005) to test alternate modes of administration but, meanwhile, interpretation of trial data should include the possible confounding nature of the dosing question.

Anecdotal evidence of benefits of cannabinoids has included relief of spasticity, pain, tremor, and bladder dysfunction (67,221). These were included among a variety of symptoms reported to be alleviated in two surveys of patients' impressions from self-medication; relief of depression and anxiety also ranked high in these reports (234,235).

With one exception, the clinical literature dealing with MS and cannabis deals with single-case studies or trials with small numbers of patients [reviewed in (67)]. Reports describing single patients included reductions in spasticity and ataxia (236) and in amplitude of nystagmus (237), in response to smoked marijuana, as well as relief of spasms, nocturia, and pain in response to oral administration of nabilone, a CB1 receptor agonist (238,239).

Results of small-scale clinical trials, involving 8 to 18 patients, have not been consistent. In a recent trial where patients self-administered cannabis medical extracts sublingually, positive effects were reported in relief of pain, bladder dysfunction, muscle spasms, and spasticity (240). Relief of pain and spasticity was seen not only with Δ^9-THC but also with CBD, suggesting that it may be possible to achieve these benefits without the psychotropic effects that accompany Δ^9-THC. In two earlier studies, administration of oral Δ^9-THC also resulted in improvement in spasticity in some patients (241,242). In contrast, oral Δ^9-THC provided no improvement in another report (243); in fact, these researchers reported a worsening global impression, a result in keeping with another report with smoked marijuana, which led to impairment of postural control in patients suffering from spasticity (244). In recent studies, oral cannabis was also found to be no better than placebo in relieving tremor in MS patients (245), and to exert a proinflammatory action (246), rather than the inhibitory effect that might have been expected from preclinical work.

In the only large, random, clinical trial published to date, patients were randomized per oral Δ^9-THC (n = 206), oral cannabis extract (n = 211), and placebo (n = 213), with treatment continuing for 15 weeks (9). The primary outcome measure was a reduction in spasticity as measured by the Ashworth scale. While both cannabis formulations led to a greater reduction than placebo in this measurement, there was no statistically significant treatment effect (p = 0.40). However, there were significant treatment benefits in patient reported symptoms associated with spasticity (pain, spasms, and sleep), and the authors argue that this may reflect some clinical benefit. These conclusions are open to question, however. On the one hand, as the Ashworth scale does not correlate with other measures of spasticity, its use may have led to an underestimate of benefits (247,248). Moreover, the interpretation of positive patient response data is also complicated by relatively high placebo response rates, as well as significant unblinding. In their commentary on this trial, Metz and Page (248) conclude that while there is now as much evidence in favor of oral cannabinoids as for many standard treatments of spasticity, including baclofen, they should be used only when other treatments have failed, until further data are available as to risks and benefits of different dosing methodologies. The situation may soon become more definitive, as more clinical trials are ongoing, with several scheduled to report over the next year (67).

Adverse Events

Overall, cannabinoids have not been reported to cause significant, acute, severe, adverse events

(67). The principal impact is psychotropic, with an initial "high" followed by a CNS depressive effect, accompanied by drowsiness and reduced motor performance as well as deficits in short-term memory. Anxiety is the most common adverse psychiatric effect and, occasionally, acute toxic psychosis has been reported. (249,250). As cognitive disorders are common in MS (105,106), it will be important to monitor the impact of long-term cannabinoid use on these symptoms. In addition to carrying the carcinogenic dangers implicit in inhalation, cannabinoids can affect a wide range of systems, including impacts on immune, cardiovascular, endocrine, reproductive, and cardiovascular systems (251), so that caution is again warranted over the long term.

CONCLUSION

While research continues apace into the fundamental physiological basis of MS and into strategies for its cure, progress is slow and the alleviation of MS symptoms remains an essential component of MS management. Given the variety and severity of the conditions that can result from demyelination, it is rare that symptoms can be relieved entirely. Nonetheless, through a combination of rehabilitative and pharmacological approaches, substantial relief can often be achieved, allowing patients to live more productively with the disease, and to minimize secondary complications that can arise if symptoms are not treated.

REFERENCES

1. Metz LM, Patten SB, McGowan D. Symptomatic therapies of multiple sclerosis. *Biomed Pharmacother* 1999;53:371–379.
2. Matthews B. Symptoms and Signs of Multiple Sclerosis. In: Compston A, Ebers GC, Lassman H, et al., eds. *McAlpine's Multiple Sclerosis*. 3rd ed. London: Churchill Livingstone, 1998: 145–190.
3. Goodin DS. Survey of multiple sclerosis in Northern California. *Mult Scler* 1999; 5:78–88.
4. Beard S, Hunn A, Wight J. Treatments for spasticity and pain in multiple sclerosis: a systematic review. *Health Technol Assess* 2003;7:iii,ix–x,1–111.
5. Aggarwal A, Parvizi J, Ganz R. Bilateral spontaneous periacetabular fracture: an unusual complication of multiple sclerosis. *J Orthop Trauma* 2004;18:182–185.
6. Ashworth, B. Preliminary trial of carisoprodol in multiple sclerosis. *Practitioner* 1964;192:540–542.
7. Bohannon RW, Smith MB. Interrater reliability of a modified Ashworth scale of muscle spasticity. *Phys Ther* 1987;67:206–207.
8. Jarrett L, Nandi P, Thompson AJ. Managing severe lower limb spasticity in multiple sclerosis: does intrathecal phenol have a role? *J Neurol Neurosurg Psychiatry* 2002;73:705–709.
9. Zajicek J, Fox P, Sanders H et al. Cannabinoids for treatment of spasticity and other symptoms related to multiple sclerosis (CAMS study): multicentre randomised placebo-controlled trial. *Lancet* 2003;362:1517–1526.
10. Satkunam LE. Rehabilitation medicine: 3. Management of adult spasticity. *CMAJ* 2003;169:1173–1179.
11. Bramanti P, Sessa E, Rifici C et al. Enhanced spasticity in primary progressive MS patients treated with interferon beta-1b. *Neurology* 1998;51:1720–1723.
12. Armutlu K, Meric A, Kirdi N, et al. The effect of transcutaneous electrical nerve stimulation on spasticity in multiple sclerosis patients: a pilot study. *Neurorehabil Neural Repair* 2003;17:79–82.
13. Kita M, Goodkin DE. Drugs used to treat spasticity. *Drugs* 2000;59:487–495.
14. Bormann J. Electrophysiology of GABAA and GABAB receptor subtypes. *Trends Neurosci* 1988;11:112–116.
15. Wagstaff AJ, Bryson HM. Tizanidine. A review of its pharmacology, clinical efficacy and tolerability in the management of spasticity associated with cerebral and spinal disorders. *Drugs* 1997;53:435–452.
16. Krause T, Gerbershagen MU, Fiege M, et al. Dantrolene–a review of its pharmacology, therapeutic use and new developments. *Anaesthesia* 2004; 59:364–373.
17. Schmidt RT, Lee RH, Spehlmann R. Comparison of dantrolene sodium and diazepam in the treatment of spasticity. *J Neurol Neurosurg Psychiatry* 1976;39:350–356.
18. Mueller ME, Gruenthal M, Olson WL, et al. Gabapentin for relief of upper motor neuron symptoms in multiple sclerosis. *Arch Phys Med Rehabil* 1997;78:521–524.
19. Cutter NC, Scott DD, Johnson JC, et al. Gabapentin effect on spasticity in multiple sclerosis: a placebo-controlled, randomized trial. *Arch Phys Med Rehabil* 2000;81:164–169.
20. Solaro C, Uccelli MM, Guglieri P, et al. Gabapentin is effective in treating nocturnal painful spasms in multiple sclerosis. *Mult Scler* 2000 6:192–193.
21. Penn RD, Savoy SM, Corcos D, et al. Intrathecal baclofen for severe spinal spasticity. *N Engl J Med* 1989;320:1517–1521.
22. Gracies JM. Physiological effects of botulinum toxin in spasticity. *Mov Disord* 2004;19[Suppl 8]:S120–S128.
23. Snow BJ, Tsui JK, Bhatt MH, et al. Treatment of spasticity with botulinum toxin: a double-blind study. *Ann Neurol* 1990;28:512–515.
24. Hyman N, Barnes M, Bhakta B, et al. Botulinum toxin (Dysport) treatment of hip adductor spasticity in multiple sclerosis: a prospective, randomised, double blind, placebo controlled, dose ranging study. *J Neurol Neurosurg Psychiatry* 2000;68:707–712.
25. Bakshi R. Fatigue associated with multiple sclerosis: diagnosis, impact and management. *Mult Scler* 2003;9:219–227.

26. Comi G, Leocani L, Rossi P, et al. Physiopathology and treatment of fatigue in multiple sclerosis. *J Neurol* 2001;248:174–179.

27. Janardhan V, Bakshi R. Quality of life in patients with multiple sclerosis: the impact of fatigue and depression. *J Neurol Sci* 2002;205:51–58.

28. Colosimo C, Millefiorini E, Grasso MG, et al. Fatigue in MS is associated with specific clinical features. *Acta Neurol Scand* 1995;92:353–355.

29. Djaldetti R, Ziv I, Achiron A, et al. Fatigue in multiple sclerosis compared with chronic fatigue syndrome: A quantitative assessment. *Neurology* 1996;46:632–635.

30. Flachenecker P, Kumpfel T, Kallmann B, et al. Fatigue in multiple sclerosis: a comparison of different rating scales and correlation to clinical parameters. *Mult Scler* 2002;8:523–526.

31. Krupp LB, Alvarez LA, LaRocca NG, et al. Fatigue in multiple sclerosis. *Arch Neurol* 1988;45:435–437.

32. Fisk JD, Pontefract A, Ritvo PG, et al. The impact of fatigue on patients with multiple sclerosis. *Can J Neurol Sci* 1994;21:9–14.

33. Ritvo PG, Fisk JD, Archibald CJ, et al. Psychosocial and neurological predictors of mental health in multiple sclerosis patients. *J Clin Epidemiol* 1996;49:467–472.

34. Bakshi R, Shaikh ZA, Miletich RS, et al. Fatigue in multiple sclerosis and its relationship to depression and neurologic disability. *Mult Scler* 2000; 6:181–185.

35. Voss WD, Arnett PA, Higginson CI, et al. Contributing factors to depressed mood in Multiple Sclerosis. *Arch Clin Neuropsychol* 2002;17:103–115.

36. Krupp LB, LaRocca NG, Muir-Nash J, et al. The fatigue severity scale. Application to patients with multiple sclerosis and systemic lupus erythematosus. *Arch Neurol* 1989;46:1121–1123.

37. Krupp LB, Rizvi SA. Symptomatic therapy for underrecognized manifestations of multiple sclerosis. *Neurology* 2002;58[8 Suppl 4]:S32–S39.

38. Costello K, Harris C. Differential diagnosis and management of fatigue in multiple sclerosis: considerations for the nurse. *J Neurosci Nurs* 2003;35:139–148.

39. Schwid SR, Covington M, Segal BM, et al. Fatigue in multiple sclerosis: current understanding and future directions. *J Rehabil Res Dev* 2002;39:211–224.

40. Schwid SR, Tyler CM, Scheid EA, et al. Cognitive fatigue during a test requiring sustained attention: a pilot study. *Mult Scler* 2003;9:503–508.

41. Schwid SR, Thornton CA, Pandya S, et al. Quantitative assessment of motor fatigue and strength in MS. *Neurology* 1999;53:743–750.

42. Petajan JH, White AT. Motor-evoked potentials in response to fatiguing grip exercise in multiple sclerosis patients. *Clin Neurophysiol* 2000;111:2188–2195.

43. Schwid SR, Petrie MD, Murray R, et al. A randomized controlled study of the acute and chronic effects of cooling therapy for MS. *Neurology* 2003; 60:1955–1960.

44. Parmenter BA, Denney DR, Lynch SG. The cognitive performance of patients with multiple sclerosis during periods of high and low fatigue. *Mult Scler* 2003;9:111–118.

45. Bakshi R, Shaikh ZA, Henschel K, et al. Fatigue in multiple sclerosis: cross-sectional correlation with brain MRI findings in 71 patients. *Neurology* 1999;53:1151–1153.

46. Mainero C, Faroni J, Gasperini C, et al. Fatigue and magnetic resonance imaging activity in multiple sclerosis. *J Neurol* 1999;246:454–458.

47. Bakshi R, Miletich RS, Kinkel PR, et al. High-resolution fluorodeoxyglucose positron emission tomography shows both global and regional cerebral hypometabolism in multiple sclerosis. *J Neuroimaging* 1998;8:228–234.

48. Roelcke U, Kappos L, Lechner-Scott J, et al. Reduced glucose metabolism in the frontal cortex and basal ganglia of multiple sclerosis patients with fatigue: a 18F-fluorodeoxyglucose positron emission tomography study. *Neurology* 1997;48:1566–1571.

49. White AT, Wilson TE, Davis SL, et al. Effect of precooling on physical performance in multiple sclerosis. *Mult Scler* 2000;6:176–180.

50. Vanage SM, Gilbertson KK, Mathiowetz V. Effects of an energy conservation course on fatigue impact for persons with progressive multiple sclerosis. *Am J Occup Ther* 2003;57:315–323.

51. Petajan JH, Gappmaier E, White AT, et al. Impact of aerobic training on fitness and quality of life in multiple sclerosis. *Ann Neurol* 1996;39:432–441.

52. Petajan JH, White AT. Recommendations for physical activity in patients with multiple sclerosis. *Sports Med* 1999;27:179–191.

53. Patti F, Ciancio MR, Reggio E, et al. The impact of outpatient rehabilitation on quality of life in multiple sclerosis. *J Neurol* 2002;249:1027–1033.

54. Scammell TE, Estabrooke IV, McCarthy MT, et al. Hypothalamic arousal regions are activated during modafinil-induced wakefulness. *J Neurosci* 2000;20:8620–8628.

55. Rammohan KW, Rosenberg JH, Lynn DJ, et al. Efficacy and safety of modafinil (Provigil) for the treatment of fatigue in multiple sclerosis: a two centre phase 2 study. *J Neurol Neurosurg Psychiatry* 2002;72:179–183.

56. Zifko UA, Rupp M, Schwarz S, et al. Modafinil in treatment of fatigue in multiple sclerosis. Results of an open-label study. *J Neurol* 2002;249:983–987.

57. Krupp LB, Coyle PK, Doscher C, et al. Fatigue therapy in multiple sclerosis: results of a double-blind, randomized, parallel trial of amantadine, pemoline, and placebo. *Neurology* 1995;45:1956–1961.

58. Rossini PM, Pasqualetti P, Pozzilli C, et al. Fatigue in progressive multiple sclerosis: results of a randomized, double-blind, placebo-controlled, crossover trial of oral 4-aminopyridine. *Mult Scler* 2001;7:354–348.

59. Gillson G, Richard TL, Smith RB, et al. A double-blind pilot study of the effect of Prokarin on fatigue in multiple sclerosis. *Mult Scler* 2002;8:30–35.

60. Tomassini V, Pozzilli C, Onesti E, et al. Comparison of the effects of acetyl L-carnitine and amantadine for the treatment of fatigue in multiple sclerosis: results of a pilot, randomised, double-blind, crossover trial. *J Neurol Sci* 2004;218:103–108.

61. Happe S. Excessive daytime sleepiness and sleep disturbances in patients with neurological diseases: epidemiology and management. *Drugs* 2003; 63:2725–2737.

62. Cheer SM, Goa KL. Fluoxetine: a review of its therapeutic potential in the treatment of depression associated with physical illness. *Drugs* 2001;61:81–110.

63. MS Society. MS Society Symptom Management Survey. London: MS Society; 1997.

64. Brochet B, Michel P, Henry P. Pain complaints in outpatients with multiple sclerosis: description and consequences on disability. *Pain Clinic* 1992; 5:157–164.

65. Archibald CJ, McGrath PJ, Ritvo PG, et al. Pain prevalence, severity and impact in a clinic sample of multiple sclerosis patients. *Pain* 1994;58:89–93.

66. Indaco A, Iachetta C, Nappi C, et al. Chronic and acute pain syndromes in patients with multiple sclerosis. *Acta Neurol (Napoli)* 1994;16:97–102.

67. Killestein J, Uitdehaag BM, Polman CH. Cannabinoids in multiple sclerosis: do they have a therapeutic role? *Drugs* 2004;64:1–11.

68. Waxman SG. Acquired channelopathies in nerve injury and MS. *Neurology* 2001;56:1621–1627.

69. Maloni HW. Pain in multiple sclerosis: an overview of its nature and management. *J Neurosci Nurs* 2000;32:139–144,152.

70. Hooge JP, Redekop WK. Trigeminal neuralgia in multiple sclerosis. *Neurology* 1995;45:1294–1296.

71. Neilson K, Field EA. Trigeminal neuralgia: a cautionary tale. *Br Dent J* 1994;176:68–70.

72. Gass A, Kitchen N, MacManus DG, et al. Trigeminal neuralgia in patients with multiple sclerosis: lesion localization with magnetic resonance imaging. *Neurology* 1997;49:1142–1144.

73. Ramsaransing G, Zwanikken C, De Keyser J. Worsening of symptoms of multiple sclerosis associated with carbamazepine. *BMJ* 2000;320:1113.

74. Minagar A, Sheremata WA. Glossopharyngeal neuralgia and MS. *Neurology* 2000;54:1368–1370.

75. Solaro C, Messmer Uccelli M, et al. Low-dose gabapentin combined with either lamotrigine or carbamazepine can be useful therapies for trigeminal neuralgia in multiple sclerosis. *Eur Neurol* 2000;44:45–48.

76. Cheshire WP. Trigeminal neuralgia: A guide to drug choice. *CNS Drugs* 1997; 7:98–110.

77. Leandri M, Lundardi G, Inglese M, et al. Lamotrigine in trigeminal neuralgia secondary to multiple sclerosis. *J Neurol* 2000;247:556–558.

78. Berk C, Constantoyannis C, Honey CR. The treatment of trigeminal neuralgia in patients with multiple sclerosis using percutaneous radiofrequency rhizotomy. *Can J Neurol Sci* 2003;30:220–223.

79. Huang E, Teh BS, Zeck O, et al. Gamma knife radiosurgery for treatment of trigeminal neuralgia in multiple sclerosis patients. *Stereotact Funct Neurosurg* 2002;79:44–50.

80. Rae-Grant AD, Eckert NJ, Bartz S, et al. Sensory symptoms of multiple sclerosis: a hidden reservoir of morbidity. *Mult Scler* 1999;5:179–183.

81. Sakurai M, Kanazawa I. Positive symptoms in multiple sclerosis: their treatment with sodium channel blockers, lidocaine and mexiletine. *J Neurol Sci* 1999;162:162–168.

82. Vermote R, Ketelaer P, Carton H. Pain in multiple sclerosis patients. A prospective study using the McGill Pain Questionnaire. *Clin Neurol Neurosurg* 1986;88:87–93.

83. Matthews WB. Paroxysmal symptoms in multiple sclerosis. *J Neurol Neurosurg Psychiatry* 1975;38:617–623.

84. Spissu A, Cannas A, Ferrigno P, et al. Anatomic correlates of painful tonic spasms in multiple sclerosis. *Mov Disord* 1999;14:331–335.

85. Solaro C, Lunardi GL, Capello E., et al. An open-label trial of gabapentin treatment of paroxysmal symptoms in multiple sclerosis patients. *Neurology* 1998;51:609–611.

86. Solaro C, Tanganelli P. Tiagabine for treating painful tonic spasms in multiple sclerosis: a pilot study. *J Neurol Neurosurg Psychiatry* 2004;75:341.

87. Moulin DE, Foley KM, Ebers GC. Pain syndromes in multiple sclerosis. *Neurology* 1988;38:1830–1834.

88. Miro J, Garcia-Monco C, Leno C, et al. Pelvic pain: an undescribed paroxysmal manifestation of multiple sclerosis. *Pain* 1988;32:73–75.

89. McCleane G. Lamotrigine can reduce neurogenic pain associated with multiple sclerosis. *Clin J Pain* 1998;14:269–270.

90. Ramirez-Lassepas M, Tulloch JW, et al. Acute radicular pain as a presenting symptom in multiple sclerosis. *Arch Neurol* 1992;49:255–248.

91. Galer BS, Lipton RB, Weinstein S, et al. Apoplectic headache and oculomotor nerve palsy: an unusual presentation of multiple sclerosis *Neurology* 1990;40:1465–1456.

92. Haas DC, Kent PF, Friedman DI. Headache caused by a single lesion of multiple sclerosis in the periaqueductal gray area. *Headache* 1993;33:452–455.

93. Leandri M, Cruccu G, Gottlieb A. Cluster headache-like pain in multiple sclerosis. *Cephalalgia* 1999;19:732–734.

94. Freedman MS, Gray TA. Vascular headache: a presenting symptom of multiple sclerosis. *Can J Neurol Sci* 1989;16:63–66.

95. Rolak LA, Brown S. Headaches and multiple sclerosis: a clinical study and review of the literature. *J Neurol* 1990;237:300–302.

96. Moulin DE. Pain in central and peripheral demyelinating disorders. *Neurol Clin* 1998;16:889–898.

97. Beck RW, Cleary PA, Anderson MM Jr, et al. A randomized, controlled trial of corticosteroids in the treatment of acute optic neuritis. The Optic Neuritis Study Group. *N Engl J Med* 1992;326:581–588.

98. Moulin DE. Pain in multiple sclerosis. *Neurol Clin* 1989;7:321–331.

99. Houtchens MK, Richert JR, Sami A, et al. Open label gabapentin treatment for pain in multiple sclerosis. *Mult Scler* 1997;3:250–253.

100. Samkoff LM, Daras M, Tuchman AJ, et al. Amelioration of refractory dysesthetic limb pain in multiple sclerosis by gabapentin. *Neurology* 1997;49:304-305.

101. Cianchetti C, Zuddas A, Randazzo AP, et al. Lamotrigine adjunctive therapy in painful phenomena in MS: preliminary observations. *Neurology* 1999;53:433.

102. Rudick RA, Goodkin DE, Ransohoff RM. Pharmacotherapy of multiple sclerosis: current status. *Cleve Clin J Med* 1992;59:267–277.

103. Browning R, Jackson JL, O'Malley PG Cyclobenzaprine and back pain: a meta-analysis. *Arch Intern Med* 2001;161:1613–1620.

104. Wei GS, Jackson JL, Hatzigeorgiou C, et al. Osteoporosis management in the new millennium. *Prim Care* 2003;30:711–741.

105. Feinstein A. The neuropsychiatry of multiple sclerosis. *Can J Psychiatry* 2004;49:157–163.

106. Fraser C, Stark S. Cognitive symptoms and correlates of physical disability in individuals with multiple sclerosis. *J Neurosci Nurs* 2003;35:314–320.

107. Amato MP, Ponziani G, Siracubi S. Cognitive dysfunction in early-onset multiple sclerosis: a reappraisal after 10 years. *Arch Neurol* 2001;58:1602–1606.

108. Rao SM, Leo GJ, Ellington L, et al. Cognitive dysfunction in multiple sclerosis. II. Impact on employment and social functioning. *Neurology* 1991;41:692–696.

109. Halper J, Kennedy P, Miller CM, et al. Rethinking cognitive function in multiple sclerosis: a nursing perspective. *J Neurosci Nurs* 2003;35:70–81.

110. Rao SM, Leo GJ, Bernardin L, et al. Cognitive dysfunction in multiple sclerosis. I. Frequency, patterns, and prediction. *Neurology* 1991;41:685–691.

111. Kujala P, Portin R, Revonsuo A, et al. Automatic and controlled information processing in multiple sclerosis. *Brain* 1994;117:1115–1126.

112. Arnett PA, Rao SM, Grafman J, et al. Executive functions in multiple sclerosis: an analysis of temporal ordering, semantic encoding, and planning abilities. *Neuropsychology* 1997;11:535–544.

113. Kidd D, Barkhof F, McConnell R, et al. Cortical lesions in multiple sclerosis. *Brain* 1999;122:17–26

114. Cifelli A, Arridge M, Jezzard P, et al. Thalamic neurodegeneration in multiple sclerosis. *Ann Neurol* 2002;52:650–653.

115. Cifelli A, Matthews PM. Cerebral plasticity in multiple sclerosis: insights from fMRI. *Mult Scler* 2002;8:193–199.

116. Comi G, Rovaris M, Leocani L, et al. Clinical and MRI assessment of brain damage in MS. *Neurol Sci* 2001;22[Suppl 2]:S123–S127.

117. Rovaris M, Filippi M, Falautano M, et al. Relation between MR abnormalities and patterns of cognitive impairment in multiple sclerosis. *Neurology* 1998;50:1601–1608.

118. Filippi M, Tortorella C, Rovaris M, et al. Changes in the normal appearing brain tissue and cognitive impairment in multiple sclerosis. *J Neurol Neurosurg Psychiatry* 2000;68:157–161.

119. Arnett PA, Rao SM, Bernardin L, et al. Relationship between frontal lobe lesions and Wisconsin Card Sorting Test performance in patients with multiple sclerosis. *Neurology* 1994;44:420–425.

120. Rao SM, Bernardin L, Leo GJ, et al. Cerebral disconnection in multiple sclerosis. Relationship to atrophy of the corpus callosum. *Arch Neurol* 1989;46:918–920.

121. Edwards SG, Liu C, Blumhardt LD. Cognitive correlates of supratentorial atrophy on MRI in multiple sclerosis. *Acta Neurol Scand* 2001;104:214–223.

122. Archibald CJ, Wei X, Scott JN, et al. Posterior fossa lesion volume and slowed information processing in multiple sclerosis. *Brain* 2004; Apr 16 [Epub ahead of print]

123. Rao SM, Glatt S, Hammeke TA, et al. Chronic progressive multiple sclerosis. Relationship between cerebral ventricular size and neuropsychological impairment. *Arch Neurol* 1985;42:678–682.

124. Benedict RH, Bakshi R, Simon JH, et al. Frontal cortex atrophy predicts cognitive impairment in multiple sclerosis. *J Neuropsychiatry Clin Neurosci* 2002;14:44–51.

125. Zivadinov R, Sepcic J, Nasuelli D, et al. A longitudinal study of brain atrophy and cognitive disturbances in the early phase of relapsing-remitting multiple sclerosis. *J Neurol Psychiatry* 2001;70:773–780.

126. Kesselring J, Klement U. Cognitive and affective disturbances in multiple sclerosis. *J Neurol* 2001;248:180–183.

127. Arnett PA, Higginson CI, Voss WD, et al. Depression in multiple sclerosis: relationship to working memory capacity. *Neuropsychology* 1999;13:546–556.

128. Benedict RH, Priore RL, Miller C, et al. Personality disorder in multiple sclerosis correlates with cognitive impairment. *J Neuropsychiatry Clin Neurosci* 2001;13:70–76.

129. Kujala P, Portin R, Ruutiainen J. The progress of cognitive decline in multiple sclerosis. A controlled 3-year follow-up. *Brain* 1997;120:289–297.

130. Goodin DS. A questionnaire to assess neurological impairment in multiple sclerosis. *Mult Scler* 1998;4:444–451.

131. Benedict RH, Munschauer F, Linn R, et al. Screening for multiple sclerosis cognitive impairment using a self-administered 15-item questionnaire. *Mult Scler* 2003;9:95–101.

132. Greene YM, Tariot PN, Wishart H, et al. A 12-week, open trial of donepezil hydrochloride in patients with multiple sclerosis and associated cognitive impairments. *J Clin Psychopharmacol* 2000;20: 350–356.

133. Jonsson A, Korfitzen EM, Heltberg A, et al. Effects of neuropsychological treatment in patients with multiple sclerosis. *Acta Neurol Scand* 1993;88:394–400.

134. Lincoln NB, Dent A, Harding J, et al. Evaluation of cognitive assessment and cognitive intervention for people with multiple sclerosis. *J Neurol Neurosurg Psychiatry* 2002;72:93–98.

135. Fischer JS, Priore RL, Jacobs LD, et al. Neuropsychological effects of interferon beta-1a in relapsing multiple sclerosis. Multiple Sclerosis Collaborative Research Group. *Ann Neurol* 2000;48:885–892.

136. Pliskin NH, Hamer DP, Goldstein DS, et al. Improved delayed visual reproduction test performance in multiple sclerosis patients receiving interferon beta-1b. *Neurology* 1996;47:1463–1468.

137. Rudick RA, Fisher E, Lee JC, et al. Use of the brain parenchymal fraction to measure whole brain atrophy in relapsing-remitting MS. Multiple Sclerosis Collaborative Research Group. *Neurology* 1999;53:1698–1704.

138. Weinstein A, Schwid SI, Schiffer RB, et al. Neuropsychologic status in multiple sclerosis after treatment with glatiramer. *Arch Neurol* 1999;56:319–324.

139. Minden SL, Schiffer RB. Affective disorders in multiple sclerosis. Review and recommendations for clinical research. *Arch Neurol* 1990;47:98–104.

140. Sadovnick AD, Remick RA, Allen J, et al. Depression and multiple sclerosis. *Neurology* 1996;46:628–632.

141. Wang JL, Reimer MA, Metz LM, et al. Major depression and quality of life in individuals with multiple sclerosis. *Int J Psychiatry Med* 2000;30:309–317.

142. Fruehwald S, Loeffler-Stastka H, Eher R, et al. Depression and quality of life in multiple sclerosis. *Acta Neurol Scand* 2001;104:257–261.

143. Janssens AC, van Doorn PA, de Boer JB, et al. Anxiety and depression influence the relation between disability status and quality of life in multiple sclerosis. *Mult Scler* 2003;9:397–403.

144. Feinstein A. An examination of suicidal intent in patients with multiple sclerosis. *Neurology* 2002;59:674–678.

145. Mohr DC, Goodkin DE, Gatto N, et al. Depression, coping and level of neurological impairment in multiple sclerosis. *Mult Scler* 1997;3:254–258.

146. Patten SB, Metz LM, Reimer MA. Biopsychosocial correlates of lifetime major depression in a multiple sclerosis population. *Mult Scler* 2000;6:115–120.

147. Lynch SG, Kroencke DC, Denney DR. The relationship between disability and depression in multiple sclerosis: the role of uncertainty, coping, and hope. *Mult Scler* 2001;7:411–416.

148. Kroencke DC, Denney DR, Lynch SG. Depression during exacerbations in multiple sclerosis: the importance of uncertainty. *Mult Scler* 2001;7:237–242.

149. Provinciali L, Ceravolo MG, Bartolini M, et al. A multidimensional assessment of multiple sclerosis: relationships between disability domains. *Acta Neurol Scand* 1999;100:156–162.

150. Bakshi R, Shaikh ZA, Miletich RS, et al. Fatigue in multiple sclerosis and its relationship to depression and neurologic disability. *Mult Scler* 2000;6:181–185.

151. Mohr DC, Hart SL, Goldberg A. Effects of treatment for depression on fatigue in multiple sclerosis. *Psychosom Med* 2003;65:542–547.

152. Haase CG, Tinnefeld M, Lienemann M, et al. Depression and cognitive impairment in disability-free early multiple sclerosis. *Behav Neurol* 2003;14:39–45.

153. Feinstein A, Roy P, Lobaugh N, et al. Structural brain abnormalities in multiple sclerosis patients with major depression. *Neurology* 2004;62:586–590.

154. Berg D, Supprian T, Thomae J, et al. Lesion pattern in patients with multiple sclerosis and depression. *Mult Scler* 2000;6:156–162.

155. Zorzon M, de Masi R, Nasuelli D, et al. Depression and anxiety in multiple sclerosis. A clinical and MRI study in 95 subjects. *J Neurol* 2001;248(5):416–21

156. Zorzon M, Zivadinov R, Nasuelli D, et al. Depressive symptoms and MRI changes in multiple sclerosis. *Eur J Neurol* 2002;9:491–496.

157. Di Legge S, Piattella MC, Pozzilli C, et al. Longitudinal evaluation of depression and anxiety in patients with clinically isolated syndrome at high risk of developing early multiple sclerosis. *Mult Scler* 2003;9:302–306.

158. Pujol J, Bello J, Deus J, et al. Beck Depression Inventory factors related to demyelinating lesions of the left arcuate fasciculus region. *Psychiatry Res* 2000;99:151–159.

159. Bakshi R, Czarnecki D, Shaikh ZA, et al. Brain MRI lesions and atrophy are related to depression in multiple sclerosis. *Neuroreport* 2000;11:1153–1158.

160. Fassbender K, Schmidt R, Mossner R, et al. Mood disorders and dysfunction of the hypothalamic-pituitary-adrenal axis in multiple sclerosis: association with cerebral inflammation. *Arch Neurol* 1998;55:66–72.

161. Mohr DC, Goodkin DE, Islar J, et al. Treatment of depression is associated with suppression of nonspecific and antigen-specific T(H)1 responses in multiple sclerosis. *Arch Neurol* 2001;58:1081–1086.

162. Kahl KG, Kruse N, Faller H, et al. Expression of tumor necrosis factor-alpha and interferon-gamma mRNA in blood cells correlates with depression scores during an acute attack in patients with multiple sclerosis. *Psychoneuroendocrinology* 2002;27:671–681.

163. Patten SB, Metz LM; SPECTRIMS Study Group. Interferon beta1a and depression in secondary progressive MS: data from the SPECTRIMS Trial. *Neurology* 2002;59:744–746.

164. Feinstein A, O'Connor P, Feinstein K. Multiple sclerosis, interferon beta-1b and depression. A prospective investigation. *J Neurol* 2002;249:815–820.

165. Mohr DC, Boudewyn AC, Goodkin DE, et al. Comparative outcomes for individual cognitive-behavior therapy, supportive-expressive group psychotherapy, and sertraline for the treatment of depression in multiple sclerosis. *J Consult Clin Psychol* 2001;69:942–949.

166. Mohr DC, Likosky W, Bertagnolli A, et al. Telephone-administered cognitive-behavioral therapy for the treatment of depressive symptoms in multiple sclerosis. *J Consult Clin Psychol* 2000;68:356–361.

167. Tesar N, Baumhackl U, Kopp M, et al. Effects of psychological group therapy in patients with multiple sclerosis. *Acta Neurol Scand* 2003;107:394–399.

168. Scott TF, Nussbaum P, McConnell H, et al. Measurement of treatment response to sertraline in depressed multiple sclerosis patients using the Carroll scale. *Neurol Res* 1995;17:421–422.

169. Barak Y, Ur E, Achiron A. Moclobemide treatment in multiple sclerosis patients with comorbid depression: an open-label safety trial. *J Neuropsychiatry Clin Neurosci* 1999;11:271–273.

170. Schapiro RT. Medications used in the treatment of multiple sclerosis. *Phys Med Rehabil Clin N Am* 1999;10:437–446,ix.

171. Feinstein A, Feinstein K, Gray T, et al. Prevalence and neurobehavioral correlates of pathological laughing and crying in multiple sclerosis. *Arch Neurol* 1997;54:1116–1121.

172. Feinstein A, O'Connor P, Gray T, et al. Pathological laughing and crying in multiple sclerosis: a preliminary report suggesting a role for the prefrontal cortex. *Mult Scler* 1999;5:69–73.

173. Feinstein A, O'Connor P, Gray T, et al. The effects of anxiety on psychiatric morbidity in patients with multiple sclerosis. *Mult Scler* 1999;5:323–326.

174. Janssens AC, van Doorn PA, de Boer JB, et al. Impact of recently diagnosed multiple sclerosis on quality of life, anxiety, depression and distress of patients and partners. *Acta Neurol Scand* 2003;108:389–395.

175. Rickels K, Rynn M. Pharmacotherapy of generalized anxiety disorder. *J Clin Psychiatry* 2002;63[Suppl 14]:9–16.

176. Mohr DC, Hart SL, Julian L, et al. Association between stressful life events and exacerbation in multiple sclerosis: a meta-analysis. *BMJ* 2004;328:731–735.

177. Andrews KL, Husmann DA. Bladder dysfunction and management in multiple sclerosis. *Mayo Clin Proc* 1997;72:1176–1183.

178. Litwiller SE, Frohman EM, Zimmern PE. Multiple sclerosis and the urologist. *J Urol* 1999;161:743–757.

179. Gallien P, Robineau S. Sensory-motor and genitosphincter dysfunctions in multiple sclerosis. *Biomed Pharmacother* 1999;53:380–385.

180. Metz LM, McGuinness SD, Harris C. Urinary tract infections may trigger relapse in multiple sclerosis. *Axone* 1998;19:67–70.

181. Fernandez O. Mechanisms and current treatments of urogenital dysfunction in multiple sclerosis. *J Neurol* 2002;249:1–8.

182. DasGupta R, Fowler CJ. Bladder, bowel and sexual dysfunction in multiple sclerosis: management strategies. *Drugs* 2003;63:153–166.

183. Abrams P, Freeman R, Anderstrom C, et al. Tolterodine, a new antimuscarinic agent: as effective but better tolerated than oxybutynin in patients with an overactive bladder. *Br J Urol* 1998;81:801–810.

184. Leippold T, Reitz A, Schurch B. Botulinum toxin as a new therapy option for voiding disorders: current state of the art. *Eur Urol* 2003;44:165–174.

185. Chartier-Kastler EJ, Thomas L, Bussel, B, et al. A urethral stent for the treatment of detrusor-striated sphincter dyssynergia. *BJU Int* 2000;86:52–57.

186. Hinds JP, Eidelman BH, Wald A. Prevalence of bowel dysfunction in multiple sclerosis. A population survey. *Gastroenterology* 1990;98:1538–1542.

187. Wiesel PH, Norton C, Glickman S, et al. Pathophysiology and management of bowel dysfunction in multiple sclerosis. *Eur J Gastroenterol Hepatol* 2001;13:441–448.

188. Chia YW, Gill KP, Jameson JS, et al. Paradoxical puborectalis contraction is a feature of constipation in patients with multiple sclerosis. *J Neurol Neurosurg Psychiatry* 1996;60:31–35.

189. Wiesel PH, Norton C, Roy AJ, et al. Gut focused behavioural treatment (biofeedback) for constipation and faecal incontinence in multiple sclerosis. *J Neurol Neurosurg Psychiatry* 2000;69:240–243.

190. Zivadinov R, Zorzon M, Locatelli L, et al. Sexual dysfunction in multiple sclerosis: a MRI, neurophysiological and urodynamic study. *J Neurol Sci* 2003;210:73–76.

191. Foley FW, LaRocca NG, Sanders AS, et al. Rehabilitation of intimacy and sexual dysfunction in couples with multiple sclerosis. *Mult Scler* 2001;7:417–421.

192. Sipski ML, Rosen RC, Alexander CJ, et al. Sildenafil effects on sexual and cardiovascular responses in women with spinal cord injury. *Urology* 2000;55:812–815.

193. Dasgupta R, Wiseman OJ, Kanabar G, et al. Efficacy of sildenafil in the treatment of female sexual dysfunction due to multiple sclerosis. *J Urol* 2004;171:1189–1193.

194. Fowler CJ, Miller J, Sharief M. Viagra® (sildenafil citrate) for the treatment of erectile dysfunction in men with multiple sclerosis. *Ann Neurol* 1999;46:497.

195. Francis SH, Corbin JD. Molecular mechanisms and pharmacokinetics of phosphodiesterase-5 antagonists. *Curr Urol Rep* 2003;4:457–465.

196. Padma-Nathan H, Hellstrom WJ, Kaiser FE, et al. Treatment of men with erectile dysfunction with transurethral alprostadil. Medicated Urethral System for Erection (MUSE) Study Group. *N Engl J Med* 1997;336:1–7.

197. Alusi SH, Glickman S, Aziz TZ, et al. Tremor in multiple sclerosis. *J Neurol Neurosurg Psychiatry* 1999;66:131–134.

198. Rice GP, Lesaux J, Vandervoort P, et al. Ondansetron, a 5-HT3 antagonist, improves cerebellar tremor. *J Neurol Neurosurg Psychiatry* 1997;62:282–284.

199. Gbadamosi J, Buhmann C, Moench A, et al. Failure of ondansetron in treating cerebellar tremor in MS patients—an open-label pilot study. *Acta Neurol Scand* 2001;104:308–311.

200. Lopez del Val LJ, Santos S. Gabapentin in the treatment of tremor. *Rev Neurol* 2003;36:322–326.

201. Schuurman PR, Bosch DA, Bossuyt PM, et al. A comparison of continuous thalamic stimulation and thalamotomy for suppression of severe tremor. *N Engl J Med* 2000;342:461–468.

202. Wishart HA, Roberts DW, Roth RM, et al. Chronic deep brain stimulation for the treatment of tremor in multiple sclerosis: review and case reports. *J Neurol Neurosurg Psychiatry* 2003;74:1392–1397.

203. Frohman EM, Kramer PD, Dewey RB, et al. Benign paroxysmal positioning vertigo in multiple sclerosis: diagnosis, pathophysiology and therapeutic techniques. *Mult Scler* 2003;9:250–255.

204. Rice GP, Ebers GC. Ondansetron for intractable vertigo complicating acute brainstem disorders. *Lancet* 1995;345:1182–1183.

205. Thompson AJ. Symptomatic management and rehabilitation in multiple sclerosis. *J Neurol Neurosurg Psychiatry* 2001;71[Suppl 2]:ii,22–27.

206. Frohman EM, Zhang H, Dewey RB, et al. Vertigo in MS: utility of positional and particle repositioning maneuvers. *Neurology* 2000;55:1566–1569.

207. Tantucci C, Massucci M, Piperno R, et al. Control of breathing and respiratory muscle strength in patients with multiple sclerosis. *Chest* 1994;105:1163–1170.

208. Rice CL, Vollmer TL, Bigland-Ritchie B. Neuromuscular responses of patients with multiple sclerosis. *Muscle Nerve* 1992;15:1123–1132.

209. Ingram DA, Thompson AJ, Swash M. Central motor conduction in multiple sclerosis: evaluation of abnormalities revealed by transcutaneous magnetic stimulation of the brain. *J Neurol Neurosurg Psychiatry* 1988;51:487–494.

210. Bever CT Jr., Anderson PA, Leslie J, et al.Treatment with oral 3,4 diaminopyridine improves leg strength in multiple sclerosis patients: results of a randomized, double-blind, placebo-controlled, crossover trial. *Neurology* 1996;47:1457–1462.

211. Solari A, Uitdehaag B, Giuliani G, et al. Aminopyridines for symptomatic treatment in multiple sclerosis. *Cochrane Database Syst Rev* 2003;(2):CD001330.

212. Calcagno P, Ruoppolo G, Grasso MG, et al. Dysphagia in multiple sclerosis—prevalence and prognostic factors. *Acta Neurol Scand* 2002;105:40–43.

213. De Pauw A, Dejaeger E, D'hooghe B, et al. Dysphagia in multiple sclerosis. *Clin Neurol Neurosurg* 2002;104:345–351.

214. Andersson PB, Goodkin DE. Glucocorticosteroid therapy for multiple sclerosis: a critical review. *J Neurol Sci* 1998;160:16–25.

215. Noseworthy JH. Treatment of multiple sclerosis and related disorders: what's new in the past 2 years? *Clin Neuropharmacol* 2003;26:28–37.

216. Barnes D, Hughes RA, Morris RW, et al. Randomised trial of oral and intravenous methylprednisolone in acute relapses of multiple sclerosis. *Lancet* 1997;349:902–906.

217. De Keyser J, Zwanikken C. Oral versus intravenous corticosteroids in acute relapses of multiple sclerosis. *Lancet* 1997;349:1696

218. Brusaferri F, Candelise L. Steroids for multiple sclerosis and optic neuritis: a meta-analysis of randomized controlled clinical trials. *J Neurol* 2000;247:435–442.

219. Hickman SJ, Kapoor R, Jones SJ, et al. Corticosteroids do not prevent optic nerve atrophy following optic neuritis. *J Neurol Neurosurg Psychiatry* 2003;74: 1139–1141.

220. Zivadinov R, Rudick RA, De Masi R, et al. Effects of IV methylprednisolone on brain atrophy in relapsing-remitting MS. *Neurology* 2001;57:1239–1247.

221. Pertwee, RG. Cannabinoids and multiple sclerosis. *Pharmacol Ther* 2002;95:165–174.

222. Baker D, Pryce G, Giovannoni G, et al. The therapeutic potential of cannabis. *Lancet Neurol* 2003;2:291–298.

223. Schlicker E, Kathmann M. Modulation of transmitter release via presynaptic cannabinoid receptors. *Trends Pharmacol Sci* 2001;22:565–572.

224. Iversen L. Cannabis and the brain. *Brain* 2003;126:1252–1270.

225. Baker D, Pryce G, Croxford JL, et al. Cannabinoids control spasticity and tremor in a multiple sclerosis model. *Nature* 2000;404:84–87.

226. Baker D, Pryce G, Croxford JL, et al. Endocannabinoids control spasticity in a multiple sclerosis model. *FASEB J* 2001;15:300–302.

227. Achiron A, Miron S, Lavie V, et al. Dexanabinol (HU-211) effect on experimental autoimmune encephalomyelitis: implications for the treatment of acute relapses of multiple sclerosis. *J Neuroimmunol* 2000;102:26–31.

228. Croxford JL, Miller SD. Immunoregulation of a viral model of multiple sclerosis using the synthetic cannabinoid R+WIN55,212. *J Clin Invest* 2003;111:1231–1240.

229. Pryce G, Ahmed Z, Hankey DJ, et al. Cannabinoids inhibit neurodegeneration in models of multiple sclerosis. *Brain* 2003;126:2191–2202.

230. Pertwee, RG. Cannabinoid receptors and pain. *Prog Neurobiol* 2001;63:569–611.

231. Walker JM, Huang SM. Cannabinoid analgesia. *Pharmacol Ther* 2002;95:127–135.

232. Hohmann AG. Spinal and peripheral mechanisms of cannabinoid antinociception: behavioral, neurophysiological and neuroanatomical perspectives. *Chem Phys Lipids* 2002;121(1–2):173–190.

233. Klein TW, Friedman H, Specter S. Marijuana, immunity and infection. *J Neuroimmunol* 1998;83:102–115.

234. Consroe P, Musty R, Rein J, et al. The perceived effects of smoked cannabis on patients with multiple sclerosis. *Eur Neurol* 1997;38:44–48.

235. Page SA, Verhoef MJ, Stebbins RA, et al. Cannabis use as described by people with multiple sclerosis. *Can J Neurol Sci* 2003;30:201–205.

236. Meinck HM, Schonle PW, Conrad B. Effect of cannabinoids on spasticity and ataxia in multiple sclerosis. *J Neurol* 1989;236:120–122.

237. Schon F, Hart PE, Hodgson TL, et al. Suppression of pendular nystagmus by smoking cannabis in a patient with multiple sclerosis. *Neurology* 1999;53:2209–2210.

238. Martyn CN, Illis LS, Thom J. Nabilone in the treatment of multiple sclerosis. *Lancet* 1995;345:579.

239. Hamann W, di Vadi PP. Analgesic effect of the cannabinoid analogue nabilone is not mediated by opioid receptors. *Lancet* 1999;353:560

240. Wade DT, Robson P, House H, et al. A preliminary controlled study to determine whether whole-plant cannabis extracts can improve intractable neurogenic symptoms. *Clin Rehabil* 2003;17:21–29.

241. Petro DJ, Ellenberger C Jr. Treatment of human spasticity with delta 9-tetrahydrocannabinol. *J Clin Pharmacol* 1981;21[8–9 Suppl]:413S–416S.

242. Ungerleider JT, Andyrsiak T, Fairbanks L, et al. Delta-9-THC in the treatment of spasticity associated with multiple sclerosis. *Adv Alcohol Subst Abuse* 1987;7:39–50.

243. Killestein J, Hoogervorst EL, Reif M, et al. Safety, tolerability, and efficacy of orally administered cannabinoids in MS. *Neurology* 2002;58:1404–1407.

244. Greenberg HS, Werness SA, Pugh JE, et al. Short-term effects of smoking marijuana on balance in patients with multiple sclerosis and normal volunteers. *Clin Pharmacol Ther* 1994;55:324–328.

245. Fox P, Bain PG, Glickman S, et al. The effect of cannabis on tremor in patients with multiple sclerosis. *Neurology* 2004;62:1105–1109.

246. Killestein J, Hoogervorst EL, Reif M, et al. Immunomodulatory effects of orally administered cannabinoids in multiple sclerosis. *J Neuroimmunol* 2003;137:140–143.

247. Hinderer SR, Gupta S. Functional outcome measures to assess interventions for spasticity. *Arch Phys Med Rehabil* 1996;77:1083–1089.

248. Metz L, Page S. Oral cannabinoids for spasticity in multiple sclerosis: will attitude continue to limit use? *Lancet* 2003;362:1513

249. Hall W, Solowij N. Adverse effects of cannabis. *Lancet* 1998;352:1611–1616.

250. Killestein J, Polman CH. Cannabis use in multiple sclerosis: excited interest. *Can J Neurol Sci* 2003;30:181–182.

251. Ashton CH. Adverse effects of cannabis and cannabinoids. *Br J Anaesth* 1999;83:637–649.

252. Tartaglia M, Narayanan S, Francis SJ, et al. The relationship between diffuse axonal damage and fatigue in MS. *Arch Neurol* 2004;61(2):176–177.

16

Use of Interferon-Beta in the Treatment of Multiple Sclerosis

Joy Derwenskus[1] and Fred D. Lublin[2]

[1]*Department of Neurology, Northwestern University, Chicago, Illinois;* [2]*Department of Neurology, Mount Sinai School of Medicine, New York, New York*

INTRODUCTION

Three beta-interferons (IFNβs) have been approved for the treatment of multiple sclerosis (MS). These disease-modifying agents (DMAs) are approved for relapsing forms of MS, but the data regarding the efficacy of these agents in secondary progressive MS are conflicting. None of the DMAs are approved for primary progressive MS. All of the IFNβ therapies are given via injection. The first agent approved by the U.S. Food and Drug Administration (FDA) to treat MS was IFNβ-1b (Betaseron, Berlex Inc., Montville, NJ) in 1993. Betaseron 0.25 mg or 8 million international units (MIU) is administered subcutaneously (SC) every other day. In 1996, IFNβ-1a (Avonex, Biogen Idec, Cambridge, MA) was approved at 30 micrograms (μg) intramuscularly (IM) once a week. Another IFNβ-1a (Rebif, Serono International S.A., Geneva) was approved in 2002 in the United States (earlier in Canada and Europe) and dosed at 22 or 44 μg subcutaneously three times a week (Table 16-1).

MECHANISM OF ACTION

Interferons (IFNs) were first described by Isaac and Lindenmann in 1957. They are thought to exhibit many effects in the body's defense of microbial, viral, and neoplastic insults by way of complex interactions with cytokines (1). Interferons have been tested with limited toxicity in many diseases. Currently, IFNs are used to treat condyloma acuminatum, hepatitis B and C, hairy-cell leukemia, Kaposi's sarcoma, chronic granulomatous disease, and MS. IFNs are produced via recombinant processes. IFNβ-1b is produced in *Escherichia coli,* while IFNβ-1a is produced in Chinese hamster ovary cells.

The exact mechanism of action of IFNβ is unknown, but it likely has multiple effects on the immune response. IFNβs are thought to inhibit

TABLE 16-1 *Three IFNβ injections approved for relapsing MS*

IFN Type	Dose	Route	Frequency	Approved in U.S.
IFNβ-1b (Betaseron)	0.25 mg	SC	Every other day	1993
IFNβ-1a (Avonex)	30 μg	IM	Once weekly	1996
IFNβ-1a (Rebif)	44 μg	SC	Three times weekly	2002

antigen presentation and, as a result, decrease T cell production of IFN gamma. There also may be a shift from T helper 1 (Th1) to T helper 2 (Th2) lymphocyte cytokine secretion that inhibits inflammation. The effect of IFNβ at the blood–brain barrier is secondary to several different mechanisms. The trafficking of T lymphocytes into the central nervous system is reduced by downregulating adhesion molecules such as intercellular adhesion molecule-1 (ICAM-1) and vascular cell adhesion molecule-1 (VCAM-1) on the surface of endothelial cells, and decreasing the production of matrix metalloproteinases. Lymphocytes must first bind to these adhesion molecules in order to migrate through the vessel endothelial wall. Access to the blood–brain barrier is gained by breaking down the basement membrane with matrix metalloproteinases. The overall effect of IFNβ is complex and not entirely elucidated. It generally affects cytokine production and alters the blood–brain barrier so T cells have reduced entry into the central nervous system (2).

PIVOTAL STUDIES

Relapsing-Remitting MS

The first pivotal trial leading to FDA approval of IFNβ in relapsing-remitting multiple sclerosis (RRMS) was reported by the IFNB Multiple Sclerosis Study Group (3,4). This was a randomized, double-blind, placebo-controlled study of 372 patients with a one year history clinically definite MS. To be eligible for the study patients had to be 18 to 50 years old, ambulatory, with an Expanded Disability Status Scale (EDSS) of 0 to 5.5, have two acute exacerbations in the previous two years, and clinically stable for 30 days prior to study entry. Patients were randomized to either 1.6 or 8 MIU IFNβ-1b or placebo given as SC injections every other day. The study duration was intended to be 2 years, but there was a third year as

part of a double-blind extension. The primary outcome measures were annual exacerbation rate and proportion of exacerbation-free patients. Secondary outcome measures included time to first exacerbation, severity of exacerbations, change from baseline EDSS, and magnetic resonance imaging (MRI) disease burden and activity.

There was a significant reduction in exacerbation rate of almost 34% for the higher-dose IFNβ-1b group (1.27 attacks per year for placebo, 1.17 attacks per year for 1.6 MIU group, and 0.84 attacks per year for 8 MIU group). There was also a significant reduction in the number of patients exacerbation-free between the placebo and 8 MIU groups at 2 years, although this did not remain significant at 3 years (Fig. 16-1). The time to first exacerbation was delayed in the 8 MIU group compared with placebo and the exacerbations were milder, requiring fewer hospitalizations. There was no significant difference in disability between the groups and EDSS increased from baseline in all three groups.

MRI scans were done at baseline and yearly in all patients (4,5). A subset of 52 patients followed at the University of British Columbia had MRI scans every 6 weeks for the first 2 years of the study. The percentage change in burden of disease was significantly different between the groups (12% increase in T2 lesion area for the placebo group compared with 1% decrease in the 8MIU group at year 1; 17% increase in placebo compared with 6% decrease in the 8 MIU group at year 3). In the group with more frequent MRI scans, there was 83% reduction in active lesions in patients receiving 8 MIU IFNβ-1b compared to placebo. The higher-dose group also demonstrated a 75% reduction in new lesion formation. Gadolinium-enhanced scans were not performed in this trial.

The pivotal study of IFNβ-1a (Avonex) that led to approval in 1996 was a randomized, double-blind, placebo-controlled study of 301 patients

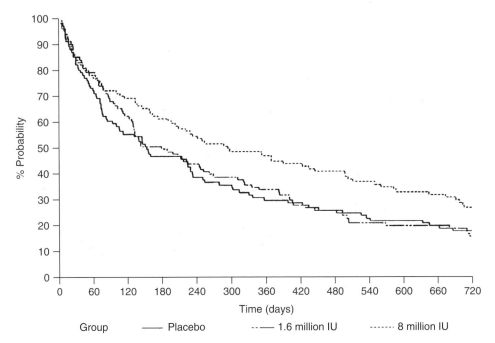

FIG. 16-1. The IFNB Multiple Sclerosis Study Group demonstrated a significant reduction in patients remaining exacerbation-free between placebo and 8 MIU IFNβ-1b during the first 2 years of the study. (From The IFNB Multiple Sclerosis Study Group. Interferon beta-1b is effective in relapsing-remitting multiple sclerosis. I. Clinical results of a multicenter, randomized, double-blind, placebo-controlled trial. *Neurology* 1993;43:655–661.)

with RRMS (6). Patients included were 18 to 55 years old, had definite MS for at least 1 year, an EDSS of 1.0 to 3.5, two exacerbations in the previous 3 years, and no exacerbations for 2 months prior to study entry. Exclusion criteria included prior immunomodulatory or IFN therapy. Patients were assigned to receive 6 million units (30 μg) IFNβ-1a or placebo given via intramuscular injection once weekly for 2 years. The primary outcome measure was time to sustained disability for 6 months as determined by an increase of 1.0 point from the baseline EDSS. Various secondary outcomes such as exacerbation rate, MRI T2 lesion volume, and gadolinium enhancement were measured. The study was terminated early, as there were fewer dropouts than anticipated. There was a significant difference in the time to disability in the actively treated group compared with placebo. Approximately 35% of the placebo group reached sustained disability compared with 22% of the IFNβ-1a group (Fig. 16-2). The annual exacerbation rate for patients in the study for 2 years was

significantly reduced (by 32% from 0.9 in the placebo group to 0.61 in the IFNβ-1a group), but for the entire intent-to-treat group the reduction was 18%. MRI gadolinium activity was also significantly reduced favoring the treated group (30% in IFNβ-1a versus 42% in placebo). The change in T2 lesion volume was not significant at year 2.

The Prevention of Relapses and Disability by Interferon β-1a Subcutaneously in Multiple Sclerosis (PRISMS) trial was the pivotal study leading to approval of IFNβ-1a (Rebif) (7). This study included 560 patients with definite RRMS for at least 1 year. Eligibility criteria included two relapses in the previous 2 years and an EDSS of 0 to 5.0. Patients were excluded if treated with IFN, cyclophosphamide, or other immunosuppressant agents for 12 months prior to study entry. The patients were randomized to receive IFNβ-1a 22 μg (6 MIU), 44 μg (12 MIU), or placebo via SC injections three times a week for 2 years. The primary outcome measure was reduction in relapse rate. The severity of relapses, time to relapse, proportion of relapse-free patients, progression in disability (determined by a 1.0 point increase in EDSS sustained for 3 months), need for steroid treatment or hospitalization, and MRI activity and disease burden were secondary outcome measures. There was a significant reduction in mean relapses in both treated groups compared with placebo (27% in the 22 μg IFNβ-1a group and 33% in the 44 μg IFNβ-1a group). Most of the secondary outcome measures were also significant in favor of the treated groups. Relapses were less severe and the time to first relapse was delayed by 3 months in the 22 μg IFNβ-1a group and 5 months in the 44 μg IFNβ-1a group. There was also less worsening by 1.0 point in EDSS, fewer courses of steroids, and fewer hospitalizations in the treated groups.

An MRI study was included as part of PRISMS (8). All patients had a baseline and semiannual MRI scans done for the duration of the study. Two hundred and five of the 560 patients had monthly MRI scans including 1 month prior to study entry, the day before starting treatment, and then monthly for 9 months. Upon study conclusion, the burden of disease increased by 10.9% in the placebo group, while it decreased 1.2% and 3.8% in the 22 μg and 44 μg IFNβ-1a groups, respectively. T2 activity and the number of new gadolinium-enhancing lesions were also decreased in both treatment groups. There was a trend for dosing effect, with better outcomes in the higher-dose IFN group.

The PRISMS study was extended to four years (PRISMS-4) (9). Patients from the original 2-year cohort were eligible for the extension if their condition was stable enough to continue in a blinded study. The extension phase did not include a placebo group. The placebo group from the initial 2-year study was randomized to receive either 22 μg or 44 μg IFNβ-1a. The previous 22 μg and 44 μg IFNβ-1a groups were continued on their same regimen. Patients were examined every 3 months in the third year and every 6 months in the fourth year. MRI scans were performed annually. The primary outcome remained the number of relapses. Additional secondary outcome measures were time to second relapse, percentage of relapse-free patients, severity of relapse, steroid use, hospitalization, and a disability measure of time to EDSS progression of 1.0 point sustained for at least 3 months. MRI scans were analyzed for disease burden and T2 activity.

There was a significant reduction in relapse rate in the patients on treatment for the full 4 years compared with the crossover groups. There was a trend for fewer relapses in the 44 μg IFNβ-1a group compared with the 22 μg IFNβ-1a group for 4 years. However, this was not significant. The effect on relapse rate was

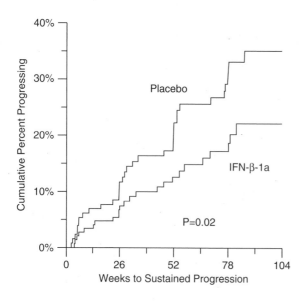

FIG. 16-2. The time to sustained disability progression of 1.0 point on EDSS during the pivotal IFNβ-1a trial given once weekly. (From Jacobs LD. Intramuscular interferon beta-1a for disease progression in relapsing multiple sclerosis. *Ann Neurol.* 1996;39:285–294.)

greatest in the group treated with 44 μg IFNβ-1a for the entire 4-year study duration. The time to confirmed EDSS progression was significantly prolonged in the high-dose group compared with the crossover group (42.1 versus 24.2 months). The Kaplan–Meier curve graphically displays the crossover group never catching up to the group on high-dose treatment for the entire 4 years. Other secondary measures were significant in favor of 4 years of treatment versus the crossover groups, with the greatest benefit occurring in the higher-dose IFN. The MRI measures detected significantly fewer new T2 lesions in the 44 μg IFNβ-1a group. The burden of disease also favored higher-dose IFN, with a demonstrable 6.2% decrease in the 44 μg IFNβ-1a group, 3.4% increase in the 22 μg IFNβ-1a group, 7.2% increase in the group on placebo crossed to 22 μg IFNβ-1a, and 9.7% increase in the group on placebo crossed to 44 μg IFNβ-1a.

Clinically Isolated Syndrome

Two studies have been done in patients with clinically isolated syndrome (CIS). Both have demonstrated benefit of IFNβ in delaying the diagnosis of definite MS. The Controlled High-Risk Subjects Avonex Multiple Sclerosis Prevention Study (CHAMPS) was a randomized, double-blind, placebo-controlled study using IFNβ-1a (Avonex) in patients with CIS (10). The 383 patients included in this study had a first episode involving demyelination of the optic nerve, spinal cord, brainstem, or cerebellum with symptoms lasting more than 48 hours. Additionally, the subjects needed at least two clinically silent lesions on brain MRI that were more than 3 mm in diameter, of which one had to be periventricular or ovoid. All patients were treated with a course of intravenous methylprednisolone followed by an oral prednisone taper. Patients were randomly assigned to receive either 30 μg IFN-β1a or placebo intramuscularly started during the prednisone taper. On a preplanned interim analysis, the results were positive and the study was terminated just before the 3-year time period. The decreased cumulative risk of defi-

nite MS, as defined by a second clinical attack, was 35% in the treated group versus 50% in the placebo group. Overall, the reduced risk of a subsequent attack was 44% in those treated with IFN-β1a (Fig. 16-3). However, it is important to note that half of the untreated group did not have a subsequent acute episode of demyelination or clinical worsening during the 3 years of follow-up.

The second trial in CIS was Early Treatment of Multiple Sclerosis Study Group (ETOMS) (11). This was a randomized, double-blind, placebo-controlled study of low-dose IFNβ-1a (Rebif) in 309 primarily CIS patients, with the primary outcome measure of conversion to clinically definite MS. To be eligible for this study, subjects needed to have a single episode of symptoms attributable to one or more parts of the nervous system within 3 months of being enrolled, plus an abnormal neurological examination and brain MRI. The MRI requirements included at least four lesions on T2-weighted images or three lesions plus either one gadolinium-enhancing or one infratentorial lesion. Only moderate or severe exacerbations were treated with steroids. Randomized patients received either 22 μg of IFNβ-1a or placebo given subcutaneously once weekly for 2 years. Thirty-four percent of the treated group compared to 45% of the placebo group converted to definite MS during this study. Overall, the risk of a subsequent attack was 24% in those treated with 22 μg of IFNβ-1a.

Both of these studies provide a rationale for treating patients with a disease-modifying agent after a single attack in the setting of an abnormal MRI scan suspicious for MS. The goal for early treatment is to delay the diagnosis of definite MS. Hopefully, this will result in a corresponding delay in disability, although this was not demonstrated in either of these short-term studies. Both studies had similar results in the primary endpoint, but there were several differences in the two protocols. CHAMPS subjects were randomized within 27 days and all were treated with intravenous steroids. ETOMS subjects were randomized within 3 months of a monosymptomatic or polysymptomatic episode for which only 70% received some form of steroids.

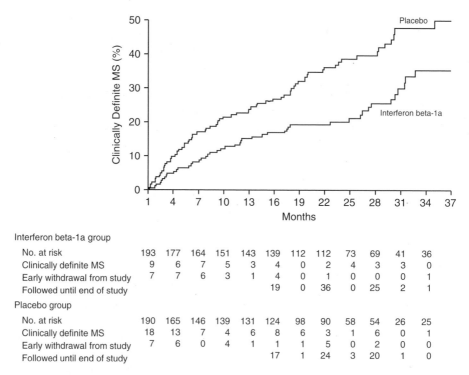

Interferon beta-1a group											
No. at risk	193	177	164	151	143	139	112	112	73	69	41	36
Clinically definite MS	9	6	7	5	3	4	0	2	4	3	3	0
Early withdrawal from study	7	7	6	3	1	4	0	1	0	0	0	1
Followed until end of study						19	0	36	0	25	2	1
Placebo group											
No. at risk	190	165	146	139	131	124	98	90	58	54	26	25
Clinically definite MS	18	13	7	4	6	8	6	3	1	6	0	1
Early withdrawal from study	7	6	0	4	1	1	1	5	0	2	0	0
Followed until end of study						17	1	24	3	20	1	0

FIG. 16-3. The CHAMPS study demonstrated a 44% reduction in subsequent attack and diagnosis of definite MS in patients with clinically isolated syndrome treated with IM IFNβ-1a given weekly compared to placebo. (From Jacobs LD. Intramuscular interferon beta-1a therapy initiated during a first demyelinating event in multiple sclerosis. *N Engl J Med.* 2000;343:898–904.)

In addition, eligible subjects were required to have four lesions on MRI in ETOMS, compared with two lesions in CHAMPS.

Secondary Progressive MS

Since the DMAs demonstrated benefit in relapsing MS, they were tested in patients with secondary progressive disease. The European Study Group on IFNβ-1b in Secondary Progressive MS (SPMS) was a multicenter, double-blind, placebo-controlled study of 718 patients published in 1998 (12). The patients were randomized to receive either 8 MIU of IFNβ-1b or placebo every other day for a planned period of 3 years. SPMS was defined as having at least 6 months of deterioration with or without superimposed relapses in a patient who initially had a relapsing-remitting course. Inclusion criteria included a baseline EDSS of 3.0 to 6.5 plus either two or more relapses or a

1.0 point increase in the EDSS during the previous 2 years. The primary outcome measure was the time to 1.0 point increase in EDSS (0.5 increase if the baseline EDSS was 6.0 to 6.5). Other outcome measures included time to first relapse, annual relapse rate, time to EDSS greater than 7.0 (wheelchair-bound), lesion volume, and gadolinium enhancement on MRI. The preplanned interim analysis was positive and the study was terminated early. There was a 22% relative reduction in confirmed disability progression in the IFNβ-1b group compared with placebo. The reduction in confirmed progression was significant at 12 months. Time to relapse was prolonged in the IFNβ-1b group (644 days) compared with placebo (403 days). Overall, the mean annual relapse rate was decreased by 30%. The time to reach an EDSS of 7.0 was also reduced by 32% in the IFNβ-1b group. The MRI results were positive, as well. T2 lesion volume was decreased by 5% in the treated group, while it increased by 8% in the placebo group. There were fewer new gadolinium lesions on MRI in the IFNβ-1b group compared with the control groups (65% reduction in the first 6 months; 78% reduction in the last 6 months).

A similar study was repeated with IFNβ-1b in North America; however, it did not yield similar results (13). This trial was also a randomized, double-blind, placebo-controlled study of 939 patients with SPMS. Subjects were randomized to receive 8 MIU IFNβ-1b, 5 MIU/m^2 IFNβ-1b (average of 9.6 MIU for the group), or placebo every other day for 3 years. As in the European study, the primary outcome was time to confirmed progression of 1.0 point on EDSS (0.5 points if baseline EDSS was ≥ 6.0). The North American SPMS study was also terminated early, but in this case it was because the study did not demonstrate a significant difference in the primary disability outcome measure. The secondary outcomes of relapse rate, MRI T2 lesion volume, and new gadolinium lesions were, however, significantly reduced in the treatment groups.

The Secondary Progressive Efficacy Clinical Trial of Recombinant Interferon-beta-1a in MS (SPECTRIMS) was a randomized, double-blind, placebo-controlled trial (14). In this study, 618 patients with definite SPMS were randomized to receive either 22 µg or 44 µg of IFNβ-1a or placebo subcutaneous injections three times a week for 3 years. Inclusion criteria included a baseline EDSS of 3.0 to 6.5 plus a pyramidal functional score of at least 2. The primary outcome in this study was also time to confirmed progression of 1.0 point on EDSS (0.5 points if baseline EDSS was 6.0 to 6.5). Secondary outcome measures included number of relapses, time to exacerbation, severity of exacerbation, and need for treatment with steroids or hospitalization. This study also failed to meet the disability primary endpoint. The secondary outcomes, such as exacerbation rate, were significantly reduced in the treatment group. On post hoc analysis it was determined that those subjects with relapses during the two years before study entry had an improved outcome. This suggests that patients earlier in the

course of secondary progressive disease, who are still having relapses, may have better response to IFN.

Additionally, an MRI substudy was conducted (15). One group had MRI scans done every 6 months while the second group had monthly scans for the first 9 months in addition to the semiannual studies. MRI scans were analyzed for burden of disease (total volume of all lesions on T2 or proton density), T2 activity, and combined unique activity. The burden of disease was decreased by 0.5% in patients on the 22 µg dose and 1.3% in patients on 44 µg, compared with a 10% increase in the placebo group. There were 67% fewer active scans in the treated versus placebo group. The combined unique activity was significantly reduced by 78% in the 22 µg group and 89% in the 44 µg group compared with placebo.

Since most of the prior studies of SPMS were negative in terms of meeting the disability primary outcome measure, the next study was the first to use the MS functional composite (MSFC) as the primary outcome. The MSFC was developed by a task force of the U.S. National Multiple Sclerosis Society (REF) in an attempt to produce a more useful measure than the EDSS. It includes testing ambulation with a timed 25-foot walk, upper extremity function with a nine-hole peg test, and cognition with the Paced Auditory Serial Addition Test (PASAT). The International MS Secondary Progressive Avonex Controlled Trial (IMPACT) was a randomized, double-blind, placebo-controlled study which included patients 18 to 60 years old with definite SPMS, an MRI consistent with MS, and an EDSS of 3.5 to 6.5 (16). Patients were excluded if they were unable to perform any portion of the MSFC or were previously treated with IFNβ. Four hundred thirty-six patients were randomized to receive either 60 µg IFNβ-1a or placebo as a weekly intramuscular injection for 2 years. The primary outcome was the reduction in disease progression as measured by MSFC. Secondary outcome measures were EDSS, relapse rate, MRI lesion load and activity, and health-related quality of life (HRQOL). There was a 40% reduction in worsening on MSFC in the treatment group compared with placebo. This effect was driven mostly by the nine-hole peg test when the individual MSFC components were compared. Like the previous SPMS studies, there was no significant difference in the treatment group in terms of worsening measured by EDSS. The remaining secondary outcomes including relapse rate, HRQOL, and MRI findings demonstrated benefit with IFNβ-1a. Despite this being a positive study, it is difficult to extrapolate these findings, as it is the first study to use MSFC as a primary outcome measure.

Primary Progressive MS

IFNβ is suspected to be more beneficial in relapsing disease with an inflammatory component, whether in RRMS or early SPMS when relapses are still occurring. The benefit of IFNβ in progressive disease such as primary progressive MS (PPMS) is unknown. There was a small, exploratory, randomized, double-blind study using IFN in PPMS (17). It was done at a single site with 50 patients. The inclusion criteria included definite PPMS as determined by a history of illness without relapses, an MRI scan with at least two lesions consistent with MS, and the presence of oligoclonal bands in the cerebrospinal fluid or abnormal visual-evoked potentials. The subjects were ages 18 to 60 and had an EDSS of 2.0 to 7.0. Exclusion criteria included treatment with an IFN or other immunosuppressant within 3 months of enrollment, pregnancy or lactation, recent seizure within 3 months, or a history of severe depression. Patients were randomized to either 30 μg or 60 μg IFNβ-1a or placebo given intramuscularly once weekly for 2 years. The primary outcome measure was confirmed disease progression of 1.0 on EDSS (or 0.5 points if the baseline EDSS was ≥ 5.5). Secondary outcome measures were the timed 10-meter walk, the nine-hole peg test, T2 lesion load, new T2 lesions in brain and spinal cord, whole-brain volume, and ventricular volume. This study did not demonstrate a significant difference between the treated and placebo groups in the primary disability outcome. Also, there was not a significant difference in the timed 10-meter walk,

nine-hole peg test, or various MRI outcome measures.

The preliminary results of a pilot study using IFNβ-1b in 49 patients with PPMS and 24 with transitional disease has been reported (18). To be included in this study, patients had to be 18 to 65 years old, have an EDSS of 3.0 to 7.0, and never received immunosuppressive therapy in the past. Patients were randomized to placebo or 8 MIU IFNβ-1b SC every other day for 2 years. The primary outcome measure was confirmed disease progression of 1.0 point on EDSS (or 0.5 points if baseline EDSS ≥ 5.5). Clinical secondary outcome measures included MSFC, the Beck depression scale, the Ashworth scale for spasticity, and the Krupp fatigue scale. MRI outcome measures included T2 lesion load, new lesions, and volume measurements of brain and spinal cord. There was a trend favoring the treated group in disease progression, but this was not significant. However, the MSFC and new T2 lesions on MRI were significantly different in the IFN group. Neither of these studies gave conclusive evidence for treating PPMS with IFN.

Dosing Comparison Studies

The optimal dose and dosing frequency of IFNβ are not known. Trials have shown that a higher dose IFNβ given more frequently is more effective. The IFNB Multiple Sclerosis Study Group demonstrated a decreased exacerbation rate in the 8 MIU compared with the 1.6 MIU of IFNβ-1b (3). The PRISMS study also revealed a dose effect with less-active MRIs in patients treated with 44 μg compared with 22 μg IFNβ-1a (7). The 4-year data demonstrated that the group switched after 2 years from placebo to IFN fared more poorly in measures of disability than the group that was on high-dose IFN for the entire 4-year duration of the study (9) (Fig. 16-4).

The Independent Comparison of Interferon (INCOMIN) Trial was a 2-year prospective, randomized, open-labeled study of 188 patients with RRMS (19). Patients were randomized to receive either 250 μg IFNβ–1b every other day or 30 μg IFNβ-1a once weekly. Primary outcomes in the study included clinical determinations of the number of relapse-free patients and

Proportion of patients free from progression

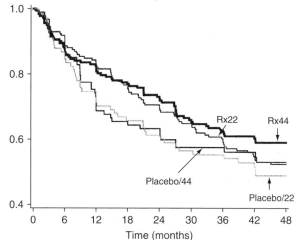

FIG. 16-4. The PRISMS-4 data demonstrated the least progression in disability occurred in the group receiving high dose IFNβ-1a three times weekly for the entire four-year duration of the study. (From the PRISMS Study Group and the University of British Columbia MS/MRI Analysis Group. PRISMS-4: Long-term efficacy of interferon-β-1a in relapsing MS. *Neurology* 2001;56:1628–1636.)

MRI determinations of new proton density or T2 lesions. There was a significant difference favoring IFNβ-1b in terms of the number of relapse-free patients (51% relapse-free in the IFNβ-1b group versus 36% in the IFNβ-1a group). Secondary outcome measures including annualized mean number of relapses, sustained disability progression on EDSS, and lower overall EDSS score at the end of the study was also found to be significant in the IFNβ-1b group. The MRI findings significantly favored the higher dose of interferon. Fifty-five percent of patients in the IFNβ-1b group did not form new proton density/T2 lesions compared with 26% of patients on IFNβ-1a. The clinical outcomes in this study were, however, not blinded, whereas the MRI results were.

In order to assess if a higher dose of IFNβ-1a is more effective, the European IFNβ –1a Dose Comparison Study investigators used 60 µg (double dose) given IM once weekly compared with the standard dose for 3 years (20). This was a randomized, double-blind study in 802 patients with relapsing forms of MS. There was no significant difference between the two doses in the primary outcome of time to disease progression, measured as an increase of 1.0 point on EDSS sustained for 6 months. Only 386 patients had annual MRI scans done. There was also no significant difference in the volume of T2 lesions or gadolinium-enhancing lesions between the two groups. Thus, doubling the dose given once weekly did not affect outcome. The potential effect of dosing more than once weekly was not studied.

The EVIDENCE (Evidence of Interferon Dose-response: European North American Comparative Efficacy) trial included 677 IFN-naive subjects (21). Patients were randomized to either IFNβ-1a 44 µg SC three times weekly or IFNβ-1a 30 µg IM once weekly for 48 weeks. The primary clinical outcome measure was the proportion of relapse-free patients at 24 weeks and the MRI outcome measure was the number of combined unique active lesions per patient. Examiners were blinded to study assignment, but patients were not blinded. At 24 weeks, there was a significant difference in the number of patients free from exacerbation (75% of patients on IFN three times weekly versus 63% of patients on weekly IFN) (Fig. 16-5). The MRI measures also demonstrated a significant difference favoring IFNβ-1a given three times weekly in combined unique active lesions (only 24-week data as gadolinium was not given for the 48-week MRI), new T2 lesions, and active lesions out to 48 weeks. This study supports the concept of higher dose and/or higher dosing frequency.

The OWIMS (Once Weekly Interferon beta-1a for Multiple Sclerosis) study included 293

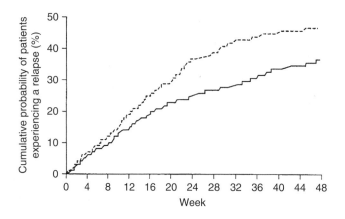

FIG. 16-5. The EVIDENCE study demonstrated a 32% relative risk reduction in proportion of patients experiencing an exacerbation on 44 μg IFNβ-1a SC three times a week compared with patients taking 30 μg IFNβ-1a IM once weekly. Solid line, IFNβ–1a 44μg tiw; dotted line, IFNβ-1a 30 μg once weekly. (From Panitch H. Randomized, comparative study of interferon β-1a treatment regimens in MS. *Neurology* 2002;59:1496–1506.)

patients with RRMS randomized to receive placebo, IFNβ-1a 22 μg, or IFNβ-1a 44 μg SC weekly (22). The primary outcome measure was MRI activity at 24 weeks and extended to 48 weeks. Clinical measures such as relapse rate, number and severity of exacerbations, and EDSS progression were secondary outcome measures. The study was extended in blinded fashion for an additional 2 years. Patients on treatment remained on current therapy, while the placebo group was randomized to either IFNβ-1a 22 μg or IFNβ-1a 44 μg. This study assessed the dosing of IFNβ-1a SC once weekly and the outcome of early compared with late treatment as patients were switched form placebo to active treatment during the extension phase. Only the higher-dose IFN group had a significantly improved MRI, while none of the other clinical measures were significantly different. Overall, no benefit was achieved from once-weekly IFNβ-1a despite the more convenient dosing schedule.

SIDE EFFECTS

Table 16-2 provides a summary of IFN side effects.

Flu-Like Symptoms

The most common side effect of IFN is flu-like symptoms. Approximately 75% of patients experience fever, chills, and myalgia with injections (23). These symptoms usually occur within 3 to 6 hours of injection and typically last 24 hours. Over time, these side effects improve and, in most cases, resolve completely within a few months. Premedication with acetaminophen or ibuprofen 4 hours before injection and every 4 hours thereafter as needed is beneficial to reduce these symptoms. A dose escalation of IFN and injecting in the evening can help minimize side effects and improve adherence to therapy. Starting therapy while patients complete a course of steroids may be helpful in reducing flu-like symptoms.

TABLE 16-2 *IFNβ side effects and treatment*

Side Effects	Treatment/Prevention
Flu-like symptoms	Premedication with acetaminophen or ibuprofen, dose escalation, injecting in evening
Injection site reactions, necrotic skin lesions (rare)	Rotation of injection sites, warm medication to room temperature, antibacterial ointment, sterile dressing, oral antibiotics
Depression	Antidepressants, psychotherapy
Laboratory abnormalities (lymphopenia, neutropenia, elevated ALT, etc.)	Monitor CBC and LFTs every 3 months and reduce dose if elevation is clinically concerning
Thyroid dysfunction	Monitor thyroid function at baseline and periodically as clinically warranted
Spasticity	Monitor tone and treat with baclofen or tizanidine as needed

Injection Site Reactions

Site reactions occur more commonly with SC injections compared to IM injections. Although uncommon with IFNβ-1a given intramuscularly, there are still reports of site reactions occurring in their pivotal trial (6). Subcutaneous IFNβ-1b or IFNβ-1a injections can cause inflammation resulting in painful injections or, in some cases, hardened lesions at the site of injection (23). The severity of this inflammatory reaction varies from individual to individual. In the IFNβ-1b pivotal trial, 69% of patients on the higher dose had inflammation at the injection site. This decreased along with the flu-like symptoms within 3 months and matched the rate of placebo by 1 year (3). The skin reactions occur more commonly in areas with less subcutaneous fat, such as the arms or thighs. Pain with injections can be lessened by applying ice to the site prior to injection, making certain that the medication has warmed to room temperature, and premedicating with a nonsteroidal anti-inflammatory drug (NSAID) (23).

Necrotic skin lesions occur with SC IFNβ in 1% to 3% of patients (3). If this occurs, the drug often may need to be discontinued. Treatment of necrotic lesions involves antibacterial ointment, sterile dressings, and in some cases antibiotics. Very rarely, surgical intervention is necessary. It is of utmost importance that patients rotate injection sites to prevent this more severe complication. Additional preventive measures such as proper injection technique and warming the solution to room temperature prior to injection may minimize necrotic lesions (23).

Depression

Depression and suicide are more common in MS patients than in age-matched controls. During the clinical trials, there was concern IFNβ may cause or worsen depression. A subanalysis in the PRISMS trial included several measures of depression, psychological distress, and hopelessness (4). There was no significant difference in any of these measures for the three treatment groups. The patients who had depression at baseline were likely to still be depressed at the end of the study. Additionally, patients with a high depression rating score were more likely to be disabled, with a higher EDSS. This difference was significant, as was the association of depression with unemployment. The SPECTRIMS subanalysis also did not reveal evidence of IFNβ causing depression (25).

Patients need to be evaluated for depression prior to instituting therapy with IFNβ. Depression does not preclude one from using IFNβ therapy, but often the depression should be treated first with an antidepressant such as a selective serotonin reuptake inhibitor (SSRI). Once IFNβ is initiated, these patients should be followed closely. Although there is no definitive evidence of IFNβ causing or exacerbating depression, if a patient develops severe depression or has worsening depression while on therapy, it should be treated and consideration given to an alternative DMA, depending on the severity of depression.

Laboratory Abnormalities

IFNβ can affect various blood counts and liver function tests (LFTs). Therefore, it is recommended to check both the complete blood count (CBC) and LFTs prior to initiating therapy, one month after starting IFN treatment, and then every 3 months while on therapy. The most common abnormality in the CBC is lymphopenia. IFN can also cause neutropenia, anemia, and thrombocytopenia. These abnormalities are significantly different from placebo and demonstrated a trend for increased dose. Fortunately, the CBC changes are typically not clinically significant and the drug rarely needs to be discontinued. If the levels reach a concerning level for the clinician, the dose should be reduced. Once the level normalizes, the patient can be rechallenged with the full dose of the drug.

Liver function can also be affected by IFN therapy. The most common liver abnormality is elevation of the transaminases. Both aspartate aminotransferase (AST) and alanine aminotransferase (ALT) are affected, but the ALT is more affected than the AST. The pivotal studies of IFNβ-1b and IFNβ-1a both demonstrated a trend for higher dose to more commonly affect the transaminases (4,5,7,9). Although the pivotal weekly intramuscular IFNβ-1a study did not report elevation in LFTs, it is nonetheless recommended to follow laboratory studies as clinical elevations do occur (6). Liver tests including ALT, AST, gamma-glutamyl transpeptidase (GGT), alkaline phosphatase, and bilirubin should be followed with the CBC. Mild elevations do not require any adjustment to the dosing. However, if the laboratory results are elevated to an uncomfortable level for the clinician, the dose should be reduced temporarily until the LFTs normalize and dosing can then be resumed. If the levels remain persistently elevated or the transaminases, alkaline phosphatase, and bilirubin elevate simultaneously, the drug should be discontinued (26). The liver abnormalities may be complicated by other liver-toxic drugs that patients may be taking. These drugs should be avoided, if possible, or more frequent monitoring of LFTs should be done in these individuals.

Tremlett et al. (27) did a retrospective chart review comparing effects on the liver in 844 patients with MS being treated with one of the three IFNβs. This study used the World Health Organization guidelines for grading elevations in transaminases: grade 0, ≤ upper limit of normal (ULN); grade 1, > ULN to 2.5 times ULN; grade 2, > 2.5 to 5 times ULN; grade 3, > 5 to 20 times ULN; and grade 4, > 20 ULN. All of the agents caused an increase in the transaminases to a higher degree than were reported in the pivotal trials. AST was elevated in 38.9% of patients on IFNβ-1b, in 27.2% of patients on IFNβ-1a given three times weekly, and in 23% of patients on once-weekly IFNβ-1a. Three-times-weekly IFNβ-1a and IFNβ-1b were more likely to have grade 2 elevations of transaminases compared to once-weekly IFNβ-1a. In addition, IFNβ-1b and IFNβ-1a three times weekly were more likely to cause elevation of the transaminases within the first 6 months compared with weekly IFNβ-1a, which affected the LFTs later (between 6 and 12 months).

Durelli et al. (28) prospectively followed 156 patients with RRMS being treated with IFNβ-1b. Twenty-three percent of these patients developed mild elevations in liver function, while 14.5% of patients had severe elevations of two to five times the upper limit of normal. The dose of IFN had to be reduced in two patients until the

enzymes normalized, within 3 months. The remaining patients with severe transaminase elevations normalized in 3 to 6 months, despite being continued on full dose of IFN. Most changes in liver function occur within 3 months of starting therapy and usually return to normal levels by 9 months. Therefore, most of these changes are transient and normalize once therapy is discontinued. However, one should continue to monitor patients for the duration of their therapy with IFN.

Thyroid Dysfunction

Thyroid function may be affected by IFNβ therapy. Durelli et al. also assessed thyroid function and thyroid autoantibodies including human thyroglobulin (TGA) and thyroid microsomal antigens (TMA) in 156 RRMS patients being treated with IFNβ-1b (28,29). Thyroid-stimulating hormone (TSH), free tri-iodothyronine (fT3), and free thyroxine (fT4) were measured twice a month for the first month, then monthly for months 2 and 3, and then every 3 months until study completion at month 12 or 15. Throughout the study 8.3% of patients developed hyperthyroidism, which was not significantly different from the 5.3% found to be hyperthyroid at baseline (29). Only one patient had subclinical hypothyroidism during the study, although this was present at baseline in this individual. Similar to the changes in the liver, the thyroid abnormalities also appear to be transient. In only one case was the IFNβ discontinued because of changes in thyroid function. This and other studies demonstrate the small increased risk for developing thyroid disease on IFNβ. Using IFNβ in patients with thyroid disease is not contraindicated, but thyroid function should be followed. Baseline thyroid function should be checked before starting IFNβ therapy and followed periodically, as clinically necessary.

Increased Spasticity

Spasticity may increase in some patients starting IFNβ injections (26). Patients may experience a worsening of symptoms such as spasticity related to an elevation of body temperature after initiating IFNβ therapy (23,26). Increased spasticity has been reported in a small (n = 19), prospective study using IFNβ in patients with PPMS. 68% of patients required starting or increasing baclofen approximately two months after initiating IFNβ therapy. Upon completion of the study, the baclofen requirements were reduced back to pre-IFNβ treatment levels. In this study, the increased spasticity was thought to be unrelated to temperature elevations because the flu-like symptoms usually resolved within a month. However, temperatures were not measured during the study. In addition, there were no new spinal cord lesions on MRI that could account for the increased spasticity (30). This was a small study of PPMS patients, but increased muscle tone was also found to be significantly different from placebo in patients treated with IFNβ-1b in the European SPMS study (12). Usually. increased spasticity is not a problem and it can be treated symptomatically. Extra caution should be taken in individuals with significant spasticity prior to treatment and who are sensitive to temperature elevations (23).

Pregnancy and Breastfeeding

It is recommended that patients discontinue IFNβ prior to attempting to conceive. During preclinical studies, rhesus monkeys treated with IFNβ developed spontaneous abortions. It is not known if there are any teratogenic effects on the fetus in humans, as there are no studies using IFN in pregnant patients (23). All three of the IFNβ agents are pregnancy category C and, therefore, patients should plan to discontinue therapy prior to trying to conceive. Before initiating IFNβ therapy, the use of birth control and family planning should be discussed with the patient.

Breastfeeding while resuming therapy with IFNβ is not recommended. It is not known if the drug is secreted into the breast milk. Because its safety in lactating women is unknown, patients should be encouraged to forgo breastfeeding and resume therapy immediately after the baby is born. This provides protection during the well-established, increased risk of exacerbations during the postpartum period.

NEUTRALIZING ANTIBODIES

Both binding antibodies (BAbs) and neutralizing anti-IFN antibodies (NAbs) form in response to IFN treatment, but only NAbs produce a clinical effect. The formation of NAbs is known to occur with IFNα and has been demonstrated with IFNβ treatment in MS. In the pivotal studies, NAbs were measured quarterly. NAbs can be measured with either a viral cytopathic effect (CPE) reduction or myxovirus protein A (MxA) synthesis reduction assay. Unfortunately, the measurement assay used and the NAb titer considered positive were not mentioned in most of these studies, making it difficult to interpret the results. Additionally, statistical methods varied between the studies.

The IFNβ MS Study Group found that NAbs formed in 35% of the 8 MIU IFNβ-1b group over 3 years (31). A test was considered positive if greater than 20 neutralizing units (NU)/mL were measured on two consecutive titers 3 months apart. The formation of NAbs appears to be an early phenomenon, detected most frequently during the first year of treatment. The 35% of patients on the higher-dose IFN who formed NAbs had an annual relapse rate similar to placebo, as well as an increased number of new lesions on MRI. However, there was less progression of disability on EDSS. This study utilized a cross-sectional statistical analysis considering a positive NAb titer as such for the remaining duration of the study. This type of analysis does not account for variations over time, especially if NAbs normalize. The IFNB MS Study Group data was reassessed using a longitudinal statistical approach, attempting to determine the difference in the response of a particular individual during NAb-positive or -negative periods (32). Again, two consecutive titers greater than 20 NU/mL were needed to be considered positive, but if a subsequent titer was negative the individual was then considered NAb-negative. Approximately 60% of NAb-positive patients reverted to NAb-negative. During the NAb-positive periods, exacerbation rates were increased, but there was no significant change in MRI lesions or progression of EDSS. The patients who reverted to NAb-negative did not have an increased rate of exacerbation.

Extensive analysis of NAbs was also done in the European SP MS trial with IFNβ-1b (33). Both statistical approaches ("once positive, always positive" and "all switches considered") were utilized. The effect of NAbs on relapse rate varied widely, depending upon which statistical method was used and the NAb titer. The relapse rate increased up to 60% in some of the NAb-positive subjects, while in other cases it appeared to actually decrease despite having NAbs. During this study, 50% of NAb-positive patients reverted to NAb-negative status. In the presence of NAbs, patients taking IFNβ-1b had an increase in T2 lesion volume on MRI, but there was still a significant difference from placebo.

NAb formation is not a significant problem with IFNβ-1a 30 µg IM weekly. Both CHAMPS and the European IFNβ-1a Dose Comparison Study demonstrated NAb formation in about 2% of individuals on standard dose IFNβ-1a (10,20). Six percent formed NAbs in the dosing study if they were on 60 µg IFNβ-1a. The EVI-DENCE study demonstrated NAbs in 2% of the 30 µg IFNβ-1a group and 24% of the group on 44 µg IFNβ-1a (21). There was not a significant effect on relapses in the individuals that developed NAbs during this 48-week study. The 44 µg IFNβ-1a group had fewer relapses than the 30 µg IFNβ-1a group, even if they were NAb-positive. MRI indicated less efficacy of the drug by increased lesion formation in the NAb-positive group. The 2-year PRISMS study demonstrated NAbs in 24% of subjects on 22 µg IFNβ-1a compared with 13% on 44 µg (7). This finding was essentially the same when carried out to 4 years (9). In patients on 44 µg IFNβ-1a, the presence of NAbs did not affect relapse count during the first 2 years. However, the PRISMS-4 data demonstrated that in years 3 and 4, NAb-positive patients had a significant increase in relapse rate compared with NAb-negative patients. The number of T2 active lesions and the burden of disease were also significantly increased in the NAb-positive patients. The burden of disease in the 44 µg IFNβ-1a group decreased by 8.5% if NAb-nega-

tive compared with 17.6% increase if NAb-positive.

The formation of NAbs is a known complication of IFN treatment. Generally, two titers greater than 1:20, 3 months apart, are considered positive. Once an individual has NAbs, the antibody reacts with and neutralizes any of the IFNβs. Controversy exists over when to check for NAbs and what to do when an individual develops NAbs. This stems from conflicting results in the studies that have demonstrated increased relapse rate and formation of new lesions on MRI, but less disability on EDSS. In addition, in more than half of the cases NAbs disappeared during the study. Higher titers, however, are less likely to normalize. The decision to check for NAbs and the consideration of changing therapy should be based on disease progression.

CONCLUSION

IFNβ has been demonstrated to be efficacious in reducing both clinical and MRI activity in individuals with RRMS. Therefore, most patients with active RRMS should be on therapy. Its use in progressive disease, such as SPMS or PPMS, remains under question. The treatment response to a disease-modifying agent is thought to be more effective earlier in the disease course, when the disease is more inflammatory, compared to later, when a more degenerative process prevails. Despite this, it is difficult to determine the benefit of therapy on disease progression in an individual once therapy is initiated, as one does not know what the course of disease would be without treatment.

REFERENCES

1. Weinstock-Guttman B, Ransohoff RM, Kinkel RP, et al. The interferons: biological effects, mechanisms of action, and use in multiple sclerosis. *Ann Neurol.* 1995;37:7–15.
2. Yong VW, Chabot S, Stuve O, et al. Interferon beta in the treatment of multiple sclerosis: mechanisms of action. *Neurology* 1998;51:682–689.
3. The IFNB Multiple Sclerosis Group. Interferon beta-1b is effective in relapsing-remitting multiple sclerosis. I. Clinical results of a multicenter, randomized, double-blind, placebo-controlled trial. *Neurology* 1993; 43:655–661.

4. Paty DW, Li DKB. Interferon beta-1b is effective in relapsing-remitting multiple sclerosis. II. MRI analysis results of a multicenter, randomized, double-blind, placebo-controlled trial. *Neurology* 1993;43:662–667.

5. The IFNB Multiple Sclerosis Study Group and the University of British Columbia MS/MRI Analysis Group. Interferon beta-1b in the treatment of multiple sclerosis: Final outcome of the randomized controlled trial. *Neurology* 1995;45:1277–1285.

6. Jacobs LD, Cookfair DL, Rudick RA, et al. Intramuscular interferon beta-1a for disease progression in relapsing multiple sclerosis. *Ann Neurol.* 1996;39:285–294.

7. PRISMS (Prevention of Relapses and Disability by Interferon β-1a Subcutaneously in Multiple Sclerosis) Study Group. Randomized double-blind placebo-controlled study of interferon β-1a in relapsing/remitting multiple sclerosis. *Lancet* 1998;352:1498–1504.

8. Li DKB, Paty DW. Magnetic resonance imaging results of the PRISMS trial: a randomized, double-blind, placebo-controlled study of interferon-β1a in relapsing-remitting multiple sclerosis. *Ann Neurol.* 1999;46:197–206.

9. The PRISMS (Prevention of Relapses and Disability by Interferon-β-1a Subcutaneously in Multiple Sclerosis) Study Group and the University of British Columbia MS/MRI Analysis Group. PRISMS-4: long-term efficacy of interferon-β-1a in relapsing MS. *Neurology* 2001;56:1628–1636.

10. Jacobs LD, Beck RW, Simon JH, et al. Intramuscular interferon beta-1a therapy initiated during a first demyelinating event in multiple sclerosis. *N Engl J Med.* 2000;343:898–904.

11. Comi G, Fillippi M, Barkhof F, et al. Effect of early interferon treatment on conversion to definite multiple sclerosis: a randomised study. *Lancet* 2001;357:1576–1582.

12. European Study Group on Interferon β-1b in Secondary Progressive MS. Placebo-controlled multicentre randomised trial of interferon β-1b in treatment of secondary progressive multiple sclerosis. *Lancet* 1998;352:1491–1497.

13. Goodkin DE. Interferon beta-1b in secondary progressive MS: clinical and MRI results of a 3-year randomized controlled trial. *Neurology* 2000;54:2350.

14. Secondary Progressive Efficacy Clinical Trial of Recombinant Interferon-beta-1a in MS (SPECTRIMS) Study Group. Randomized controlled trial of interferon-beta-1a in secondary progressive MS. *Neurology* 2001;56:1496–1504.

15. Secondary Progressive Efficacy Clinical Trial of Recombinant Interferon-beta-1a in MS (SPECTRIMS) Study Group. Randomized controlled trial of interferon-beta-1a in secondary progressive MS: MRI results. *Neurology* 2001;56:1505–1513.

16. Cohen JA, Cutter GR, Fischer JS, et al. Benefit of interferon β-1a on MSFC progression in secondary progressive MS. *Neurology* 2002;59:679–687.

17. Leary SM, Miller DH, Stevenson VL, et al. Interferon β-1a in primary progressive MS: an exploratory, randomized, controlled trial. *Neurology* 2003;60:44–51.

18. Montalban X. Overview of European pilot study in interferon β-1b in primary progressive multiple sclerosis. *Mult Scler* 2004;10:S62-S64.

19. Durelli L, Verdun E, Barbero P, et al. Every-other-day interferon beta-1b versus once-weekly interferon beta-1a for multiple sclerosis: results of a 2-year prospective randomized multicentre study (INCOMIN). *Lancet* 2002;359:1453–1460.

20. Clanet M, Radue EW, Kappos L, et al. A randomized, double-blind, dose-comparison study of weekly interferon β-1a in relapsing MS. *Neurology* 2002;59:1507–1517.

21. Panitch H, Goddin DS, Francis G, et al. Randomized, comparative study of interferon β-1a treatment regimens in MS: the EVIDENCE trial. *Neurology* 2002;59:1496–1506.

22. Freedman MS, Francis GS, Sanders EACM, et al. Randomized study of once-weekly interferon β-1a therapy in relapsing multiple sclerosis: three-year data from the OWIMS study. *Multiple Sclerosis* 2005;11: 41–45.

23. Walther EU and Hohfeld R. Multiple sclerosis side effects of interferon beta therapy and their management. *Neurology* 1999;53:1622–1627.

24. Patten SB, Metz LM. Interferon β-1a and depression in relapsing-remitting multiple sclerosis: an analysis of depression data from the PRISMS clinical trial. *Mult Scler* 2001;7:243–248.

25. Patten SB, Metz LM for the SPECTRIMS study group. Interferon β1a and depression in secondary progressive MS: data from the SPECTRIMS trial. *Neurology* 2002;59:744–746.

26. Lublin FD, Whitaker JN, Eidelman BH, et al. Management of patients receiving interferon beta-1b for multiple sclerosis: report of a consensus conference. *Neurology* 1996;46:12–18.

27. Tremlett HL, Yoshida EM, Oger J. Liver injury associated with the β-interferons for MS: a comparison between the three products. *Neurology* 2004;62:628–631.

28. Durelli L, Ferrero B, Oggero A, et al. Liver and thyroid function and autoimmunity during interferon-β1b treatment for MS. *Neurology* 2001;57:1363–1370.

29. Durelli L, Ferrero B, Oggero A, et al. Thyroid function and autoimmunity during interferon β-1b treatment: a multicenter prospective study. *J of Clin Endocrinology & Metabolism.* 2001;86:3525–3532.

30. Bramanti P, Sessa E, Rifici C, et al. Enhanced spasticity in primary progressive MS patients treated with interferon beta-1b. *Neurology* 1998;51:1720–1723.

31. The INFB Multiple Sclerosis Study Group and the University of British Columbia MS/MRI Analysis Group. Neutralizing antibodies during treatment of multiple sclerosis with interferon beta-1b: experience during the first three years. *Neurology* 1996;47:889–894.

32. Petkau AJ, White RA, Ebers GC, et al. Longitudinal analyses of the effects of neutralizing antibodies on interferon beta-1b in relapsing-remitting multiple sclerosis. *Mult Scler* 2004;10:126–138.

33. Polman C, Kappos L, White R, et al. Neutralizing antibodies during treatment of secondary progressive MS with interferon β-1b. *Neurology* 2003;60:37–43.

17

The Use of Glatiramer Acetate in the Treatment of Multiple Sclerosis

Jerry S. Wolinsky

Bartels Family and Opal Rankin Professorships in Neurology, University of Texas Health Science Center at Houston, Texas

ABSTRACT

Glatiramer acetate is a collection of synthetic polypeptides indicated as therapy for relapsing a remitting multiple sclerosis (MS). Current understanding of the immunological and neuroprotective mechanisms of action of GA makes it unique among current MS therapies. The clinical efficacy of GA appears similar to that of the recombinant beta interferons. GA has a favorable side effect profile with excellent patient compliance and long-term acceptance. The results of pivotal controlled clinical trials and long-term data derived from organized extension studies are reviewed. Supportive data from open-label comparison, combination treatment and therapeutic switch studies are also provided to enable informed decisions on the appropriate place for GA among other immunomodulatory treatments for relapsing MS.

INTRODUCTION

Multiple sclerosis (MS) is a central nervous system (CNS) disease characterized pathologically by an inflammatory destruction of myelin with variable axonal loss. It is the most common, nontraumatic, disabling neurological disorder in young adults. The etiology of MS remains unknown, but its pathogenesis likely includes altered immune reactivity to myelin components, placing it among the organ-specific autoimmune diseases. The clinical course of relapsing-remitting MS (RRMS) includes exacerbations or episodic neurologic worsening followed by complete or partial remissions. These attacks, or relapses, are followed within weeks to a few months by resolution of clinical symptoms. However, recovery from up to 40% of all relapses is incomplete, leaving measurable, residual neurologic deficits, sometimes including functional disability (1). After a variable interval of relapsing-remitting disease, a substantial proportion of RRMS patients begin to exhibit more continuous deterioration [secondary progressive MS (SPMS)] with or without continued attacks. Less commonly, more purely progressive forms of MS are encountered that begin with gradual neurological deterioration, often insidious in onset, continuing over many months to years without remission. These patients acquire increasing clinical deficits in the absence of any discernible attacks [primary progressive MS (PPMS)], or with an occasional defined attack after the progressive disease is well-established [progressive relapsing MS (PRMS)] (2).

Currently approved immunomodulator therapies for RRMS include glatiramer acetate (GA) and the recombinant interferons (IFN), (IFNβ-1a, Avonex, Biogen, Inc., Cambridge, MA; IFNβ-1a, Rebif, Serono, Inc., Geneva; IFNβ-1b, Betaseron, Berlex Laboratories, Montville, NJ), with natalizumab (Antegren, Biogen Idec, Inc., Cambridge, MA) possibly on the near horizon (3). All immunomodulatory treatments reduce disease activity and the accumulation of disability in RRMS. The National Multiple Sclerosis Society recommends initiation of therapy with an immunomodulator as soon as possible following diagnosis of RRMS. Mitoxantrone (Novantrone), an antineoplastic agent, is also approved for treatment of relapsing MS, but is generally reserved for secondary progressive and severe relapsing-remitting forms of the disease (4,5).

GA (formerly known as copolymer 1 or Cop 1), the subject of this chapter, is indicated for the reduction of the frequency of relapses in RRMS. The drug is approved in 42 countries worldwide, including the United States, Canada, Australia, Europe, and Israel. A number of excellent reviews of GA are available (6,7). GA is the acetate salt of a synthetic mixture of polypeptides that consists of random sequences of four naturally occurring amino acids: L-glutamic acid, L-lysine, L-alanine, and L-tyrosine in racemic form (molar ratio of 1.4:3.4:4.2:1.0). The copolymer was first synthesized in 1967 by Drs. Arnon and colleagues at the Weizmann Institute of Science in an attempt to simulate some of the then-known physicochemical properties of myelin basic protein (MBP) to induce and then dissect experimental allergic encephalomyelitis (EAE) (8). EAE is a laboratory animal model of organ-specific autoimmune CNS inflammatory disease with some similarities to MS. GA was incapable of inducing EAE, but had a marked effect in suppressing EAE when animals were subsequently challenged with MBP.

MECHANISMS OF ACTION

The immunopharmacology of GA in humans remains incompletely understood, but substantial preclinical and clinical data support immunomodulatory and neuroprotective effects that may contribute to the activity of the drug. At least five interdependent processes are thought to contribute to the effects of GA (Fig. 17-1): (a) high-affinity binding to the major histocompatibility complex (MHC) within the antigen binding pocket; (b) competition with MBP at the antigen-presenting cell (APC) level for binding to MHC and subsequent inhibition of MBP-specific T cell activation through competition with MBP/MHC complexes for the T cell receptor; (c) induction of a shift in GA-reactive T cells

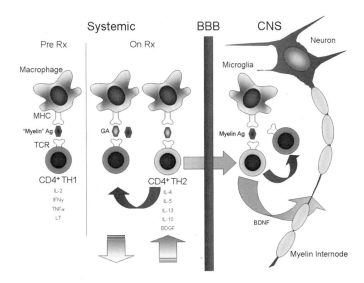

FIG. 17-1 Simplified diagrammatic representation of the immunopharmacology of GA in MS thera-peutics. The pretreatment *(Pre-Rx)* portion of the panel emphasizes the baseline state in MS with CD4+ TH1 myelin antigen-reactive cells being activated by systemic antigen processing cells, includ-ing macrophages that present foreign antigens that are myelin-like ("myelin" Ag) in the context of sur-face major histocompatibility complex (MHC) to the T cell receptor (TCR); invoking the concept of molecular mimicry. Stimulated CD4+ TH1 "myelin" Ag-reactive cells secrete a number of proinflamma-tory cytokines (IL-2, IFNγ, TNFα, LT). On GA therapy, GA may displace some "myelin" Ag. More important, on presentation and stimulation of GA and "myelin" Ag-reactive CD4+ TH1 cells, GA silences cross-reacting CD4+ TH1 "myelin" Ag-reactive cells through anergy, apoptosis, or antigen-specific mechanisms. Concomitantly, GA stimulates and expands a population of GA-reactive CD4+ TH2 cells that secrete anti-inflammatory cytokines (IL-4, IL-5, IL-13, IL-10) to systemically inhibit "myelin" Ag-reactive CD4+ TH1 cells *(red arrow)*. With continued therapy, the net result is a reduced proportion of CD4+ TH1 and an increased proportion of GA and "myelin" cross-reactive CD4+ TH2 cells. When these GA and "myelin" cross-reactive CD4+ TH2 cells gain access to the central nervous system (CNS) by trafficking across the blood–brain barrier (BBB), they are restimulated by true myelin antigens processed and presented by microglia, a brain-resident macrophage. On restimula-tion, the GA-reactive CD4+ TH2 cells secrete anti-inflammatory cytokines to inhibit "myelin" Ag reac-tive CD4+ TH1 cells within the CNS, and also secrete trophic factors such as brain-derived neurotrophic factor (BDNF) that may facilitate neuronal survival *(green arrow)*. (From Wolinsky JS. Glatiramer acetate for the treatment of multiple sclerosis. *Expert Opin Pharmacother.* 2004;5:875–891,with permission.)

from a TH1 to a TH2 phenotype; (d) migration of GA-specific T cells into the CNS; and (e) neuroprotection induced via promotion of neu-rotrophic factors. Immunization with GA also consistently induces GA antibodies.

High-Affinity Binding to MHC

Before any antigen-specific, T-cell-dependent immune response can take place, there must be processing and presentation of a fragment of the antigen by an APC to a T cell precursor. Ordinarily, the appropriately processed antigen is bound by physicochemical interactions to the antigen-binding cleft of the MHC within an APC, and the resulting unique structure cycled to the cell surface for presentation where it can interact with complementary, hypervariable por-tions of the T cell receptors of appropriate T cells. The resulting trimolecular complex is essential, but not necessarily sufficient to acti-vate and condition subsequent T cell "educa-tion" and behavior.

Intact GA can directly bind to MHC. This can be blocked by anti-DR, but not anti-DQ or anti-class I antibodies. The binding of GA to class II occurs at, or very near to, the peptide-binding cleft (9). This is a high-avidity interaction demonstrated to occur for all common MS-associated DR haplotypes. The molecular structure of the immunodominant peptide of MBP and DR2 has been resolved by crystallography (10). Based on that information, it is likely that the repeated alanines and tyrosines in GA facilitate its anchoring within binding pockets of class II molecules. The inherent variation in amino acid sequence of GA could account its binding to different class II haplotypes. The high-affinity interaction between GA and class II antigen is probably central to its in vivo activity, as it would seem to ensure that some of the drug will interact with any available APC at the subcutaneous site of injection. However, this alone cannot explain the drug's mechanism of action, as the immunobiologically inert dextrorotatory form of GA binds with similar avidity to DR.

Competition with MBP

The substantial MHC-binding affinity of GA allows it to compete with MBP and other myelin-associated proteins at the level of APC binding in vitro (11). GA efficiently displaces MBP, proteolipid protein (PLP), and myelin oligodendrocyte glycoprotein (MOG)-derived peptides from the MHC binding site, but is not displaced by these antigens once it is bound (12). GA isomers behave similarly, but do not suppress EAE (13). Once bound, the GA/MHC complex competes with available MBP/MHC molecules for binding to T cell receptors, rendering some of the myelin-specific pathogenic T cells anergic or otherwise altered (14).

TH1 to TH2 Lymphocyte Shift

Exposure to GA induces a relative anti-inflammatory state by causing a shift in the GA-reactive lymphocyte population from a dominant type-1 T helper (TH1) state to a type-2 (TH2) dominant state (15,16). TH1 cells produce interleukin (IL)-2, IL-12, IFN-γ, and tumor necrosis factor (TNF)-α, which generally are proinflammatory cytokines, while TH2 cells produce IL-4, IL-5, IL-6, IL-10, and IL-13 with anti-inflammatory

effects. GA-reactive peripheral blood lymphocytes from untreated MS patients express mostly TNF-α mRNA, while those harvested from GA-treated patients mainly express IL-10, transforming growth factor (TGF)-β, and IL-4 mRNA (17). The shift toward a TH2 bias is reflected by diminished ratios of IFN-γ/IL-5 secretion of GA-reactive T cell lines isolated from MS patients on therapy (16,18). The GA-reactive TH2 cells presumably are regulatory cells that modulate myelin antigen-directed pathogenic immune reactions. Many T cell lines reactive to a number of potentially encephalitogenic myelin proteins, when stimulated in vitro with GA, do not proliferate but predominantly secrete anti-inflammatory cytokines (19).

Naive and memory GA-reactive CD4$^+$ T cells are part of the resident T cell repertory (20). Two phenomena occur in concert on initiating GA therapy. First, after a transient increase within the first month, the number of GA-reactive T cells found using proliferation assays falls within 3 to 6 months, is substantial at 12 months, and decreases by 75% from baseline to 24 months (21). Those without an in vitro proliferative response to GA increased from 5% at baseline to 40% at two years. Second, GA therapy results in increased apoptosis of a substantial percentage of activated (CD69$^+$) CD4$^+$ T cells (22), and long-term treatment showed a 2.9-fold decrease in the estimated precursor frequency of GA-reactive T cells (23). Nevertheless, the ex vivo assayed response to GA remained TH2-biased and, in part, cross-reactive with MBP and MBP (83–99) for up to nine years following initiation of GA (23). Thus, as the shift from a TH1 to a TH2 state develops, TH1 GA-reactive cells are also lost. These ex vivo observed effects likely occur systemically in the MS treated patient, with the result that there is a diminished systemic pool of autoaggressive cells; an effect that appears quite sustained.

Activated T Cell Migration into the CNS

White matter plaques with active CNS demyelination and axonal loss contain numerous inflammatory cells. GA is unlikely to directly inhibit the transmigration of inflammatory cells into the brain. TH2 cells can penetrate the brain endothelium in vitro (24). Syngeneic GA-reactive murine TH2 cells, when systemically administered in adoptive transfer experiments, will enter the CNS (25,26). Once in the brain, these cells are postulated to decrease local inflammation through so-called bystander suppression. Presumably, products of normal myelin turnover or active demyelination are presented by local APCs to locally restimulated, transmigrating, GA-specific TH2. The presented antigen within-brain cannot be GA, since the drug is rapidly metabolized at the site of administration and does not circulate systemically as a free molecule. Local reactivation of GA-specific T cells in brain stimulates the release of anti-inflammatory cytokines such as IL-4, IL-6, IL-10, TGF-β and brain-derived neurotrophic factor (BDNF), but not IFN-γ (26,27). Proinflammatory cytokine production is then inhibited through this bystander effect (28). Bystander suppression could make GA useful in other CNS diseases where TH1 cells might contribute to the disorder (29,30).

Neuroprotection

Subsets of autoreactive TH1 and TH2 cells have neuroprotective effects in models of axonal injury. In a rodent optic nerve crush injury model with predictable retinal-ganglion neuron loss, injection of MBP-reactive T cells immediately after the injury resulted in an attenuated loss of retinal ganglion neurons, but also the expected undesired consequence of adoptive transfer EAE (31). However, when similarly injured rats were injected with GA-specific T cells they showed improved retinal ganglion neuron survival without developing EAE (32). In related experiments, intraocular injection of glutamate destroyed mouse retinal ganglion neurons. Here, glutamate toxicity was reduced by GA preimmunization, but not in mice immunized with MBP or MOG (33). Reduced axonal damage in C57/bl mice with chronic EAE may reflect the neuroprotective rather than a more conventional anti-inflammatory effect of GA (34).

Several possible mechanisms could account for the neuroprotective effect of GA. Nitric oxide (NO) is an inflammatory mediator that affects regulation immune responses, permeability of the blood–brain barrier, and neural trafficking of cells. It is implicated in primary demyelination via nonspecific damage to the myelin sheath of axons, and may directly promote oligodendrocyte death (35). NO is markedly increased in murine EAE, and GA therapy leads to a significant decrease in NO secretion by encephalitogen stimulated splenocytes (36).

BDNF is a neurotrophic factor that plays a prominent role in CNS development and plasticity (28,37). Some GA-specific TH2 and TH1 T cell lines on stimulation produce BDNF (38). Others have shown that secreted BDNF levels of GA-specific T cells generated on GA therapy were higher than those generated before treatment was started (27), and that high levels of BDNF were secreted by TH2 biased T cell lines. Tyrosine kinase receptor (trk) B is the signal transducing receptor for BDNF and trk B is expressed on neurons and astrocytes in MS lesions (39). Thus, BDNF secreted by GA-reactive TH2 cells in the CNS might exert neurotrophic effects directly in target tissues.

Alternatively, the GA-reactive TH2 cells may induce BDNF within the lesions indirectly by other cytokine-mediated effects on astrocytes, and may limit damage that might otherwise be orchestrated by activated microglia. In an intriguing murine model of 1-methyl-4-phenyl-1,2,3,6-tetrahydropyridine (MPTP) nigrostriatal toxicity, adoptive transfer of GA-TH2 cells attenuated neuronal loss and dopamine depletion. In this model, the extent of microglia activation was markedly reduced and BDNF increased in the substantia nigra pars compacta, which was a site of accumulation of transferred T cells. However, it appeared that astrocytes (and not the transferred cells) were the dominant source of BDNF (30). It is of interest that in vitro, GA-reactive T cells also have a reduced ability to transform bipolar microglia into morphologically activated forms (40). Recent observations on cells harvested from treated patients also show both indirect reciprocal effects of GA-reactive T cells on APCs (41) and direct effects of GA on APCs (42).

GA-specific Antibody Induction

Immunization with GA results in polyclonal anti-GA antibody formation with little evidence that these cross-react with MBP or other myelin proteins. However, some murine IgM monoclonal antibodies (mAb) generated to GA or MBP show substantial cross-reactivity in binding and competition assays (43). In a murine model of virus-associated inflammatory demyelination, polyclonal murine GA IgG antibodies stimulated remyelination (44).

Patients develop demonstrable levels of GA-binding antibodies within 1 month of starting treatment that peak within 3 months, reaching levels 8- to 20-fold higher than baseline and greatly exceeding background levels in controls. Titers decrease by month 6 of therapy, but are detected to persist with continued treatment (21). Consistent with a TH2-driven response, the antibodies are IgG class restricted, with IgG_1 levels several-fold higher than IgG_2 and with low IgG_4 (45). Patients who were relapse-free at 18 and 24 months of therapy had statistically higher GA antibody titers than those treated patients with one or more on-trial relapses (21).

Extended attempts failed to show that IgG class GA mAbs inhibit cellular responses to GA either in vitro or in vivo (46). These included various in vitro and in vivo approaches attempting to block the binding of GA to isolated MHC molecules, to inhibit the proliferative and secretory responses of GA-specific T cell lines to stimulation by GA, and to inhibit GA protection in EAE. Negative results also occurred with high-titer human GA-antibody sera, and sera from 34 GA-treated patients failed to reduce the proliferative response of a murine GA-specific T cell clone to GA, or reduce the competitive inhibition of proliferation of an MBP-specific human T cell clone by GA. In a small study, GA antibodies were found in only 48% of 42 GA-treated RRMS patients, with most antibody-positive patients seen after 1 year on therapy (47). Six of 14 high-titer sera inhibited the proliferation of normal donor peripheral blood cells to GA and, at low dilution, these six sera variably inhibited the proliferate responses of a panel of GA-specific T cell lines. However, the predominance of available data does not suggest GA antibodies influence the drug's therapeutic effect.

CLINICAL EFFICACY IN CONTROLLED TRIALS

Bornstein Single-Center RRMS Study (1980–1985)

The first double-blind, randomized, placebo-controlled trial of GA was done in the 1980s as a single-center study at Albert Einstein College of Medicine in the Bronx, NY (48). Fifty relatively young, clinically active, and modestly disabled RRMS patients were recruited (ages 20 to 35, mean 30.5 years; ≥ 2 relapses in the 2 years before entry, average 3.9 relapses; Kurtzke Disability Status Scale (DSS) score ≤ 6, mean score 3) and assigned to subcutaneously (SC) daily GA 20 mg or placebo (PBO) for 2 years. The treatment groups were matched for sex, prior relapses, and disability (DSS 0 to 2 or 3 to 6). The proportion of relapse-free patients was selected as the primary endpoint; secondary endpoints included relapse frequency, change in DSS score from baseline, and time to progression (defined as ≥ 1 DSS point increase maintained for ≥ 3 months).

Relapse-free patients were significantly more common with GA treatment (14/25 or 56% GA versus 6/23 or 26% PBO; p = 0.045). The overall two-year relapse frequencies were 0.6 in the GA and 2.7 in the PBO groups. A lower entry disability score increased the likelihood of remaining relapse-free on study (p = 0.003). By study's end, 84.6% of GA-treated patients in the lower DSS stratum (0 to 2) were stable or improved versus 30% of the PBO-treated group. Mean improvement was 0.5 DSS units with GA, while those on PBO worsened by 1.2 DSS units (p = 0.012). At the higher DSS stratum (3 to 6), similar proportions of patients were stable, improved, or worsened.

The Pivotal Multicenter American Trial [1991–Present (2005)]

This study had three phases: a randomized, PBO-controlled, 24-month, double-blind treatment phase (core study); a blinded extension phase of up to 36 months that preserved the original treatment assignments; and an open-label extension phase in which patients received GA. In 2005, the latter phase is ongoing into its twelfth year. The primary endpoint (for all study phases) was relapse number. Secondary endpoints included the proportion of relapse-free patients, time to first relapse, change in Expanded Disability Status Scale (EDSS) score from entry, and proportion of patients with sustained disease progression (defined as ≥ 1 point increase in EDSS persisting for ≥ 3 months). EDSS evaluations were made every three months during the blinded core and extension phases and every six months thereafter. Patients were seen within seven days of each suspected relapse. When possible, the same neurologist and nurse coordinator completed the assessments of each patient.

Core Study (1991–1994)

Two hundred fifty-one RRMS patients, ages 18 to 45 (mean age 34 years), were enrolled and randomized to GA or PBO (49). Eligible patients had $\geq$ two relapses in the 2 years before entry (mean 2.9), and an EDSS score of ≤ 5 (mean 2.5). At 24 months there was a 29% relapse rate reduction in favor of GA (1.19 ± 0.13 GA, 1.68 ± 0.13 PBO, p = 0.007; annualized rates were 0.59 and 0.84, respectively). A total of 33.6% of GA-treated patients and 27.0% of PBO patients were relapse-free (p = 0.098). The proportions of patients improved, unchanged, or worsened by ≥ 1 EDSS steps from entry to 2 years of treatment favored GA (p = 0.037). A post hoc analysis suggested a better therapeutic effect of GA in patients with lower entry EDSS scores (≤ 2).

Double-Blind Extension Phase (1991–1994)

Two hundred and three core patients entered the blinded extension (50). After approximately 35 months of treatment there was a 32% relapse rate reduction with GA (mean 1.34 GA, 1.98 PBO, p = 0.002; annualized rates were 0.58 and 0.81, respectively). More

GA-treated patients remained relapse-free over the extended trial (33.6% GA-treated, 24.6% PBO-treated, p = 0.035). No GA-treated patient who was relapse-free during the core relapsed during the extension. The median time to first relapse was prolonged by active treatment (287 days with GA, 198 days with PBO, p = 0.057). Placebo-assigned subjects experienced more multiple relapses (p = 0.008). The proportion of patients who improved by ≥ 1 EDSS steps from entry favored GA (27.2% GA, 12.0% PBO, p = 0.001). Worsening by ≥ 1.5 EDSS steps was more frequent with PBO (21.6% GA, 41.6% PBO, p = 0.001). The mean EDSS score improved by -0.11 on GA and worsened by $+0.34$ with PBO (p = 0.006).

Open-Label Extension [1991–Present (2005)]

All patients who were enrolled in the pivotal trial were invited into the open-label study as long as they had not violated the original study's exclusion criteria; 208 of the original 251 patients chose to do so. At ≥ 6 years of continuous GA therapy from randomization, 26 of 101 (25.7%) remained relapse-free. The relapse rate of all patients treated from the beginning of the study dropped annually, with an overall annualized relapse rate from randomization of 0.42 (95% CI: 0.34 to 0.51), which reached 0.23 during year 6 (51,52). 69.3% of those on GA from study inception were neurologically unchanged (within 0.5 EDSS steps of baseline), or had improved.

Data beyond 6 years remains published only as abstracts. One hundred forty two patients (56.6% of the original cohort) remained on study at eight years (51). The annual relapse rate had declined to 0.2 with a mean EDSS 3.14, reflecting an increase of 0.5 steps from randomization. Patient attrition and the lack of a true placebo group complicate drawing firm conclusions from this long-term cohort. Still, natural history studies predict a higher level of neurological disability within 12 years of disease onset, with 50% of RRMS patients reaching EDSS 6 (53). When the 72 patients always on GA were compared to those originally randomized to PBO (oPBO), the disability differences seen at the end of the controlled extension phase were still evident at year 6.

Of the 208 patients who entered the open-label study, 133 began year 10 (64 always on GA and 69 oPBO). Before randomization, their annualized relapse rates were comparable at 1.52 and 1.46, respectively; by year 10, these had fallen to 0.22 and 0.23. The mean EDSS score for the group always on GA was 3.67; an increase from randomization of 0.9. However, 64.4% remained stable or improved (54). When oPBO patients on active treatment were compared to those always on GA, the proportions with confirmed progression over the entire 10 years differed significantly (50 always GA, 72 oPBO, p = 0.015).

European/Canadian MRI Study (1997–1998)

This multicenter, double-blind, randomized, placebo-controlled study sought to study RRMS subjects similar to those enrolled in the pivotal American trial, but was designed specifically to define the onset, magnitude, and durability of the effect of GA on MRI-monitored disease (55). Major entry criteria differences were that only one relapse was required in the 2 years before study entry, and all randomized subjects had at least one enhancing lesion on a screening cranial MRI scan after administration of gadolinium (Gd). Altogether, 485 subjects were screened to accumulate 252 meeting all entry criteria, and most were randomized into the initial nine-month placebo-controlled phase of the study (119 to GA and 120 to PBO). Thus, these RRMS subjects were enriched for the primary outcome variable of interest. At entry, these patients were of similar age (mean 34.1 years), but shorter disease duration (mean 4.9 years), lower prior 2-year relapse rates (mean 2.6), and slightly lower entry neurological deficits (mean EDSS 2.3) than in the pivotal American trial. The primary MRI outcomes will be provided below. Clinically, at 9 months there was a 33% relapse rate reduction in favor of GA (0.51 GA, 0.76 PBO, p = 0.012; annualized rates were 0.81 and 1.21, respectively). There was little change in EDSS over the short study.

Meta-analysis of the Double-blind, Placebo-controlled Clinical Trials in RRMS

Data was pooled from all 540 patients in the above randomized, PBO-controlled trials over the double-blind phase of each (56). Estimates of the annualized relapse rate, total number of on-trial relapses, and time to first relapse were based on regression models. Also explored were the effect of GA on accumulated disability and the potential role of clinical variables as predictors of relapse rate and treatment efficacy (57). The average annualized relapse rate reduction was 28% in the pooled data set (mean adjusted annual relapse rate 1.14 ± 0.09 PBO, 0.82 ± 0.09 GA, treatment effect 0.31, 95% CI: 0.10 to 0.52, p = 0.004). A 36% reduction in on-trial relapses occurred with GA therapy (risk ratio = 0.64, CI: 0.52 to 0.78, p < 0.0001). Median time to first relapse favored GA (GA = 322 days, CI: 243 to 433, PBO = 219 days, CI: 170 to 255, p = 0.01). Entry patient demographic predictors of on-trial relapse rate included drug assignment (p = 0.004), baseline EDSS score (p = 0.02), and the number of relapses during the two years prior to study entry (p = 0.002) (56).

The risk of accumulating disability was reduced with GA therapy (risk ratio 0.57, CI: 0.39 to 0.91, p = 0.02). Accumulation of disability was more rapid among male patients (the proportion with increased disability over the placebo-controlled duration of the pooled data) with a similar magnitude of the treatment effect size for both sexes (Fig. 17-2). A Kaplan–Meier estimate of the time 25% of PBO patients accumulated sustained disability ($\geq$ 1 EDSS step sustained for 90 days) was 521 days; GA-treated patients did not reach this milestone (p = 0.03). GA nearly doubled the time to confirmed progression (ratio estimate 1.88; p = 0.02) (57). Independent of treatment assignment, patients with on-trial relapses were more likely to accumulate deficits (odds ratio 4.3, CI: 2.4 to 7.6, p < 0.0001). This finding reemphasizes that relapse reduction limits accumulating disability in RRMS. Age, as a categorical variable, was also associated with accumulation of disability, supporting the concept of early initiation of immunomodulatory therapy to maximize benefit.

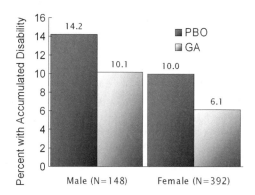

FIG. 17-2 Effect of gender on accumulated disability in RRMS. A meta-analysis was conducted of data from three PBO-controlled trials of GA in RRMS. When stratified by gender, the analysis suggests that the risk of RRMS patients accumulating new disability is greater for male patients regardless of treatment assignment (Wolinsky and Ladkani, unpublished data). However, both male and female patients appeared to benefit from glatiramer acetate therapy (male odds ratio = 0.62, 95% CI: 0.29 to 1.32; female odds ratio = 0.58, 95% CI: 0.33 to 1.00).

Another meta-analysis was communicated based on data in published reports that considered a different selection of trials for inclusion in their analysis. The authors' dissection of the data was constrained by the lack of access to primary data. Nevertheless, were relatively comparable, they reported generally similar relative risk ratios to those just provided that were developed on the primary data, but they ignored all favorable analyses in their conclusions (58).

Bornstein Chronic Progressive Trial (1981–1988)

This trial was conducted through the Albert Einstein College of Medicine in the Bronx, NY, with the aid of Baylor College of Medicine in Houston, TX. The two centers enrolled 169 subjects who would now be classified as having a mix of SPMS and PPMS. Recruitment extended over nearly a 4-year screening interval. The trial was both unique and groundbreaking; it was unique in that it required direct observation and confirmation of sustained progression over an interval of at least 6 to a maximum of 15 months by the investigators prior to randomization to the double-blind, placebo-controlled, treatment phase of the study. Consequently, only 106 of the recruited and followed subjects were randomized. It was groundbreaking in that it defined time to sustained progression of disability as a primary endpoint of an MS trial (59). In this case patients were required to advance ≥ 1.5 EDSS steps when entered at EDSS < 5, and ≥ 1 if entered a level of ≥ 5.0 that was sustained for 3 months; this was a more substantial extent of worsening than that used in subsequent SPMS trials. Subjects injected 15 mg GA twice daily in the only controlled trial that deviated from the 20-mg daily dose. Deterioration occurred in 9 GA and 14 PBO patients, but the overall survival curves did not significantly differ. Two-year progression rates for the secondary outcomes of unconfirmed progression, and progression of 0.5 EDSS units, were significant (p = 0.03). A subsequent post hoc analysis suggested that patients retrospectively classified as PPMS or transitional MS (a PPMS course developing at least a decade after a single, isolated attack) were significantly delayed in progressing when on GA rather than PBO; this helped to launch a subsequent, large trial in PPMS.

Oral Copaxone in RRMS (Coral Study, 2000–2001)

Dosing GA by mouth either before or after induction of EAE protects or attenuates clinical disease in a variety of animal models (60,61). Based on these observations and the highly inviting concept of oral tolerance as a potential means of controlling many organ-specific autoimmune diseases, a global, multicenter, double-blind, placebo-controlled trial testing the effects of enteric-released oral formulations of 5 mg and 50 mg GA was mounted. Altogether 1,651 RRMS patients were recruited and MRI was performed in a subset of 486 subjects. The results, which have yet (2005) to be formally communicated, showed that while the drug was safe when administered as formulated, no statistically significant clinical or MRI effect could be found at either dose. It remains uncertain whether the discrepancy between the effects of GA in the animal model and in humans reflects some aspect of trial design (e.g., dosing, site of drug release), or a flaw in the translation of the concept of oral tolerance to humans.

PROMISE Study (1999–2003)

This was a double-blind, placebo-controlled trial of GA in PPMS that enrolled 943 patients (460 male patients) with progressive disease, the absence of relapse, and EDSS scores between 3 and 6.5, to receive either GA or PBO at a 2:1 allocation ratio. The study's objective was to determine whether GA could slow confirmed disease progression in the absence of the confounding effects of relapses (62). The primary endpoint was the time to confirmed progression (increase of 1 EDSS point sustained for three months for entry EDSS 3.0 to 5.0, or 0.5 EDSS for entry EDSS 5.5 to 6.5). This was originally conceived as a 3-year trial with quarterly clinical evaluations and annual MRI monitoring. Early after enrollment was completed, a blinded extension on assigned study medication until the last subject completed 3 years of study, and drug exposure and data were locked and analyzed, was added.

The Data Safety Monitoring Committee (DSMC) for the trial convened as part of a pre-planned second-interim analysis when at least 600 subjects had completed ≥ 2 years of therapy or had prematurely withdrawn from study. Safety data were available for all patients and intention-to-treat (ITT) efficacy data were available for 757 subjects, of whom 620 had completed ≥ 2 years of treatment. The DSMC found no safety concerns. However, their unblinded review of the efficacy data and the results of a futility analysis led them to conclude it was improbable that the study would reach statistical significance for its primary outcome. Based on the conclusions and recommendations of the DSMC, and recognizing the scientific importance of this large cohort of PPMS subjects, all patients remaining in the trial were taken off study medication in an organized fashion and offered entry into a natural history study until the originally projected conclusion of the trial in October 2003; all investigators and patients remained blinded to the original study medication assignments.

An ITT analysis was performed following closure of the study in October, 2004, using all available trial data, and thus far (2005) published only in abstract form (63). A trend was found for a delay in the time to progression and there was a lower proportion with progression for those randomized to GA compared to the PBO-assigned group [hazard ratio (HR) = 0.860, 95% CI: 0.699 to 1.057, p = 0.152]. Most sensitivity and subcohort analyses supported the trend. The survival curve for male patients assigned to GA diverged early and widened over time from that of the group assigned to PBO (HR = 0.695, CI: 0.523 to 0.924, p = 0.012). Analyses of MRI-monitored enhancements and plaque burden favored GA treatment for both genders. The results suggest different time-dependent effects of GA on the endpoints.

The premature stopping of study medication and unanticipated low progression rates greatly complicate interpretation of the trial. Nevertheless, it appears that GA has benefit in retarding progression in the absence of relapses, an effect most evident in the subcohort of PPMS patients where the PBO group had the most rapid progression.

MRI Studies

MRI provides a noninvasive estimate of ongoing pathologic change within the brains of MS patients. The first indication of the effect of GA on MRI was from a small crossover trial of 10 RRMS patients in whom monthly Gd-enhanced MRI scans were obtained over 9 to 27 months before initiation of GA therapy, and then for 10 to 14 months on therapy. There were overall trends found in the frequency of new Gd-enhanced lesions (0.92 versus 2.20 lesions/month; p = 0.10), and in the rate of T2-weighted lesion volume increase for a subset of six patients with the longer pretreatment observations of 25 to 27 months (p = 0.05) compared to the interval on GA treatment (64).

American Multicenter Study

MRI was not included in the original multicenter study design. However, a cohort of 14 GA and 13 PBO patients followed at the University of Pennsylvania was studied as part of a National Multiple Sclerosis Society pilot program to explore MRI as an adjunct outcome measure for clinical trials (65). Annual decreases from baseline to 24 months in Gd-enhanced lesion number (GA = −1.2, PBO = 0.5; p = 0.03) and Gd-enhanced tissue volume (GA = −83.5 mm^3, PBO = 147.5 mm^3; p = 0.003) were found. Annualized brain volume loss was also three-fold lower (GA = −0.6%, PBO = −1.8%; p < 0.008). No significant differences were found the number of new T2 lesions or percentage increase in T2 volumes.

Cross-sectional MRI data were obtained on 135 of the 147 patients available in the open-label phase of the American Multicenter Study (66). At imaging, 66 oPBO patients had taken GA for 1,467 ± 63 days, and 69 always-GA patients were on the drug for 2,433 ± 59 days. The annualized relapse rate in the two years just prior to beginning the drug was, as expected, higher in oPBO patients (oPBO = 0.93 ± 0.89, GA = 0.51 ± 0.64; p = 0.002), but similar for both groups during open-label treatment (oPBO = 0.27 ± 0.45, GA = 0.28 ± 0.40). The rate reduction was greater for those crossed over from PBO (oPBO reduced by 0.66 ± 0.71, GA reduced 0.23 ± 0.58; p = 0.0002). Consistent with these clinical findings, the proportion of patients with Gd-enhancements was higher in the oPBO cohort (oPBO = 36.4%, GA = 18.8%, p = 0.02). The risk of having an enhancement, regardless of original treatment assignment, was higher in those with open-label phase relapses (odds ratio 4.65, 95% CI: 2.0 to 10.7; p = 0.001), and 2.5 times higher for the oPBO group (CI: 1.1 to 5.4; p = 0.02). Atrophy was worse for those originally on PBO.

European/Canadian MRI Study

This study had two prospectively defined stages: a 9-month, PBO-controlled phase with monthly imaging, and a 9-month, open-label phase with quarterly MRI. The open-label phase was designed to determine if any MRI-related treatment effects found in the first 9 months were reproduced on initiation of GA in the PBO sub-jects, and to learn whether they were sustained with continued active therapy (55,67).

Controlled Phase

The treatment groups were comparable at baseline for all demographic, clinical, and MRI variables. Mean baseline enhancing lesion numbers (PBO = 4.4, GA = 4.2) were relatively high, reflecting enrichment for this activity. Results of the 9-month, double-blind phase (Fig. 17-3) showed that GA reduced total enhancements (−10.8, CI: −18.0 to −3.7; p = 0.003). Treatment effects increased over the 9-month period (55). The cumulative number of Gd-enhanced lesions was highly correlated with clinical relapses in both treatment groups (Spearman rank correlation coefficient in PBO = 0.35, p = 0.001 and in GA = 0.24, p = 0.01). Differences favoring GA were found for all secondary outcomes: number of new enhancements (−33%, p < 0.003), change in enhanced lesion volumes (−57%, p = 0.01), new T2 lesion numbers (−30%; p < 0.003), and change in T2 lesion volumes (−36%; p = 0.006).

Newly detected T2 lesions are nearly always accompanied by T1 enhancements, and ~65% of these new lesions appear hypointense on unenhanced T1 images. Once enhancement ceases, nearly one-third of new lesions remain hypointense lesions on T1-weighted images. These so-called black holes indicate more severe and permanent tissue damage, with better correlations found between the extent of black holes in the brain and MS-related disability than for the total T2-defined disease burden. In a post hoc analysis, newly formed T2 lesions (defined as a T2 lesion arising from an area of previously normal white matter with associated T1 enhancement) were identified from scans taken between study months 1 and 6 that could be followed over at least three to up to eight subsequent monthly scans to evaluate new lesion evolution (68). GA treatment reduced the proportion of new MS lesions that evolved into black holes and the recurrence of enhancements (Fig. 17-4). A total 1,251 new lesions (515 GA, 736 PBO) were found suitable for serial evaluation over a mean follow-up of 5.6 months. The proportion of persisting black holes on follow-

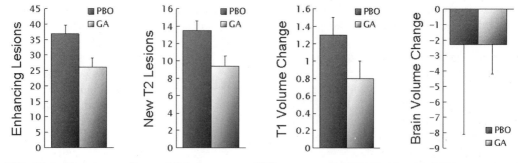

FIG. 17-3 Short-term effects of GA therapy on MRI measures in RRMS. Monthly MRI scans were obtained for 119 GA- and 120 PBO-randomized RRMS patients who were required to have at least one enhanced lesion documented on an MRI done within 30 days of randomization and initiation of study drug. The *far left panel* shows the mean number of total enhancing lesions per subject over the entire nine-month study; a 29% difference that favored GA (p = 0.003). The *left middle panel* displays the mean number of new T2 lesions per subject over the nine-month study, a 30% difference that favored GA (p < 0.003). The *middle right panel* displays the mean change from baseline in total T1 hypointense lesion volume per subject (in mL) from baseline to nine months (p = 0.14). (After data in Comi G, Filippi M, Wolinsky JS. European/Canadian multicenter, double-blind, randomized, placebo-controlled study of the effects of glatiramer acetate on magnetic resonance imaging—measured disease activity and burden in patients with relapsing multiple sclerosis. European/Canadian Glatiramer Acetate Study Group. *Ann Neurol.* 2001;49:290–297.) The *far right panel* shows the mean change from baseline in central brain volume per subject (in mL) from baseline to nine months (not significant). (Developed from Rovaris M, Comi G, Rocca MA, et al. Short-term brain volume change in relapsing-remitting multiple sclerosis: effect of glatiramer acetate and implications. *Brain* 2001;124:1803–1812.)

up scans was lower in GA-treated patients at all times, became significant at month 7, and by month 8 was nearly half that of the PBO group (GA = 15.6%, PBO = 31.4%, p = 0.002). The frequency of re-enhancing lesions was also lower in GA-treated patients (GA = 5.0%, PBO = 8.5%, p = 0.002).

Open-label Phase

Fully 94% of randomized patients began or continued GA for an additional 9 months (67). There were 35% fewer enhancements (p = 0.03) over the entire 18-month trial for those always on GA (Fig. 17-5), or six enhancing lesions per oPBO patient that might have been preventable. The intent-to-treat (with the last observation carried forward) imputation analysis favored patients always on GA over the entire study and its two phases. Enhanced lesion numbers on quarterly imaging were always lower for those always on GA, with a trend seen at 3 months that strengthened by months 6 and 9 (both p < 0.001) during the double-blind phase, and with the pro-

portion of enhanced-lesion-free patients increasing to 63% at month 18. Within 3 months of crossover to GA, the proportion of enhanced-lesion-free oPBO patients increased from 31% to 45% and rose to 60% by the end of the trial.

The T2 disease burden showed little change during the open-label phase for either group, but was greatest in the oPBO group. An increase in T1 hypointense volume was found for both groups over both trial phases. However, the 9-month delay in the initiation of GA treatment was associated with a 2.2-fold increase in the accumulated hypointense lesion volume over the entire 18-month study (67).

Initially, a semiautomated segmentation method based on local thresholding was used to estimate brain volume—seven contiguous, periventricular slices from the MRI obtained at entry and at the end of the placebo-controlled and open-label phases of the study. With this measure, brain volume correlated significantly with the patients' disability at each timepoint; while there was a trend for a reduced rate of brain volume loss for those always on GA over the last

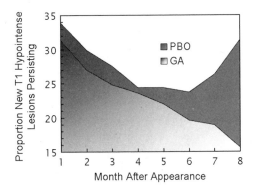

FIG. 17-4 Effect of GA on newly formed T1 hypointense lesion evolution. Monthly MRI scans were reviewed for evolution over at least three to eight months of all newly formed T1 hypointense lesions (defined as a low-signal-intensity region on a T1-weighted image that had appeared one month earlier with enhancement in a previously normal-appearing white matter region, but no longer enhanced and was not already isointense at month 1). A total of 1,722 lesions among 239 patients were available for serial evaluation. Between 31% and 34% of newly enhanced lesions persisted for 30 days as T1 hypointensities; this proportion fell progressively on GA therapy. For those treated with PBO, the decline stabilized at four months and began to rise again after six months. Difference in the evolution of these lesions between the groups was significant at months 7 and 8 (p = 0.04 and p = 0.002, respectively). (Modified from Filippi M, Rovaris M, Rocca MA, et al. Glatiramer acetate reduces the proportion of new MS lesions evolving into "black holes." *Neurology* 2001;57:731–733.)

nine months of the entire trial, it was not statistically significant (69). When the analysis was repeated using an automated technique that measured the entire intracranial contents with less variability than the prior study, the differences in loss of brain parenchyma over time were statistically significant, favoring treatment with GA at nine months (p = 0.015) and over the entire 18-month trial (p = 0.037). The overall proportional magnitude of the effect was similar with the two analytic measurement systems (70).

UNCONTROLLED CLINICAL STUDIES

The relative efficacy of currently approved, disease-modifying therapies for use in RRMS is contentious, but of considerable practical con-

cern. Randomized, blinded, direct comparison clinical trials pose methodological, logistical, and cost problems (71). While several industry-sponsored trials are now underway to directly look at the efficacy of subcutaneous interferon (IFN) β-1a and IFNβ-1b relative to GA, these studies are not fully blinded and the results will not be available for several years. Until they are completed and reported, nonrandomized, open-label prospective and retrospective observational studies, and therapeutic "switch" studies provide the only insight into this issue for physicians and patients to judge therapeutic choice in the day-to-day clinical setting.

Comparative Studies

Khan et al. organized a prospective, nonrandomized, open-label trial of 156 RRMS patients to compare the effects of various regimens on annualized relapse rates and disability status (72), as follows: 30 µg IFNβ-1a intramuscularly and weekly (n = 40); 250 µg IFNβ-1b every other day (n = 41); GA 20 mg daily (n = 42); and no treatment (n = 33). The treating physicians and patients were directly involved in selecting treatment choices. Eligible patients were treatment-naive with at least one relapse in the previous 2 years and had a Kurtzke EDSS score ≤ 4 when starting therapy. Relapses were defined as in the pivotal American trial of GA. Mean annualized relapse rates in the 2 years similar before starting therapy (untreated = 1.08; IFNβ-1a = 1.20; IFNβ-1b = 1.21; GA = 1.10). Twelve months after initiating or declining treatment, relapse rates were 0.97 without therapy, and 0.85 [not significant, (NS)], 0.61 (p = 0.002), and 0.62 (p = 0.003) in the IFNβ-1a, IFNβ-1b, and GA groups compared to untreated patients, respectively. At 18 months of follow-up, 122 of 156 patients remained on their original treatments with similar results on relapse rate declines compared to those untreated (GA = 0.49, p < 0.0001; IFNβ-1b = 0.55, p = 0.001; IFNβ-1a = 0.81, p = 0.11). Mean EDSS increased in untreated patients (0.60) and those on IFNβ-1a (0.19, NS), but decreased for those on the GA (–0.44, p = 0.003) and IFNβ-1b (–0.25, p = 0.01); all inferences relative to the untreated cohort (73).

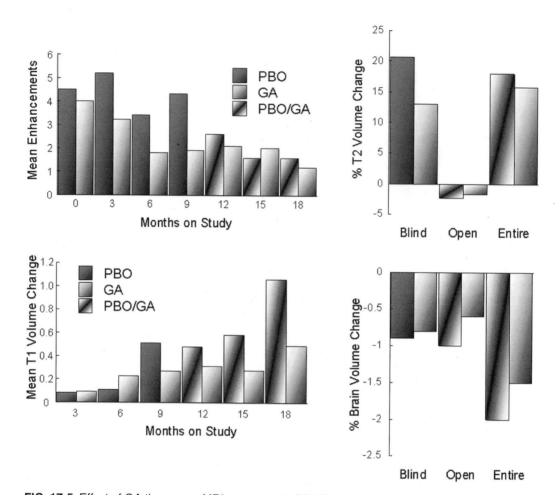

FIG. 17-5 Effect of GA therapy on MRI measures in RRMS. Following nine months of placebo-controlled study, all patients in the European/Canadian study were offered continued quarterly follow-up on open-label glatiramer acetate (67). The *upper left panel* shows the mean change from baseline in the number of enhanced lesions found on quarterly images, with significant differences noted in favor of active treatment at months 6 and 9. When switched to active treatment, a significant reduction in enhancements for those previously treated with placebo was seen within three months. Similarly, a reduction in percentage change from baseline that favored treatment was seen during the controlled phase for patients on glatiramer acetate that was reproduced during the open-label treatment phase, as seen in the *upper right panel.* In the *lower left panel,* the change in mean T1-hypointense lesion volume from baseline was significantly retarded by glatiramer acetate treatment during the controlled phase (p = 0.035), a finding that was reproduced over the next nine months for those with a late initiation of therapy. The *lower right panel* shows that the rate of atrophy was significantly reduced over the open label and entire study for those continuously exposed to glatiramer acetate compared to those initially randomized to placebo when total brain contents were measured (70).

Generally, similar results were found in an observational, retrospective analysis of outcomes in a sequential cohort of Argentine RRMS patients (71). Here patients were treated for 16 months with 30 μg IFNβ-1a weekly (n = 26), 44 μg IFNβ-1a three times per week (n = 20), 250 μg IFNβ-1b every other day (n = 20), or GA (n = 30), and compared with a group of untreated patients (n = 38). Socioeconomic factors influenced the latter choice, but most other demographic and clinical variables were otherwise similar between the groups. There was considerable variation in baseline annual relapse rates between the groups (IFNβ-1a weekly = 0.77; IFNβ-1a = 1.28; IFNβ-1b = 1.13; GA = 1.02; untreated = 0.54), likely reflecting substantial selection bias. Significant declines in annual relapse rate were seen for all treated patients (IFNβ-1a weekly = 49.4%; IFNβ-1a = 65.6%; IFNβ-1b = –64.6%; GA = –81.4%), but rose for those not on therapy (131.5%). The proportion of patients who remained relapse-free over the entire treatment period varied from 37% of untreated to 83% of GA treated patients. Slight differences in EDSS score changes over the study were found, but none was significant.

Haas communicated results from a 24-month prospective, controlled, open-label clinical trial comparing the efficacy of 30 µg IFNβ-1a IM weekly (n = 79), 22 µg IFNβ-1a SC three times weekly (n = 48), 250 µg IFNβ-1b SC every other day (n = 77), and GA (n = 79) (74). RRMS patients with EDSS < 3.5 who were treated for ≥ 6 months were included an ITT-like analysis, with missing values handled as "last observation carried forward." The effect of GA on relapse reduction from prestudy rates was significant at six months (–0.71, p < 0.001), and remained similar at months 12 and 24. Significant reductions from prestudy to on-study relapse rates for all of the IFN preparations tested were also found, but the reduction in relapse rate with GA appeared to be superior to all beta-interferons at month 24 (p < 0.05).

All of the above studies must be regarded with caution. Nevertheless, the treatment effects seen were generally comparable with those found in randomized clinical trials. All of the studies confirm the importance of treatment in reducing relapse rates in RRMS and suggest possible differences in efficacy among immunomodulatory treatments worthy of rigorous study.

Dose Comparison Studies

The optimal dose or frequency of dosing of GA is relatively unexplored. In one study, 58 consecutive RRMS patients were randomly assigned to 20 mg GA daily, 20 mg GA on alternate days, or alternate-day INFβ-1b (75). After 2 years of therapy, all three cohorts showed a similar significant reduction of relapses compared to their prior 2-year relapse rates. Mean disability scores worsened by the study's end for all three cohorts—significantly so for both GA-treated groups. In another study, 68 RRMS patients were followed over two years on open-label, alternate-day GA therapy with no comparator group (76). The mean relapse rate declined by 80.8% with treatment (before = 2.91 ± 1.10; after = 0.56 ± 1.02, p < 0.0001). No firm conclusions can be drawn from this limited view of alternative-day GA therapy, but it does provide some guidance for alternatives for patients on GA therapy whose injection site reactions are problematic.

Therapeutic "Switch" Studies

Preliminary data were presented based on 85 RRMS patients who received 30 µg IFNβ-1a weekly over a mean of 19.7 months before switching to GA; 73% for a lack of efficacy, the rest for intolerable side effects (77). Their annual relapse rates while on IFNβ-1a declined 53% over 18 months of GA. Most of the relapse rate reduction could be attributed to those subjects who switched to GA therapy for a perceived lack of IFNβ-1a efficacy. After 3 years of follow-up from the start of GA, the mean EDSS of the group had slightly improved (78).

In a postmarketing study, the Copaxone Treatment IND Study Group developed data from 805 RRMS patients, 247 of whom had been initially treated with IFNβ-1b, the remainder being treatment naive (79). The subjects with prior exposure to IFNβ-1b had somewhat more disability on entry. All patients received GA and were clinically evaluated every 6 months and within 7 days of any relapse. The mean duration of GA exposure was 20 months. Annualized relapse rates were similar in both treatment-naive (0.3) and prior IFNβ-1b-treated patients (0.4), with both cohorts achieving a 75% relapse rate reduction. The safety and tolerability of GA therapy were similar regardless of prior treatment status.

Combination Therapy

Recombinant interferons have mechanisms of action that include antagonism of proinflammatory cytokines, reduction in T cell activation, and inhibition of blood–brain barrier transmigration and leakage that differ from those of GA (80–82). It is justified to pursue the potential effectiveness of combination therapy. The combination has an additive effect on reducing proliferation of MBP-specific T cells in vitro (83). A 12-month safety study monitored the clinical and MRI effects of adding GA after a three-month run-in period in 33 RRMS patients already taking 30 μg IFNβ-1a IM weekly for ≥ 6 months (84). The combination was safe and a decline in number and volume of Gd-enhanced lesions suggested possible increased effectiveness. Study of the behavior of GA-reactive T cell lines isolated from subjects at one participating site found no evidence to suggest that IFNβ-1a interfered with the immune response to GA. A definitive National Institutes of Health-sponsored trial is underway (2005) to confirm these observations.

Observational Biomarker Studies as Potential Clinical Response Predictors

In MS, where clinical indicators of success (reductions in relapses and accumulated disability and contained MRI activity) are relatively infrequent, delayed or difficult to quantitate), and where available therapies may be only partially effective, prediction or early identification of responders and nonresponders to therapy is a noble goal. In what may prove to have been a signal retrospective study, 44 RRMS patients (29 GA-treated, the rest with weekly 30 μg IFNβ-1a), the subject's MHC haplotype had little, if any, influence on the apparent clinical response to IFNβ-1a. In stark contrast, while all patients on GA had an apparent response to therapy, those who were DRB1*1501+ had a far greater reduction of relapses (twice as many were retrospectively classified as responders than those on GA, who lacked this haplotype). GA binds promiscu-

ously to all common MHC haplotypes. However, the efficiency of presentation of GA complexed to different haplotypes to T cells of appropriate specificity is not well-known. If independently confirmed, this observation would establish that host genetic factors can condition the extent of responsiveness to GA.

In preliminary work requiring prospective confirmation, a highly selected cohort of MS patients failing therapy with GA differed in their in vitro immune response profile to GA compared with GA clinical responders (85). Clearly, there is the suggestion that a combination of genetic profiling, early drug immune response, and sentinel MRI parameters might differentiate those unlikely to respond to GA from the potential responders. Such relative risk response profiles could lead to rational drug selection and knowledge-based decisions on switching therapy before clinical failure becomes obvious.

Experience in Childhood MS

The pivotal trials of GA excluded subjects under 18 years of age. Childhood- and juvenile-onset cases account for only about 5% to 7% of all MS cases, but there is little evidence to suggest that they differ in immunopathogenesis from adult-onset cases. A preliminary communication (86) and other published anecdotal experience suggests that the drug is well-tolerated in children (87); no conclusions on efficacy can be drawn from these anecdotal reports.

TOLERABILITY

Preclinical Studies

Preclinical toxicology indicates that GA is safe, nonmutagenic, and not carcinogenic at up to 15 times the human therapeutic dose. No toxic fetal loss, fetal abnormalities, or postnatal developmental abnormalities occurred in animal reproduction studies at doses up to 36 times the human equivalent. In vivo studies showed only hypotensive effects following high-dose intravenous GA boluses.

Clinical Safety

Safety data on > 3,500 subjects (70% female patients) collected from controlled and uncontrolled studies show adverse experiences leading to therapy withdrawal in 8.4%. Most often cited were dyspnea and vasodilation (~2% each). No patients withdrew for laboratory abnormalities. Local injection site reactions are the most common adverse experiences, described as erythema (41.6%), pain (37%), inflammation (24.5%), pruritus (19.5%), and swelling (12.8%), without skin necrosis. Localized lipoatrophy occurs after a year or more of treatment in some cases (88,89). In a recent review of 76 prior or current GA users identified by chart review and then follow-up examination in a single clinic, 43% had evidence of some regional lipoatrophy, which was rated severe in five women (90). Other adverse events reported by more than 5% of patients include vasodilation (14%), dyspnea (10%), pain (10%), headache (10%), asthenia (10%), urinary infections (8%), paresthesia (7%), rash (7%), depression (6%), nausea (5%), anxiety (5%), backache (5%), and fever (5%).

A postinjection systemic reaction happens in 10% to 15% of GA-treated patients. Affected patients report a variable combination of flushing, chest tightness, palpitations, dyspnea, tachycardia, and anxiety within seconds or minutes of the injection. Portions of or the entire symptom complex last several minutes to several hours, and resolve spontaneously. Most patients who experience this reaction have a single episode, but some have additional episodes at irregular intervals. The cause of the reaction is unknown.

Two of 3,736 patients treated with GA in clinical trials experienced drug-related, nonfatal anaphylactic reactions (data on file, Teva Pharmaceutical Industries, Nordau, Netanya, Israel). There is no evidence of relevant drug interactions.

GA does not induce hematological abnormalities, elevation of hepatic enzymes, flu-like symptoms, depression, or abnormalities of blood pressure. Fatigue may even decrease for some on GA therapy (91). Overall, adverse events observed during GA treatment are few and mild. No medication guide is required by the U.S. Food and Drug Administration (FDA) to accompany its use. Extensive experience with GA in > 40,000 patients shows that it is well-tolerated and local adverse events rarely limit treatment (92).

Pregnancy

Among 253 of 421 reported pregnancies with exposure to GA and known outcome were 187 healthy births, 47 spontaneous abortions, 11 elective abortions, one ectopic pregnancy, and one stillbirth (86). Six cases involved congenital anomalies including failure to thrive, finger anomaly, cardiomyopathy, urethrostenosis, anencephaly, and left adrenal cyst. The remaining 168 cases had not yet reached their due date or were lost to follow-up. Major congenital anomalies occur in 3% of the general population and spontaneous abortion in 15% to 20%. Thus, the rate of these outcomes in women exposed to GA for varying intervals surrounding conception and gestation is within that of the general population. However, GA is viewed as a Pregnancy Category B drug (93).

CONCLUSIONS

MS typically begins with symptoms that can resolve completely or leave residual deficits, with a clinical course that spans years; untreated, it is usually a progressively disabling disease. While the immunopharmacology of GA is complex and not completely understood, the drug appears to have both anti-inflammatory and neuroprotective effects. Controlled studies demonstrate the benefits of GA therapy on the clinically relevant outcomes of reduced relapse rate, delayed accumulation of disability, and on major MRI-monitored measures of disease pathology, with some indication that it may retard the progression of clinical disability that occurs in the absence of defined relapses. The drug has a favorable side effect profile. GA may be most effective when begun in the early phases of the disease and its effects appear to persist over long-term treatment. GA appears a reasonable first-choice therapy for relapsing MS, and a logical alternative for patients who must switch from a beta-interferon due to intolerable side effects or apparent lack of efficacy.

REFERENCES

1. Lublin FD, Baier M, Cutter G. Effect of relapses on development of residual deficit in multiple sclerosis. *Neurology* 2003;61:1528–32.
2. Lublin FD, Reingold SC. Defining the clinical course of multiple sclerosis: results of an international survey. National Multiple Sclerosis Society (USA) Advisory Committee on Clinical Trials of New Agents in Multiple Sclerosis. *Neurology* 1996;46:907–911.
3. Miller DH, Khan OA, Sheremata WA, et al. A controlled trial of natalizumab for relapsing multiple sclerosis. *N Engl J Med* 2003;348:15–23.
4. Hartung H-P, Gonsette R, König N, et al. Mitoxantrone in progressive multiple sclerosis: a placebo-controlled, double-blind, randomised, multicentre trial. *Lancet* 2002;360:2018–2025.
5. Goodin DS, Arnason BG, Coyle PK, et al. The use of mitoxantrone (Novantrone) for the treatment of multiple sclerosis: report of the Therapeutics and Technology Assessment Subcommittee of the American Academy of Neurology. *Neurology* 2003;61:1332–1338.
6. Dhib-Jalbut S. Glatiramer acetate (Copaxone) therapy for multiple sclerosis. *Pharmacol Ther* 2003;98:245–255.
7. Wolinsky JS. Glatiramer acetate for the treatment of multiple sclerosis. *Expert Opin Pharmacother* 2004;5:875–891.
8. Arnon R. The development of Cop 1 (Copaxone), an innovative drug for the treatment of multiple sclerosis: personal reflections. *Immunol Lett* 1996;50:1–15.
9. Fridkis-Hareli M, Neveu JM, Robinson RA, et al. Binding motifs of copolymer 1 to multiple sclerosis- and rheumatoid arthritis-associated HLA-DR molecules. *J Immunol* 1999;162:4697–4704.
10. Gauthier L, Smith KJ, Pyrdol J, et al. Expression and crystallization of the complex of HLA-DR2 (DRA, DRB1*1501) and an immunodominant peptide of human myelin basic protein. *Proc Natl Acad Sci USA* 1998;95:11828–11833.
11. Aharoni R, Teitelbaum D, Arnon R, et al. Copolymer 1 acts against the immunodominant epitope 82–100 of myelin basic protein by T cell receptor antagonism in addition to major histocompatibility complex blocking. *Proc Natl Acad Sci USA* 1999;96:634–639.
12. Sela M, Teitelbaum D. Glatiramer acetate in the treatment of multiple sclerosis. *Expert Opin Pharmacother* 2001;2:1149–1165.
13. Arnon R, Sela M, Teitelbaum D. New insights into the mechanism of action of copolymer 1 in experimental allergic encephalomyelitis and multiple sclerosis. *J Neurol* 1996;243:S8–S13.
14. Neuhaus O, Farina C, Wekerle H, et al. Mechanisms of action of glatiramer acetate in multiple sclerosis. *Neurology* 2001;56:702–708.
15. Neuhaus O, Farina C, Yassouridis A, et al. Multiple sclerosis: comparison of copolymer-1-reactive T cell lines from treated and untreated subjects reveals

cytokine shift from T helper 1 to T helper 2 cells. *Proc Natl Acad Sci USA* 2000;97:7452–7457.
16. Chen M, Gran B, Costello K, et al. Glatiramer acetate induces a Th2-biased response and crossreactivity with myelin basic protein in patients with MS. *Mult Scler* 2001;7:209–219.
17. Miller A, Shapiro S, Gershtein R, et al. Treatment of multiple sclerosis with copolymer-1 (Copaxone): implicating mechanisms of Th1 to Th2/Th3 immune-deviation. *J Neuroimmunol* 1998;92:113–121.
18. Duda PW, Schmied MC, Cook SL, et al. Glatiramer acetate (Copaxone) induces degenerate, Th2-polarized immune responses in patients with multiple sclerosis. *J Clin Invest* 2000;105:967–976.
19. Dhib-Jalbut S, Chen M, Said A, et al. Glatiramer acetate-reactive peripheral blood mononuclear cells respond to multiple myelin antigens with a Th2-biased phenotype. *J Neuroimmunol* 2003;140:163–171.
20. Duda PW, Krieger JI, Schmied MC, et al. Human and murine CD4 T cell reactivity to a complex antigen: recognition of the synthetic random polypeptide glatiramer acetate. *J Immunol* 2000;165:7300–7307.
21. Brenner T, Arnon R, Sela M, et al. Humoral and cellular immune responses to Copolymer 1 in multiple sclerosis patients treated with Copaxone(R). *J Neuroimmunol* 2001;115:152–160.
22. Rieks M, Hoffmann V, Aktas O, et al. Induction of apoptosis of CD4+ T cells by immunomodulatory therapy of multiple sclerosis with glatiramer acetate. *Eur Neurol* 2003;50:200–206.
23. Chen M, Conway K, Johnson KP, et al. Sustained immunological effects of Glatiramer acetate in patients with multiple sclerosis treated for over 6 years. *J Neurol Sci* 2002;201:71–7.
24. Biernacki K, Prat A, Blain M, et al. Regulation of Th1 and Th2 lymphocyte migration by human adult brain endothelial cells. *J Neuropathol Exp Neurol* 2001;60:1127–1136.
25. Aharoni R, Teitelbaum D, Arnon R, et al. Copolymer 1 inhibits manifestations of graft rejection. *Transplantation* 2001;72:598–605.
26. Aharoni R, Kayhan B, Eilam R, et al. Glatiramer acetate-specific T cells in the brain express T helper 2/3 cytokines and brain-derived neurotrophic factor in situ. *Proc Natl Acad Sci USA* 2003;100:14157–14162.
27. Chen M, Valenzuela RM, Dhib-Jalbut S. Glatiramer acetate-reactive T cells produce brain-derived neurotrophic factor. *J Neurol Sci* 2003;215:37–44.
28. Yong VW. Differential mechanisms of action of interferon-beta and glatiramer acetate in MS. *Neurology* 2002;59:802–808.
29. Angelov DN, Waibel S, Guntinas-Lichius O, et al. Therapeutic vaccine for acute and chronic motor neuron diseases: implications for amyotrophic lateral sclerosis. *Proc Natl Acad Sci USA* 2003;100:4790–4795.
30. Benner EJ, Mosley RL, Destache CJ, et al. Therapeutic immunization protects dopaminergic neurons in a mouse model of Parkinson's disease. *Proc Natl Acad Sci USA* 2004;101:9435–9440.
31. Moalem G, Leibowitz-Amit R, Yoles E, et al. Autoimmune T cells protect neurons from secondary degeneration after central nervous system axotomy. *Nat Med* 1999;5:49–55.
32. Kipnis J, Yoles E, Porat Z, et al. T cell immunity to copolymer 1 confers neuroprotection on the damaged

optic nerve: possible therapy for optic neuropathies. *Proc Natl Acad Sci USA* 2000;97:7446–451.

33. Schori H, Kipnis J, Yoles E, et al. Vaccination for protection of retinal ganglion cells against death from glutamate cytotoxicity and ocular hypertension: implications for glaucoma. *Proc Natl Acad Sci USA* 2001;98:3398–3403.

34. Gilgun-Sherki Y, Panet H, Holdengreber V, et al. Axonal damage is reduced following glatiramer acetate treatment in C57/bl mice with chronic-induced experimental autoimmune encephalomyelitis. *Neurosci Res* 2003;47:201–207.

35. Parkinson JF, Mitrovic B, Merrill JE. The role of nitric oxide in multiple sclerosis. *J Mol Med* 1997;75:174–186.

36. Kayhan B, Aharoni R, Arnon R. Glatiramer acetate (Copaxone) regulates nitric oxide and related cytokine secretion in experimental autoimmune encephalomyelitis *Immunol Lett* 2003;88:185–192.

37. Thoenen H. Neurotrophins and neuronal plasticity. *Science* 1995;270:593–598.

38. Ziemssen T, Kumpfel T, Klinkert WE, et al. Glatiramer acetate-specific T-helper 1- and 2-type cell lines produce BDNF: implications for multiple sclerosis therapy. Brain-derived neurotrophic factor. *Brain* 2002;125:2381–2391.

39. Stadelmann C, Kerschensteiner M, Misgeld T, et al. BDNF and gp145trkB in multiple sclerosis brain lesions: neuroprotective interactions between immune and neuronal cells? *Brain* 2002;125:75–85.

40. Chabot S, Yong FP, Le DM, et al. Cytokine production in T lymphocyte-microglia interaction is attenuated by glatiramer acetate: a mechanism for therapeutic efficacy in multiple sclerosis. *Mult Scler* 2002;8:299–306.

41. Kim HJ, Ifergan I, Antel JP, et al. Type 2 monocyte and microglia differentiation mediated by glatiramer acetate therapy in patients with multiple sclerosis. *J Immunol* 2004;172:7144–153.

42. Weber MS, Starck M, Wagenpfeil S, et al. Multiple sclerosis: glatiramer acetate inhibits monocyte reactivity in vitro and in vivo. *Brain* 2004;127:1370–1378.

43. Teitelbaum D, Aharoni R, Sela M, et al. Cross-reactions and specificities of monoclonal antibodies against myelin basic protein and against the synthetic copolymer 1. *Proc Natl Acad Sci USA* 1991;88:9528–9532.

44. Ure DR, Rodriguez M. Polyreactive antibodies to glatiramer acetate promote myelin repair in murine model of demyelinating disease. *FASEB J* 2002;16:1260–1262.

45. Farina C, Vargas V, Heydari N, et al. Treatment with glatiramer acetate induces specific IgG4 antibodies in multiple sclerosis patients. *J Neuroimmunol* 2002;123:188–192.

46. Teitelbaum D, Brenner T, Abramsky O, et al. Antibodies to glatiramer acetate do not interfere with its biological functions and therapeutic efficacy. *Mult Scler* 2003;9:592–599.

47. Salama HH, Hong J, Zang YC, et al. Blocking effects of serum reactive antibodies induced by glatiramer acetate treatment in multiple sclerosis. *Brain* 2003;126:2638–2647.

48. Bornstein MB, Miller A, Slagle S, et al. A pilot trial of Cop 1 in exacerbating-remitting multiple sclerosis. *N Engl J Med* 1987;317:408–414.

49. Johnson KP, Brooks BR, Cohen JA, et al. Copolymer 1 reduces relapse rate and improves disability in relapsing-remitting multiple sclerosis: results of a phase III multicenter, double-blind placebo-controlled trial. The Copolymer 1 Multiple Sclerosis Study Group. *Neurology* 1995;45:1268–1276.

50. Johnson KP, Brooks BR, Cohen JA, et al. Extended use of glatiramer acetate (Copaxone) is well tolerated and maintains its clinical effect on multiple sclerosis relapse rate and degree of disability. Copolymer 1 Multiple Sclerosis Study Group. *Neurology* 1998;50:701–708.

51. Johnson KP, Brooks BB, Ford CC, et al. Results of the long term (eight-year) prospective, open-label trial of glatiramer acetate for relapsing multiple sclerosis. *Neurology* 2002;58:A458.

52. Johnson KP, Brooks BR, Ford CC, et al. Glatiramer acetate (Copaxone): comparison of continuous versus delayed therapy in a six-year organized multiple sclerosis trial. *Mult Scler* 2003;9:585–591.

53. Weinshenker BG. The natural history of multiple sclerosis. *Neurol Clin* 1995;13:119–146.

54. Ford C, Johnson K, Brooks B, et al. Sustained efficacy and tolerability of Copaxone (glatiramer acetate) in relapsing-remitting multiple sclerosis patients treated for over 10 years. *Mult Scler* 2003;9:120.

55. Comi G, Filippi M, Wolinsky JS. European/Canadian multicenter, double-blind, randomized, placebo-controlled study of the effects of glatiramer acetate on magnetic resonance imaging—measured disease activity and burden in patients with relapsing multiple sclerosis. European/Canadian Glatiramer Acetate Study Group. *Ann Neurol* 2001;49:290–297.

56. Boneschi FM, Rovaris M, Johnson KP, et al. Effects of glatiramer acetate on relapse rate and accumulated disability in multiple sclerosis: meta-analysis of three double-blind, randomized, placebo-controlled clinical trials. *Mult Scler* 2003;9:349–355.

57. Wolinsky JS, Johnson KP, Comi G, et al. The effects of glatiramer acetate on sustained accumulated disability in relapsing multiple sclerosis are evident within one year: meta-analysis results of three double-blind, placebo-controlled clinical trials. *Mult Scler* 2003;9:120.

58. Munari L, Lovati R, Boiko A. Therapy with glatiramer acetate for multiple sclerosis. *Cochrane Database Syst Rev* 2004;CD004678.

59. Bornstein MB, Miller A, Slagle S, et al. A placebo-controlled, double-blind, randomized, two-center, pilot trial of Cop 1 in chronic progressive multiple sclerosis. *Neurology* 1991;41:533–539.

60. Aharoni R, Meshorer A, Sela M, et al. Oral treatment of mice with copolymer 1 (glatiramer acetate) results in the accumulation of specific Th2 cells in the central nervous system. *J Neuroimmunol* 2002;126:58–68.

61. Maron R, Slavin AJ, Hoffmann E, et al. Oral tolerance to copolymer 1 in myelin basic protein (MBP) TCR transgenic mice: cross-reactivity with MBP-specific TCR and differential induction of anti-inflammatory cytokines. *Int Immunol* 2002;14:131–138.

62. Wolinsky JS. The diagnosis of primary progressive multiple sclerosis. *J Neurol Sci* 2003;206:145–152.

63. Wolinsky JS, Pardo L, Stark Y, et al. Effect of glatiramer acetate on primary progressive multiple sclerosis: initial analysis of the completed PROMiSe Trial. *Neurology* 2004;62:A97–A98.

64. Mancardi GL, Sardanelli F, Parodi RC, et al. Effect of copolymer-1 on serial gadolinium-enhanced MRI in

relapsing remitting multiple sclerosis. *Neurology* 1998;50:1127–1133.

65. Ge Y, Grossman RI, Udupa JK, et al. Glatiramer acetate (Copaxone) treatment in relapsing-remitting MS: quantitative MR assessment. *Neurology* 2000;54:813–817.

66. Wolinsky JS, Narayana PA, Johnson KP. United States open-label glatiramer acetate extension trial for relapsing multiple sclerosis: MRI and clinical correlates. Multiple Sclerosis Study Group and the MRI Analysis Center. *Mult Scler* 2001;7:33–41.

67. Wolinsky JS, Comi G, Filippi M, et al. Copaxone's effect on MRI-monitored disease in relapsing MS is reproducible and sustained. *Neurology* 2002;59:1284–1286.

68. Filippi M, Rovaris M, Rocca MA, et al. Glatiramer acetate reduces the proportion of new MS lesions evolving into "black holes." *Neurology* 2001;57:731–733.

69. Rovaris M, Comi G, Rocca MA, et al. Short-term brain volume change in relapsing-remitting multiple sclerosis: effect of glatiramer acetate and implications. *Brain* 2001;124:1803–1812.

70. Sormani MP, Rovaris M, Valsasina P, et al. Measurement error of two different techniques for brain atrophy assessment in multiple sclerosis. *Neurology* 2004;62:1432–1434.

71. Carra A, Onaha P, Sinay V, et al. A retrospective, observational study comparing the four available immunomodulatory treatments for relapsing-remitting multiple sclerosis. *Eur J Neurol* 2003;10:671–676.

72. Khan OA, Tselis AC, Kamholz JA, et al. A prospective, open-label treatment trial to compare the effect of IFN beta-1a (Avonex), IFNbeta-1b (Betaseron), and glatiramer acetate (Copaxone) on the relapse rate in relapsing-remitting multiple sclerosis. *Eur J Neurol* 2001;8:141–148.

73. Khan OA, Tselis AC, Kamholz JA, et al. A prospective, open-label treatment trial to compare the effect of IFNbeta-1a (Avonex), IFNbeta-1b (Betaseron), and glatiramer acetate (Copaxone) on the relapse rate in relapsing–remitting multiple sclerosis: results after 18 months of therapy. *Mult Scler* 2001;7:349–353.

74. Haas J. Onset of clinical benefit of glatiramer (Copaxone) acetate in 255 patients with relapsing-remitting multiple sclerosis. *Neurology* 2003;60:A480.

75. Flechter S, Vardi J, Pollak L, et al. Comparison of glatiramer acetate (Copaxone) and interferon beta-1b (Betaseron) in multiple sclerosis patients: an open-label 2-year follow-up. *J Neurol Sci* 2002;197:51–55.

76. Flechter S, Kott E, Steiner-Birmanns B, et al. Copolymer 1 (glatiramer acetate) in relapsing forms of multiple sclerosis: open multicenter study of alternate-day administration. *Clin Neuropharmacol* 2002;25:11–15.

77. Khan O, Caon C, Zvartau-Hind M, et al. Clinical course before and after change of immunomodulating therapy in relapsing remitting MS. *Neurology* 2001;56:A355.

78. Caon C, Din M, Zvartau-Hind M, et al. Three-year follow-up and clinical course after change of immunomodulatory therapy in relapsing-remitting MS. *J Neurology* 2003;250[Suppl 2]:190.

79. Zwibel H, for the Copaxone Treatment IND Study Group. Benefit of Copaxone demonstrated in patients with relapsing-remitting multiple sclerosis (RRMS) previously treated with interferon. *J Neurology* 2001;248[Suppl 2]:P521.

80. Dhib-Jalbut S. Mechanisms of action of interferons and glatiramer acetate in multiple sclerosis. *Neurology* 2002;58:S3–S9.

81. Yong VW. Differential mechanisms of action of interferon-a and glatiramer acetate in MS. *Neurology* 2002;59:802–808.

82. Simpson D, Noble S, Perry C. Glatiramer acetate: a review of its use in relapsing-remitting multiple sclerosis. *CNS Drugs* 2002;16:825–850.

83. Milo R, Panitch H. Additive effects of copolymer-1 and interferon beta-1a on the immune response to myelin basic protein. *J Neuroimmunol* 1995;61:185–193.

84. Lublin F, Cutter G, Elfont R, et al. A trial to assess the safety of combining therapy with interferon beta-1a and glatiramer acetate in patients with relapsing MS. *Neurology* 2001;56:A148.

85. Farina C, Wagenpfeil S, Hohlfeld R. Immunological assay for assessing the efficacy of glatiramer acetate (Copaxone) in multiple sclerosis. A pilot study. *J Neurol* 2002;249:1587–1592.

86. Coyle PK, Johnson KP, Pardo L, et al. Pregnancy outcomes in patients with multiple sclerosis treated with glatiramer acetate (Copaxone). *Mult Scler* 2003; 9:P160.

87. Kornek B, Bernert G, Balassy C, et al. Glatiramer acetate treatment in patients with childhood and juvenile onset multiple sclerosis. *Neuropediatrics* 2003;34: 120–126.

88. Mancardi GL, Murialdo A, Drago F, et al. Localized lipoatrophy after prolonged treatment with copolymer 1. *J Neurol* 2000;247:220–221.

89. Hwang L, Orengo I. Lipoatrophy associated with glatiramer acetate injections for the treatment of multiple sclerosis. *Cutis* 2001;68:287–288.

90. Edgar CM, Brunet DG, Fenton P, et al. Lipoatrophy in patients with multiple sclerosis on glatiramer acetate. *Can J Neurol Sci* 2004;31:58–63.

91. Metz LM, Patten SB, Archibald CJ, et al. The effect of immunomodulatory treatment on multiple sclerosis fatigue. *J Neurol Neurosurg Psychiatry* 2004;75:1045–1047.

92. Ziemssen T, Neuhaus O, Hohlfeld R. Risk-benefit assessment of glatiramer acetate in multiple sclerosis. *Drug Saf* 2001;24:979–990.

93. Ferrero S, Pretta S, Ragni N. Multiple sclerosis: management issues during pregnancy. *Eur J Obstet Gynecol Reprod Biol* 2004;115:3–9.

18

Mitoxantrone in Multiple Sclerosis

Oliver Neuhaus, Bernd C. Kieseier and Hans-Peter Hartung

Department of Neurology, Heinrich Heine University, Düsseldorf, Germany

INTRODUCTION

The results of the Phase III MIMS study (Mitoxantrone In Multiple Sclerosis) provide clear evidence for the use of mitoxantrone in patients with active relapsing-remitting multiple sclerosis (RRMS) or secondary progressive multiple sclerosis (SPMS), a fact acknowledged by the approval of several health authorities. This chapter discusses the putative mechanisms of action of mitoxantrone, provides an outline of relevant preclinical as well as clinical studies, discusses relevant side effects of the compound, and places mitoxantrone in the context of other therapeutic approaches available against this disabling disorder.

Therapeutic Approaches in Multiple Sclerosis

Until the early 1990s, corticosteroids were the sole proven therapy, but they were active only in shortening acute MS attacks; effective long-term drug treatment was not available. In addition, a number of immunosuppressive agents (i.e., inhibitors of crucial components of the immune system causing generalized immune dysfunction) were used off-label, but their potential beneficial effects in MS were limited by systemic adverse effects, such as increased risk of cancer or infection. Examples are azathioprine (licensed for MS treatment in some countries) or cyclophosphamide. More recently, two classes of immunomodulatory agents have been approved for the treatment of RRMS, namely interferon-β (IFN-β1a or IFN-β1b) and glatiramer acetate (GA). Immunomodulators—without generally suppressing immunological properties—shift immune responses from proinflammatory autoimmune conditions (mediated by T-helper (TH)-1 cytokines released from autoreactive T cells) toward a more beneficial anti-inflammatory environment (mediated through TH2 cytokines secreted by regulatory T cells). Both IFN-β and GA have been proven to be at least partially effective in RRMS as assessed in pivotal and subsequent trials (1–4).

Treatment options in SPMS are limited. All IFN-β preparations have been investigated in Phase III clinical trials, but only IFN-β1b, as administered in the European Trial of Betaferon in SPMS (EUSP) (5), convincingly delayed time to onset of sustained progression of disability as measured by the Expanded Disability Status Scale (EDSS) (6). Thus, recent approval of mitoxantrone in MS gave clinicians another evidence-based therapeutic tool for treatment of active RRMS and SPMS.

For PPMS patients, treatment options are even more limited. So far, no immunomodulatory or immunosuppressive agents have been proven effective in PPMS. Currently, the therapeutic focus of PPMS is based on symptomatic measures. Other therapeutic strategies are reviewed elsewhere (8,9).

Mitoxantrone

Mitoxantrone (Fig. 18-1) was developed in the 1970s and is an antineoplastic agent. It is an anthracenedione derivative related to the anthracyclins doxorubicin and daunorubicin. It interacts with topoisomerase-2 and causes single- and double-strand breaks by intercalating the DNA (10), and is used to effectively treat various malignancies such as breast and advanced prostate cancer, lymphoma, and leukemia (11). Furthermore, strong immunosuppressive properties of mitoxantrone have been observed, providing a rationale for its use in autoimmune disorders such as MS (12–15).

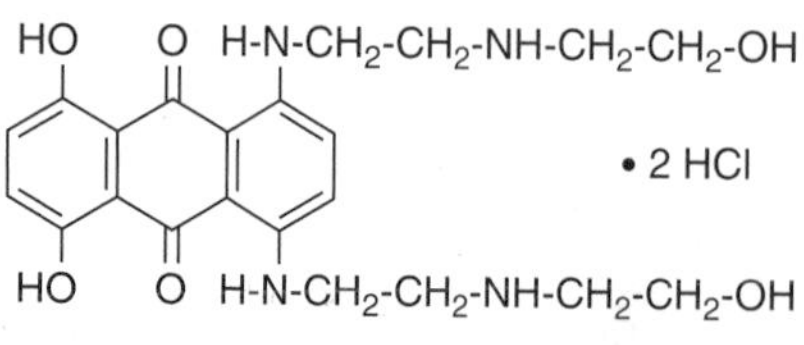

FIG. 18-1. Structure of mitoxantrone: Mitoxantrone, 1,4-Dihydroxy-5,8-bis-[[2-[(2-hydroxyethyl)-amino]-ethyl]-amino]-anthraquinone dihydrochloride, $C_{22}H_{28}N_4O_6$ ● 2HCl; molecular mass: 517.4 Da.

Putative Mechanisms of Action of Mitoxantrone in Multiple Sclerosis

Apart from the cytotoxic efficacy of mitoxantrone, immunosuppressive effects and even antiviral and antibiotic effects have been observed. More recently, immunomodulatory properties have been suggested, as a number of distinct immunological effects have been described (12,16,17). Possible action sites of mitoxantrone in the putative pathogenesis of MS are shown in Figure 18-2. Still, more research is warranted to illuminate the immunological effects of mitoxantrone in MS, as its specific mechanisms of action targeting the immune system still remain unclear.

Immunosuppressive Properties

As has been well-established for decades, mitoxantrone is a potent immunosuppressive agent targeting proliferating immune cells (18–21). It inhibits proliferation of macrophages, B lymphocytes and T lymphocytes (18,20,22).

Effects on Helper and Suppressor T Cells

In an in vitro system testing an anti-sheep red blood cell response, mitoxantrone was observed to inhibit T helper activity and, conversely, to enhance T suppressor functions (19). In contrast, in an in vivo mouse model, the induction of suppressor T cells was also abrogated by mitoxantrone (19). T helper cells were indirectly inhibited by mitoxantrone-induced macrophages.

Induction of Cell Death—Apoptosis and Cell Lysis

Mitoxantrone was shown to induce apoptosis of B lymphocytes (23) and other types of antigen-presenting cells (24). Comparison of peripheral blood mononuclear cells (PBMC) obtained from MS patients before and immediately after application of mitoxantrone exhibited a decreased proliferation of PBMC based on necrotic cell death (22). Thus, there may be a bimodal mechanism of cell death induced by

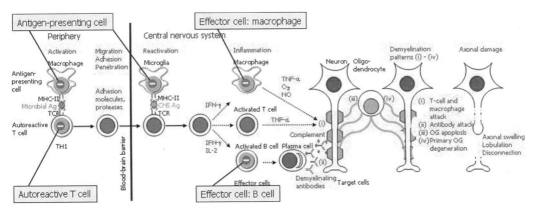

FIG. 18-2. Action sites of mitoxantrone in the hypothetical pathogenesis of MS. Via their T cell receptor (TCR), proinflammatory T cells are activated in the periphery by foreign or self antigens (Ag) presented on major histocompatibility complex class II (MHC-II) by antigen-presenting cells. The activated T cells migrate to, adhere at, and penetrate through the blood–brain barrier, a step mediated by adhesion molecules, proteases, and chemokines. Inside the central nervous system (CNS), the T cells are reactivated by CNS Ag presented on MHC-II by other antigen-presenting cells, predominantly microglia cells. The reactivated T cells secrete proinflammatory cytokines, such as interferon (IFN)-γ or interleukin (IL)-2 and induce CNS inflammation by subsequent activation of macrophages, other T cells, and B cells as effector cells. Macrophages and T cells attack the oligodendrocytic myelin sheath by cytotoxic mediators, mainly tumor necrosis factor (TNF)-α, oxygen (O_2) radicals, and nitric oxide (NO). B cells differentiate to plasma cells that secrete demyelinating antibodies. They can guide and activate macrophages or ignite the complement cascade with assembly of the membrane attack complex, which causes pore formation in myelin membranes. Mitoxantrone exerts inhibitory effects on autoreactive T cells, B cells, macrophages, and other antigen-presenting cells. (Modified, with permission, from Neuhaus O, Archelos JJ, Hartung HP. Immunomodulation in multiple sclerosis: from immunosuppression to neuroprotection. *Trends Pharmacol Sci.* 2003;24:131–138.)

mitoxantrone: apoptosis at lower concentrations and cell lysis at higher concentrations. Previous pharmacokinetic studies in oncology revealed maximum serum concentrations of mitoxantrone between 308 and 839 ng/mL and terminal half-lifes between 38.4 and 71.5 hours (25–28). Thus, in the first approximately 10 days after infusion, maximum serum concentrations are higher than 20 ng/mL (a putative threshold between induction of necrosis and apoptosis) (24), whereas the following time after infusion (approximately 80 days at a 3-month dosage regime), the concentrations are below 20 pg/mL. Thus, mitoxantrone apparently may act via short-term immunosuppressive effects by the induction of cell lysis leading both to leukocyte reduction in the blood post infusion and to inhibition of proliferation of all types of immune cells in vitro (18,19,22). In addition, a long-term immuno-

logical impact of mitoxantrone is considered to occur at lower and lowest concentrations by induction of programmed cell death in antigen-presenting cells (24). Consistent with this hypothesis, the clinical effects of mitoxantrone in MS have been suggested to last up to one year posttreatment (29).

Effects on the Cytokine Network

In the 1980s, Fidler et al. reported a decreased secretion of the proinflammatory cytokines interferon-γ, tumor necrosis factor (TNF)-α, and interleukin (IL)-2 (18). In contrast, recent ex vivo analysis of the cytokine profile of immune cells obtained from patients before and during treatment with mitoxantrone revealed a decrease of IL-10 (an anti-inflammatory cytokine) expressing monocytes and of IL-2R-β1 expressing T cells after six months of treatment (30).

Mitoxantrone in Experimental Autoimmune Encephalomyelitis

Also in the 1980s, mitoxantrone was proven effective in experimental autoimmune encephalomyelitis (EAE), an animal model of MS (31–33). Ridge et al. observed an inhibitory effect as determined by clinical evaluation and histopathology in rat EAE (31). Interestingly, in an adoptive transfer model, encephalitogenic T cells treated with mitoxantrone prior to injection were no longer able to induce the disease, indicating an inhibitory effect of mitoxantrone on T cells. Clinical relapses could be prevented or ameliorated (32,33).

Clinical Studies of Mitoxantrone in Multiple Sclerosis

In a number of small, open trials, positive effects of mitoxantrone in MS were documented [overview in (13) and Table 18-1]. In a randomized, magnetic resonance imaging (MRI)-controlled but clinically unblinded and non-placebo-controlled trial in France and the United Kingdom, the effects of mitoxantrone were assessed in patients with very active MS, defined as frequent, severe relapses without clinical remittance (34). Forty-two patients were included and randomized to receive monthly infusions of either 20 mg mitoxantrone (irrespective of the body surface) plus 1 g methylprednisolone (MP) or 1 g MP alone for six months. The primary endpoint was the percentage of patients without new, active MRI lesions. At study entry the percentages were: mitoxantrone plus MP, 10%; MP alone, 4.8%. After 6 months, the numbers were: mitoxantrone plus MP, 90%; MP alone, 31% (p < 0.001).

In an Italian trial, the efficacy of mitoxantrone was assessed in 51 patients with RRMS (35). Inclusion criteria were an EDSS between 2 and 5 (6) and at least two relapses within the previous two years. The patients were randomized and received either mitoxantrone (8 mg/m^2 body surface) or placebo. Clinical assessment was performed by blinded physicians. The primary endpoint was the percentage of patients with clinical progression, defined as an EDSS increase by 1 point. After 24 months of observation, 9 out of 24 patients with placebo (37%) and 2 out of 27 patients with mitoxantrone (7%) deteriorated clinically by 1 EDSS point (p = 0.02). Regarding the secondary endpoints, mitoxantrone was partially superior to placebo.

A comparative double-blind trial of mitoxantrone (13 infusions of 12 mg/m^2 body surface) versus MP (13 infusions of 1 g, both groups over 32 months) performed in Belgium on 49 patients with SPMS revealed both a significant improvement of the EDSS and a significant decrease of the total number of gadolinium-enhancing lesions in the mitoxantrone group (36).

The largest and most definitive Phase III study, the MIMS study (Mitoxantrone In Multiple Sclerosis) (37) was a randomized, placebo-controlled, investigator-blinded, multicenter trial in patients with worsening RRMS and SPMS. One hundred ninety-four patients with an EDSS between 3 and 6 were randomized and divided into three groups: (a) mitoxantrone 12 mg/m^2 body surface, (b) mitoxantrone 5 mg/m^2, and (c) placebo (methylene blue). All patients received mitoxantrone or placebo intravenously every 3 months for 2 years. The primary study endpoint was a multivariate analysis of five different clinical parameters (change from three neurological baseline scores, including

TABLE 18-1 *First clinical studies of mitoxantrone in MS*

Author	Number of Patients	MS Course	Dosage
Gonsette and	16	Relapsing	14 mg/m^2 body surface every 3 weeks for 3
Demonty (65)	6	Progressive	cycles followed by 14 mg/m^2 every 3 months for up to 2 years
Kappos et al. (66)	14	Rapidly progressing	10 mg/m^2 every 3 weeks
Mauch et al. (20)	6	Relapsing	12 mg/m^2 every 3 months
	4	Progressive	
Noseworthy et al. (67)	13	Progressive	8 mg/m^2 every 3 weeks

EDSS after 24 months, time to first treated relapse, and number of relapses treated with steroids). After 2 years, 188 patients still participated in the study. In all five parameters (making up the predefined multivariate endpoint), the mitoxantrone 12 mg/m^2 group was significantly superior compared to the other groups. Progression of disability and relapse rate were significantly reduced. This therapeutic effect still was measurable 12 months after the final infusion. In a subgroup of 110 patients, in addition to the clinical investigation, MRI assessment was performed and analyzed in a central laboratory. Significantly fewer patients receiving 12mg/m^2 mitoxantrone demonstrated enhancing lesions at 24 months relative to placebo (0% versus 15.6%, p = 0.02). The mean increase in the number of T2-weighted lesions was 0.29 in 12 mg/m^2 mitoxantrone and 1.94 in placebo recipients (p = 0.03). In both mitoxantrone groups, a significant reduction of new lesions and a reduced burden of disease were observed. Table 18-2 summarizes the most important aspects of the controlled clinical trials.

CURRENT CLINICAL ASPECTS OF MITOXANTRONE IN MULTIPLE SCLEROSIS

Several national and international medical advisory boards to MS societies recommend the use of mitoxantrone in patients with RRMS with frequent relapses and incomplete remissions, and with SPMS with rapid progression (by at least one EDSS point per year). Indication of treatment should be given by experienced clinical MS centers. Although the following treatment recommendations have no definite evidence base (but do reflect expert opinions), three groups of MS patients are recommended for treatment with mitoxantrone (15,38,39):

1. RRMS patients with two or more relapses per year, incomplete remission (EDSS ≥ 3), and insufficient response to IFN-β or GA
2. SPMS patients with marked progression of disability (≥ 1 EDSS point per year) and/or high relapse rate (≥ 2 relapses per year)
3. SPMS patients with rapid progression (≥ 1 EDSS point per year) without relapses

According to the primary endpoints of the different clinical studies with mitoxantrone, the therapeutic goal is the clinical and MRI stabilization of the disease. The characterization criteria of responders or nonresponders and the treatment duration before the evaluation of a clinical response are not yet defined. A suggested but not evidence-based marker to detect a clinical nonresponder is the deterioration of one EDSS point after 1 year of treatment.

Before onset of therapy a number of laboratory exams are recommended, including pregnancy test (during pregnancy and nursing, mitoxantrone is contraindicated), chest x-ray, electrocardiography, and echocardiography with quantitative assessment of the left ventricular

TABLE 18-2 *Mitoxantrone in MS–controlled clinical trials*

	French–British Trial (34)	Italian Trial (35)	MIMS Trial (37)
Number of Patients	42	51	194
Clinical Course of MS	Active RRMS/SPMS	RRMS	Active RRMS/SPMS
Dosage	Mitoxantrone 20 mg (absolute dose) + methylprednisolone 1 g	8 mg/m^2 body surface	12 mg/m^2 body surface
Treatment Frequency	Monthly	Monthly	Every 3 months
Treatment Duration	6 months	12 months	24 months
Observation Duration	6 months	24 months	24 months
Reduction of Progression of Disability[*]	84%	79%	64%
Reduction of Relapse Rate	77%	60%	60%
Reduction of New MRI Lesions	84%	52%	85%
Reduction of Active MRI Lesions	86%	n.d.	100%

[*]Deterioration by 1 EDSS point. RRMS, relapsing-remitting MS; SPMS, secondary progressive MS; n.d., not determined.

ejection fraction (LVEF). Due to the risk of infertility, male patients should be offered the opportunity to cryopreserve their sperm. According to the approvals based on the clinical trials, the currently recommended mitoxantrone dose is 12 mg/m^2 body surface administered intravenously every 3 months. In some countries, the dosage regimen of the French–British trial are approved (i.e., 20 mg monthly for 6 months, irrespective of the body surface) (15,34). Patients with aggressive MS can be considered for treatment with an induction therapy with mitoxantrone 10 to 12 mg/m^2 monthly for the first 3 months, followed by the regular trimester scheme (38). The optimal dosage regimen remains to be evaluated and is currently (2005) being assessed in a European clinical trial comparing three different doses (5, 9, and 12 mg/m^2 body surface) (15). According to the laboratory results (white blood count, thrombocytes, and liver enzymes), dose adjustments should be performed as shown in Table 18-3. Antiemetic protection in parallel with the mitoxantrone infusion may be helpful. The clinically most-relevant interactions of mitoxantrone are with phenytoin (decreased plasma concentration) and with angiotensin-converting enzyme (ACE) inhibitors (increased bone marrow toxicity). Due to the increased risk of infections, patients treated with mitoxantrone should not receive vital vaccines. Patients with hepatic disturbances require reduced doses of mitoxantrone (Table 18-3), whereas for patients with renal disturbances there are no restrictions.

Safety and Tolerability

The MIMS trial and preceding studies exhibited a generally good safety profile of mitoxantrone (Table 18-4) (37). Adverse events were rare, and mild to moderate. However, long-term follow-up data are still pending for final evaluation of the safety profile of mitoxantrone. To this end, a large, open-label, multicenter study of mitoxantrone in MS with a five-year observation period and a broad number of outcome measures [the RENEW study (Registry to Evaluate Novantrone Effects in Worsening MS)] is currently (2005) underway (40).

Cardiotoxicity

Treatment with mitoxantrone is restricted to a cumulative total life dose of 140 mg/m^2 body surface (i.e., when using the standard dose of 12 mg/m^2, the treatment must be discontinued after approximately 12 infusions). The reason of this restriction is the increased risk of an irreversible congestive cardiomyopathy beyond the threshold of 140 mg/m^2 body surface, as observed in cancer patients treated with mitoxantrone (29,41). A recently published retrospective study has investigated the risk of mitoxantrone-induced cardiotoxicity in patients with MS (42).

TABLE 18-3 *Recommended dose adjustment of mitoxantrone (37)*

Event	Recommended Dose (mg/m^2 body surface)
WBC 1.0–1.99 T/l and/or thrombocytes 25–49 T/L 3 weeks after last infusion	10
WBC < 1.0 T/l and/or thrombocytes < 25 T/L 3 weeks after last infusion	8
WBC 3.0–3.99 T/l and/or thrombocytes 75–99 T/L 1 week before infusion	9
WBC 2.0–2.99 T/l and/or thrombocytes 50–74 T/L 1 week before infusion	6
WBC < 2.0 T/l and/or thrombocytes < 50 T/L 1 week before infusion	No infusion
Non-hematological toxicity (WHO grade 2 or 3)*	10
Non-hematological toxicity (WHO grade 4)	No infusion

*Nausea: WHO grade 2, transient nausea; WHO grade 3, nausea requiring therapy; WHO grade 4, intractable vomiting. Liver enzymes: WHO grade 2, 2.6–5.0 × upper reference value; WHO grade 3, 5.1–10.0 × upper reference value. WHO grade 4, > 10.0 × upper reference value. Alopecia: WHO grade 2, moderate alopecia, alopecia areata; WHO grade 3, complete but reversible alopecia; WHO grade 4, complete, non-reversible alopecia. WBC, white blood count.

TABLE 18-4 *Freqencies of adverse events in the MIMS trial (12 mg/m² treatment group) (37)*

Adverse Event	Frequency (%)
Nausea	76*
Alopecia	61*
Menstrual disorder	61*
Upper respiratory tract infection	53
Urinary tract infections	32*
Secondary amenorrhea (absence of menses for ≥ 6 months)	25*
Stomatitis	19
Leukopenia	19*
Arrhythmia	18
Diarrhea	16
Increased liver enzymes	15*
Urine abnormal	11
Electrocardiography abnormal	11
Constipation	10
Rhinitis	8
Back pain	8
Pharyngitis	6
Sinusitis	6
Viral infection	6
Headache	6
Anemia	6

*Significantly more common in active drug recipients (p < 0.05).

In this study, data obtained from 1,378 patients from three clinical trials were analyzed: the MIMS trial (124 patients) (37); a French open, multicenter trial (802 patients) (43); and a retrospective German trial (452 patients) (44). The mean treatment duration was 29 months and the mean cumulative dose was 61 mg/m² body surface. One hundred forty-one patients had received a cumulative mitoxantrone dose of more than 100 mg/m² body surface. Two of the 1,378 patients developed a lethal congestive heart failure after onset of therapy with mitoxantrone. One of the two patients had received a cumulative dose of 162 mg/m² body surface. The other patient had received only one single dose of 9 mg/m²; after 1 year, her LVEF was > 50%, and four years after treatment with mitoxantrone she died of congestive heart failure. However, the relationship between that outcome and the previous mitoxantrone therapy remains uncertain. Seven hundred seventy-nine patients were examined by echocardiography before and during treatment. In 17 of these 779 patients, a reduction of the LVEF below 50% was observed. All 17 patients had received a cumulative dose of more than 100 mg/m². More recently, one more mitoxantrone-treated MS patient with congestive heart failure was documented in a case report (45).

The pathomechanisms of the mitoxantrone-associated cardiotoxicity remain elusive. Matters of discussion are (a) free radicals (46), (b) oxidative stress (47), (c) altered function of myocardial adrenergic receptors (48), (d) disturbed calcium transport in the cardiac sarcolemma (49), and (e) cytokines such as TNF-α or IL-2 (50). Currently, several strategies are being pursued to circumvent the problem of mitoxantrone-associated cardiotoxicity. There are approaches to give pulses of reduced doses of mitoxantrone in order to prolong its application. Furthermore, animal data revealed that the combination of mitoxantrone with the cardioprotector dexrazoxane may be useful to ameliorate or even prevent the mitoxantrone-associated cardiotoxicity (51–53). Interestingly, in a recent publication, dexrazoxane was shown to increase the efficacy of mitoxantrone in EAE (54). An alternative would be the development of other anthracenedione derivatives with lower cardiotoxicity (55).

Induction of Leukemia

The risk of mitoxantrone-associated acute leukemia cannot be ruled out. In the retrospective study with 1,392 patients mentioned above, one case was observed (0.07%) (56). Another seven case reports have been published (57–63). However, valid evaluation of the risk of mitoxantrone-associated acute leukemia and its dose-dependency will need a longer follow-up in more patients.

CONCLUSION

For treatment of MS, immunosuppressive drugs, including mitoxantrone, have been used off-label for decades. Approval of immunomodulatory agents in the mid-1990s shifted the market toward IFN-β and GA. However, worsening forms of RRMS, and especially SPMS, could often not be treated satisfactorily with these new therapeutics. Thus, mitoxantrone, which has immunosuppressive and apparently also immunomodulatory effects, returned to the focus of interest; based on its proven efficacy in Phase III trials, it has recently been approved.

The positive experiences with mitoxantrone open further questions:

1. Can dose and frequency of administration be optimized?
2. Due to cardiotoxicity, can the dose be reduced after an induction phase without impairing the clinical effect?
3. Is there a rationale for a combination of mitoxantrone with IFN-β or GA?
4. What is the optimal subsequent therapy after discontinuation with mitoxantrone?
5. What are the treatment options for clinical nonresponders to mitoxantrone? In this circumstance, is there a rationale for the use of other immunosuppressants such as azathioprine or cyclophosphamide?

These and other questions are matters of intensive discussion. Preclinical and clinical studies, including combination trials of mitoxantrone plus IFN-β, GA, or dexrazoxane, have been initiated to address some of these issues. Furthermore, as the encouraging experience with mitoxantrone induced a revival of immunosuppressive agents, new immunosuppressants are currently being tested in clinical trials (64).

REFERENCES

1. The IFNB Multiple Sclerosis Study Group. Interferon beta-1b is effective in relapsing-remitting multiple sclerosis: I. Clinical results of a multicenter, randomized, double-blind, placebo-controlled trial. *Neurology* 1993;43:655–661.
2. Jacobs LD, Cookfair DL, Rudick RA, et al. Intramuscular interferon beta-1a for disease progression in exacerbating-remitting multiple sclerosis. The Multiple Sclerosis Collaborative Research Group (MSCRG). *Ann Neurol* 1996;39:285–294.
3. PRISMS (Prevention of Relapses and Disability by Interferon beta-1a Subcutaneously in Multiple Sclerosis) Study Group. Randomised double-blind placebo-controlled study of interferon beta-1a in relapsing/remitting multiple sclerosis. *Lancet* 1998;352:1498–1504.
4. Johnson KP, Brooks BR, Cohen JA, et al. Copolymer 1 reduces relapse rate and improves disability in relapsing-remitting multiple sclerosis: results of a phase III multicenter, double-blind, placebo-controlled trial. The Copolymer 1 Multiple Sclerosis Study Group. *Neurology* 1995;45:1268–1276.
5. European Study Group on Interferon beta-1b in Secondary Progressive MS. Placebo-controlled multicentre randomised trial of interferon beta-1b in treatment of secondary progressive multiple sclerosis. *Lancet* 1998;352:1491–1497.
6. Kurtzke JF. Rating neurological impairment in multiple sclerosis: an expanded disability status scale (EDSS). *Neurology* 1983;33:1444–1452.
7. Stüve O, Kita M, Pelletier D, et al. Mitoxantrone as a potential therapy for primary progressive multiple sclerosis. *Mult Scler* 2004;10:1–4.
8. Wiendl H, Kieseier BC. Disease-modifying therapies in multiple sclerosis: an update on recent and ongoing trials and future strategies. *Exp Opin Invest Drugs* 2003;12:689–712.
9. Neuhaus O, Archelos JJ, Hartung HP. Immunomodulation in multiple sclerosis: from immunosuppression to neuroprotection. *Trends Pharmacol Sci* 2003;24:131–138.
10. Smith IE. Mitoxantrone (Novantrone): a review of experimental and early clinical studies. *Cancer Treat Rev* 1983;10:103–115.
11. Shenkenberg TD, von Hoff D. Mitoxantrone: a new anticancer drug with significant clinical activity. *Ann Intern Med* 1986;105:67–81.
12. Jain KK. Evaluation of mitoxantrone for the treatment of multiple sclerosis. *Exp Opin Invest Drugs* 2000;9:1139–1149.
13. Edan G, Morrissey SP, Hartung HP. Use of Mitoxantrone to Treat Multiple Sclerosis. In: Cohen JA, Rudick RA, eds. *Multiple Sclerosis Therapeutics*. London, New York: Martin Dunitz, 2003:403–426.
14. Neuhaus O, Kieseier BC, Hartung HP. Mitoxantrone (Novantrone) in multiple sclerosis—new insights. *Exp Rev Neurotherapeutics* 2004;4:17–26.
15. Edan G, Morrissey S, Le Page E. Rationale for the use of mitoxantrone in multiple sclerosis. *J Neurol Sci* 2004;223:35–39.
16. Stüve O, Cree BC, von Büdingen HC, et al. Approved and future pharmacotherapy for multiple sclerosis. *Neurologist* 2002;8:290–301.
17. Neuhaus O, Kieseier BC, Hartung HP. Mechanisms of mitoxantrone in multiple sclerosis—what is known? *J Neurol Sci* 2004;223:25–27.
18. Fidler JM, de Joy SQ, Gibbons JJ. Selective immunomodulation by the antineoplastic agent mitoxantrone. I. Suppression of B lymphocyte function. *J Immunol* 1986;137:727–732.
19. Fidler JM, de Joy SQ, Smith FR, et al. Selective immunomodulation by the antineoplastic agent mitoxantrone. II. Nonspecific adherent suppressor cells derived from mitoxantrone treated mice. *J Immunol* 1986;136:2747–2754.
20. Mauch E, Kornhuber HH, Krapf H, et al. Treatment of multiple sclerosis with mitoxantrone. *Eur Arch Psychiatry Clin Neurosci* 1992;242:96–102.
21. Gbadamosi J, Buhmann C, Tessmer W, et al. Effects of mitoxantrone on multiple sclerosis patients' lymphocyte subpopulations and production of immunoglobulin, TNF-alpha and IL-10. *Eur Neurol* 2003;49:137–141.
22. Chan A, Weilbach FX, Koyka KV, et al. Mitoxantrone induces cell death in peripheral blood leucocytes of

multiple sclerosis patients. *Clin Exp Immunol* 2005; 139:152–158.

23. Bellosillo B, Colomer D, Pons G, et al. Mitoxantrone, a topoisomerase II inhibitor, induces apoptosis of B-chronic lymphocytic leukaemia cells. *Br J Haematol* 1998;100:142–146.

24. Neuhaus O, Wiendl H, Kieseier BC, et al. Multiple sclerosis: mitoxantrone promotes differential effects on immunocompetent cells in vitro. In press.

25. Hu OY, Chang S, Law C, et al. Pharmacokinetic and pharmacodynamic studies with mitoxantrone in the treatment of patients with nasopharyngeal carcinoma. *Cancer* 1992;69:847–853.

26. Repetto L, Vannozzi MO, Balleari E, et al. Mitoxantrone in elderly patients with advanced breast cancer: pharmacokinetics, marrow and peripheral hematopoietic progenitor cells. *Anticancer Res* 1999;19:879–884.

27. Canal P, Attal M, Chatelut E, et al. Plasma and cellular pharmacokinetics of mitoxantrone in high-dose chemotherapeutic regimen for refractory lymphomas. *Cancer Res* 1993;53:4850–4854.

28. Ballestrero A, Ferrando F, Garuti A, et al. High-dose mitoxantrone with peripheral blood progenitor cell rescue: toxicity, pharmacokinetics and implications for dosage and schedule. *Br J Cancer* 1997;76:797–804.

29. Gonsette RE. Mitoxantrone immunotherapy in multiple sclerosis. *Mult Scler* 1996;1:329–332.

30. Khoury SJ, Bharanidharan P, Bourcier K, et al. Immunologic effects of mitoxantrone therapy in patients with multiple sclerosis. *Neurology* 2002;58[Suppl 3]:A245–A246.

31. Ridge SC, Sloboda AE, McReynolds RA, et al. Suppression of experimental allergic encephalomyelitis by mitoxantrone. *Clin Immunol Immunopathol* 1985;35:35–42.

32. Levine S, Saltzman A. Regional suppression, therapy after onset and prevention of relapses in experimental allergic encephalomyelitis by mitoxantrone. *J Neuroimmunol* 1986;13:175–181.

33. Lublin FD, Lasvasa M, Viti C, et al. Suppression of acute and relapsing experimental allergic encephalomyelitis with mitoxantrone. *Clin Immunol Immunopathol* 1987;45:122–128.

34. Edan G, Miller D, Clanet M, et al. Therapeutic effect of mitoxantrone combined with methylprednisolone in multiple sclerosis: a randomised multicentre study of active disease using MRI and clinical criteria. *J Neurol Neurosurg Psychiatry* 1997;62:112–118.

35. Millefiorini E, Gasperini C, Pozzilli C, et al. Randomized placebo-controlled trial of mitoxantrone in relapsing-remitting multiple sclerosis: 24-month clinical and MRI outcome. *J Neurol* 1997;244:153–159.

36. Van de Wyngaert FA, Beguin C, D'Hooge MB, et al. A double-blind clinical trial of mitoxantrone versus methylprednisolone in relapsing, secondary progressive multiple sclerosis. *Acta Neurol Belg* 2001;101: 210–216.

37. Hartung HP, Gonsette R, König N, et al. A placebo-controlled, double-blind, randomised, multicentre trial of mitoxantrone in progressive multiple sclerosis. *Lancet* 2002;360:2018–2025.

38. Gonsette RE. Mitoxantrone in progressive multiple sclerosis: when and how to treat? *J Neurol Sci* 2003;206:203–208.

39. Jeffery DR. The argument against the use of cyclophosphamide and mitoxantrone in the treatment of multiple sclerosis. *J Neurol Sci* 2004;223:41–46.

40. Smith CH, Lopez-Bresnahan MV, Beagan J. Safety and tolerability of Novantrone (mitoxantrone) in clinical practice: status report from the Registry to Evaluate Novantrone Effects in Worsening MS (RENEW) Study. *Neurology* 2004;62[Suppl 5]:A489.

41. De Castro S, Cartoni D, Millefiorini E, et al. Noninvasive assessment of mitoxantrone cardiotoxicity in relapsing-remitting multiple sclerosis. *J Clin Pharmacol* 1995;35:627–632.

42. Ghalie RG, Edan G, Laurent M, et al. Cardiac adverse effects associated with mitoxantrone (Novantrone) therapy in patients with MS. *Neurology* 2002;59:909–913.

43. Edan G, Brochet B, Clanet M, et al. Safety profile of mitoxantrone in a cohort of 800 multiple sclerosis patients. *Mult Scler* 2001;7[Suppl 1]:S14.

44. Mauch E, Eisenman S, Hahn A, et al. Mitoxantrone (MITOX) in the treatment of patients with multiple sclerosis: a large single center experience. American Neurological Association, 1999.

45. Gbadamosi J, Munchau A, Weiller C, et al. Severe heart failure in a young multiple sclerosis patient. *J Neurol* 2003;250:241–242.

46. Doroshow JH. Anthracycline antibiotic-stimulated superoxide, hydrogen peroxide, and hydroxyl radical production by NADH dehydrogenase. *Cancer Res* 1983;43:4543–4551.

47. Singal PK, Deally CM, Weinberg LE. Subcellular effects of adriamycin in the heart: a concise review. *J Mol Cell Cardiol* 1987;19:817–828.

48. Robison TW, Giri SN. Effects of chronic administration of doxorubicin on myocardial beta-adrenergic receptors. *Life Sci* 1986;39:731–736.

49. Singal PK, Pierce GN. Adriamycin stimulates low-affinity Ca^{2+} binding and lipid peroxidation but depresses myocardial function. *Am J Physiol* 1986;250:H419–H425.

50. Ehrke MJ, Maccubbin D, Ryoyama K, et al. Correlation between adriamycin-induced augmentation of interleukin 2 production and of cell-mediated cytotoxicity in mice. *Cancer Res* 1986;46:54–60.

51. Weilbach FX, Toyka KV, Gold R. Combination therapy with the iron chelator dexrazoxane augments therapeutic efficacy of mitoxantrone in experimental autoimmune encephalomyelitis in Lewis rats. *Rev Neurol* 2000;156:S127.

52. Herman EH, Zhang J, Rifai N, et al. The use of serum levels of cardiac troponin T to compare the protective activity of dexrazoxane against doxorubicin- and mitoxantrone-induced cardiotoxicity. *Cancer Chemother Pharmacol* 2001;48:297–304.

53. Mikol DD, Bernitsas E. Novantrone plus dexrazoxane therapy in multiple sclerosis patients: a safety and tolerability pilot study. *Mult Scler* 2001;7[Suppl:S14.

54. Weilbach FX, Chan A, Toyka KV, et al. The cardioprotector dexrazoxane augments therapeutic efficacy of mitoxantrone in experimental autoimmune encephalomyelitis. *Clin Exp Immunol* 2004;135:49–55.

55. Gonsette RE. Pixantrone (BBR2778): a new immunosuppressant in multiple sclerosis with a low cardiotoxicity. *J Neurol Sci* 2004;223:81–86.

56. Ghalie RG, Mauch E, Edan G, et al. A study of therapy-related acute leukaemia after mitoxantrone therapy for multiple sclerosis. *Mult Scler* 2002;8:441–445.

57. Vicari AM, Ciceri F, Folli F, et al. Acute promyelocytic leukemia following mitoxantrone as single agent for the treatment of multiple sclerosis. *Leukemia* 1998;12:441–442.

58. Brassat D, Recher C, Waubant E, et al. Therapy-related acute myeloblastic leukemia after mitoxantrone treatment in a patient with MS. *Neurology* 2002;59:954–955.

59. Heesen C, Bruegmann M, Gbadamosi J, et al. Therapy-related acute myelogenous leukaemia (t-AML) in a patient with multiple sclerosis treated with mitoxantrone. *Mult Scler* 2003;9:213–214.

60. Jaster JH, Niell HB, Dohan FCJ, et al. Therapy-related acute myeloblastic leukemia after mitoxantrone treatment in a patient with MS. *Neurology* 2003;60:1399–1400.

61. Cattaneo C, Almici C, Borlenghi E, et al. A case of acute promyelocytic leukaemia following mitoxantrone treatment of multiple sclerosis. *Leukemia* 2003;17:985–986.

62. Mogenet I, Simiand-Erdociain E, Canonge JM, et al. Acute myelogenous leukemia following mitoxantrone treatment for multiple sclerosis. *Ann Pharmacother* 2003;37:747–748.

63. Voltz R, Starck M, Zingler V, et al. Mitoxantrone therapy in multiple sclerosis and acute leukaemia: a case report out of 644 treated patients. *Mult Scler* 2004;10:472–474.

64. Gonsette RE. New immunosuppressants with potential implication in multiple sclerosis. *J Neurol Sci* 2004;223:87–93.

65. Gonsette RE, Demonty L. Immunosuppression with mitoxantrone in multiple sclerosis: a pilot study for 2 years in 22 patients. *Neurology* 1990;40[Suppl 1]:S261.

66. Kappos L, Gold R, Künstler E, et al. Mitoxantrone (Mx) in the treatment of rapidly progressive MS: a pilot study with serial gadolinium (Gd)-enhanced MRI. *Neurology* 1990;40[Suppl 1]:261.

67. Noseworthy JH, Hopkins MB, Vandervoort MK, et al. An open-trial evaluation of mitoxantrone in the treatment of progressive MS. *Neurology* 1993;43:1401–1406.

19

Acute Disseminated Encephalomyelitis: Distinction from Multiple Sclerosis and Treatment Issues

Dean M. Wingerchuk

Department of Neurology, Mayo Clinic, Scottsdale, Arizona

INTRODUCTION

Adult and pediatric neurologists frequently face difficult diagnostic, treatment, and counseling decisions when evaluating a patient with new-onset idiopathic inflammatory demyelinating disease of the central nervous system (CNS). This term encompasses several diagnostic considerations, including clinically isolated syndromes (optic neuritis, brain stem inflammation, or myelitis) that may herald future multiple sclerosis (MS), acute disseminated encephalomyelitis (ADEM), acute transverse myelitis (TM), neuromyelitis optica (NMO), and miscellaneous focal demyelinating syndromes (Baló's concentric sclerosis; Marburg variant of MS). Each of these diagnoses carries different prognostic and treatment implications; there are now established treatments for typical MS, even at the time of the first clinical attack (1–3).

A diagnosis of ADEM is often tentative for several reasons, including the lack of validated diagnostic criteria for the syndrome and the implication that there will be no future clinical relapses. Pathological features, though not validated, appear to be more specific and reasonably consistent in cases diagnosed clinically as ADEM (see also Chapter 3 by Morales et al.); better clinicopathological, neuroimaging, and immune biomarker correlations will advance the state of the art. Until that time, ADEM will remain a clinical construct, at least for clinicians who elect not to biopsy affected nervous tissue (4,5). This review will summarize the clinical, laboratory, and pathological evidence supporting the existence of ADEM (including idiopathic, postinfectious, and postvaccinial types) and features that assist in differentiating ADEM from MS, emphasizing the limitations clinicians must appreciate due to overlap of these syndromes.

What Is the Clinical Definition of ADEM?

There are no universally applied diagnostic criteria for ADEM (4,5). Usually, reported cases are children (especially infants) or young adults with focal or multifocal neurological symptoms and signs in conjunction with an acute meningoencephalitic syndrome. Pediatric cases are usually preceded by a febrile illness or exanthem (postinfectious ADEM) or an immunization (postvaccinial ADEM). However, these antecedent events are not necessary to establish the diagnosis, and even when an infection is suspected, objective evidence defining a specific agent is often absent.

Recent retrospective case series (6–9) and one prospective study (10) used quite varied ADEM case definitions (Table 19-1), none of which required a prodromal or triggering illness. The most inclusive of these criteria required acute neurological symptoms in association with undefined brain magnetic resonance imaging (MRI) white matter abnormalities "compatible with ADEM," or no MRI at all. More recent series in children and adults specifically required first-ever neurological events with white matter lesions and no evidence of prior white matter involvement (although this is not well-defined). The results of these studies suggest that the broad spectrum of clinical and MRI findings in ADEM and their significant overlap with MS may hinder the development of any more precise diagnostic criteria until the discovery of a biological marker for either entity.

Associations with Infectious Agents

Postinfectious ADEM is associated with an antecedent or concomitant viral infection. Table 19-2 lists several infection and vaccine associations; many of these represent single case reports or small case series and cannot be considered causative (4). However, the association of ADEM with measles, varicella-zoster, and rubella viruses appears quite firm. Recent associations include parainfluenza virus, Pontiac fever, *Chlamydia pneumoniae*, *Legionella pneumophila*, dengue fever, *Pasteurella multocida*, Leptospira, and the vaccinia, hepatitis B,

tetanus, and meningococcus A and C immunizations (11–21). Noninfectious causes such as bee stings and parenteral use of herbal extracts have also recently been implicated (22,23).

Post-measles ADEM occurs at a rate of about 1 per 1,000 infections and was historically associated with high rates of mortality (up to 25%) and permanent neurological injury in survivors (25% to 40%) (24,25). The incidence has fallen markedly in industrialized nations due to childhood measles immunization programs; prior to measles, varicella, and rubella vaccination programs, ADEM was estimated to account for up to 30% of all encephalitis cases (26). Postinfectious ADEM is much less common with the other virus types and in many instances the diagnosis is made without documenting a specific infectious illness.

Clinical Presentation: Pediatric Population

The diagnosis of ADEM is a more common consideration in children than adults. The slight male predominance (58%), based on aggregate data from recent case series, requires confirmation (6–8,10). About two-thirds of patients experience an infectious illness during the month preceding neurological symptoms, often in the form of a typical childhood exanthem.

ADEM presents in a myriad of ways because it depends upon the lesion number and distribution as well as the severity of the inflammatory and demyelinating process (Tables 19-3 and 19-4) (6–8,10,27,28). Symptoms and signs generally evolve subacutely and reach their nadir after several days. Polysymptomatic neurological events, consisting of some combination of focal or multifocal pyramidal signs and ataxia, are very common, as are cranial neuropathies, including unilateral or bilateral optic neuritis. Myelitis, usually recognized by paraparesis or quadriparesis and urinary dysfunction, may be evident in about 25% of cases. Less-common focal features include aphasia and involuntary movement disorders.

Impairment of consciousness, sometimes progressing to coma, is the most common meningoencephalitic presentation. Headache, fever, seizures, confusion, or behavioral disturbances

TABLE 19-1 *Definitions of ADEM in recent case series*

	Dale et al., 2000	Hynson et al., 2001	Murthy et al., 2002	Tenembaum et al., 2002	Schwarz et al., 2001
Study Sample Age Clinical Inclusion	Pediatric Monophasic event of disseminated CNS demyelination	Pediatric Acute neurological disturbance	Pediatric Acute neurological signs and symptoms	Pediatric Presumed inflammatory demyelinating event with acute or subacute onset affecting multifocal areas of the CNS; polysymptomatic	Adult Acute neurological symptoms
Clinical Exclusion	Preceding neurological abnormality Isolated ON or TM Infection/other inflammatory disease	Not stated	Not stated	History of symptoms suggesting earlier demyelinating episode Isolated acute ON or TM	Preceding unexplained neurological symptoms Isolated TM or unilateral ON
MRI Inclusion	None	Brain MRI white matter changes in a distribution consistent with ADEM	MRI evidence of multifocal, hyperintense lesions on FLAIR and T2-weighted MRI	White matter changes on brain-spinal imaging without radiologic evidence of a previous destructive white matter process	One or multiple supra- or infratentorial demyelinating lesions and absence of T1 black holes
Laboratory	None	None	None	None	CSF analysis excludes infection, vasculitis, autoimmune disease

CNS, central nervous system; ON, optic neuritis; TM, transverse myelitis; MRI, magnetic resonance imaging; FLAIR, fluid-attenuated inversion recovery (MRI technique).

(Modified, with permission, from Wingerchuk DM. Postinfectious encephalomyelitis. *Current Neurology & Neuroscience Reports* 2003;3:256–264.)

TABLE 19-2 *Infections and immunizations associated with ADEM*

Viral Infections

Measles	Hepatitis A or B
Mumps	Herpes simplex
Rubella	Human herpes virus-6
Varicella	Epstein–Barr virus
Influenza A or B	Cytomegalovirus
Rocky Mountain Spotted Fever	Vaccinia
HTLV-1	Parainfluenza
Dengue Fever	

Bacterial or Spirochetal Infections

Mycoplasma pneumoniae	Campylobacter
Chlamydia	Streptococcus
Legionella	*Pasteurella multocida*
Pontiac fever	Leptospira

Immunizations

Rabies	Measles
Diphtheria, tetanus, polio	Japanese B encephalitis
Smallpox	Hog vaccine
Vaccinia	Hepatitis B
Meningococcus A and C	Tetanus

may also be prominent (29). Several case reports document adolescents or young adults with psychosis (30–32). Hypersomnia and narcolepsy have both been described (33,34). Respiratory failure secondary to suppressed level of consciousness or cervical myelitis occurs in 11% to 16% of patients (6,10).

Although in most instances there is no compelling association between the clinical phenotype and the infectious agent, there are some exceptions, such as varicella-associated cerebellar ataxia. Recently, a unique childhood ADEM phenotype was reported in association with Group A beta-hemolytic streptococcal infection and the presence of elevated antibasal ganglia antibody titers (35). Ten children aged 3 to 14 years developed consciousness or pyramidal weakness but with prominent additional features of a dystonic extrapyramidal syndrome (70%) or behavioral disorders such as emotional lability or inappropriate speech (50%). The syndrome was preceded by acute infectious pharyngitis but was distinct from rheumatic fever or Sydenham chorea. This finding suggests that certain recognizable clinical and imaging phenotypes may be associated with specific infectious agents, but even these subgroups remain somewhat heterogeneous.

Clinical Presentation: Adult Population

Cumulative data from most case series suggest that adult ADEM generally parallels that of children (31,36–38). Recently Schwarz et al., in the largest contemporary series of adult-onset ADEM, confirmed that the frequency of individual neurological symptoms and signs is remarkably similar in each age group (Tables 19-3 and 19-4) (9). These include preponderance of female patients (65%), less likelihood of clinically evident antecedent infection (46% versus 62% to 77% in children), and less-common accompanying acute meningoencephalitic syndrome. Notably, these features are also more characteristic of typical MS.

A potentially distinct ADEM-related phenotype was described by Modi et al. (39). Eight black South Africans (seven adults) experienced a multiphasic disorder usually consisting of attacks of optic neuritis (ON) and myelitis suggestive of neuromyelitis optica (NMO) but their brain MRI demonstrated diffuse white matter abnormalities compatible with ADEM. These cases argue for a genetic- or environmentally-determined phenotypic expression of diffuse, ADEM-like pathology.

Does Diagnostic Testing Assist in the Diagnosis of ADEM?

Cerebrospinal Fluid (CSF)

Cerebrospinal fluid results are summarized in Table 19-4. Most often, a lymphocytic pleocytosis of several hundred cells is detected in conjunction with an elevated total protein level. The frequency of unique CSF oligoclonal bands is generally low in children (3% to 29%) but more common in adult ADEM, even after prolonged follow-up (58%), and those who have their diagnosis revised to clinically definite MS (80%) (9).

MRI Features

Early descriptions of brain MRI abnormalities in ADEM emphasized the presence of large, reasonably symmetric, multifocal, primarily

TABLE 19-3 *Study and patient sample features from five ADEM series*

	Dale et al., 2000	Hynson et al., 2001	Murthy et al., 2002	Tenembaum et al., 2002	Schwarz et al., 2001
Study Sample	Pediatric	Pediatric	Pediatric	Pediatric	Adult
Country of Origin	United Kingdom	Australia	United States	Argentina	Germany
Patients (N)	35	31	18	84	26
Age Range, y	3–15	2–16	2.5–22	0.4–16	19–61
Female sex (%)	16 (46)	18 (58)	7 (39)	30 (36)	17 (65)
Antecedent Infection (%)	22 (63)	24 (77)	13 (72)	52 (62)	12 (46)
Antecedent Vaccination (%)	2 (6)	2 (6)	0	10 (12)	0
Prodrome to Onset of ADEM Mean (Range) Days	13 (2–31)	Not stated	10 (range not stated)	12 (2–30)	Not stated
Seasonal Occurrence	Winter	No	Winter and spring	Not stated	Not stated
ADEM Onset to Nadir Mean (Range) Days	7.1 (1–31)	4.2 (1–42)	<1 week from hospitalization	4.5 (1–45)	4* (0–14)

* Value represents median time from prodrome until hospital admission. (Reproduced, with permission, from Wingerchuk DM. Postinfectious encephalomyelitis. *Current Neurology & Neuroscience Reports* 2003;3:256–264.)

TABLE 19-4 *Clinical and laboratory features from five ADEM series*

Study Sample	Dale et al., 2000	Hynson et al., 2001	Murthy et al., 2002	Tenembaum et al., 2002	Schwarz et al., 2001
	Pediatric	Pediatric	Pediatric	Pediatric	Adult
Meningoencephalitic Features (%)					
Fever	43	52	39	Not stated	15
Headache	58	45	23	32	Not stated
Meningism	31	26	6	43	15
Alteration of Consciousness	69	74	45	69	19 (loss of consciousness)
Focal Neurological Features (%)					
ON	23 (all bilateral)	13	Unclear	23	Not stated
Cranial Neuropathy	51	45	23 (includes ON)	44	Not stated
Pyramidal/Focal Motor Signs	71	23	39	85	77
Sensory Deficit	17	3	28	Unclear	65
Aphasia/Language Disturbance	0	26	6	21	8
Seizure	17	13	17	35	4
Ataxia	49	65	39	50	38
Movement Disorder	3	Not stated	Not stated	12	Not stated
Spinal Cord Syndrome	23	Not stated	Unclear	24	15
Cerebrospinal Fluid (%)					
Pleocytosis	64	62	39	28 (combined with protein)	81
Elevated Protein Level	60	48	55	28 (combined with pleocytosis)	Not stated
Oligoclonal Bands Present	29	3	13	4	58

(Reproduced, with permission, from Wingerchuk DM. Postinfectious encephalomyelitis. *Current Neurology & Neuroscience Reports* 2003; 3:256–264.)

subcortical cerebral white matter lesions that uniformly enhanced with gadolinium. Exceptional case reports describe unusual imaging characteristics such as normal initial brain scan (40), normal scan followed by the development of lesions during clinical recovery (41), lesions in the deep gray matter (42) or thalami (43,44), a solitary lesion restricted to an area such as the brainstem (45), or the presence of multiple cystic lesions (46) or ring-enhancing lesions with mass effect (47).

The recent large case series clarified the relative frequency of MRI characteristics of ADEM (Table 19-5). First, brain MRI findings overlap significantly in cases diagnosed as ADEM compared with MS at follow-up. Up to 60% of ADEM cases have periventricular lesions and up to 29% demonstrate evidence of callosal abnormalities. Uniform and multifocal lesion enhancement sometimes occurs, but approximately half of cases present with no enhancing lesions. Bilateral symmetric thalamic or basal ganglia lesions, present in perhaps 15% of patients, are more suggestive of ADEM than of MS or acute hemorrhagic leukoencephalomyelitis (AHLE) and are even more common (80%) in those children with the Group A streptococcus-associated subtype (35,48). In monophasic cases, serial brain MRI studies performed several months after clinical improvement usually reveal partial or complete resolution of the original lesions without new lesion development (49).

Neuroimaging findings characteristic of ADEM were reported in a group of black South Africans with a clinical course resembling relapsing NMO (39). These cases demonstrate that the imaging findings and clinical phenotype are often incongruent; therefore, diagnostic criteria relying on the presence of specific findings for each will likely prove unsuccessful.

Advanced Neuroimaging Techniques

Quantitative proton MR spectroscopy revealed low levels of N-acetyl aspartate (NAA) (but normal choline levels) within regions of T2-weighted signal abnormality during an acute ADEM relapse in a 4-year-old child (50). Follow-up studies 6 months later, after complete clinical recovery, were normal, suggesting that reduced NAA levels may not always be associated with neuronal loss and poor neurological prognosis.

Diffusion- and perfusion-weighted MRI and MR spectroscopy showed elevated lactate levels and abnormal diffusion (reduced, normal, or increased) and perfusion (reduced or normal) characteristics within ADEM lesions (51,52). Recent diffusion tensor MR studies confirm that the basal ganglia are affected in ADEM but not MS (53), and that normal-appearing white matter in ADEM is indeed spared (54). Positron emission tomography (55) and coregistration of single-positron emission computed tomography (SPECT) and MRI (56) demonstrated metabolic abnormalities within lesions. It is unclear whether any of these modalities will prove useful in discriminating ADEM from MS and other idiopathic demyelinating syndromes.

What is the Pathological Basis of the ADEM Syndrome?

Fulminant ADEM causes gross brain swelling, congestion, and may cause signs of herniation. The freshly sliced brain may reveal only swelling and scattered petechial hemorrhages; in contrast, acute MS lesions are usually visible to the unaided eye. The core pathological feature of ADEM is perivenous, macrophage-predominant, inflammatory infiltration with an associated sleeve-like pattern of demyelination within the white matter. Multiple lesions are usually present and may be concentrated in a particular area such as a lobe (especially the occipital lobe), brainstem, or spinal cord (57). Lesions may involve the deeper layers of the cerebral cortex, thalamus, hypothalamus, and basal ganglia and as well as vasculature within the walls of the lateral and third ventricle. The lesion distribution has prompted synonyms such as perivenous encephalomyelitis and acute perivascular myelinoclasis. Refer also to Chapter 3 by Luchinetti et al.

Microscopic abnormalities may include the presence of lymphocytes and, to a lesser degree, neutrophils outside the Virchow–Robin spaces; vessel wall invasion by inflammatory cells;

TABLE 19-5 *MRI characteristics of ADEM*

	Dale et al., 2000	Hynson et al., 2001	Murthy et al., 2002	Tenembaum et al., 2002	Schwarz et al., 2001
Number with MRI (% of total)	32 (91)	31 (100)	15 (83)	79 (94)	26 (100)
Lesion site (% of those with MRI)					
White Matter	91	90	93	Not stated	100
Periventricular	44	29	60	Not stated	54
Corpus Callosum	Not stated	29	7 (splenium)	Not stated	23
Subcortical/Deep	91	80	93	Not stated	38
Cortical Gray Matter	12	Not stated	80	Not stated	8
Brainstem	56	42	47	Not stated	57
Cerebellum	31	Not stated	13	Not stated	31
Thalamus	41	32	27	13 (bilateral, symmetric)	15 (includes basal ganglia)
Basal Ganglia	28	39	20	Not stated	15 (includes thalamus)
Spinal Cord	n not stated (28)	4/6 (67)	5/7 (71)	Not stated	Not stated
Gadolinium Enhancement (%)	Not stated	8/28 (29)	7/15 (47)	10/27 (37)	20/21 (95)
Follow-up Brain MRI (%)	19/32 (59)	8/31 (26)	14/15 (93)	Not stated	20/26 (77)
Mean MRI Follow-up, y (range)	1.5 (0.2–9)	0.2–2 (range only)	0.04–1.5 (range only)	Not stated	Not stated
Original Brain Lesion Change (%)					
Complete Resolution	37	Unclear	7	Not stated	30
Partial Resolution	53	n=6	57	Not stated	55
No Change	10	Unclear	21	Not stated	0
New Lesions	0	n=3 (all relapsed clinically)	14 (all within 8 weeks)	0 (denominator not stated)	15 (no clinical relapses)

(Reproduced, with permission, from Wingerchuk DM. Postinfectious encephalomyelitis. *Current Neurology & Neuroscience Reports* 2003;3:256–264.)

perivascular edema; petechial hemorrhage; and endothelial swelling. Axons are relatively preserved and but those affected are often tortuous and swollen. Narrow zones of subpial demyelination in the spinal cord and brainstem may be present. There is no convincing evidence of inflammatory cells in spinal roots, ganglia, or peripheral nerves. The neuropathology of so-called relapsing ADEM has also been described; these rare cases show scattered, sleeve-like, perivenous demyelinating lesions with little or no similarities with MS pathology.

Acute hemorrhagic leukoencephalitis (AHL) is a hyperacute, severe, and often fatal form of ADEM, though successful recovery has been described (58–61). It is characterized by predominantly neutrophilic infiltrates with pericapillary ball and ring hemorrhages surrounding necrotic venules. Occasionally, fibrinous exudates may be seen within the vessel or extending into adjacent tissue.

Other uncommon idiopathic demyelinating CNS syndromes demonstrate pathological features that differ from those of ADEM. Neuromyelitis optica, a humorally-mediated syndrome, can usually be readily differentiated from ADEM on clinical and imaging grounds and is considered in Chapter 20. Baló's concentric sclerosis consists of large demyelinating plaques that show alternating rings of myelin preservation and loss, giving the lesions the macroscopic and microscopic appearance of onion bulbs. These changes may be visible on brain MRI. The Marburg variant of MS is characterized by lesions that are more destructive than typical MS or ADEM, with massive macrophage infiltration, acute axonal injury, and necrosis.

Most importantly, the pathological pattern of MS usually differs substantially from that of ADEM, allowing more precise diagnosis in cases where brain biopsy material is available. The results of standardized pathological examination of MS biopsy and autopsy specimens implicate four different immunopathological patterns of disease (62); Chapter 3 provides an in-depth discussion of these patterns.

Similar detailed immunopathological study will clarify the common and differentiating characteristics of ADEM and typical forms of MS. Table 19-6 summarizes current understanding of the differences between MS and ADEM, using standard pathological techniques. This represents a general guide; expert neuropathological advice is always warranted and it should be noted that some patients have lesions with immunopathological features of both ADEM and MS. The presence of these transitional forms suggests a spectrum of inflammatory demyelinating diseases that share a common pathogenic relationship.

What is the Pathogenesis of ADEM?

A viral infection or vaccination is often recognized to have occurred prior to the clinical onset of ADEM. However, unlike confirmed cases of infectious encephalitis or meningoencephalitis, viral proteins and RNA are virtually never recovered from cerebrospinal fluid or brain biopsies. The implication of this finding is that ADEM is an autoimmune disorder triggered by an infectious agent (63–65). A cell-mediated autoimmune response to myelin proteins triggered by infection or immunization is a possible etiological factor. Autoimmunity may be triggered by several mechanisms, including molecular mimicry, bystander activation, epitope spreading, and mistaken self (66,67).

Animal models of experimental allergic encephalomyelitis (EAE) may be relevant to some of the mechanisms underlying human ADEM. Lesions induced by Theiler virus in a murine EAE model closely resemble ADEM lesions and, to a lesser extent, those of MS. The initial injury caused by the virus is followed by a secondary autoimmune response. In this virus model, CD4 and CD8 cells each express postinfectious reactivity to myelin autoantigens, and mice with severe combined immunodeficiency do not develop demyelination (68–72).

The neuropathology of other EAE models induced by exposure to myelin antigens such as myelin basic protein (MBP), proteolipid protein (PLP), or myelin oligodendrocyte glycoprotein (MOG) in complete Freund's adjuvant results in a diffuse white matter encephalomyelitis that also has greater similarity to ADEM than to MS.

TABLE 19-6 *Pathological features: comparison of ADEM, AHLE, and acute MS*

	ADEM	AHLE	MS
Macroscopic examination			
Number and location of lesions	Lesions inconspicuous or multiple small perivenous lesions throughout white and gray matter of brain, spinal cord, and optic nerves	Lesions in centrum ovale, internal capsule, and cingulate gyrus extending to corpus callosum with spread to involve gray and white matter in brainstem and cerebellar peduncles. Spinal cord rarely involved.	Variably sized lesions throughout white >> gray matter of brain, spinal cord and optic nerves
Microscopic examination			
Perivascular infiltrates	Prominent, perivenular	Variable	Scant, variable
macrophages	+	++	+
lymphocytes	++	++	++
polymorphs	±	++ (also often in leptomeninges)	±
eosinophils	–	–	– (rare)
Perivascular IgG/complement	–	–	+
Perivascular hemorrhage	– –	++	–
Perivascular demyelination	++	+	±
Astrocytic reaction	Less prominent than MS	Less prominent than MS	Large, numerous Creutzfeldt cells
Acute axonal injury	++	+++	+
Necrosis of blood vessel walls ± fibrinous exudates	±	++	–

Table courtesy of Dr. S. Pittock, Mayo Clinic, Rochester, MN.

(73–77). MBP-reactive T cells have previously been reported in patients with ADEM (78), and patients with post-measles encephalomyelitis have increased immune responses to MBP (73). Tissue destruction in EAE is associated with predominance of myelin reactive Th1-type T cells, whereas in the recovery phase, Th2-type T cells may play a protective role (79–81). Patients recovering from ADEM have a significantly higher frequency of MBP-reactive T cells than patients with viral encephalitis and normal subjects (76). These cells were interleukin-4-secreting Th2 cells, further supporting the similarity between ADEM and EAE. In some cases, GM1 and GD1a antibodies may play an additional role (82).

Cytokine profiles and apoptotic mechanisms have been extensively studied in MS but only have only recently received attention in ADEM (83–88). In the acute phase, cytokines such as tumor necrosis factor-α, soluble tumor necrosis factor receptor 1, interleukin-6, and interleukin-10 have been implicated. Apoptotic cells make up a large proportion of T lymphocytes in ADEM lesions, similar to what is found in EAE (89). Although these are very preliminary results, they support the concept that T cell-mediated autoimmune responses are operative in ADEM.

Can ADEM be Differentiated from MS in Children at Disease Onset?

Dale et al. compared 13 children with MS to 35 children with either ADEM or MDEM (multiphasic disease; still considered a form of ADEM but with early relapse within eight weeks of discontinuing corticosteroid treatment) (6). The ADEM/MDEM group more commonly experienced an antecedent infection, polysymptomatic presentation, pyramidal signs, and encephalopathy. Seizures, bilateral ON, and CSF pleocytosis were also more common but the rate difference was not statistically significant. Unilateral ON occurred only in the MS group. Periventricular brain MRI lesions were common in the MS group but present in 44% of the ADEM/MDEM patients. Therefore, some clinical features appear to be more suggestive of ADEM but the

clinical phenotypes still overlap significantly (27,28).

Can ADEM be Differentiated from MS in Adults at Disease Onset?

Many, if not most, cases of ADEM-like presentation in adults will eventually evolve into rather typical MS. Nevertheless, some cases do remain monophasic, both clinically and by neuroimaging criteria, for many years (49). The maintenance of a monophasic course does not, of course, prove that these patients have a different disease than MS. However, it serves as a reminder that despite the often-worrisome polysymptomatic clinical presentation, some patients will enjoy a prolonged clinical remission.

Schwarz et al. reported that 14/40 (35%) adults with ADEM developed clinically definite MS during a mean follow-up period of 38 months (9). Group comparisons did not reveal any useful clinical or laboratory predictors of disease course. Almost half of the monophasic ADEM group had brain MRI findings (periventricular or callosal lesions) compatible with prototypic MS. Notably, some patients developed new, asymptomatic MRI lesions after relatively brief periods of follow-up, thus providing additional uncertainty about the validity of the ADEM diagnosis. This suggests that attempts to diagnose MS or ADEM based on the initial brain MRI scan stand a significant chance of being erroneous. The McDonald diagnostic criteria for MS reflect these concerns (90). They recommend that an initial diagnostic judgment be suspended and that MS may be confirmed should new clinical or MRI abnormalities occur more than three months after the onset of the sentinel event (an arbitrary interval). This recommendation seems quite sensible, although it remains to be validated.

The aggregate results of the retrospective and prospective studies of children and adults with ADEM suggest that there are clinical, laboratory, and MRI characteristics that may assist the clinician in judging the relative likelihood, at least in qualitative terms, that a patient has ADEM versus MS (Table 19-7). However, these features overlap enough that it

TABLE 19-7 *Features useful in discriminating ADEM from MS*

	Favors ADEM	Favors MS
• Age	Pediatric, especially infant	Adult
• Symptom and Signs		
Antecedent infection	Yes	No
Antecedent immunization	Yes	No
Onset	Fulminant/acute	Subacute
Severity	More severe	Less severe
Presentation	Polysymptomatic	Monosymptomatic
Type	Fever	Unilateral optic neuritis
Headache/meningism		
Alteration of consciousness		
Aphasia		
Seizures		
Bilateral optic neuritis		
• CSF		
Cell count	> 50 WBC/mm^3	< 50 WBC/mm^3
Total protein	Increased	Normal
Oligoclonal bands	Absent	Present
• Brain MRI		
Lesion size	Larger	Small to medium
Lesion distribution (predominant)	Subcortical	Periventricular
Mass effect and edema	Present	Absent
Gray matter involvement	Present	Absent
Gadolinium enhancement	Uniform (all lesions)	Heterogeneous (some lesions)
T1 "black holes"	Absent	Present
Serial MRI scanning	No new lesions	New lesions

seems sensible, especially in adult cases, to temper the diagnosis of ADEM with caution and to emphasize the clarity that observation over time usually delivers.

What is the Clinical Course of ADEM?

The outcome of ADEM is, not surprisingly, quite variable. Significant long-term neurological abnormalities persist in 15% to 33% of patients. Dale et al. followed 35 children for 5.8 years (range 1.0 to 15.4 years) and noted that all patients survived the acute illness and most completely recovered within a few weeks (6). Fifty-seven percent had no long-term impairment, but motor dysfunction (17%; half of these severe), cognitive impairment (11%), visual loss (11%), and behavioral problems (11%) persisted in the remainder. Recurrent seizures developed in 9% but resolved in two-thirds on extended follow-up.

Adults with monophasic ADEM had more severe initial symptoms but better overall recovery than those ultimately diagnosed with MS (9). At last follow-up, a greater proportion of ADEM patients were asymptomatic (46% versus 14% in the MS group). Moderate neurological deficits persisted in 12% of ADEM patients, whereas 43% of the MS group accrued moderate to severe deficits after mean follow-up of 38 months.

What is Recurrent or Relapsing ADEM?

The concept of ADEM as a monophasic disease is generally accepted, but there are several descriptions of relapsing or recurrent forms (91–93). One series reported that 10% of cases had biphasic disease with a single relapse occurring between two months and eight years (median two years) after ADEM onset; all were oligoclonal band-negative (10). The patients who relapsed early (within the first 2 months) may have been considered by some to have MDEM (6), whereas other clinicians may have diagnosed MS. One potential differentiating factor that was not clarified was whether the recurrence occurred at the same site as the original event. Cohen et al. studied this carefully and found that 5/21 (24%) ADEM patients developed between two and four relapses (92). These relapses occurred in the same brain region in 6/9 recurrences in 3/5 patients. Some of the relapses were recurrent events of large, tumor-like lesions and most were corticosteroid-responsive. The investigators confirmed the diagnosis of ADEM using brain biopsy, which demonstrated diffuse demyelination and perivascular mononuclear cell infiltration, loosening of white matter, and foamy macrophages. These reports illustrate that there are rare instances in which cases that have clinical and pathological features of ADEM experience relapses but lack features characteristic of typical forms of MS.

What Treatments are Available for ADEM?

There have been no controlled clinical therapeutic trials for ADEM. Most children are initially treated empirically for infectious meningoencephalitis until the diagnosis of ADEM is established, whereupon the mainstay of treatment is corticosteroids (6–8,10,94). This usually consists of high-dose intravenous methylprednisolone (10 to 30 mg/kg/day for children under 30 kg; 1,000 mg/day for those over 30 kg), or dexamethasone (1 mg/kg/day) for 3 to 10 days followed by an oral corticosteroid taper over two to six weeks. In one study (10), neurological status was better (Expanded Disability Status Scale score 1 versus 3; p = 0.029) in a group of 21 children who received pulsed intravenous methylprednisolone versus 25 others treated with intravenous dexamethasone. Treatment of adults is similar, generally using pulse intravenous methylprednisolone, 1,000 mg/day for 5 days, followed by a tapering dose of oral prednisone over several weeks.

Plasma exchange represents second-line therapy and is indicated for patients who clinically worsen or fail to improve from severe deficits despite parenteral corticosteroid therapy. A randomized, controlled, crossover trial of true versus sham plasma exchange for corticosteroid-refractory attacks of severe CNS demyelination (including patients with established MS, neuromyelitis optica, acute transverse myelitis, Marburg MS variant, and ADEM) showed that 42% of patients had a clinically meaningful response to true plasma exchange compared with only 6% of those in the sham treatment arm (95). This study confirmed prior uncontrolled observations, and case reports of response in steroid-refractory ADEM still appear (38,96–98). Currently, it seems most reasonable to treat ADEM with parenteral corticosteroids followed by a parenteral or oral taper; refractory or severe deficits should then be treated with plasma exchange (7 treatments administered over 14 days).

Many other approaches have been used empirically to treat refractory or severe ADEM. Case reports and uncontrolled experience suggest that intravenous immune globulin may be useful in children and adults (99–105). Intravenous cyclophosphamide has been used in steroid-refractory cases (9) and hypothermia was reported to be effective in one adult case (106). The role of chronic immunosuppression or immunomodulation (for example, with current MS therapies such as beta-interferon) in the rare relapsing ADEM cases is not known.

CONCLUSION

ADEM remains a poorly understood, heterogeneous syndrome. It is usually monophasic and has a good prognosis in many cases. Current clinical, laboratory, and neuroimaging modalities do not allow precise discrimination of ADEM from MS or other clinical phenotypes of idiopathic CNS demyelinating disease, especially at disease onset. Despite the use of the clinical, CSF, and MRI features summarized above, there is often lingering diagnostic uncertainty and clinicians are often faced with waiting to determine if the disorder relapses, "behaves like MS," and results in new imaging abnormalities. This is especially problematic in adults, in whom a diagnosis of MS is statistically more likely and for whom early treatment with immunomodulatory drugs is widely promoted, including after the first attack. Advances in diagnosis and treatment will require careful, longitudinal study utilizing standardized clinicopathological correlation and identification and validation of biological markers.

REFERENCES

1. Noseworthy JH, Lucchinetti C, Rodriguez M, et al. Multiple sclerosis. *N Engl J Med*. 2000;343:938–952.
2. Jacobs LD, Beck RW, Simon JH, et al. Intramuscular interferon beta-1a therapy initiated during a first demyelinating event in multiple sclerosis. *N Engl J Med*. 2000;343:898–904.
3. Comi G, Filippi M, Barkhof F, et al. Effect of early interferon treatment on conversion to definite multiple sclerosis: a randomised study. *Lancet* 2001; 357:1576–1582.
4. Wingerchuk DM. Postinfectious encephalomyelitis. *Current Neurology & Neuroscience Reports* 2003; 3:256–264.
5. Bennetto L, Scolding N. Inflammatory/post-infectious encephalomyelitis. *J Neurol Neurosurg Psychiatry*. 2004;75[Suppl I]:I22–I28.
6. Dale RC, de Sousa C, Chong WK, et al. Acute disseminated encephalomyelitis, multiphasic encephalomyelitis and multiple sclerosis in children. *Brain* 2000;123:2407–2422.
7. Hynson JL, Kornberg AJ, Coleman LT, et al. Clinical and neuroradiologic features of acute disseminated encephalomyelitis in children. *Neurology* 2001; 56:1308–1312.
8. Murthy SN, Faden HS, Cohen ME, et al. Acute disseminated encephalomyelitis in children. *Pediatrics* 2002;110:e21.
9. Schwarz S, Mohr A, Knauth M, et al. Acute disseminated encephalomyelitis. A follow-up study of 40 adult patients. *Neurology* 2001;56:1313–1318.
10. Tenembaum S, Chamoles N, Fejerman N. Acute disseminated encephalomyelitis. A long-term follow-up study of 84 pediatric patients. *Neurology* 2002; 59:1224–1231.
11. Au WY, Lie AK, Cheung RT, et al. Acute disseminated encephalomyelitis after para-influenza infection post bone marrow transplantation. *Leukemia & Lymphoma* 2002;43:455–457.
12. Spieker S, Petersen D, Rolfs A, et al. Acute disseminated encephalomyelitis following Pontiac fever. *Eur Neurol*. 1998;40:169–172.
13. Heick A, Skriver E. Chlamydia pneumoniae-associated ADEM. *Eur J Neurol*. 2000;7:435–438.
14. Sommer JB, Erbguth FJ, Neundorfer B. Acute disseminated encephalomyelitis following Legionella pneumophila infection. *Eur Neurol*. 2000;44: 182–184.
15. Yamamoto Y, Takasaki T, Yamada K, et al. Acute disseminated encephalomyelitis following dengue fever. *J Infection Chemotherapy*. 2002;8:175–177.
16. Proulx NL, Freedman MS, Chan JW, et al. Code CC. Acute disseminated encephalomyelitis associated with Pasteurella multocida meningitis. *Can J Neurol Sci*. 2003;30:155–158.
17. Alonso-Valle H, Munoz R, Hernandez JL, et al. Acute disseminated encephalomyelitis following Leptospira infection. *Eur Neurol*. 2001;46:104–105.
18. Centers for Disease Control and Prevention. Vaccinia (smallpox) vaccine: recommendations of the Advisory Committee on Immunization Practices 2001. *MMWR Morb Mortal Wkly Rep*. 2001;50:1–24.
19. Ascherio A, Zhang SM, Hernan MA, et al. Hepatitis B vaccination and the risk of multiple sclerosis. *N Engl J Med*. 2001;344:327–332.
20. Py MO, Andre C. Acute disseminated encephalomyelitis and meningococcal A and C vaccine: case report. *Arquivos de Neuro-Psiquiatria*. 1997; 55:632–635.
21. Bolukbasi O, Ozemenoglu M. Acute disseminated encephalomyelitis associated with tetanus vaccination. *Eur Neurol*. 1999;41:231–232.
22. Schwarz S, Knauth M, Schwab S, et al. Acute disseminated encephalomyelitis after parenteral therapy with herbal extracts: report of two cases. *J Neurol Neurosurg Psychiatry*. 2000;69:516–518.
23. Boz C, Velioglu S, Ozmenoglu M. Acute disseminated encephalomyelitis after bee sting. *Neurol Sci*. 2003;23:313–315.
24. Miller HG, Evans MJL. Prognosis in acute disseminated encephalomyelitis; with a note on neuromyelitis optica. *Q J Med*. 1953;22:347–349.
25. Litvak AM, Sands IJ, Gibel H. Encephalitis complicating measles: report of 56 cases with follow-up studies in 32. *Am J Dis Child*. 1943;65:265–295.
26. Scott TFM. Post infectious and vaccinal encephalitis. *Med Clin North Am*. 1867;51:701–716.
27. Anlar B, Basaran C, Kose G, et al. Acute disseminated encephalomyelitis in children: outcome and prognosis. *Neuropediatrics* 2003;34:194–199.
28. Brass SD, Caramanos Z, Santos C, et al. Multiple sclerosis vs acute disseminated encephalomyelitis in childhood. *Ped Neurol*. 2003;29:227–231.
29. Patel SP, Friedman RS. Neuropsychiatric features of acute disseminated encephalomyelitis: a review. *J Neuropsychiatr Clin Neurosci*. 1997;9:534–540.
30. Moscovich DG, Singh MB, Eva FJ, et al. Acute disseminated encephalomyelitis presenting as an acute psychotic state. *J Nerv Ment Dis*. 1995;183:116–117.
31. Wang PN, Fuh JL, Liu HC, et al. Acute disseminated encephalomyelitis in middle-aged or elderly patients. *Eur Neurol*. 1996;36:219–223.
32. Nasr JT, Andriola MR, Coyle PK. ADEM: literature review and case report of acute psychosis presentation. *Pediatr Neurol*. 2000;22:8–18.
33. Kubota H, Kanbayashi T, Tanabe Y, et al. A case of acute disseminated encephalomyelitis presenting hypersomnia with decreased hypocretin level in cerebrospinal fluid. *J Child Neurol*. 2002; 17:537–539.
34. Gledhill RF, Bartel PR, Yoshida Y, et al. Narcolepsy caused by acute disseminated encephalomyelitis. *Arch Neurol*. 2004;61:758–760.
35. Dale RC, Church AJ, Cardoso F, et al. Poststreptococcal acute disseminated encephalomyelitis with basal ganglia involvement and auto-reactive antibasal ganglia antibodies. *Ann Neurol*. 2001;50:588–595.
36. Ziegler DK. Acute disseminated encephalitis: some diagnostic and therapeutic considerations. *Arch Neurol*. 1966;14:476–488.
37. Atlas SW, Grossman RK, Goldberg HI, et al. Diagnosis of acute disseminated encephalomyelitis. *J Comput Assist Tomogr*. 1986;10:798–801.
38. Kanter DS, Horensky D, Sperling RA et al. Plasmapheresis in fulminant acute disseminated encephalomyelitis. *Neurology* 1995;45:824–827.
39. Modi G, Mochan A, Modi M, et al.. Demyelinating disorder of the central nervous system occurring in black South Africans. *J Neurol Neurosurg Psychiatry*. 2001;70:500–505.
40. Murray BJ, Apetauerova D, Scammell TE. Severe acute disseminated encephalomyelitis with normal MRI at presentation. *Neurology* 2000;55:1237–1238.

41. Honkaniemi J, Dastidar P, Kähärä V, et al. Delayed MR imaging changes in acute disseminated encephalomyelitis. *Am J Neuroradiol.* 2001;22:1117–1124.

42. Baum PA, Barkovich AJ, Koch TK, et al. Deep gray matter involvement in children with acute disseminated encephalomyelitis. *Am J Neuroradiol.* 1994;15:1275–1283.

43. Olivero WC, Deshmukh P, Gujrati M. Bilateral enhancing thalamic lesions in a 10 year old boy: case report. *J Neurol Neurosurg Psychiatry.* 1999;66:633–635.

44. Hamed LM, Silbiger J, Guy J, et al. Parainfectious optic neuritis and encephalomyelitis. A report of two cases with thalamic involvement. *J Clin Neuro-ophthalmol.* 1993;13:18–23.

45. Miller DH, Scaravilli F, Thomas DCT, et al. Acute disseminated encephalomyelitis presenting as a solitary brainstem mass. *J Neurol Neurosurg Psychiatry.* 1993;56:920–922.

46. De Recondo A, Guichard JP. Acute disseminated encephalomyelitis presenting as multiple cystic lesions. *J Neurol Neurosurg Psychiatry.* 1997;63:15.

47. van der Meyden CH, de Villiers JFK, Middlecote BD, et al. Gadolinium ring enhancement and mass effect in acute disseminated encephalomyelitis. *Neuroradiol.* 1994;36:221–223.

48. Kuperan S, Ostrow P, Landi MK, et al. Acute hemorrhagic leukoencephalitis vs ADEM: FLAIR MRI and neuropathology findings. *Neurology* 2003;60:721–722.

49. O'Riordan JI, Gomez-Anson B, Moseley IF, et al. Long term MRI follow-up of patients with post infectious encephalomyelitis: evidence for a monophasic disease. *J Neurol Sci.* 1999;167:132–136.

50. Bizzi A, Ulug AM, Crawford TO, et al. Quantitative proton MR spectroscopic imaging in acute disseminated encephalomyelitis. *Am J Neuroradiol.* 2001;22:1125–1130.

51. Harada M, Hisaoka S, Mori K, et al. Differences in water diffusion and lactate production in two different types of postinfectious encephalopathy. *J Mag Res Imag.* 2000;11:559–563.

52. Bernarding J, Braun J, Koennecke H-C. Diffusion- and perfusion-weighted MR imaging in a patient with acute disseminated encephalomyelitis (ADEM). *J Mag Res Imag.* 2002;15:96–100.

53. Holtmannspotter M, Inglese M, Rovaris M, et al. A diffusion tensor MRI study of basal ganglia from patients with ADEM. *J Neurol Sci.* 2003;206:27–30.

54. Inglese M, Salvi F, Iannucci G, et al. Magnetization transfer and diffusion tensor MR imaging of acute disseminated encephalomyelitis. *Am J Neuroradiol.* 2002;23:267–272.

55. Tan TXL, Spigos DG, Mueller CF. Abnormal cortical metabolism in acute disseminated encephalomyelitis. *Clin Nucl Med.* 1998;23:629–630.

56. Itti E, Huff K, Cornford ME, et al. Postinfectious encephalitis. A coregistered SPECT and magnetic resonance imaging study. *Clin Nucl Med.* 2002; 27:129–130.

57. Prineas JW, McDonald, WI, Franklin, RJM. Demyelinating Diseases. In: Graham DI and Lantos PL, eds. *Greenfield's Neuropathology*, 7th ed. London: Arnold, 2002: 471–535.

58. Hurst EW. Acute hemorrhagic leukoencephalitis: a previously undefined entity. *Med J Aust.* 1941;1:1–6.

59. Klein C, Wijdicks EFM, Earnest IVF. Full recovery after acute hemorrhagic leukoencephalitis (Hurst's disease). *J Neurol.* 2000;247:977–979.

60. Rosman NP, Gottlieb SM, Bernstein CA. Acute hemorrhagic leukoencephalitis: recovery and reversal of magnetic resonance imaging findings in a child. *J Child Neurol.* 1997;12:448–454.

61. Seales D, Greer M. Acute hemorrhagic leukoencephalitis: a successful recovery. *Arch Neurol.* 1991; 48:1086–1088.

62. Lucchinetti C, Bruck W, Parisi J, et al. Heterogeneity of multiple sclerosis lesions: implications for the pathogenesis of demyelination. *Ann Neurol.* 2000; 47:707–717.

63. Johnson RT. Pathogenesis of acute viral encephalitis and post infectious encephalomyelitis. *J Infect Dis.* 1987;155:359–364.

64. Johnson RT. Postinfectious Demyelinating Diseases. In: Johnson RT. *Viral Infections of the Nervous System.* 2nd ed. Philadelphia: Lippincott-Raven, 1998: 181–210.

65. Cherry, JD, Shields WD. Encephalitis and Meningoencephalitis. In: Feigin RD, Cherry JD, eds. *Textbook of Pediatric Infectious Diseases.* Philadelphia: W.B. Saunders, 1992: 445–454.

66. Stocks M. Genetics of childhood disorders: XXIX. Autoimmune disorders, part 2: molecular mimicry. *J Am Acad Child Adolescent Psychiatry.* 2001; 40:977–980.

67. Miller SD, Vanderlugt CL, Begolka WS, et al. Persistent infection with Theiler's virus leads to autoimmunity via epitope spreading. *Nat Med.* 1997; 3:1133–1136.

68. Murray PD, Pavelko KD, Leibowitz J, et al. CD4+ and CD8+ T cells make discrete contributions to demyelination and neurologic disease in a viral model of multiple sclerosis. *J Virol.* 1998; 72:7320–7329.

69. Lin X, Pease LR, Murray PD, et al. Theiler's virus induced infection of genetically susceptible mice induces central nervous system-infiltrating CTLs with no apparent viral or major myelin antigenic specificity. *J Immunol.* 1998; 160:5661–5668.

70. Rodriguez M, Dunkel AJ, Thiemann RL, et al. Abrogation of resistance to Theiler's virus-induced demyelination in H-2b mice deficient in beta 2-microglobulin. *J Immunol.* 1993;151:266–276.

71. Rivera-Quinones C, McGavern D, Schmelzer JD, et al. Absence of neurologic deficits following extensive demyelination in a class I-deficient murine model of multiple sclerosis. *Nat Med.* 1998;4:187–193.

72. Njenga MK, Murray PD, McGavern D, et al. Absence of spontaneous central nervous system remyelination in class II-deficient mice infected with Theiler's virus. *J Neuropathol Exp Neurol.* 1999; 58:78–91.

73. Johnson RT, Griffin DE, Hirsch RL, et al. Measles encephalomyelitis: clinical and immunologic studies. *N Engl J Med.* 1984;310:137–141.

74. Gold R, Hartung HP, Toyka KV. Animal models for autoimmune demyelinating disorders of the nervous system. *Mol Med Today.* 2000;62:88–91.

75. Ben-Nun A, Wekerle H, Cohen IR. The rapid isolation of clonable antigen specific T lymphocyte lines capable of mediating autoimmune encephalomyelitis. *Eur J Immunol.* 1981;11:195–199.

76. Pohl-Koppe A, Burchett SK, Thiele EA, et al. Myelin basic protein reactive Th2 T cells are found in acute disseminated encephalomyelitis. *J Neuroimmunol.* 1998;19–27.

77. Kuchroo VK, Sobel RA, Yamamura T, et al. Induction of experimental allergic encephalomyelitis by myelin proteolipid-protein-specific T cell clones and synthetic peptides. *Pathobiology* 1991;59:305–312.

78. Hafler DA, Benjamin DS, Burks J, et al. Myelin basic protein and proteolipid protein reactivity of brain and cerebrospinal fluid derived T cell clones in multiple sclerosis and post infectious encephalomyelitis. *J Immunol.* 1987;139:69–72.

79. Miller A, Al-Sabbagh A, Santos LMB, et al. Epitopes of myelin basic protein that trigger TGF-β release after oral tolerization are distinct from encephalitogenic epitopes and mediate epitope-driven bystander suppression. *J Immunol.* 1993;151:7307–7315.

80. Wucherpfennig KW, Weiner HL, Hafler DA. T cell recognition of myelin basic protein. *Immunol Today.* 1991; 12:277–282.

81. Kuchroo VK, Prabhu-Das M, Brown JA, et al. B7–1 and B7–2 costimulatory molecules activate differentially the Th1/Th2 developmental pathways: application to autoimmune disease therapy. *Cell* 1995; 80:707–718.

82. Laouini D, Kennou MF, Khoufi S, et al. Antibodies to human myelin proteins and gangliosides in patients with acute neuroparalytic accidents induced by brain-derived rabies vaccine. *J Neuroimmunol.* 1998;91:63–72.

83. Wingerchuk DM, Lucchinetti CF, Noseworthy JH. Multiple sclerosis: current pathophysiological concepts. *Lab Invest.* 2001;81:263–281.

84. Ichiyama T, Shoji H, Kato M, et al. Cerebrospinal fluid levels of cytokines and soluble tumour necrosis factor receptor in acute disseminated encephalomyelitis. *Eur J Pediatr.* 2002;161:133–137.

85. Kadhim H, De Prez C, Gazagnes MD, et al. In situ cytokine immune responses in acute disseminated encephalomyelitis: insights into pathophysiologic mechanisms. *Human Pathol.* 2003; 34:293–297.

86. Ichiyama T, Shoji H, Kato M, et al. Cerebrospinal fluid levels of cytokines and soluble tumour necrosis factor receptor in acute disseminated encephalomyelitis. *Eur J Pediatr.* 2002;161:133–137.

87. Dale RC, Morovat A. Interleukin-6 and oligoclonal IgG synthesis in children with acute disseminated encephalomyelitis. *Neuropediatrics* 2003;34:141–145.

88. Kadhim H, De Prez C, Gazagnes MD, et al. In situ cytokine immune responses in acute disseminated encephalomyelitis: insights into pathophysiologic mechanisms. *Human Pathol.* 2003;34:293–297.

89. Bauer J, Stadelmann C, Bancher C, et al. Apoptosis of T lymphocytes in acute disseminated encephalomyelitis. *Acta Neuropathologica.* 1999;97:543–546.

90. McDonald WI, Compston A, Edan G, et al. Recommended diagnostic criteria for multiple sclerosis: guidelines from the International Panel on the Diagnosis of Multiple Sclerosis. *Ann Neurol.* 2001;50:121–127.

91. Durston JHJ, Milnes JN. Relapsing encephalitis. *Brain* 1970;93:715–730.

92. Cohen O, Steiner-Birmanns B, Biran I, et al. Recurrence of acute disseminated encephalomyelitis at the previously affected brain site. *Arch Neurol.* 2001;58:797–801.

93. Hartel C, Schilling S, Gottschalk S, et al. Multiphasic disseminated encephalomyelitis associated with streptococcal infection. *Eur J Paed Neurol.* 2002;6:327–329.

94. Straub J, Chofflon M, Delavelle J. Early high-dose intravenous methylprednisolone in acute disseminated encephalomyelitis: a successful recovery. *Neurology* 1997;49:1145–1147.

95. Weinshenker BG, O'Brien PC, Petterson TM, et al. A randomized trial of plasma exchange in acute central nervous system inflammatory demyelinating disease. *Ann Neurol.* 1999;46:878–886.

96. Rodriguez M, Karnes WE, Bartleson JD, et al. Plasmapheresis in acute episodes of fulminant CNS inflammatory demyelination. *Neurology* 1993; 43:1100–1104.

97. Balestri P, Grosso S, Acquaviva A, et al. Plasmapheresis in a child affected by acute disseminated encephalomyelitis. *Brain Devel.* 2000;22:123–126.

98. Miyazawa R, Hikima A, Takano Y, et al. Plasmapheresis in fulminant acute disseminated encephalomyelitis. *Brain & Development* 2001;23:424–426.

99. Kleiman M, Brunquell P. Acute disseminated encephalomyelitis: response to intravenous immunoglobulin? *J Child Neurol.* 1995;10:481–483.

100. Hahn JS, Siegler DJ, Enzmann D. Intravenous gamma-globulin therapy in recurrent acute disseminated encephalomyelitis. *Neurology* 1996;46:1173–1174.

101. Pradhan S, Gupta RP, Shashank S, et al. Intravenous immunoglobulin therapy in acute disseminated encephalomyelitis. *J Neurol Sci.* 1999;165:56–61.

102. Apak RA, Anlar B, Saatci I. A case of relapsing acute disseminated encephalomyelitis with high dose corticosteroid treatment. *Brain Dev.* 1999;21:279–282.

103. Sahlas DJ, Miller SP, Guerin M, et al. Treatment of acute disseminated encephalomyelitis with intravenous immunoglobulin. *Neurology* 2000;54:1370–1372.

104. Marchioni E, Marinou-Aktipi K, Uggetti C, et al. Effectiveness of intravenous immunoglobulin treatment in adult patients with steroid-resistant monophasic or recurrent acute disseminated encephalomyelitis. *J Neurol.* 2002;249:100–104.

105. Andersen JB, Rasmussen LH, Herning M, et al. Dramatic improvement of severe acute disseminated encephalomyelitis after treatment with intravenous immunoglobulin in a three-year-old boy. *Devel Med Child Neurol.* 2001;43:136–138.

106. Takata T, Hirakawa M, Sakurai M, et al. Fulminant form of acute disseminated encephalomyelitis: successful treatment with hypothermia. *J Neurol Sci.* 1999;165:94–97.

20

Neuromyelitis Optica

Dean M. Wingerchuk

Department of Neurology, Mayo Clinic, Scottsdale, Arizona

INTRODUCTION

Neuromyelitis optica (NMO; also known as Devic syndrome or Devic disease) is an idiopathic inflammatory disorder of the central nervous system (CNS) that preferentially affects the optic nerves and spinal cord while virtually sparing the brain (1). Accumulating evidence suggests that idiopathic NMO, which has long been categorized as a probable multiple sclerosis variant, is a distinct clinical entity and perhaps a separate disease. This chapter summarizes the clinical, genetic, laboratory, neuroimaging, and immunopathological data that support this contention.

HISTORY AND NOMENCLATURE

In 1870, Albutt described a patient with a "sympathetic disorder of the eye" that came on "twelve or thirteen weeks at least" after an acute episode of myelitis (2). Erb, in 1880, described *myelitis transversa dorsalis with neuritis descendens opticorum* in a patient with a prolonged clinical course but eventual good visual and motor recovery, although he considered the association to be a coincidence (3). Achard and Guinon presented the first pathological account of NMO in 1889 and described complete loss of the myelin sheath from the optic nerves (4).

In 1894, Devic summarized 16 cases from the literature as well as a fatal case from his own clinical experience (5). He used the terms *neuro-myélite* and *neuroptico-myélite* to describe cases of either papillitis or retrobulbar neuritis in conjunction with acute myelitis. His student Gault summarized these cases in his doctoral thesis and used the term *neuromyélite optic aiguë* (acute optic neuromyelitis) (6). Subsequently, Devic became the eponym for the disorder.

In 1914, Goulden concluded that the pathological findings of NMO were likely due to an infection based upon his review of 51 case reports and a personal case studied at autopsy (7). In 1927, Beck noted a case with a relapsing course and he concluded that NMO was a distinct disorder often confused with multiple sclerosis (MS) or Schilder disease (8). In 1935, Berliner discussed MS, acute disseminated encephalomyelitis (ADEM), NMO, and encephalitis periaxialis diffusa as clinical variants of one disease (9). Throughout the remainder of the twentieth century, investigators published case reports and series, with or without pathological data, and continued to debate the nosology of the syndrome, especially its relationship to MS (10–13). The question is incompletely resolved but increasingly compelling clinical, laboratory, neuroimaging, and immunopathological evidence suggests that NMO should be considered a distinct disorder and that its spectrum may be broader than previously recognized (14).

CLINICAL DEFINITION AND DIAGNOSTIC CRITERIA

The sine qua non of NMO is the coexistence of ON and myelitis. However, this clinical combination is not specific for the disorder. It also occurs commonly in typical MS and has been reported in association with many systemic autoimmune disorders including systemic lupus erythematosus, Sjögren syndrome, and mixed connective tissue disease. An opticospinal syndrome may also occur as a parainfectious phenomenon, similar to acute disseminated encephalomyelitis, in association with infectious diseases (pulmonary tuberculosis and a myriad of viral illnesses) and immunizations

(11,15,16). What differentiates most cases of NMO from these other disorders is the severity of individual clinical attacks, its tendency to recur, and its persisting restriction, almost exclusively, to the optic nerves and spinal cord.

The diagnostic term NMO is currently applied when a patient experiences optic neuritis (unilateral or bilateral) and myelitis without clinical evidence of demyelination affecting brain white matter. Incremental revisions in admittedly arbitrary but clinically very useful diagnostic criteria attempt to discriminate NMO from MS by emphasizing several apparent clinical, laboratory, and neuroimaging differences; criteria in wide use are summarized in Table 20-1 (17–19). Results of magnetic resonance imaging (MRI) studies of the brain and spinal cord and cerebrospinal fluid (CSF) examination are integral to the NMO diagnostic algorithm. Brain MRI is usually normal or reveals only scattered, nonspecific white matter lesions that fail to meet imaging criteria for MS. Spinal cord MRI demonstrates that virtually all patients have one or more longitudinally extensive lesions extending over three or more vertebral segments. Analysis of CSF, especially close to the time of a myelitis attack, often reveals pleocytosis of more than 50 leukocytes, with or without the presence of neutrophils, but without accompanying unique oligoclonal bands. As diagnostic criteria have been refined and applied to groups of patients with what most would agree is a disease course most compatible with NMO rather than typical MS, several key findings have gained acceptance.

TABLE 20-1 *Proposed diagnostic criteria for neuromyelitis optica*

Diagnosis requires all absolute criteria AND one major supportive criterion OR two minor supportive criteria.

Absolute criteria
1. Optic neuritis
2. Acute myelitis
3. No clinical disease outside of the optic nerves and spinal cord

Major Supportive Criteria
1. Negative brain MRI at disease onset (normal or not meeting radiological diagnostic criteria for MS)
2. Spinal cord MRI with T2 signal abnormality extending over ≥ 3 vertebral segments
3. CSF pleocytosis (> 50 WBC/mm^3) OR > 5 neutrophils/mm^3

Minor Supportive Criteria
1. Bilateral optic neuritis
2. Severe ON with fixed visual acuity worse than 20/200 in at least one eye
3. Severe, fixed, attack-related weakness (MRC grade 2 or less) in one or more limbs

These include: (a) the interval between the initial events of ON and myelitis is quite variable (occasionally several years); (b) some patients experience unilateral rather than bilateral optic neuritis; and (c) the course may be monophasic or relapsing. Although the diagnostic criteria have not been formally validated in the strictest sense, they have clearly improved the ability of define a relatively homogeneous group of patients whose natural history differs significantly from those with typical forms of MS and are consistent with results obtained by independent investigators (15,20,21). The core characteristics of the diagnostic criteria will be described in greater detail below.

EPIDEMIOLOGY AND GENETICS

Neuromyelitis optica is predominantly a disorder of women. The female-to-male ratio is greater than 4:1 for the more common relapsing disease course, whereas it is approximately 1:1 in reports detailing monophasic cases. Contemporary series suggest that the median age of onset is late in the fourth decade, about 10 years later than for typical MS, but new-onset NMO has been reported in infants and octogenarians (19,22).

The role of genetic factors in NMO is not clear (12,23). Most patients do not have a family history of typical MS or CNS demyelinating disease of any type, but there are reports of familial cases, including a set of identical twins with a similar age of disease onset (24–27). Shared genetic influence is implicated in these cases, especially with monozygotic twin concordance, but environmental influences, such as the common intrauterine and early childhood environment, cannot be excluded. In Japan, where Asian-type "opticospinal MS" is a common phenotype, less than 1% of families contained more than one affected individual (28). Neuromyelitis optica may differ genetically from typical MS in that most studies do not find an association with the HLA-DRB1*1501 allele that is associated with typical MS (29–31).

The incidence and prevalence of NMO are unknown. In Western nations, it has generally been considered a rare disorder but is almost certainly under-recognized, in part due to the lack of clear diagnostic criteria and confusion with MS. Racial or ethnic background appears significant because there is a clear overrepresentation of non-Caucasians (such as those with Asian, African, or Hispanic ancestry or ethnicity) compared with typical MS, even in North American patients (19,32–37). Demyelinating disease in Asia is much more commonly restricted to, or has a strong predilection for, the optic nerves and spinal cord. In fact, Japanese investigators often distinguish an "opticospinal" form of MS from a "Western-type" MS; recent discovery of an autoantibody that may discriminate NMO from MS suggests that Asian opticospinal MS and NMO are the same disorder (30,31,38,39). A Japanese national survey determined that 7.6% of patients with demyelinating disease had NMO, but this rate may be declining with a concomitant increase in the frequency of Western-type MS (28,40). Up to 6% of demyelinating disease cases in India are NMO (41).

Certain human leukocyte antigen (HLA) alleles are also associated with opticospinal forms of MS. The HLA-DPB1*0501 allele was present in a higher frequency of patients with opticospinal MS than prototypic MS in Japanese patients, whereas the DPB1*0301 allele may be underrepresented (28,42–46). These HLA associations differ from those described in patients with Western-type MS, which is most consistently associated with HLA-DRB1*1501. One study of Caucasians did not show that opticospinal MS was associated with the HLA-DPB1*0501 allele (47,48). More studies of patients from different racial backgrounds are needed to clarify the results of these initial results. Finally, mutations found in Leber hereditary optic neuropathy have been described in some MS patients who have particularly prominent and severe optic nerve involvement, but searches for these mutations, as well as other mitochondrial abnormalities, in patients with NMO were negative (49,50).

CLINICAL PRESENTATION

Onset and Concomitant Illnesses

The NMO syndrome may occur as a parainfectious phenomenon antedated by a viral prodrome (headache, pyrexia, myalgias, and respiratory or gastrointestinal complaints). Disease associations, including connective tissue disorders, are summarized in Table 20-2 (11,12). Systemic autoimmune disorders such as hypothyroidism and Sjögren syndrome are overrepresented in relapsing NMO (19).

Optic neuritis attacks are usually severe and may be unilateral or bilateral (19). A minority of patients experience simultaneous bilateral ON but the frequency is significantly higher than in MS. Acute optic neuritis in NMO is usually severe and may or may not be associated with retro-orbital pain. Visual field defects are variable and include central and paracentral scotomata as well as altitudinal and chiasmatic patterns. It is likely that asymptomatic optic nerve involvement occurs in some people with incompletely developed clinical NMO. Some patients with recurrent myelitis were shown at autopsy to have optic nerve or chiasm lesions that appeared consistent with chronic demyelination.

During the first episode of ON in NMO, nearly 40% of affected eyes become completely blind (no light perception) at the nadir of the event. Most patients experience some improvement in vision, especially if their disease course is monophasic; relapsing cases accumulate visual impairment with successive recurrences of ON (19,20,22).

Acute myelitis attacks typically cause complete transverse myelitis, defined as severe, bilateral inflammatory spinal cord injury with neurological dysfunction worsening over several hours to days and involving motor, sensory, and sphincter function. This pattern is rare in prototypic MS. Motor weakness rapidly evolves to paraplegia or quadriplegia, and occasionally spinal shock occurs with flaccidity and absent muscle stretch reflexes, and plantar responses. Fewer patients develop asymmetric lesions presenting as Brown–Sequard or central cord syndromes. L'hermitte symptom, paroxysmal tonic spasms, and radicular pain are relatively common occurrences in patients with relapsing disease. Partial recovery is common following the initial myelitis event. Between 78% and 88% of patients improved by one or more levels on a seven-point ordinal scale of motor function regardless of eventual disease course (19,22).

Myelitis may cause severe morbidity or death. Acute cervical myelitis is associated with respiratory failure and death, especially in relapsing NMO (19,22). The immobility that results following myelitis places patients at risk for thromboembolic disease, urinary tract infections, decubitus ulcerations, and pneumonia.

Current clinical diagnostic criteria for NMO have allowed better diagnostic differentiation from MS. Patients with typical MS do not have a clinical phenotype comparable to NMO but may experience both ON and spinal cord exacerbations at some time during their disease course. The inclusion of patients who have experienced clinical symptoms outside of the opticospinal axis early in the disease course probably led to the inclusion of patients with otherwise typical MS in NMO case series. Is it now clear that in NMO, symptoms outside of the optic nerves and spinal cord are rare, usually minor or subjective, tend to occur later in the disease course, and are plausibly due to causes other than NMO. This includes symptoms such

TABLE 20-2 *Infectious agents and diseases associated with NMO*

Infections and Immunizations	Other Diseases
Varicella	Systemic lupus erythematosus
Infectious mononucleosis	Autoimmune thyroid disease
Influenza A	Sjögren syndrome
Streptococcal pharyngitis	Pernicious anemia
Human herpes virus types 6 and 8	Behcet disease
Human immunodeficiency virus	Mixed connective tissue disease
Mycobacterium tuberculosis	Disseminated cholesterol emboli
Chlamydia pneumoniae	Ulcerative colitis
Rubella vaccine	Primary sclerosing cholangitis
Smallpox vaccine	Idiopathic thrombocytopenic purpura

as vertigo, facial numbness, nystagmus, headache, and postural tremor. Rare findings reported in NMO include extraocular palsies, seizures, ataxia, dysarthria, encephalopathy, dysautonomia (51), and peripheral neuropathy (52). As for most clinical criteria, there are always exceptions, and the Mayo Clinic group has identified a number of patients with cerebral or brain stem symptoms at some time during the disease course, even at onset, yet the subsequent disease course seemed highly compatible with NMO and met other components of the diagnostic criteria. Further evaluation of large datasets and development of diagnostic biomarkers will clarify these issues.

Diagnostic Evaluation

In most instances, diagnostic testing is utilized to attempt to differentiate NMO from typical multiple sclerosis. Features that assist in this clinical decision are summarized in Table 20-3.

Brain MRI is diagnostically helpful for patients with suspected NMO (18–20). Normal results or the presence of nonspecific white matter lesions that do not meet radiological criteria for MS in a patient with recurrent optic neuritis and myelitis should raise suspicion for NMO.

Some patients with relapsing disease accumulate white matter lesions over time, but these lesions tend to be nonspecific punctate foci that fail to meet radiological criteria for MS (19). As with all idiopathic demyelinating syndromes, there are exceptions to clinical rules and some cases that otherwise appear highly consistent with NMO will have MS-like cerebral or brainstem lesions. Therefore, this finding should not negate the possibility of NMO in an otherwise typical case.

During acute ON, MR imaging with attention to the orbits may demonstrate swelling and/or gadolinium enhancement of the affected optic nerve or the chiasm (Fig. 20-1). In some patients, the lesions appear more extensive than those of MS but the range of abnormality is so great that it does not distinguish between the disorders.

Spinal cord MRI is probably the most useful discriminative test. During acute myelitis, the affected region of the cord is usually expanded and swollen and may enhance with gadolinium (Fig. 20-2). Heterogeneous T2-weighted signal abnormality within the lesion suggests cavitation or necrosis and lesions are often centered within the cord. Most patients with NMO have a contiguous, longitudinally extensive, gadolinium-enhancing cord lesion that

TABLE 20-3 *Features that assist in discriminating NMO from MS*

	Favors NMO	Favors MS
Age of Onset	Median: late 30s	Median: 29
Clinical Features		
Optic neuritis	More severe/poor recovery	Less severe/better recovery
	Sometimes bilateral and simultaneous	Rarely bilateral and simultaneous
Myelitis	Often bilateral, more symmetric	Usually unilateral, more asymmetric
Brain or brain stem	Not clinically involved	Usually involved
MRI		
Brain	Normal or nonspecific at onset	Usually abnormal at onset
	Nonspecific abnormalities not meeting MS criteria	Increasing number of typical MS lesions
Spinal cord: acute lesions	Cord expansion	Rarely cord expansion
	Lesion(s) extend over three or more vertebral segments	Lesion(s) less than one vertebral segment
Spinal cord: chronic lesions	Focal atrophy common	Focal atrophy uncommon
CSF		
Pleocytosis	Sometimes > 50 WBC/mm³	Rarely > 50WBC/mm³
Cell differential	Sometimes neutrophilic	Lymphocytic
Oligoclonal banding	About 30%	About 85%
Associated autoimmunity		
Clinical disease	Substantial minority	Uncommon except hypothyroidism
Autoimmune serology	Common, multiple autoantibodies	Minority, usually one autoantibody

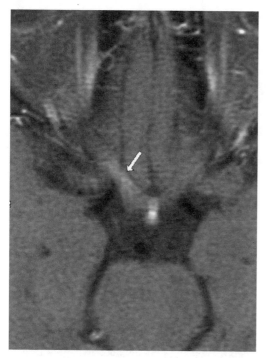

FIG. 20-1. Orbital MRI in NMO. T1-weighted, post-gadolinium orbital MRI demonstrates an enhancing right optic nerve lesion in a patient with relapsing NMO and acute optic neuritis.

spans three or more vertebral segments (19). In contrast, spinal cord plaques in MS uncommonly exceed two segments in length and are located more peripherally (52). Cord lesions in NMO evolve over time such that the swelling and enhancement give way to persistent intramedullary T2-weighted signal abnormality and segmental cord atrophy.

Magnetization transfer (MT) brain and spinal cord imaging, currently used as a research tool, detects abnormalities in brain tissue that appears normal by conventional MRI techniques. In NMO, Filippi et al. demonstrated that MT brain images were not different from controls (53). Furthermore, despite the more longitudinally extensive cord lesions in NMO, MT imaging characteristics of spinal lesions were similar in NMO and MS. Recently, however, Rocca et al. used MT and diffusion tensor imaging to study MT ratios of white and grey matter separately in NMO patients and healthy controls (54). White matter results were normal, but grey matter was not. This unexpected finding is of uncertain significance and worthy of further study.

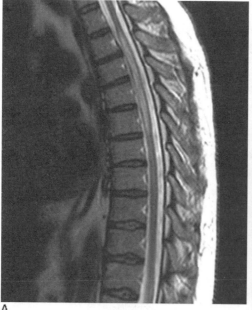

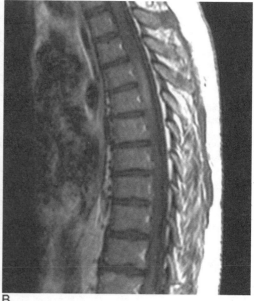

A   B

FIG. 20-2. Spinal cord MRI in NMO. Sagittal T2-weighted imaging performed shortly after the onset of an acute myelitis attack demonstrates abnormal signal extending over four vertebral segments and associated cord swelling **(A)**. The lesion enhances with gadolinium **(B)**.

Cerebrospinal fluid analysis may assist in NMO diagnosis because perhaps 30% of patients will have a pleocytosis of greater than 50 WBC/mm^3 in the setting of an acute myelitis exacerbation; this degree of CSF cellularity is very rare in typical MS (19). The CSF leukocyte differential may also reveal the presence of neutrophils, another finding rarely seen in MS.

Approximately 85% of patients with MS have more than one unique oligoclonal band detectable by electrophoresis or immunofixation techniques (55,56). The frequency of CSF oligoclonal band positivity (20% to 40%) and other immunoglobulin (IgG) abnormalities, such as increased rate of IgG synthesis, are also much less common in NMO (17–19,20,57).

Electrophysiological studies are of little diagnostic use in NMO with the exception of the scenario where visual-evoked potentials may detect a subclinical optic nerve lesion in a patient with isolated, recurrent myelitis. This finding suggests NMO, although current diagnostic criteria do not account for subclinical optic nerve pathology and may require revision.

One or more autoantibodies, including antinuclear antibody, anti-double-stranded DNA antibody, extractable nuclear antigen, and antithyroid antibodies are commonly present in the serum of patients with NMO (19). The incidence of each of these antibodies has not been assessed by an appropriate study design, but perhaps 50% of patients appear to have at least one positive test result.

Mayo Clinic investigators reported the discovery of a novel serum autoantibody that appears to discriminate NMO from typical multiple sclerosis (38,39). This indirect immunofluorescence assay reveals a distinct staining pattern (termed NMO-IgG) that appears to selectively bind a target associated with CNS microvessels, pia, subpia, and Virchow–Robin space (38). With the NMO diagnostic criteria as the gold standard, the assay was reasonably sensitive (73%; 95% CI: 60% to 86%) and highly specific (91%; 95% CI: 79% to 100%) for NMO in 45 North American patients who presented with either optic neuritis or myelitis and in whom NMO was considered possible (39). The assay was also positive in 58% of 12 Japanese opticospinal MS patients and was negative in five Japanese patients with Western-type MS. This finding represents the first specific biological marker for NMO and, if validated, may be a powerful diagnostic tool available at disease onset. It also suggests that Asian opticospinal MS and NMO may be the same entity and that some cases of idiopathic recurrent optic neuritis or recurrent myelitis represent incompletely evolved NMO (58–62).

NATURAL HISTORY OF NMO: DISEASE COURSES

Neuromyelitis optica remains a clinically defined entity with diagnostic criteria derived from the clinical, imaging, and laboratory testing that appear to identify a group of patients with a different disease course than those with typical MS (19–22). Patients who meet NMO diagnostic criteria proceed along either a monophasic or a relapsing course (Table 20-4) (19,22). A *monophasic* course, which probably

TABLE 20-4 *Characteristics of monophasic and relapsing NMO*

	Monophasic	Relapsing
Frequency	Less common	More common
Age of Onset (median)	29	39
Sex Ratio	About 50% female	80% to 90% female
History of Autoimmune Disease	Uncommon	About 50%
Index (Presenting) Events:		
ON or myelitis only	48%	90%
Bilateral ON	17%	8%
Simultaneous ON + myelitis	31%	0%
Severity at nadir	More severe	Less severe
Recovery	Good	Fair
Respiratory Failure	Rare	About one-third
Mortality Rate (5 years)	10%	32%

occurs in fewer than 25% of all NMO cases, is defined by co-occurrence of either unilateral or bilateral ON and a single episode of myelitis and extended follow-up (several years) during which no further exacerbations emerge. Most patients experience *relapsing* disease, in which the index events of ON and myelitis may be many weeks or even years apart but attacks of ON, myelitis, or both recur over the next months to years. In most instances, the relapsing course is established quite early in the disease. After fulfilling NMO diagnostic criteria, the cumulative proportion of patients who experience another attack that defines relapsing disease is 55% at one year, 78% at three years, and 90% at five years (19).

The relapsing nature of NMO was recognized earlier in Japan, where such cases were diagnosed as opticospinal or Asian variants of MS, distinguishing it clearly from Western-type or typical MS. The Asian opticospinal form appears to have the same demographic, clinical, neuroimaging, and pathological characteristics as cases of relapsing NMO reported from North America, with the exception that systemic autoimmunity is recognized much more commonly in the West (23). The characteristics of a "pure" subgroup of opticospinal MS (clinical opticospinal disease, normal head MRI except for optic nerve abnormalities, and more than five years of clinical follow-up) are virtually identical to cases of relapsing NMO (31). Finally, a serum autoantibody that appears to discriminate MS from NMO is also positive in most Japanese opticospinal MS patients (39).

Clinical and laboratory features that are available early in the disease course and have the ability to discriminate between the relapsing and monophasic NMO varieties would be very useful to provide prognostic information and assist with treatment planning. Initial studies showed that MRI and CSF variables did not predict disease course or severity (19,22). The observation that patients who present with a combination of near-simultaneous bilateral ON and myelitis are much more likely have a monophasic course was recently confirmed by observational data utilizing a longitudinal database of 80 NMO patients (22). The median interval between the first clinical event and the development of bila-

teral ON and myelitis (traditional definition of NMO) was 5 days (range 0 to 151 days) in the monophasic group versus 166 days (range 2 to 730 days) for the relapsing group (19). The relative risk of relapsing disease is increased by 2.16 *for every month increase* in the first interattack interval (22). In other words, patients who present with ON and myelitis attacks several weeks or months apart are highly likely to have relapsing disease.

Additional independent predictors of a relapsing course include female sex (relative risk = 10.0 female versus male) and less severe motor impairment with the initial myelitis event (relative risk = 0.48 for every point decrease on a motor weakness scale). Complete paraplegia occurs with the first myelitis attack in 70% of monophasic patients, compared with only 31% of those who later develop relapsing disease. Initial ON attack severity was not an independent risk factor for disease course prediction. These prognostic variables may be useful when considering the use of preventive immunosuppressant therapies early in the disease course and in planning epidemiological and therapeutic studies.

Patients with monophasic NMO have a better long-term prognosis than those with relapsing disease because, although their index attacks are usually more severe, they achieve a permanent remission and are faced with static residual neurological impairments. Although 22% of patients with monophasic disease remained functionally blind (20/200 vision or worse) in at least one affected eye, more than 50% of ON episodes recovered visual acuity to a level of 20/30 or better. However, most patients experience at least a moderate degree of permanent limb weakness and sphincter dysfunction from myelitis; permanent monoplegia or paraplegia occurs in 31%. Five-year survival of this group is approximately 90% and cause of death is usually unrelated to NMO or a medical complication of immobility (19,22).

Like typical MS, relapsing NMO follows an unpredictable course consisting of clusters of attacks months or years apart. When attack severity and cumulative disability are considered, however, the natural history of relapsing

NMO is markedly different from that of a typical MS cohort. More than half of people with relapsing NMO have permanent and severe visual impairment in at least one eye or are nonambulatory due to attack-related paraplegia or quadriplegia within 5 years of NMO onset. This compares unfavorably to MS, in which most patients recover well (or completely) from early attacks and tolerate relatively mild impairment until evolution of the secondary progressive phase of the disease. Progressive disease is an uncommon feature of NMO.

Relapse frequency in NMO is highly variable. Remissions may last only weeks or extend for more than a decade. In one patient cohort followed over a median of 16.9 years, the median number of relapses was 5 (range 1 to 18) (19).

Relapsing NMO reduces survival. In one longitudinal series, 5-year survival was 68% with all deaths secondary to myelitis-related respiratory failure (19). The true incidence of myelitis-associated respiratory failure is probably lower as diagnostic criteria are revised and some milder cases, which would have previously been classified as MS, are confirmed to be NMO. Predictors of mortality in relapsing NMO include a history of systemic autoimmune disease (relative risk = 4.15), greater exacerbation frequency during the first 2 years of disease (relative risk = 1.21 per attack) and better motor recovery following the first myelitis attack (22).

When bilateral ON and myelitis occur simultaneously or in rapid succession, it usually predicts a monophasic course; in these instances, the NMO syndrome may represent a restricted form of acute disseminated encephalomyelitis (ADEM). More commonly, however, the index events (those that signal NMO onset) occur weeks to months apart and consist of unilateral ON, myelitis, bilateral ON, or a combination of unilateral ON and myelitis. It is now well-established, however, that patients with unilateral ON pursue a course indistinguishable from those with bilateral ON (19). In one series, the initial presentation was an isolated event of either ON or myelitis in 90% of patients destined for a relapsing course, compared with only 48% of those who had a monophasic illness (19).

The original concept of NMO as a severe, monophasic disease probably applies only to a minority of patients with the disease. The natural history is best understood when patients with monophasic and relapsing disease courses are considered separately, as there are significant differences between these two groups (Table 20-3). Wingerchuk et al. found that 48 of 71 (68%) patients experienced at least one optic nerve or spinal cord relapse after meeting NMO diagnostic criteria in a mainly retrospective series (19). Attacks of NMO are more severe than those in MS; therefore, it would be desirable to institute long-term disease-suppressing treatment early in the course of disease. Thus, it is important to be able to distinguish the patient destined to relapse from the one with a monophasic course as early as possible following disease onset.

PATHOLOGY AND IMMUNOPATHOGENESIS

Optic nerve pathology in NMO consists of demyelination with modest inflammatory infiltrates (10). Congruent with orbital MRI abnormalities, lesions are typically more extensive than those of MS. Brain parenchyma is usually normal or reveals small areas of patchy demyelination, gliosis, or perivascular infiltrates.

Acute spinal cord lesions contain more distinctive characteristics. Gross spinal cord expansion, softening, and cavitation may be noted (7,8,10,63). Microscopic findings range from modest perivascular inflammatory demyelination to complete hemorrhagic and necrotic destruction of both gray and white matter. In many cases, large numbers of polymorphonuclear cells, including neutrophils and eosinophils, are present (63). The severe, polymorphonuclear pattern of inflammation is very different from the generally mild, lymphocyte-predominant inflammatory lesions found in typical MS. The etiologic role of eosinophils in NMO is unknown; their presence may be a primary response or reflect secondary activation by the C5a component of complement (63).

Several groups have described a distinctive hyalinized appearance of medium-sized arteries supplying the spinal cord in NMO biopsy and autopsy material (63–65). Spinal cord necrosis and a mild, macrophage-predominant infiltrate were associated with the vascular changes. The cause and significance of this vascular pathology is unknown.

Recent immunopathological study of biopsy and autopsy spinal cord material strongly implicates humoral pathogenic mechanisms in NMO. Lucchinetti et al. discovered prominent deposition of IgG and C9 neoantigen (a marker of complement activation) in areas of active myelin destruction. These deposits were also present in vessel walls accompanying vascular proliferation and fibrosis (63).

The recent discovery of the NMO-IgG serum autoantibody marker described above, together with the immunopathological support for humoral disease mechanisms, implicates one or more autoantigens in NMO pathogenesis, but these remain unidentified (38,39). Interestingly, one can mimic the restricted lesional pattern of NMO in a particular form of the putative animal model of MS, experimental allergic encephalomyelitis (EAE), using the provocative antigen myelin oligodendrocyte glycoprotein (MOG). Depending upon the genetic strain of the animal and the type and timing of antigen administration, anti-MOG animal models may also produce patterns comparable to prototypic MS, optic neuritis, and the acute Marburg variant of MS (66,67). These findings suggest that one autoantigen, influenced by environmental and genetic factors, may result in several alternative clinical and pathological phenotypes. The identification of pathogenic autoantigen(s) in NMO therefore may have widespread implications toward the understanding of many demyelinating phenotypes.

Immunological studies in NMO are otherwise limited. Analysis of peripheral CD4+ T cells demonstrated a shift toward a Th1 phenotype (increased intracellular ratio of interferon-γ to interleukin-4) during both the relapse and remission phases of opticospinal MS. In contrast, this Th1 shift occurred only in the relapse phase in conventional MS (68,69). Increased interferon-γ from CD8+ T cells and upregulation of chemokine receptors (a Th-1 type response)

have been detected in both the relapse and remission phases in opticospinal MS (69,70). Again, conventional MS differed in that chemokine upregulation occurred only in the relapse stage. Such Th1 shifts were associated with decreased serum IgE concentrations were interpreted as possibly contributing to relapse generation in opticospinal MS (23,68). These results require replication in Japanese and non-Japanese populations and it is unclear how to place them in context with the pathological findings of Th2-predominance.

Cerebrospinal fluid studies consistently show that oligoclonal banding is less prevalent in NMO (about 20% to 40%) and Japanese opticospinal MS (35% to 45%) than in conventional MS in Europeans (85% to 90%) (23). This association is revealed even when consecutive MS patients in Japan were compared based on their oligoclonal banding status; of those who were band-negative, 50% had opticospinal MS and 78% had no or few MRI lesions (71). The reason for oligoclonal band absence in most NMO and Japanese opticospinal MS cases is not clear. Nakashima et al. recently found that both NMO and MS patients have higher CSF IgG concentrations than controls; the IgG1% and IgG1 index were elevated only in the MS cases (72). Since oligoclonal bands were usually restricted to IgG, the investigators speculated that lack of IgG1 response might explain the absence of oligoclonal banding in NMO. Furthermore, since IgG1 is associated with Th1 autoimmunity, this finding is congruent with immunological and immunopathological findings that suggest that Th2 mechanisms are operative. Other investigators found that higher CSF interleukin-10 levels were associated with the presence of oligoclonal banding and that these levels were much lower in NMO than in MS (73). An early report on CSF chemokines found no significant difference between levels of CXCL10/IP-10, CCL17/TARC, CCL2/MCP-1, and CCL11/Eotaxin in patients with NMO and MS (74).

Matrix metalloproteinases are potential markers of inflammation. One type, MMP-9, is elevated in CSF during the acute phase of MS but reduced in NMO (75). Furthermore, tissue inhibitor of metalloproteinases (TIMP-1) was reduced in CSF from relapsing-remitting MS patients but not in NMO CSF. These differences in inflammatory markers suggest that the basic inflammatory reaction differs in MS and NMO.

Immunological or biochemical CSF biomarkers that correlate with clinical outcome would be clinically useful. The degree of pleocytosis, total protein level, and presence or absence of CSF oligoclonal bands are not independent predictors of disease course or outcome (19,22). The level of 14–3-3 protein was associated with disability and other CSF abnormalities suggestive of severe CNS tissue injury in Japanese opticospinal and myelitis patients (76), similar to what was found in studies of patients with isolated transverse myelitis and MS (77,78). Further study of such markers is an area of active study in all CNS demyelinating syndromes.

THERAPY

All therapeutic recommendations to date consist of either anecdotal experience with single cases or small, uncontrolled case series. The areas of therapeutic emphasis in monophasic NMO and for the recurrent exacerbations that characterize the relapsing form include treatment of acute attacks, prevention of medical complications, and rehabilitation. Chronic immunotherapy is required for patients with relapsing NMO.

Treatment of Acute Exacerbations

Optic neuritis and myelitis exacerbations are typically treated with intravenous corticosteroids, usually methylprednisolone 1000 mg/day or dexamethasone 200mg/day, for 5 consecutive days (16,19). Clinical experience suggests that this approach speeds attack recovery but it is not clear whether the ultimate clinical outcome is favorably influenced. Oral prednisone is often started after the parenteral corticosteroid course is complete, usually as part of an attack prevention strategy for relapsing NMO (see below).

For severe, steroid-refractory exacerbations, a frequent occurrence in NMO, plasmaphere-

sis is the treatment of choice (19). A double-blind crossover study of plasmapheresis versus sham exchanges showed that plasmapheresis (seven exchanges of approximately 55 mL/kg administered every other day) results in a greater proportion of patients achieving a clinically meaningful improvement (42.1% versus 5.9%) (79). Plasmapheresis seems to be especially useful in patients with NMO; a recent report of uncontrolled experience at Mayo Clinic described moderate or marked improvement associated with plasmapheresis in 6/10 patients (80). Early treatment initiation, male sex, and preserved muscle stretch reflexes independently predicted a favorable response. These findings suggest early intervention with plasmapheresis in scenarios where patients treated with high-dose corticosteroid therapy either worsen or fail to improve substantially within a few days of treatment initiation.

Prevention and treatment of medical complications has probably contributed to improved survival, especially for patients who have suffered respiratory failure due to ascending, severe cervical myelitis (19,22). Patients at risk for this complication require intensive care unit observation with frequent evaluation of respiratory and bulbar status to determine the need for ventilatory support. Medical measures to prevent thromboembolic complications, aspiration pneumonia, decubiti, and urinary tract infections are also necessary for patients who become immobilized.

Preventive Immunotherapy

Patients with relapsing NMO accrue disability in a stepwise fashion as a result of cumulative, attack-related neurological injury. Therefore, successful attack prevention strategies can reasonably be expected to preserve long-term neurological function for these patients. Since a secondary progressive disease course seems to be a rare phenomenon, achievement of prolonged clinical remissions may significantly alter the natural history of relapsing NMO. Unfortunately, there are not yet randomized, controlled studies upon which to make therapeutic decisions.

Many NMO patients first receive a diagnosis of MS and are treated with standard MS immunomodulatory therapies such as beta-interferon or glatiramer acetate (81). A recent Japanese study found that interferon-β-1b seemed to favorably influence the course of both the opticospinal and Western forms of MS (82). A case report suggested that glatiramer acetate (GA) was associated with reduced NMO attack frequency in one individual (83). Despite these findings, there is sentiment amongst many North American neurologists who treat NMO patients that current standard MS therapies are ineffective. Quite frequently, patients receive a diagnosis of NMO only after they have tried one or more standard immunotherapies for presumed MS and had persistent breakthrough disease. This remains a clinical observation, albeit a consistent one.

Mandler et al. prospectively treated seven newly diagnosed NMO patients with azathioprine and oral prednisone for at least 18 months (84). After an initial course of intravenous methylprednisolone, oral prednisone (1 mg/kg/day) was started. Three weeks later, patients received azathioprine (2 mg/kg/day). At two months, the prednisone dose was gradually tapered (by 10 mg every 3 weeks to 20 mg/day, then an even slower reduction to a maintenance dose of 10 mg/day). Most patients were maintained on prednisone 10 mg/day and azathioprine 75 to 100 mg/day. During the 18-month follow-up period, no exacerbations occurred and Expanded Disability Status Scale scores improved modestly. Based upon this experience and similar anecdotal reports of success, together with the postulated humoral mechanisms summarized above, I usually employ a similar combination of azathioprine and prednisone as first-line preventative therapy for patients with relapsing NMO. Azathioprine is typically initiated at 50 mg/day and the dose is increased in 50-mg increments over several weeks to a target of 3 mg/kg/day. Prednisone, at doses of 60 to 80 mg/day, is continued until there is laboratory evidence of azathioprine effect (persistent mild reduction in leukocyte count and elevation in mean corpuscular volume). It is then gradually tapered over several months. This combination requires ongoing monitoring of complete blood count (CBC) and liver function, surveillance for infection, consideration of measures to limit loss of bone calcium, and avoidance of live vaccinations.

We have observed that at low doses of prednisone (5 to 15 mg daily or every other day), some patients experience breakthrough symptoms when further dose lowering is attempted. Sometimes the symptoms represent a clear, new attack of optic neuritis or myelitis, while in other cases patients perceive worsening of lower extremity function and it is difficult to document clinical or imaging evidence of a new exacerbation. In these cases, a slower taper to accomplish alternate-day dosing before discontinuing prednisone completely is sometimes successful. Some patients seem to require long-term prednisone, however, something shown not to be helpful in typical MS. In this instance, use of the lowest possible dose on alternate days may help to limit adverse effects.

Some initial success with the use of the chimeric monoclonal antibody rituximab, which targets CD20+ immune cells, has been reported in abstract form (85). The rationale for this approach is that rituximab therapy results in persistent B cell clearance and this should affect antibody production in a humorally-mediated disorder (86). Rituximab appears to be quite well-tolerated. It represents a logical choice for a second-line agent in patients who continue to experience objective breakthrough disease activity despite immunosuppression. Its rapid onset of action also suggests that it may be appropriate as a first-line agent in some patients with very severe and active disease, but experience to date remains quite limited.

Various other immunosuppressive drugs have been used, but in limited numbers and outside the realm of a structured study. Mycophenolate mofetil (1,000 mg BID orally) is not associated with the idiosyncratic gastrointestinal symptoms that can occur with azathioprine but its onset of action may be no more rapid. Two patients, one having failed azathioprine therapy, remained attack-free for at least one year using monthly infusions of intravenous immunoglobulin (87). Mitoxantrone, a chemotherapeutic agent approved for use in rapidly worsening secondary progressive or relapsing-remitting MS (88,89), is worthy of investigation. Cyclophosphamide, used occasionally in severe, treatment-refractory MS, has a significant effect on B cells and may be reasonable to consider in situations where other therapies have failed. The emergence of the data supporting humoral mechanisms may allow more focused interventions and clinical investigations in future studies of this uncommon disorder.

CONCLUSION

Exciting findings from modern immunopathology, together with careful clinical observation, provide compelling evidence to support the contention that Asian opticospinal MS and NMO are the same entity and that they are not multiple sclerosis. Critical questions concerning the identity of the autoantigen(s), genesis of the humoral response, role of eosinophils and vascular hyalinization, genetic factors, restricted lesion topography, and many others remain to be answered. Better diagnostic techniques, perhaps including the novel NMO-IgG autoantibody assay, will facilitate valid clinical studies aimed at more accurate differentiation of NMO from MS, early diagnosis of NMO after presentation with a first event of optic neuritis or myelitis, and prediction of a relapsing disease course following the first attack. Ultimately, that will lead to more effective therapies for those afflicted with this fascinating disease that has puzzled neurologists for more than a century.

REFERENCES

1. Weinshenker BG, Miller D. MS: One Disease or Many? In: Siva A, Kesselring J, Thompson A, eds. *Frontiers in Multiple Sclerosis*. London: Martin Dunitz, 1999: 37–46.
2. Allbutt TC. On the ophthalmoscopic signs of spinal disease. *Lancet* 1870;1:76–78.
3. Erb W. Ueber das zusammenvorkommen von neuritis optica und myelitis subacuta. *Arch f Psychiatr*. 1880; 10:146–157.
4. Achard C, Guinon L. Sur un cas de myelite aigue diffuse avec double nevrite optique. *Arch de Med Exper er d'Anat Path*. 1889; 1:696–710.
5. Devic E. Myélite subaiguë compliquée de néurite optique. *Bull Med*. 1894; 8.
6. Gault F. De la neuromyelite optique aigue. Lyon: Thesis. 1894.
7. Goulden C. Optic neuritis and myelitis. *Trans Ophthal Soc UK*. 1914; 34:229–252.
8. Beck GM. A case of diffuse myelitis associated with optic neuritis. *Brain* 1927; 50:687–703.
9. Berliner M. Acute optic neuritis in demyelinating diseases of the nervous system. *Arch Ophthalmol*. 1939; 13:83–98
10. Stansbury FC. Neuromyelitis optica (Devic's disease). Presentation of five cases with pathological study and review of the literature. *Arch Ophthalmol*. 1949;42:292–335.
11. Cree BA, Goodin DS, Hauser SL. Neuromyelitis optica. *Semin Neurol*. 2002;22:105–122.
12. Wingerchuk DM, Weinshenker BG. Neuromyelitis Optica. In: McDonald WI, Noseworthy JH, eds. *Multiple Sclerosis 2*. Woburn, MA: Butterworth-Heinemann, 2003: 243–258.
13. de Seze J. Neuromyelitis optica. *Arch Neurol*. 2003;60:1336–1338.
14. Weinshenker BG. Neuromyelitis optica: what it is and what it might be. *Lancet* 2003;361:889–890.
15. Papais-Alvarenga, RM, Miranda-Santos CM, Puccioni-Sohler M, et al. Optic neuromyelitis syndrome in Brazilian patients. *J Neurol Neurosurg Psychiatry*. 2002;73:429–435.
16. Wingerchuk DM. Neuromyelitis optica: current concepts. *Front Biosci*. 2004;9:834–840.
17. Mandler RN, Davis LE, Jeffery DR, et al. Devic's neuromyelitis optica: a clinicopathological study of 8 patients. *Ann Neurol*. 1993;34:162–168.
18. O'Riordan JI, Gallagher HL, Thompson AJ, et al. Clinical, CSF, and MRI findings in Devic's neuromyelitis optica. *J Neurol Neurosurg Psychiatry*. 1996;60:382–387.
19. Wingerchuk DM, Hogancamp WF, O'Brien PC, et al. The clinical course of neuromyelitis optica (Devic's syndrome). *Neurology* 1999;53:1107–1114.
20. de Seze J, Stojkovic T, Ferriby D, et al. Devic's neuromyelitis optica: clinical, laboratory, MRI and outcome profile. *J Neurol Sci*. 2002;197:57–61.
21. de Seze J, Lebrun C, Stojkovic T, et al. Is Devic's neuromyelitis optica a separate disease? A comparative study with multiple sclerosis. *Mult Scler*. 2003; 9:521–525.
22. Wingerchuk DM, Weinshenker BG. Neuromyelitis optica: clinical predictors of a relapsing course and survival. *Neurology* 2003;60:848–853.
23. Kira J. Multiple sclerosis in the Japanese population. *Lancet Neurology* 2003;2:117–127.
24. McAlpine D. Familial neuromyelitis optica: its occurrence in identical twins. *Brain* 1938;61:430–438.
25. Ch'ien LT, Medeiros MO, Belluomini JJ, et al. Neuromyelitis optica (Devic's syndrome) in two sisters. *Clinical Electroencephalography* 1982;13:36–39.
26. Keegan BM, Weinshenker B. Familial Devic's disease. *Can J Neurol Sci*. 2000;27[Suppl 2]:S57–S58.
27. Yamakawa K, Kuroda H, Fujihara K, et al. Familial neuromyelitis optica (Devic's syndrome) with late onset in Japan. *Neurology* 2000;55:318–320.
28. Kuroiwa Y, Igata A, Itahara K, et al. Nationwide survey of multiple sclerosis in Japan: clinical analysis of 1,084 cases. *Neurology* 1975;25:845–851.
29. Ono T, Zambenedetti MR, Yamasaki K, et al. Molecular analysis of HLA class (HLA-A and -B) and HLA class II (HLA-DRB1) genes in Japanese patients with multi-

ple sclerosis (Western type and Asian type). *Tiss Antigens*. 1998;52:539–542.

30. Yamasaki K, Horiuchi I, Minohara M, et al. HLA-DPB1*0501-associated opticospinal multiple sclerosis: clinical, neuroimaging and immunogenetic studies. *Brain* 1999;122:1689–1696.

31. Misu T, Fujihara K, Nakashima I, et al. Pure opticospinal form of multiple sclerosis in Japan. *Brain* 2002;125:2460–2468.

32. Okinaka S, Tsubaki K Kuroiwa Y, et al. Multiple sclerosis and allied diseases in Japan: clinical characteristics. *Neurology* 1958;8:756–763.

33. Osuntokun BO. The pattern of neurological illness in tropical Africa: experience at Ibadan, Nigeria. *J Neurol Sci*. 1971;12:417–442.

34. Jain S, Maheshwari MC. Multiple sclerosis: Indian experience in the last thirty years. *Neuroepidemiology* 1985;4:96–107.

35. Phillips PH, Newman NJ, Lynn MJ. Optic neuritis in African Americans. *Arch Neurol*. 1998;55:186–192.

36. Mirsattari SM, Johnston JB, McKenna R, et al. Aboriginals with multiple sclerosis: HLA types and predominance of neuromyelitis optica. *Neurology* 2001;56:317–323.

37. Cabre P, Heinzlef O, Merle H, et al. MS and neuromyelitis optica in Martinique (French West Indies). *Neurology* 2001;56:507–514.

38. Lennon VA, Lucchinetti CF, Weinshenker BG. Identification of a marker autoantibody of neuromyelitis optica. *Neurology* 2003;60[Suppl 1]:A519–A520.

39. Lennon VA, Wingerchuk DM, Kryzer TJ, et al. A serum autoantibody marker of neuromyelitis optica. *Lancet* 2004; in press.

40. Kira J, Yamasaki K, Horiuchi I, et al. Changes in the phenotypes of multiple sclerosis over the last 50 years in Japan. *J Neurol Sci*. 1999; 166:53–57.

41. Singhal BS. Multiple sclerosis—Indian experience. *Annals of the Academy of Medicine, Singapore* 1985; 14:32–36.

42. Ono T, Zambenedetti MR, Yamasaki K, et al. Molecular analysis of HLA class (HLA-A and -B) and HLA class II (HLA-DRB1) genes in Japanese patients with multiple sclerosis (Western type and Asian type). *Tiss Antigens*. 1998;52:539–542.

43. Yamasaki K, Horiuchi I, Minohara M, et al. HLA-DPB1*0501-associated opticospinal multiple sclerosis: clinical, neuroimaging and immunogenetic studies. *Brain* 1999;122:1689–1696.

44. Fukazawa T, Kikuchi S, Sasaki H, et al. Genomic HLA profiles of MS in Hokkaido, Japan: important role of DPB1*0501 allele. *J Neurol*. 2000;247:175–178.

45. Fukazawa T, Yamasaki K, Ito H, et al. Both the HLA-DPB1 and -DRB1 alleles correlate with risk for multiple sclerosis in Japanese: clinical phenotypes and gender as important factors. *Tiss Antigens*. 2000;55:199–205.

46. Kikuchi S, Fukazawa T, Niino M, et al. HLA-related subpopulations of MS in Japanese with and without oligoclonal IgG bands. *Neurology* 2003;60:647–651.

47. Herrera BM, Ebers GC. Progress in deciphering the genetics of multiple sclerosis. *Curr Opin Neurol*. 2003;16:253–258.

48. Hensiek AE, Sawcer SJ, Feakes R, et al. HLA-DR 15 is associated with female sex and younger age at diagnosis in multiple sclerosis. *J Neurol Neurosurg Psychiatry*. 2002;72:184–187.

49. Cock H, Mandler R, Ahmed W, et al. Neuromyelitis optica (Devic's syndrome): no association with the primary mitochondrial DNA mutations found in Leber hereditary optic neuropathy. *J Neurol Neurosurg Psychiatry*. 1997;62:85–87.

50. Kalman B, Mandler RN. Studies of mitochondrial DNA in Devic's disease revealed no pathogenic mutations, but polymorphisms also found in association with multiple sclerosis. *Ann Neurol*. 2002;51:661–662.

50. Baudoin D, Gambarelli D, Gayraud D, et al. Devic's neuromyelitis optica: a clinicopathological review of the literature in connection with a case showing fatal dysautonomia. *Clin Neuropathol*. 1998; 17:175–183.

51. Aimoto Y, Ito K, Moriwaka F, et al. Demyelinating peripheral neuropathy in Devic disease. *Japanese Journal of Psychiatry & Neurology* 1991; 45: 861–864.

52. Thielen KR, Miller GM. Multiple sclerosis of the spinal cord: magnetic resonance appearance. *J Comput Assist Tomogr*. 1996;20:434–438.

53. Filippi M, Rocca MA, Moiola L, et al. MRI and magnetization transfer imaging changes in the brain and cervical cord of patients with Devic's neuromyelitis optica. *Neurology* 1999;53:1705–1710.

54. Rocca MA, Agosta F, Mezzapesa DM, et al. Magnetization transfer and diffusion tensor MRI show gray matter damage in neuromyelitis optica. *Neurology* 2004;62: 476–478.

55. Andersson M, Alvarez-Cermeno J, Bernardi G, et al. Cerebrospinal fluid in the diagnosis of multiple sclerosis: a consensus report. *J Neurol Neurosurg Psychiatry*. 1994;57:897–902.

56. Rudick RA, Cookfair DL, Simonian NA, et al. Cerebrospinal fluid abnormalities in a phase III trial of Avonex (IFNbeta-1a) for relapsing multiple sclerosis. The Multiple Sclerosis Collaborative Research Group. *J Neuroimmunol*. 1999;93:8–14.

57. Bergamaschi RS, Tonietti S, Franciotta D, et al. Oligoclonal bands in Devic's neuromyelitis optica and multiple sclerosis: differences in repeated cerebrospinal fluid abnormalities. *Mult Scler*. 2004;10:2–4.

58. Kidd D, Burton B, Plant, GT, et al. Chronic relapsing idiopathic optic neuropathy. *Brain* 2003;126:276–284.

59. Tippett DS, Fishman PS, Panitch HS. Relapsing transverse myelitis. *Neurology* 1991;41:703–706.

60. Pandit L, Rao S. Recurrent myelitis. *J Neurol Neurosurg Psychiatry*. 1996;60:336–338.

61. Kim K. Idiopathic recurrent transverse myelitis. *Arch Neurol*. 2003;60:1290–1294.

62. Wingerchuk DM. Delayed evolution of recurrent transverse myelitis into relapsing neuromyelitis optica. *Can J Neurol Sci*., 2002:29[Suppl 1]:S87.

63. Lucchinetti CF, Mandler RN, McGavern D, et al. A role for humoral mechanisms in the pathogenesis of Devic's neuromyelitis optica. *Brain* 2002;125:1450–1461.

64. Ortiz de Zarate JC, Tamaroff L, Sica RE, et al. Neuromyelitis optica versus subacute necrotic myelitis. II. Anatomical study of two cases. *J Neurol Neurosurg Psychiatry*. 1968;31:641–645.

65. Lefkowitz D, Angelo JN. Neuromyelitis optica with unusual vascular changes. *Arch Neurol*. 1984;41: 1103–1105.

66. Stefferl A, Brehm U, Storch M, et al. Myelin oligodendrocyte glycoprotein induces experimental autoimmune encephalomyelitis in the 'resistant' Brown Norway rat: disease susceptibility is determined by MHC and MHC-

linked effects on the B cell response. *J Immunol.* 1999;163:40–49.

67. Storch MK, Stefferl A, Brehm U, et al. Autoimmunity to myelin oligodendrocyte glycoprotein in rats mimics the spectrum of multiple sclerosis pathology. *Brain Pathol.* 1998;8:681–694.

68. Horiuchi I, Kawano Y, Yamasaki K, et al. Th1 dominance in HAM/TSP and the optico-spinal form of multiple sclerosis versus Th2 dominance in mite antigen-specific IgE myelitis. *J Neurol Sci.* 2000;172:17–24.

69. Ochi H, Wu X-M, Osoegawa M, et al. Tc1/Tc2 and Th1/Th2 balance in Asian and Western types of multiple sclerosis, HTLV-I-associated myelopathy/tropical spastic paraparesis and hyperIgEaemic myelitis. *J Neuroimmunol.* 2001;119:297–305.

70. Wu X-M, Osoegawa M, Yamasaki K, et al. Flow cytometric differentiation of Asian and Western types of multiple sclerosis, HTLV-1-associated myelopathy/tropical spastic paraparesis (HAM/TSP) and hyperIgEaemic myelitis by analyses of memory CD4 positive T cell subsets and NK cell subsets. *J Neurol Sci.* 2000;177:24–31.

71. Nakashima I, Fujihara K, Misu T, et al. A comparative study of Japanese multiple sclerosis patients with and without oligocolonal IgG bands. *Mult Scler.* 2002;8:459–462.

72. Nakashima I, Fujihara K, Fujimori J, et al. Absence of IgG1 response in the cerebrospinal fluid of relapsing neuromyelitis optica. *Neurology* 2004;62:144–146.

73. Nakashima I, Fujihara K, Misu T, et al. Significant correlation between IL-10 levels and IgG indices in the cerebrospinal fluid of patients with multiple sclerosis. *J Neuroimmunol.* 2000;111:64–67.

74. Narikawa K, Misu T, Fujihara K, et al. Cerebrospinal fluid chemokine levels in relapsing neuromyelitis optica and multiple sclerosis. *J Neuroimmunol.* 2004; 149:182–186.

75. Mandler RN, Dencoff JD, Midani F, et al. Matrix metalloproteinases in cerebrospinal fluid differ in multiple sclerosis and Devic's neuromyelitis optica. *Brain* 2001;124:493–498.

76. Satoh J, Yukitake M, Kurohara K, et al. Detection of the 14–3-3 protein in the cerebrospinal fluid of Japanese multiple sclerosis patients presenting with severe myelitis. *J Neurol Sci.* 2003;212:11–20.

77. Irani DN, Kerr DA. 14–3-3 protein in the cerebrospinal fluid of patients with acute myelitis. *Lancet* 2000;355:901.

78. Martinez-Yelamos A, Saiz A, Sanchez-Valle R, et al. 14–3-3 protein in the CSF as a prognostic marker in early multiple sclerosis. *Neurology* 2001;57:722–724.

79. Weinshenker BG, O'Brien PC, Petterson TM, et al. A randomized trial of plasma exchange in acute central nervous system inflammatory demyelinating disease. *Ann Neurol.* 1999;46:878–886.

80. Keegan M, Pineda AA, McClelland RL, et al. Plasma exchange for severe attacks of demyelination: predictors of response. *Neurology* 2001;58:143–146.

81. Noseworthy JH, Weinshenker BG, Lucchinetti C, et al. Multiple sclerosis. *N Engl J Med.* 2000;343:938–952.

82. Itoyama Y, Saida T, Tashiro K, et al. The Interferon-beta Multiple Sclerosis Research Group in Japan. Japanese multicenter, randomized, double-blind trial of interferon beta-1b in relapsing-remitting multiple sclerosis: two year results. *Ann Neurol.* 2000;48:487.

83. Bergamaschi R, Uggetti C, Tonietti S, et al. A case of relapsing neuromyelitis optica treated with glatiramer acetate. *J Neurol.* 2003;250:359–361.

84. Mandler RN, Ahmed W, Dencoff JE. Devic's neuromyelitis optica: a prospective study of seven patients treated with prednisone and azathioprine. *Neurology* 1998;51:1219–1220.

85. Silverman GJ, Weisman S. Rituximab therapy and autoimmune disorders. Prospects for anti-B cell therapy. *Arthritis Rheum.* 2003;48:1484–1492.

86. Cree B, Lamb S, Chin A, et al. Tolerability and effects of rituximab (anti-CD20 antibody) in neuromyelitis optica (NMO) and rapidly worsening multiple sclerosis (MS). *Neurology* 2004;62[Suppl 5]:A492.

87. Bakker J, Metz L. Devic's neuromyelitis optica treated with intravenous gamma globulin (IVIG). *Can J Neurol Sci.* 2004;31:265–267.

88. Hartung HP, Gonsette R, Konig N, et al. Mitoxantrone in progressive multiple sclerosis: a placebo-controlled, double-blind, randomized, multicenter trial. *Lancet* 2002;360:2018–2025.

89. Goodin DS, Arnason BG, Coyle PK, et al. The use of mitoxantrone (Novantrone) for the treatment of multiple sclerosis: Report of the Therapeutic and Technology Assessment Subcommittee of the American Academy of Neurology. *Neurology* 2003;61:1332–1338.

21

Other Demyelinating Diseases

Alex C. Tselis and Robert P. Lisak

*Department of Neurology, Wayne State University School of Medicine,
Detroit, Michigan*

INTRODUCTION

The most common central nervous system (CNS) demyelinating disease is multiple sclerosis (MS). In most forms of MS, there occur discrete clinical relapses and remissions, roughly corresponding to episodes of demyelination, with subsequent varying degrees of remyelination. In most cases, the course eventually becomes smoothly and progressively worse. In the primary progressive form of MS (PPMS), the deficits progress smoothly from the very beginning of the disease, without individual attacks. However, there exist several other inflammatory central demyelinating diseases of unclear relation to MS. These diseases are quite rare and not especially well-characterized. We discuss them in this chapter.

SCHILDER'S DISEASE

Schilder's disease is a subacute progressive neurologic illness characterized by a simultaneous multifocal inflammatory demyelination at all levels of the central nervous system, including cortex, subcortical white matter, basal ganglia, cerebellum, and brainstem. Signs and symptoms include some combination of headache, confusion, emotional lability, seizures, optic neuritis, brainstem involvement (ocular motor palsies, dysarthria, dysphagia), facial palsies, hemiparesis, quadriparesis, aphasia, bladder and bowel dysfunction, and movement disorders. There appears to be relatively more cortical involvement in Schilder's disease than in MS, even though the main inflammatory pathology occurs in the white matter in both diseases. The disease can affect all ages, but is more common in late childhood and young adulthood, although this is based on only a small number of cases (1). The disease in adolescents and young adults can present as a psychosis, with the diagnosis only suspected when examination reveals neurologic abnormalities (1).

Schilder's disease was first described early in the last century by Paul Schilder, who published three separate reports of a progressive neurologic illness leading to death and characterized by diffuse inflammatory demyelination in the brain (2). The cases were published in 1912, 1913, and 1924. Two of these cases were personally evaluated by him, but only one (1912) appears to be a true example of the disease that bears his name. The 1913 report consisted only of an analysis of the brain of a young patient seen elsewhere. Since this patient had a sibling who had also died of a similar illness, the nature of his disease is in doubt, and one of the genetic leukodystrophies (probably adrenoleukodystrophy) appears to be a likelier diagnosis than true Schilder's disease. The other (1924) was most likely a case of subacute sclerosing panencephalitis, since there were perivascular inflammatory infiltrates in the cortex as well as the white matter (1,3,4), and inflammation is not pronounced in MS cortical lesions (5). A number of original publications describing the pathological findings in chronic neurological diseases referred to "diffuse sclerosis," which encompassed a number of disease entities, since this is a common pathological endpoint of chronic progressive white matter disease (3). Thus, some cases of diffuse sclerosis were due to adrenoleukodystrophy, subacute sclerosing panencephalitis, Krabbe disease, metachromatic leukodystrophy, Pelizaeus–Merzbacher disease, and so forth (1,3,6). The initial confusion is mirrored in the many obsolete names of the disease, such as encephalitis periaxialis diffusa, centrolobar sclerosis, progressive degenerating subcortical encephalopathy, leukoencephalopathia myeloclastica primitive, and encephaloleukopathia scleroticans (6).

Clinical Presentation

Clinically, the illness is subacute in onset and tends to be progressive, occasionally with plateaus, and was usually thought to lead to complete disability or death within a few months or years (1). However, this conclusion is based on case series, which likely have an ascertainment bias, since only the most severe and fulminant cases would be referred to major academic centers and published. This is illustrated by the fact that modern cases seem to be more likely to have a relatively benign outcome. Thus, patients occasionally improve on corticosteroid therapy, with return to baseline or near-baseline functioning (7–10). Occasionally, the disease appears in a very focal manner. In one case, a 7-year-old child presented with a unilateral optic neuritis; an MRI of the brain showed lesions typical of Schilder's disease in both the brain and a lesion in the optic nerve (see below) (11). A biopsy showed inflammatory infiltrates with demyelination and reactive gliosis. The patient improved on oral prednisone.

Pathology and Pathogenesis

Pathologically, the disease is characterized by diffuse inflammatory demyelination, very similar (if not identical) to MS, although the demyelination may be more severe than that seen in MS. The areas of demyelination are usually grossly much more extensive than in MS, however, leading to the term "diffuse sclerosis" (12). There are perivascular inflammatory infiltrates, with lymphocytes and foamy macrophages, loss of myelin and reactive astrocytosis (7). The macrophage contents stain positive for myelin fragments (13). The perivascular infiltrates consist mostly of T cells. Axon stains show relative preservation of axons (7,14). Some involved areas have been described as having microcystic changes (7). Electron microscopy shows no nuclear or cytoplasmic inclusions (7,8).

The relationship of Schilder's disease to MS is unclear, but cases of Schilder's disease have developed relapsing-remitting courses, typical of MS (15). At autopsy, some patients with Schilder's disease have been found to harbor undoubted MS plaques (4). This was termed "transitional sclerosis" by Poser and Van Bogaert and considered a disease "in transition" between Schilder's disease and MS. Some authorities view Schilder's disease as a subtype of MS (4). There are points of similarity between Schilder's disease and MS, including the inflammatory central demyelination, with relapses and remissions in at least in some cases of Schilder's disease. Differences include the apparently more severe and often progressive course, and lack of pleocytosis and oligoclonal bands in the CSF, of patients with Schilder's disease. However, the distinction between MS and Schilder's disease is probably not so clear-cut, and at least a subset of Schilder's cases is MS. In a review of 105 cases reported in the literature, Poser divided them into "pure" Schilder's disease and transitional sclerosis (16). He found that the former were almost exclusively childhood cases, while the distribution of the age of onset of the latter was very similar to that of MS. In another series of 31 patients with large, inflammatory demyelinating lesions, presenting clinically as tumors and responding to corticosteroids, three had relapses over a period of 9 months to 12 years (17). These patients were not tested to allow the criteria proposed by Poser (see below) for the diagnosis of Schilder's disease, but otherwise resembled it very closely.

Diagnosis

In order to separate true cases of Schilder's disease from other diseases that mimic it, particularly the degenerative metabolic diseases such as metachromatic leukodystrophy and adrenoleukodystrophy, the following criteria were proposed by Poser et al. (18):

- One or two symmetrical bilateral plaques measuring at least 3 cm by 2 cm in two of three dimensions, involving the centrum semiovale.
- These must be the only lesions that can be detected on the basis of clinical, paraclinical (e.g., evoked potentials), or imaging studies.
- There must be no involvement of the peripheral nervous system.
- Adrenal function must be normal.
- Serum fatty acids must have normal carbon-chain lengths.
- Histology must be identical to that of MS.

These criteria include features required to make the diagnosis and exclude other entities in the differential diagnosis. This includes progressive multifocal leukoencephalopathy, subacute sclerosing panencephalitis, and various other degenerative and neoplastic diseases of the white matter, such as Krabbe globoid leukoencephalopathy, metachromatic leukodystrophy, adrenoleukodystrophy, Pelizaeus–Merzbacher disease, gliomatosis cerebri and others. The criteria may well be too restrictive, since undoubtedly cases have occurred with unilateral lesions (7). Note that this definition also excludes optic neuritis and spinal cord lesions, which may also be too restrictive.

Neuroimaging

Imaging studies show large lesions that may be difficult to distinguish from tumors or abscesses. On computed tomography (CT), the lesions are large and hypodense, often with some mass effect, and generally display a thin ring enhancement (Fig. 21-1). On magnetic resonance imaging (MRI), there are large lesions, often bilateral, with no or mild mass effect, bright on T2-weighted and dark on T1-weighted images, displaying ring enhancement, which may be incomplete and irregular (7,13). The lesions often appear cystic, and indeed in some cases xanthochromic fluid has been aspirated from these lesions during biopsy (7). The fluid shows the expected macrophages and lymphocytes (7).

Cerebrospinal Fluid and EEG

Ancillary studies are usually unremarkable. Cerebrospinal fluid (CSF) is generally normal, with no pleocytosis, and no oligoclonal bands and normal immunoglobulin (IgG) index and synthesis rate (8–10,13,14,19). Electroencephalography (EEG) shows only nonspecific slowing (13,19).

Treatment

There is no established standard treatment for Schilder's disease, but corticosteroids have been used, in analogy with the treatment of multiple sclerosis, which is known to respond (at least in

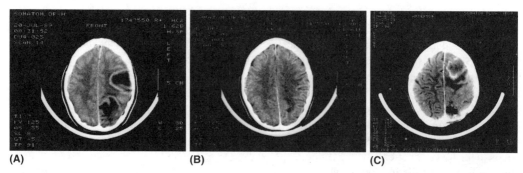

(A) **(B)** **(C)**

FIG. 21-1. **(A)** Schilder's diffuse sclerosis in a 13-year-old girl with a one-month history of speech difficulty and hand clumsiness. Biopsy of the lesion was initially interpreted as showing an astrocytoma, but reevaluation several years later showed inflammatory demyelination. **(B)** Complete resolution of the lesions after biopsy (which was initially incorrectly read as a grade III astrocytoma) and two short courses of chemotherapy ("8 in 1" regimen, cyclophosphamide, vincristine, cisplatin, methylprednisolone, carmustine, hydroxyurea, procarbazine and cytarabine, all given in one 24-hour period) and six weeks of radiation therapy. **(C)** Four-and-a-half years later, progressive right hemiparesis recurred, beginning with right-hand clumsiness. Repeat CT of the brain showed an enhancing mass lesion in the left hemisphere. Repeat biopsy showed inflammatory demyelination.

the short term) to these agents. Several patients have responded to high-dose, intravenous methylprednisolone, both clinically and radiologically, as mentioned previously. In one case, a prolonged oral prednisone taper, along with azathioprine, were used. A child with a progressive course of clumsiness and behavioral abnormality was put on adrenocorticotropic hormone (ACTH), but nevertheless progressed to left-sided hemiplegia. Cyclophosphamide 300 mg/m²/day was added to the ACTH and 7 days later the patient was able to lift his left arm. On the next day, he was able to ambulate independently and 2 months later he had only abnormal reflexes and cognitive difficulties. The ACTH and cyclophosphamide were continued for a total of 12 days, until the white blood cell count fell below 4,500. Nine months later, a relapse with a right hemiparesis occurred and was successfully treated with ACTH and cyclophosphamide (20). Other possible therapeutic modalities used in multiple sclerosis, including mitoxantrone, intravenous immunoglobulin, plasmapheresis, would be reasonable to try in a rapidly progressive case unresponsive to corticosteroids. In patients worsening when tapering off corticosteroids or cytotoxic agents after initial improvement, or who become dependent on plasmapheresis or

intravenous immunoglobulin, it would be reasonable to start on interferon therapy or glatiramer acetate.

BALÓ'S CONCENTRIC SCLEROSIS

Baló's concentric sclerosis is another inflammatory CNS demyelinating disease of uncertain relationship to MS. The clinical presentation of Baló's concentric sclerosis (or Baló's disease) is similar to that of Schilder's disease.

The disease was first fully reported by Joseph Baló from Hungary in 1927, although there were previous reports by Marburg and by L'hermitte. Baló's original case was published in a Romanian medical journal, but a year later he published a more elaborate report in the *Archives of Neurology and Psychiatry* (21). The patient was a 23-year-old law student who noted difficulty using his right hand for writing. Over the next several weeks, he experienced right-sided weakness and numbness, along with headaches, nausea, and vomiting. He became bedfast, incontinent, and developed right-sided spasms, and died two months after the initial onset of the illness. Examination of the brain postmortem revealed an unusual type of lesion in the white matter consisting of alternating, concentric gray and white stripes. Baló's description of the gross appearance of the lesion is elegant and perspicacious: "The white stripes were the same color as the white matter, while the gray stripes, which were depressed, corresponded to the gray softening" (21). These concentrically demyelinated laminae are the pathological hallmark of the disease.

Clinical Presentation

The disease presents with acute or subacute progressive neurologic deficits. These can be multifocal, and may include behavioural abnormalities. Clinical reports have described presentations with acute hemiparesis resembling a stroke; quadriparesis with confusion and seizures; headache, euphoria and hemiparesis (22); ataxia, hemiparesis and agitation; sensory aphasia; and dysarthria, dysphagia, and fatigue (23). The disease tends to be more severe and monophasically progressive than MS, clinically resembling the Marburg variant of MS (see below).

This disease is quite rare, with 36 cases reported between Baló's original publication and a review published in 1970 (24). In that review, it was noted that only 25% of patients survived longer than a year. The disease was thought to be monophasic, leading to severe disability or death within a few months (24). However, as in the case of Schilder's disease discussed earlier, there is an ascertainment bias in the old literature in that only cases coming to autopsy could be diagnosed and this give a picture of the disease which is misleading. Indeed, several mild and almost self-limited cases have been reported (23).

A case seen at our institution illustrates several important points. Both the clinical presentation and imaging studies can be atypical and suggest an infectious, neoplastic, or even vascular pathology. The patient was a 43-year-old woman presenting with Jacksonian seizures involving the right side of the body. She had previously had a progressive difficulty in gait with left-sided weakness and numbness. A CT scan of the brain showed a nonenhancing mass lesion in the right parietooccipital region. MRI of the brain showed an area of partially concentric decreased signal intensity on T1-weighted images in the right parietooccipital region; this did not enhance. MRI of the cervical cord was normal. A brain biopsy showed active inflammatory demyelination (details below). The CSF showed oligoclonal bands. She was treated with intravenous methylprednisolone, without significant improvement.

Pathology and Pathogenesis

The hallmark lesion of Baló's concentric sclerosis is a discrete lesion consisting of concentrically alternating layers of myelinated and demyelinated bands (Figs. 21-2 to 21-4). There may be several such lesions in the brain simultaneously (25). In the actively demyelinating layers, there are perivascular lymphocytic infiltrates, foamy macrophages, loss of myelin, and reactive astrocytes (25,26). The loss of myelin is demonstrated by lack of uptake of a myelin-staining dye, luxol fast blue (Figs. 21-5 and 21-6). The inflammatory process that causes demyelination may not always spare axons, and axonal damage may be prominent in areas of active disease (Fig. 21-7). The cellular infiltrates consist of T cells and macrophages, as shown in Figures 21-8 and 21-9. Note that both CD4 and CD8 T lymphocytes are present in the demyelinated lesions. This is as in MS, in which the cells are thought to arise sequentially with CD4 cells followed by CD8 cells (27). These lesions are usually located in the centrum semiovale, but rarely can be found in the spinal cord and in optic chiasm (in a lamellated but nonconcentric form) (28). Studies show decreased transcription of myelin protein-associated specific mRNAs (myelin basic protein, proteolipid protein, cyclic nucleotide phosphodiesterase), loss of oligodendrocytes (as measured by staining for carbonic anhydrase type II) in regions of demyelination, and preserved axons in the demyelinated areas (29). Perivascular inflammatory infiltrates, typical of MS plaques, were noted in actively demyelinating areas (29).

The evolution of the concentric lesions is of interest, and might shed light on the pathogenesis of the disease, but limited data are available. An interesting report of serial MRI studies of five patients with Baló's concentric sclerosis is pertinent (25). The lesions were noted to enhance in all the layers, in two or three outer layers only, at the outer margin of the lesions, or not at all. In some cases, new rings of enhancing demyelination were noted to form a wrap around the existing lesions, somewhat like annual tree rings (25). This is in accord with the findings in a pathological study of a patient who died after a four-month course of Baló's disease, in which the rings of concentric lesions were noted to have less gliosis and myelin breakdown the farther they were placed from the central core, indicating that they were younger lesions than those closer to the center (28).

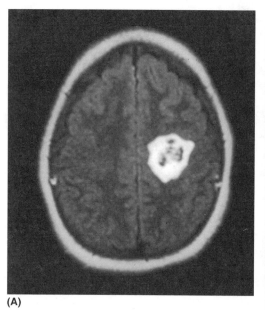

(A)

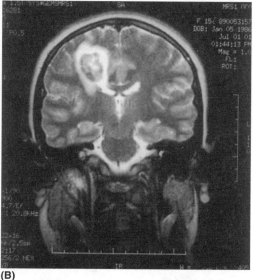

(B)

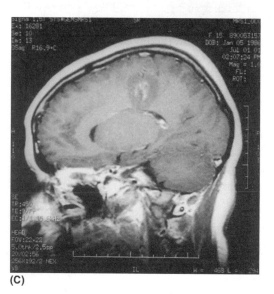

(C)

FIG. 21-2. A–C, Example of Baló's concentric sclerosis. The patient was a woman with subacute hemiparesis. A biopsy showed inflammatory demyelination. She went on to have a typical case of relapsing-remitting multiple sclerosis, so that this is really a form of transitional Baló's concentric sclerosis. (Courtesy of Dr. A. Shah, Department of Neurology, Wayne State University/Detroit Medical Center, Detroit, MI.)

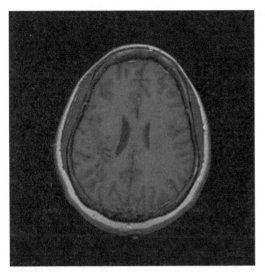

FIG. 21-3. MRI of the lesion in the right parieto-occipital white matter, having a partially concentric appearance with decreased intensity on this T1-weighted image.

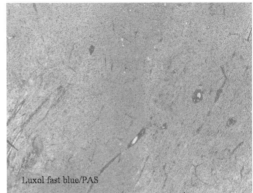

FIG. 21-5. Luxol fast blue stain of a sample from the case shown in Figs. 21-3 and 21-4. Note the lack of myelin available for staining (thus showing demyelination), at the *right* and *left* of the figure. (Courtesy of Dr. William Kupsky, Division of Neuropathology, Department of Pathology, and Dr. S Thankappan, Department of Neurology, Harper University Hospital, Wayne State University/Detroit Medical Center, Detroit, MI.)

The relation between Baló's concentric sclerosis and MS is uncertain. There are patients who have the characteristic concentric lesions, along with demyelinating plaques typical of MS, as in the transitional sclerosis cases of Schilder's disease described above. Those patients often have relapsing and remitting courses typical of MS, and probably can be placed in the spectrum of manifestations of MS. This is further illustrated by the fact that undoubted cases of MS have developed concentric lesions during the course of their disease (30). Some patients seem to have improved spontaneously (23).

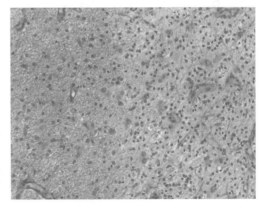

FIG. 21-6. Higher magnification of a Luxol fast blue-stained specimen, again showing loss of myelin (lack of staining) on the *right* side of the figure (same patient as in Figs. 21-3 and 21-4). (Courtesy of Dr. William Kupsky, Division of Neuropathology, Department of Pathology, and Dr. S Thankappan, Department of Neurology, Harper University Hospital, Wayne State University/Detroit Medical Center, Detroit, MI.)

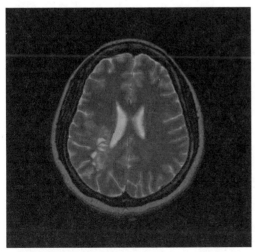

FIG. 21-4. A T2-weighted image of the brain in a case of Baló's concentric sclerosis. Same patient as in Fig. 21-3.

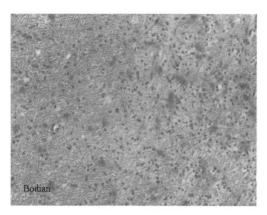

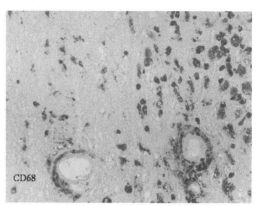

FIG. 21-7. Same patient as in Figs. 21-3 and 21-4. This figure shows depletion of axons on the *right* side of the figure, using Bodian stain, which is specific for axons. Compare with Fig. 21-6, which shows depletion of myelin. These figures together show destruction of both myelin and axons. (Courtesy of Dr. William Kupsky, Division of Neuropathology, Department of Pathology, and Dr. S Thankappan, Department of Neurology, Harper University Hospital, Wayne State University/Detroit Medical Center, Detroit, MI.)

FIG. 21-8. Same patient as in Figs. 21-3 and 21-4. Specimen specifically stained for macrophages (CD68), showing these cells to be centered perivascularly and scattered in the parenchyma. Note the perivascular preference. (Courtesy of Dr. William Kupsky, Division of Neuropathology, Department of Pathology, and Dr. S Thankappan, Department of Neurology, Harper University Hospital, Wayne State University/Detroit Medical Center, Detroit, MI.)

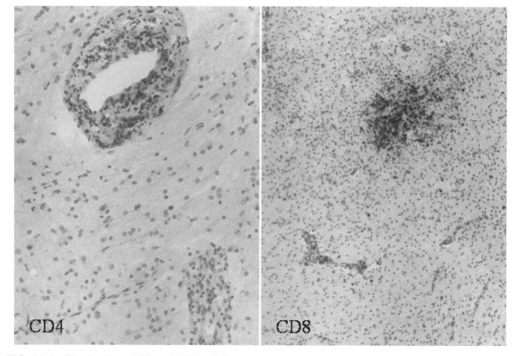

FIG. 21-9. Distribution of CD4+ (*left*) and CD8+ (*right*) T lymphocytes in the brain of the patient with Balό's sclerosis, shown in Figs. 21-3 and 21-4. These are immune active cells whose presence suggests the presence of a specific antigen (or antigens).

Neuroimaging

The neuroimaging appearance of Baló's concentric sclerosis is quite characteristic (see Fig. 21-2) and, in fact, MRI was used to make the first reported antemortem diagnosis of the disease in 1986 (31). A somewhat atypical imaging study is shown in Figures 21-3 and 21-4, in which the concentric nature of the lesion is only partly developed. Magnetic resonance spectroscopy (MRS) of a concentric lesion has revealed increased choline and decreased *N*-acetyl aspartate peaks, as well as lipid peaks, typical of active MS plaques (26). Follow-up MRS showed a decrease in the amplitudes of the lipid peaks, an increase in the myoinositol peak (a marker for astrocytes), and no changes in the choline and *N*-acetyl aspartate signals (26).

Cerebrospinal Fluid and Electrophysiologic Studies

Most cases of Baló's have a normal cerebrospinal fluid formula, with no pleocytosis and no oligoclonal bands. Rarely, patients have shown mild pleocytosis and oligoclonal bands (22,23). An increased IgG index has been reported in one case (23). There are a few reports of evoked potential abnormalities, in visual- and somatosensory-evoked potentials, as would be expected with any multifocal disease of the white matter (23).

Therapy

There is no specific therapy established for Baló's concentric sclerosis but, as with Schilder disease, the analogy with multiple sclerosis mandates consideration of corticosteroids as first-line therapy. There are numerous case reports of clinical improvement coincident with high-dose intravenous corticosteroids (22,23,26,32). Clinical improvement may not necessarily be mirrored in resolution of lesions on MRI. In one case, the patient improved clinically but the active lesion had increased in size (26). There are little data on other modalities. A 28-year-old with a rapidly progressive encephalopathy due to Baló's disease clearly improved after treatment with immunoadsorption plasmapheresis after not immediately

responding to corticosteroids (33). However, whether this improvement was due to the pheresis or a delayed response to the steroids cannot be determined or even correlated to therapy.

MARBURG VARIANT OF MS

The Marburg variant of MS is a rapidly progressive demyelinating disease of the central nervous system which was first reported by Marburg in 1906, in the case of a 30-year-old woman who developed headache, confusion, vomiting, gait ataxia with left-sided weakness, and progressed to death within a month. At autopsy, she had inflammatory demyelination.

Only a few similar cases have since been reported in detail, although some number of such cases undoubtedly go unreported (34–36). In all cases reported there is a rapid progression of disease, with little or no response to therapy. This is well illustrated in a report of a 27-year-old woman presented with headache, dizziness, nausea, and visual loss, and progressed to dysarthria, dysphagia, and hemiparesis. Despite treatment with high-dose intravenous methylprednisolone, plasmapheresis, and cyclophosphamide, she progressed to coma, lost brainstem reflexes, and her EEG became flat (36). In another case, a 25-year-old man developed vertigo, nausea, headache, confusion, and focal weakness, and progressed to coma with decerebration and focal seizures. He died despite methylprednisolone (80 mg/day) followed by dexamethasone (20 mg/day) as well as ACTH and azathioprine. Occasionally, there may be some response to therapy, as in the case of a 37-year-old woman who had good response to ACTH during two exacerbations 9 months apart, but no response at the next exacerbation 6 months later (37). She had a progressive unremitting deterioration to death in 9 more months.

Imaging studies are scarce, but generally show deep white matter lesions, some of which may be periventricular, with increased T2 signal and mass effect. There may be a dramatic enlargement in the size of the lesions in just a few days (36). The cerebrospinal fluid is often abnormal, but in a nonspecific way. There may be only a slight increase in total protein and no pleocytosis (35), or only a mild pleocytosis (34). Grossly, the brain is frequently swollen with tonsillar and uncal herniation (34,35). The microscopic pathology consists of inflammatory demyelination, with lymphocytic perivascular infiltrates (consisting mostly of T cells), macrophages containing myelin breakdown products, astrocytosis, and relative preservation of axons (34–36).

There may be subtle differences in the myelin of patients with the Marburg variant of MS. In one study, myelin basic protein (MBP) isolated from the white matter of a Marburg patient had a higher molecular weight, because of the conversion of 18 of 19 arginine residues to citrulline, than MBP from normal or chronic MS brain but was similar to that in the brain of an infant (36). Such MBP may result in a looser arrangement of myelin-ensheathing axons, and thus modify the antigenicity of myelin (38).

RECURRENT CLINICALLY ISOLATED SYNDROMES (OPTIC NEURITIS AND TRANSVERSE MYELITIS)

Optic neuritis and transverse myelitis are inflammatory diseases of the optic nerve and spinal cord, respectively, and have a rather broad differential diagnosis, which would include various infectious and autoimmune diseases (39,40). Transverse myelitis implies complete loss of all modalities below the lesions, while myelitis implies loss of only some modalities (e.g., numbness with a sensory level with only mild weakness in the legs). The distinction may be important, since transverse myelitis is only rarely the first episode of MS, whereas myelitis can be (39).

In many cases, however, there is a purely inflammatory demyelination in the optic nerve or spinal cord, with lesions identical to typical demyelinating plaques as seen in multiple sclerosis or acute disseminated encephalomyelitis (ADEM), but with no lesions elsewhere in the central nervous system (39,40). These illnesses are typically monophasic and generally have a moderate to good prognosis (39). They may be the initial manifestation of MS, with the risk being higher in patients with multiple white matter lesions on brain MRI. Occasionally, there can be recurrences of optic neuritis or myelitis (41), although these appear to be rather rare since so few cases are published. However, recurrent optic neuritis may not be as uncommon as once thought.

In the Optic Neuritis Treatment Trial (ONTT), 457 patients with acute unilateral optic neuritis with no other disease (except for MS) present, were treated with either intravenous methylprednisolone, oral prednisone or placebo, and followed (42). At the 5-year time point, there were 397 patients for evaluation, and 28% of these had recurrent optic neuritis in either eye (43). However, some of these patients had MS, but of 118 patients with recurrent optic neuritis, 36 had no evidence of MS (43). Recurrent and progressive optic neuritis has been reported, as well, without any other evidence of MS or autoimmune disease (except for some laboratory abnormalities) (44). In a series of 15 patients, 12 of whom were women, there was severe visual loss, which only improved with megadose corticosteroid therapy in 11 out of 12 (44). The visual improvement required long-term prednisone and cytotoxic drugs for its maintenance (44). This requirement for prolonged immunosuppressive therapy has also been noted in a series of patients with bilateral recurrent optic neuritis (see below).

Usually, optic neuritis is unilateral, but occasionally bilateral optic neuritis can be seen. Again, this has a broad differential diagnosis, including inflammatory demyelination, sarcoidosis, vitamin B_{12} deficiency, neoplastic compression or infiltration, infection, and mitochondrial disease (39). The risk of progression from bilateral optic neuritis to MS is relatively small, but not negligible. A few cases of bilateral optic neuritis have also been reported in the context of acute disseminated encephalomyelitis (39). Recurrent bilateral optic neuritis has rarely been reported. Over a 10-year period, 15 cases of recurrent bilateral optic neuritis were seen at several large referral centers in England (45). The patients responded well to corticosteroids, but tended to relapse when the drug was decreased, and most required long-term immunosuppression. The nature of the bilateral optic neuritis was not ascertained.

There is also a combined version of optic neuropathy and myelopathy, known as variously as Devic's neuromyelitis optica, Devic's disease, Devic's syndrome, or neuromyelitis optica (46). The differential diagnosis of Devic's syndrome is broad, as it is in optic neuritis or myelitis, but there is a group of patients with idiopathic inflammatory demyelinating and necrotizing lesions affecting the optic nerves and spinal cord, fairly closely together in time, with no lesions elsewhere in the nervous system. This latter entity is neuromyelitis optica, and can be monophasic or recurrent (46). The recurrent form of neuromyelitis optica is more likely to occur in patients with a longer interval between successive involvement of the optic nerve and spinal cord, in women, in those older at onset, and in milder disease of the cord (47). The recurrent form of neuromyelitis optica is more likely to occur in those with a longer interval between successive involvement of the optic nerve and spinal cord, in women, in those older at onset and in milder disease of the cord (47). Some of these patients may respond to immunosuppression, particularly with prednisone and azathioprine in combination (47). The recurrent form of the disease can be difficult to distinguish from multiple sclerosis, and the lack of lesions in the white matter of the brain is the key support for the diagnosis of Devic's disease. This is discussed in more detail in Chapter 20 by Dr. Wingerchuk.

ACUTE DISSEMINATED ENCEPHALOMYELITIS AND RECURRENT ACUTE DISSEMINATED ENCEPHALOMYELITIS

Acute disseminated encephalomyelitis (ADEM) is an acute, multifocal, inflammatory demyelinating disease of the central nervous system characterized by an abrupt onset of fever, headache, confusion, seizures, drowsiness, and delirium (often with concurrent focal neurological deficits, such as hemiparesis, myelopathy, and optic neuritis) (39). A rare form of ADEM, acute hemorrhagic leukoencephalitis (AHLE) involves the development of hemorrhagic white matter lesions and is generally thought to be more severe, with higher morbidity and mortality. Both forms of the disease mimic viral encephalitis very closely, and it is the MRI that usually suggests the correct diagnosis, with areas of abnormal signal in the white matter (39).

Generally speaking, the disease is monophasic and recurrences appear to be very rare, at least in adults (48–51). A recurrence of ADEM, defined as a recurrence of the original clinical presentation of ADEM immediately after a full or partial resolution, is denoted as multiphasic disseminated encephalomyelitis (MDEM) (52). In a series of 52 Taiwanese patients diagnosed with ADEM, only one (2%) had MDEM (53). Most cases of recurrence in adults turn out to be MS. Thus, of 40 adults with ADEM seen at the University of Heidelberg, 14 (35%) had relapses, but all of these were thought to be MS relapses rather than MDEM (54). The authors stated that the recurrent episodes in their patients would satisfy the Poser criteria for MS. The difficulty in classifying these cases is that there are no precise criteria to differentiate MDEM from MS.

In children, however, clear relapses of ADEM may not be quite as rare. The risk of recurrence can be estimated from reported case series of ADEM in children from large centers, although this is subject to ascertainment bias. Thus, the proportion of childhood ADEM that becomes MDEM has been reported (in various series) as 15% of cases at Great Ormond Street in England (52), 10% in Buenos Aires, Argentina (55), 13% at the Royal Children's Hospital in Australia (56), and 32% in a multicenter series in the United States (57). In the Argentinian series, the relapsing illness was described as biphasic, since only a single relapse occurred in this group (55). The follow-up of these cases was limited however, and some clinical details are lacking so that some of these MDEM cases may in reality have been multiple sclerosis. Four out of 31 patients (13%) seen at the Royal Children's Hospital in Australia had definite relapses, one of whom apparently had three relapses; the others had only two (56). In a large series of 121 pediatric patients, 39 (32%) had relapses, 17 of which were eventually diagnosed as multiple sclerosis (57).

RECURRENT BELL'S PALSY

Bell's palsy is a weakness of the facial muscles caused by disease of the facial nerve. The lesion responsible for Bell's palsy involves either the nuclear (i.e., involving the facial nucleus in the brainstem) or infranuclear part of the nerve within the brainstem parenchyma, or the peripheral nerve beyond. It is characterized by a inability to smile, close the eye, and corrugate the forehead on the affected side. Lesions in the peripheral part of the nerve therefore result in a mononeuropathy simplex form of peripheral neuropathy. Usually, Bell's palsy is due to this type of peripheral involvement. There is little evidence for involvement of the brain parenchyma in most cases of Bell's palsy. Most patients have no clinical evidence of CNS involvement, and in the few imaging studies of Bell's palsy that examine the CNS, usually no such lesions are found. Thus, in an MRI study of the facial nerve in 39 patients with Bell's palsy, in no case were there lesions in the brain or brainstem to account for the facial palsy (58). The affected facial nerves enhance in most cases of Bell's palsy, while unaffected nerves usually do not (59).

Brainstem lesions resulting in peripheral facial palsy are certainly not impossible, on the other hand, and have occasionally been documented. A lesion within the substance of the brainstem, affecting only the facial nucleus or intraparenchymal part of the facial nerve, would be clinically indistinguishable from a lesion affecting the peripheral part of the nerve. The easiest way to make the distinction is by imaging of the facial nerve and brainstem.

Thus, cases of multiple sclerosis presenting as a peripheral facial palsy, with pontine lesions involving the facial nucleus and infranuclear part of the facial nerve on MRI, have been reported (60,61). An interesting case of a pontine hemorrhage giving rise to an isolated Bell's palsy has been reported as well (62). A patient with a cavernous angioma of the brainstem presented with a slowly progressive facial paralysis (63). Finally, in a series of 18 patients with acute Bell's palsy, five reportedly had lesions in the cerebral white matter to suggest a central vascular or demyelinating cause. Many of these MRIs had nonspecific abnormalities and some of the patients were elderly, so that the clinical--imaging correlation was not tight. Although details are scarce, however, one of the patients had a transitory abnormal signal in the pons which accounted for her symptoms (64).

Reports of the pathological examination of the facial nerve in Bell's palsy are scarce. Because most pathologic specimens are small, sampling error limits the interpretability of the results, which include degenerative changes such as axonal degeneration, myelin fragmentation, and phagocytosis, as well as intraneural hemorrhages and lymphocytic infiltrations (65,66).

Occasionally, Bell's palsy can be present with other cranial neuropathies. In one study of 51 consecutive patients with Bell's palsy, four (8%) had symptoms of other cranial nerve involvement. However, with careful examination, 40% had abnormalities in other cranial nerves, most frequently the trigeminal nerve (13 patients, 25% of the total) (67). It has been proposed that Bell's palsy is but one manifestation of a spectrum of multiple cranial nerve involvement—benign cranial polyneuritis—with an acute but self-limited and spontaneously resolving involvement of multiple cranial nerves (68).

Bell's palsy is usually monophasic but, rarely, can be recurrent. The differential diagnosis is broad and includes viral disease, particularly due to one of the herpes viruses, (a *forme fruste* of) acute inflammatory demyelinating polyneuropathy, acute human immunodeficiency virus (HIV) seroconversion syndrome, syphilis, sarcoidosis, Lyme disease, tubercular meningitis, and other forms of chronic meningitis. Most of these are easily diagnosed clinically. Most cases of Bell's palsy are labelled idiopathic but, while there is undoubtedly inflammation affecting the nerve, a nagging question is whether one of the herpes viruses is infecting the nerve (69). There is certainly evidence (mostly serological) to implicate herpes simplex and varicella zoster virus in the pathogenesis of the disease (69). This translates into the dilemma of whether to treat such patients with corticosteroids (for the inflammation) or acyclovir (for a putative viral infection), or both.

An evidence-based review of the use of corticosteroids and acyclovir in Bell's palsy concluded that corticosteroids were probably beneficial and acyclovir was possibly beneficial in its treatment (70). Doses of prednisone in the different studies summarized in the review ranged from 216 to 760 mg total, given over 10 to 17 days. For acyclovir, the doses ranged from 1,000 mg a day in 5 days to 2,000 mg a day (400 mg five times a day) over 10 days.

Cases of recurrent Bell's palsy are very infrequent, reportedly occurring in 10% to 15% of patients in case series reports (71,72). Many of these patients have had family members with recurrent Bell's palsy. A case with a total number of 11 episodes is probably the record (73). There are no data on imaging or pathological results in such cases, and their relationship to other central inflammatory demyelinating diseases is unknown.

UNIFIED VIEW OF DEMYELINATING DISEASES OF THE CENTRAL NERVOUS SYSTEM

There are enough common features in the inflammatory demyelinating diseases of the central nervous system to suggest a shared pathogenesis, with host-specific, perhaps genetic and maturational, variations on a theme. In three conditions discussed here, Schilder's disease, Baló's concentric sclerosis, and the Marburg variant of MS, the inflammatory demyelination is microscopically indistinguishable from that of multiple sclerosis. In many cases of Schilder disease and Baló's concentric sclerosis, classical demyelinating plaques are seen, identical to those of MS, in addition to the unique lesions defining these diseases. Also, with experience and more sensitive diagnostic modalities such as MRI, we have learned that in many cases the clinical course of these diseases is remitting and relapsing. The diseases may respond in some cases to immunomodulation with corticosteroids, immunosuppressants, or plasmapheresis, although no definitive controlled studies have been reported. These diseases are similar to each other but differ clinically from MS in that the clinical presentation tends to be dominated initially by vague constitutional symptoms such as

headache, vertigo, nausea, and confusion, with a rapid progression to severe neurological deficits, while MS is more indolent, has more specifically neurological symptoms, and the deficits are much less severe and much more easily controlled.

We believe that the case can be made for categorizing these diseases together rather than splitting them. All of them can be mild or severe, apparently responsive or refractory to immunosuppression and immunomodulation, and relapsing-remitting or relentlessly progressive. The histopathologies are very similar, if not identical. There may or may not be common triggers, such as mild febrile illnesses. Also, as we have seen, in transitional sclerosis, lesions typical of Schilder diffuse sclerosis can coexist with typical MS plaques. Similarly, concentric lesions of Baló's sclerosis can coexist with typical MS plaques. This is also the case in other central inflammatory demyelinating diseases; some cases of acute disseminated encephalomyelitis (with perivenular demyelination) and acute hemorrhagic leukoencephalitis (with polymorphonuclear infiltration and hemorrhages) can each have lesions characteristic of the other(s) (39,74,75). Furthermore, many of these diseases can have monosymptomatic manifestations (optic neuritis and transverse myelitis) that may be superimposed on otherwise typical acute disseminated encephalomyelitis (40). Acute disseminated encephalomyelitis is well-known to progress to MS, although uncommonly (39). Finally, there are animal models in which different forms of mild or severe, diffuse or localized disease can be produced by appropriately modifying the triggering factors (dose and route of myelin antigen, addition of pertussis as adjuvant, and so forth) (76). Thus, almost all central inflammatory demyelinating diseases have some overlap with each other, and a unified view of them is reasonable and heuristic.

REFERENCES

1. Poser C. Myelinoclastic Diffuse Sclerosis. In: *Demyelinating Diseases.* Koetsier J, ed. New York: Elsevier, 1985: 419–428.
2. Schilder P. Zur kenntnis der sogennanten diffusen Sklerose. *Z Gesamte Neurol Psychiatr.* 1912; (10):1–60.

3. Poser C. Myelinoclastic Diffuse and Transitional Sclerosis. In: *Multiple Sclerosis and Other Demyelinating Diseases*. Vinken PJ, Bruyn GW, eds. Amsterdam: North Holland Publishing Co., 1970: 469–484.

4. Poser C, Van Bogaert L. Natural history and evolution of the concept of Schilder's diffuse sclerosis. *Acta Psychiatr Neurol Scand*. 1956;(31):285–331.

5. Peterson JL, Bo S, Mork A, et al. Transected neurites apoptotic neurons and reduced inflammation in cortical multiple sclerosis lesions. *Ann Neurol*. 2001;(50): 389–400.

6. Christensen A, Fog M. A case of Schilder's disease in an adult with remarks to the etiology and pathogenesis. *Acta Psychiatr Neurol Scand*. 1955;(30): 141–154.

7. Afifi A, Bell W, Menezes A, et al. Myelinoclastic diffuse sclerosis (Schilder's disease): report of a case and review of the literature. *J Child Neurol*. 1994; (9):398–403.

8. Garell P, Menezes A, Baumbach G, et al. Presentation management and follow-up of Schilder's disease. *Pediatr Neurosurg*. 1998;(29):86–91.

9. Pretorius M, Loock D, Ravenscroft A, et al. Demyelinating disease of Schilder's type in three young South African children: dramatic response to corticosteroids. *J Child Neurol*. 1998;(13):197–201.

10. Leuzzi V, Lyon G, Cilio M, et al. Childhood demyelinating diseases with a prolonged remitting course and their relation to Schilder's disease: report of two cases. *J Neurol Neurosurg Psych*. 1999;(66):407–408.

11. Afifi A, Follett K, Greenlee J, et al. Optic neuritis: a novel presentation of Schilder's disease. *J Child Neurol*. 2001;(16):693–696.

12. Lassmann H. Pathology of Multiple Sclerosis. In: *McAlpine's Multiple Sclerosis*. Compston A, Ebers G, Lassman H, et al., eds. London: Churchill Livingstone, 1998: 323–358.

13. Eblen F, Poremba M, Grodd W, et al. Myelinoclastic diffuse sclerosis (Schilder's disease): cliniconeuroratiologic correlations. *Neurology* 1991;(41):589–591.

14. Dresser L, Tourian A, Anthony D. A case of myelinoclastic diffuse sclerosis in an adult. *Neurology* 1991;(41):316–318.

15. Sastre-Garriga J, Rovira A, Rio J, et al. Clinically definite multiple sclerosis after radiological Schilder-like onset. *J Neurology*. 2003;(250):871–873.

16. Poser C. Diffuse-disseminated sclerosis in the adult. *J Neuropathol Exp Neurol*. 1957;(16):61–78.

17. Kepes J. Large focal tumor-like demyelinating lesions of the brain: intermediate entity between multiple sclerosis and acute disseminated encephalomyelitis? A study of 31 patients. *Neurology* 1993;(33):18–27.

18. Poser C, Goutieres F, Carpentier MA, et al. Schilder's myelinoclastic diffuse sclerosis. *Pediatrics* 1986;(77): 107–112.

19. Mehler M, Rabinowich L. Inflammatory myelinoclastic diffuse sclerosis. *Ann Neurol*. 1988;(23):413–415.

20. Konkol R, Bousounis D, Kuban K. Schilder's disease: additional aspects and a therapeutic option. *Neuropediatrics* 1987;(18):149–152.

21. Baló BJ. Encephalitis periaxialis concentrica. *Arch Neurol Psych*. 1928;(19):242–264).

22. Gu J, Wang R, Lin J, et al. Concentric sclerosis: imaging diagnosis and clinical analysis of 3 cases. *Neurology India* 2003;(51):528–530.

23. Kararslan E, Altintas A, Senol U, et al. Baló's concentric sclerosis: clinical and radiologic features of five cases. *AJNR Am J Neuroradiol*. 2001;(22):1362–1367.

24. Courville C. Concentric Sclerosis. In: *Multiple Sclerosis and Other Demyelinating Diseases*. Vinken PJ, Bruyn GW, eds. Amsterdam: North Holland Publishing Co., 1970: 437–451.

25. Chen C, Chu N, Lu C, et al. Serial magnetic resonance imaging in patients with Baló's concentric sclerosis: natural history of lesion development. *Ann Neurol*. 1999;(46):651–656.

26. Kim M, Lee S, Choi C, et al. Baló's concentric sclerosis: a clinical study of brain MRI biopsy and proton magnetic resonance spectroscopic findings. *J Neurol Neurosurg Psych*. 1997;(62):655–658.

27. Traugott U, Reinherz E, Raine C. Multiple sclerosis: distribution of T cell subsets within active chronic lesions. *Science* 1983;(219):308–310.

28. Moore G, Neumann K, Suzuki H, et al. Baló's concentric sclerosis: new observations on lesion development. *Ann Neurol*. 1985;(17):604–611.

29. Yao D, Webster H, Hudson L, et al. Concentric sclerosis (Baló): morphometric and in situ hybridization study of lesions in six patients. *Ann Neurol*. 1994;(35):18–30.

30. Iannucci G, Mascalchi M, Salvi F, et al. Vanishing Baló-like lesions in multiple sclerosis. *J Neurol Neurosurg Psych*. 2000;(69):399–400.

31. Garbern J, Spence A, Alvord EJ. Baló's concentric demyelination diagnosed premortem. *Neurology* 1986;(36):1610–1614.

32. Murakami Y, Matsuishi T, Yamashita STY, et al. Baló's concentric sclerosis in a 4-year-old Japanese infant. *Brain Devel*. 1998;(20):250–252.

33. Sekijima Y, Tokuda T, Hashimoto T, et al. Serial magnetic resonance imaging (MRI) study of a patient with Baló's concentric sclerosis treated with immunoadsorption plasmapheresis. *Mult Scler*. 1997;(2):291–294.

34. Mendez M, Pogacar S. Malignant monophasic multiple sclerosis or "Marburg's disease." *Neurology* 1988;(38):1153–1155.

35. Banerjee A, Chopra J, Kumar B. Acute multiple sclerosis. Report of a case with neuropathological and neurochemical studies. *Neurology India* 1977; (25):233–237.

36. Wood DD, Bilbao JM, O'Connors P, et al. Acute multiple sclerosis (Marburg type) is associated with developmentally immature myelin basic protein. *Ann Neurol*. 1996;(40):18–24.

37. Dubois-Dalcq M, Schumacher G, Sever J. Acute multiple sclerosis: electron microscopic evidence for and against a viral agent in the plaques. *Lancet* 1973):1408–1411.

38. Beniac D, Wood D, Palaniyar N, et al. Marburg's variant of multiple sclerosis correlates with a less compact structure of myelin basic protein. *Mol Cell Biol Res Comm*. 1999;(1):48–51.

39. Tselis A, Lisak R. Acute Disseminated Encephalomyelitis. In: Antel J, Birnbaum G, Hartung H, eds. *Clinical Neuroimmunology*. Oxford: Blackwell Science, 1998: 116–147.

40. Tselis A, Lisak R. Acute disseminated encephalomyelitis and isolated central nervous system demyelinative syndromes. *Current Opinion in Neurology* 1995;(8): 227–229.

41. Tippett DS, Fishman PS, Panitch HS. Relapsing transverse myelitis. *Neurology* 1991;41(5):703–706.
42. Beck RW, Cleary PA, Anderson MM Jr., et al. A randomized, controlled trial of corticosteroids in the treatment of acute optic neuritis. The Optic Neuritis Study Group. *N Engl J Med.* 1992;326(9):581–588.
43. The Optic Neuritis Study Group. Visual function 5 years after optic neuritis. *Arch Ophthalmol.* 1997; 115:1545–1552.
44. Kupersmith M, Burde R, Warren F, et al. Autoimmune optic neuropathy: evaluation and treatment. *J Neurol Neurosurg Psych.* 1988;(52):1381–1386.
45. Kidd D, Burton B, Plant G, et al. Chronic relapsing inflammatory optic neuropathy (CRION). *Brain* 2003;(126):276–284.
46. Weinshenker B. Neuromyelitis optica: what it is and what it might be. *Lancet* 2003;(361):889–890.
47. Wingerchuk D, Weinshenker B. Neuromyelitis optica. Clinical predictors of a relapsing course and survival. *Neurology* 2003;(60):848–853.
48. Poser C, Roman G, Emery E. Recurrent disseminated vasculomyelinopathy. *Arch Neurol.* 1978;(36):166.
49. Alcock N, Hoffman H. Recurrent encephalomyelitis in childhood. *Arch Dis Child.* 1962;(37):40.
50. Durston J, Milnes J. Relapsing encephalomyelitis. *Brain* 1970;(93):715–730.
51. Lamarche J. Recurrent acute necrotizing hemorrhagic encephalopathy. *Acta Neuropath (Berlin).* 1972; (22):79–87.
52. Dale R, de Sousa C, Chong W, et al. Acute disseminated encephalomyelitis multiphasic disseminated encephalomyelitis and multiple sclerosis in children. *Brain* 2000;(123):2407–2422.
53. Hung K, Liao H, Tsai M. The spectrum of postinfectious encephalomyelitis. *Brain Devel.* 2001;(23):42–45.
54. Schwartz S, Mohr A., Knauth M, et al. Acute disseminated encephalomyelitis. A follow-up study of 40 adult patients. *Neurology* 2001;(56):1313–1318.
55. Tenembaum S, Chamoles N, Fejerman N. Acute disseminated encephalomyelitis. A long-term follow-up study of 84 pediatric patients. *Neurology* 2002; (59):1224–1231.
56. Hynson J, Kornberg A, Coleman L, et al. Clinical and neuroradiologic features of acute disseminated encephalomyelitis in children. *Neurology* 2001;(56): 1308–1312.
57. Rust R, Dodson W, Presnky A, et al. Classification and outcome of acute disseminated encephalomyelitis. *Ann Neurol.* 1997;(42):491.
58. Kress B, Griesbeck F, Stippich F, et al. Bell palsy: quantitative analysis of MR imaging data as a method of predicting outcome. *Radiology* 2004;(230):504–509.
59. Korzec K, Sobol S, Kubal W, et al. Gadolinium-enhanced magnetic resonance imaging of the facial nerve in herpes zoster oticus and Bell's palsy: clinical implications. *Amer J Otol.* 1991;(12):163–168.
60. Jonsson L, Thuomas K, Stenquist M, et al. Acute peripheral facial palsy simulating Bell's palsy in a case of probable multiple sclerosis with a clinically correlated transient pontine lesion on magnetic resonance imaging. *J Otolaryngol Relat Spec.* 1991;(53):362–365.
61. LaBagnara Jr. J, Jahn A, Habif D, et al. MRI findings in two cases of acute facial paralysis. *Otolaryngol Head Neck Surg.* 1989;(101):562–565.
62. Martinez-Garcia FA, Salmeron P, Morales-Ortiz A, et al. Pontine hemorrhage as a cause of peripheral facial paralysis. *Rev Neurol.* 1996;(132):984–986.
63. Hoffmann D, May M, Kubal W. Slowly progressive facial paralysis due to vascular malformation of the brainstem. *Am J Otol.* 1990;(11):357–159.
64. Jonsson L, Hemmingsson A, Thomander L, et al. Magnetic resonance imaging in patients with Bell's palsy. *Acta Otolaryngol Suppl.* 1989;(468):403–405.
65. Proctor B, Corgill D, Proud G. The pathology of Bell's palsy. *Trans Am Acad Ophthal Otol.* 1976;(82):70–80.
66. Matsumoto Y, Patterson M, Pulec J, et al. Facial nerve biopsy for etiologic clarification of Bell's palsy. *Ann Otol Rhinol Laryngol.* 1988;(97):22–27.
67. Benatar M, Edlow J. The spectrum of cranial neuropathy in patients with Bell's palsy. *Arch Intern Med.* 2004;(164):2382–2385.
68. Adour K. Cranial polyneuritis and Bell palsy. *Arch Otolaryngol.* 1976;(102):262–264.
69. Morgan M, Nathwani D. Facial palsy and infection: the unfolding story. *Clin Infect Dis.* 1992;(14):263–271.
70. Grogan PM, Gronseth GS. Practice parameter: steroids, acyclovir, and surgery for Bell's palsy (an evidence-based review): report of the Quality Standards Subcommittee of the American Academy of Neurology. *Neurology* 2001;56(7):830–836.
71. Pitts DB, Adour KK, Hilsinger RL Jr. Recurrent Bell's palsy: analysis of 140 patients. *Laryngoscope* 1988;98(5):535–540.
72. English J, Stommel E, Bernat J. Recurrent Bell's palsy. *Neurology* 1996;(47):604–605.
73. Kurca E, Drobny M, Vosko M, et al. Unique case of eleven Bell's palsy episodes. *Int J Neurosci.* 2001;(111):55–66.
74. Russell D. The nosologic unity of acute hemorrhagic leucoencephalitis and acute disseminated encephalomyelitis. *Brain* 1955;(78):369–376.
75. Adams R, Kubik C. The morbid anatomy of the demyelinating diseases. *Amer J Med.* 1952;(12):510–546.
76. Levine S. Hyperacute neutrophilic and localized forms of experimental allergic encephalomyelitis: a review. *Acta Neuropath (Berlin).* 1974;(28):179–189.

Subject Index